T0212024

Urinary Stents

Federico Soria • Duje Rako • Petra de Graaf
Editors

Urinary Stents

Current State and Future Perspectives

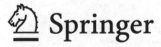 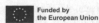 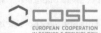

Funded by the European Union

COST
EUROPEAN COOPERATION
IN SCIENCE & TECHNOLOGY

Editors
Federico Soria
Foundation
Jesús Usón Minimally Invasive
Surgery Center
Cáceres, Spain

Duje Rako
Croatia PolyClinic
Zagreb, Croatia

Petra de Graaf
University Medical Center Utrecht
Utrecht, The Netherlands

This book is an open access publication.

ENIUS. CA16217. European Network of multidisciplinary research to Improve the Urinary Stents

ISBN 978-3-031-04486-1   ISBN 978-3-031-04484-7   (eBook)
https://doi.org/10.1007/978-3-031-04484-7

This Springer imprint is published by the registered company Springer Nature Switzerland AG
The registered company address is: Gewerbestrasse 11, 6330 Cham, Switzerland

We would like to dedicate this book to the people who are the main reason for our daily work in our different areas of knowledge such as R&D, healthcare and innovation….. the patients. The aim of all health technological developments should be to improve the quality of life of patients. We would also like to thank Dr. Mónica Pérez-Cabero, Milena Stoyanova and Fernanda Carrizosa for their support, and also express our gratefulness to all the authors involved in this book for sharing their wide-ranging knowledge.

Preface

The aim of this book is to provide a multidisciplinary overview of an area of knowledge that affects a multitude of patients worldwide on a daily basis and that unfortunately shows a slow technological development. The main reasons for the lack of innovation in the development of urinary stents and catheters are, on the one side, the characteristics of the urinary tract, urine and the particularities of the research groups involved. The urinary tract shows challenging characteristics for the placement of urinary stents and catheters, both at the level of the upper and lower urinary tract. The peristalsis, the urinary microbiome, the ease of biofilm formation on the surface of urinary medical devices, as well as the changes that occur when placing a ureteral stent such as invalidation of the anti-reflux system of the ureterovesical junction, and the high sensitivity of the bladder trigone cause manifest drawbacks in patients. On the other hand, urine is a fluid supersaturated with mineral salts, which represents a very hostile environment for biomaterials, both polymeric and metallic, leading to a series of side effects with stents and catheters that favour encrustation and bacterial contamination. This leads to the failure of these medical devices in daily clinical practice. In addition to all these limitations, which make the urinary tract a complicated area for innovation in indwelling medical devices, the research groups involved in the improvement of these devices are composed of a small number of researchers and are groups generally isolated from each other. It is logical to think that the possibility of improving urinary stents and catheters will come from a wider and mainly multidisciplinary approach, as many different disciplines are needed to overcome the current pitfalls. Not only urologists are important, because although they are the ones who know the limitations of the current urological armamentarium, technological development is also the responsibility of other areas of knowledge. These include bioengineering, chemical engineering, microbiology, experts in coatings, in new polymers, in biomaterials, translational researchers, experts in new metal alloys, etc. And to this large group of researchers it is also necessary to include physicists, mathematicians and experts in an area that affects the urinary tract and the medical devices that are placed inside it, which is fluid dynamics.

This is precisely the proposal of the COST Action (CA16217) that has developed this book. ENIUS, European network of multidisciplinary research to improve the urinary stents, is a multidisciplinary network of experts whose aim is to work towards overcoming the current limitations in this area of knowledge. The enhancements in the collaboration through a multidisciplinary network allow the detection of the most important factors that cause urinary stent failure. Not only from a clinical point of view, but concerning also aspects as industrial design and the use of different biomaterials and new antimicrobial coatings. Therefore, the great difference of our proposal with regard to the current books on urinary stents is the multidisciplinary approach that allows a broad view of the current limitations, but above all of the lines of development and innovation that are being worked on today. As well as the proposal of new lines of research and future technological development that we believe will be implemented in the next few years, to improve the characteristics of the stents and mainly to improve the quality of life of patients, which is the aim of all technological development. This multidisciplinary feature broadens the interest of the book not only to urologists or medical students interested in increasing their knowledge, but also integrates a wide group of researchers who dedicate their efforts to biomaterials, new designs, and coatings of urinary devices.

The European Cooperation in Science and Technology is an EU programme funding interdisciplinary research networks in Europe and beyond. These networks, called COST Actions, provide open spaces where researchers and innovators can connect, collaborate, and grow their ideas together. COST is dedicated to the creation of pan-European research networks in all science and technology fields. Their strategic priorities are very accurate: Promoting and spreading excellence; fostering interdisciplinary research for breakthrough science; empowering and retaining young researchers and innovators. Therefore, COST Actions is a network, open for young and experienced researchers and innovators collaborating in all fields of science and technology of common interest, based on a joint work programme lasting 4 years.

The aims and scope of work of the multidisciplinary ENIUS network are described in the COST Memorandum of Understanding of 23/06/2017 (cost.eu/actions/CA16217/). The first aim of this Action is to create a multidisciplinary group to identify the inherent pitfalls in current urinary stents, related to its design, composition, biomaterials, coatings, encrustation, interactions between urinary tract stents and fluid dynamics, morbidity of urinary stents and assessing the drawbacks from different points of view. And of course, propose consensus recommendations from our experts on the current weaknesses of urinary stents. Our capacity goals have been consolidated into a multidisciplinary network actively involved in urinary stents research to facilitate scientific knowledge exchange; to create a cohort of skilled bioengineer/researchers with experience in stents by providing training courses and supporting exchange visits between Research Centres or Hospitals. Finally, ENIUS has played a key role in providing links between researchers and industrial communities/partners. The transfer of technological knowledge to industry is a major factor in bringing basic and translational research to industry. *From bench to bedside and beyond.*

ENIUS was launched in September 2017 and has been composed of up to 204 researchers from different disciplines such as medicine, bioengineering, biomaterials, translational research, coatings, etc. A total of 30 European countries as well as Canada, USA, Republic of Korea and India joined the network. During the 4.5 years of its lifetime, our network has developed up to 24 activities of dissemination of scientific activities related to its aims, mainly in face-to-face mode, but also with the use of videoconference tools to overcome movement restrictions due to the severe COVID pandemic. A total of 590 registered participants have attended our dissemination of scientific and technological activities. During these years, up to 28 STSM (Short Term Scientific Missions Grants) have been carried out between different organisations in different countries, with the aim of training young researchers in new techniques, not available in their workplaces. This exchange reduces the weaknesses of the research groups that make up ENIUS, as well as strengthening research links in urinary stents. Also noteworthy is the production of 15 scientific papers describing current and future lines of research in urinary stents, which are the result of the collaboration of the multidisciplinary groups that join in the COST Actions. The scientific production, as well as scientific dissemination activities, can be found at www.enius.org.

The Action is organised in six multidisciplinary Working Groups. State of art of Urinary stents (WG1) is led by D. Rako (Croatia) and P. de Graaf (Netherlands); this WG will focus its work in analysing the current literature on ureteral, urethral and prostatic stents. Computational simulation, Biomedical fluid dynamics, Biomechanical characterization (WG2) led by S. Waters (UK) and F. Clavica (Switzerland) focused on exploring the *in silico* assessment and flow dynamics in a stented ureter. Methodology for the development and validation of new stent designs (WG3) led by S. Stavridis (North Macedonia) and W. Kram (Germany) has been responsible for developing the methodology and validation protocols for future urinary tract stents. Biomaterials and stent coatings (WG4) led by A. Barros (Portugal) and E. O'Cearbhaill (Ireland) has worked on the search of new biomaterials-nanomaterials and coatings with improved behaviour at urinary tract when used for developing urinary stents. Drug Eluting Stents (WG5), led by G. Ciardelli (Italy) and E. Tofail (Ireland), follows the idea to add drugs onto the urinary stent surface to reduce stent-related adverse effects and release drugs locally in the urinary tract. And finally, New research lines (WG6) is dedicated exclusively to proposing forward-looking solutions such as Bioactive-Antibody, Biocovered stents, Biodegradable, Nanotechnology and Bioprinting, led by N. Buchholz (UK), A. Abou-Hassan (France) and I. Skovorodkin (Finland).

The work carried out in the preparation of this book has been distributed in six sections that mainly correspond to the six ENIUS WGs. The first group of chapters focuses on "Current state and clinical applications"; the second is dedicated to the research groups that make up WG2, "Fluid dynamics and urinary stents". The next section of chapters is dedicated to "Design assessment and validation methods", managed by WG3. The last chapters describe the innovative research in "Urinary biomaterials" and "Coatings to reduce the biofilm formation" along with other that focus in "new designs and future developments", carried out the members of WG6.

Therefore, the book that we present represents the work of more than 40 research and clinical groups that provide a multidisciplinary update of great importance by focusing on the problems and above all the solutions from different points of view, which allows a deeper understanding of the current weaknesses of urinary stents, but also addresses the improvement of stents from a multidisciplinary perspective, necessary to reduce the adverse effects of urinary stents, to provide new therapeutic devices to urologist, and as a result improve the quality of life of patients.

We hope that the information provided in this book will be useful to researchers and clinicians and that it will inspire the development of new urinary stents.

Cáceres, Spain   Federico Soria

Acknowledgments

This publication is based upon work from COST Action ENIUS-European Network of Multidisciplinary Research to Improve the Urinary Stents, CA16217, supported by COST (European Cooperation in Science and Technology).

COST (European Cooperation in Science and Technology) is a funding agency for research and innovation networks. Our Actions help connect research initiatives across Europe and enable scientists to grow their ideas by sharing them with their peers. This boosts their research, career and innovation.

www.cost.eu

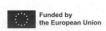

Contents

Present and Future of Urinary Stents

Federico Soria

1 Introduction

Urinary catheters or stents are medical devices widely used in daily urological practice. Their indications are widespread, although they are mainly used to allow internal drainage of urine, either at the ureteral or urethral area. Its use as an internal scaffold is also widely used in patients to promote both first and second intention healing at the urinary tract, after a large number of surgical techniques. It is also widely used in oncology patients to mitigate extrinsic compression and obstructive uropathy, in which case both plastic stents and mainly metallic stents are used. The metal stents have a greater mechanical strength to compression and provide a more appropriate drainage than plastic stents.

Their use is currently very common, reaching more than 80% in patients who have undergone endourological intervention for the resolution of renal or ureteral lithiasis [1]. This gives us an idea of its implantation in lithiasis disease which, as is well known, is increasing its appearance due to the change in dietary habits of the population, mainly in Western countries, although the rates in countries such as China have increased significantly in the last two decades [2].

Unfortunately, urinary stents are associated with high rates of side effects and complications that significantly decrease the quality of life of patients [3]. Therefore, despite their evident usefulness in urological clinical practice, their use should be subject to an important medical evaluation to balance the benefits against the side effects, as well as the possible complications associated with current urinary stents.

F. Soria (✉)
Foundation, Jesús Usón Minimally Invasive Surgery Center, Cáceres, Spain

© The Author(s) 2022
F. Soria et al. (eds.), *Urinary Stents*,
https://doi.org/10.1007/978-3-031-04484-7_1

More than 80% of patients with ureteral stents have significant adverse effects affecting their quality of life, sex life and compromising their labor life [4]. In the case of metallic, ureteral or urethral stents, despite the improvements in design and biomaterials that have appeared in the last decade, their use is essentially reduced to oncological patients with short life expectancy [5]. In the latter case, that of metallic stents in urology, their residual use differs from the widespread and successful use of metallic stents in areas such as cardiology or vascular diseases. This huge difference between such similar devices in different anatomical regions is related to two aspects that differentiate both areas of knowledge, on the one hand, the resources devoted to research and on the other hand, the peculiarities that differentiate the blood vessels of the urinary tract. With regard to the peculiarities of the urinary tract, the first major difference between blood and urine is its relationship with biomaterials. Due to the use of anticoagulants, the interactions of the components that make up the blood with the biomaterials that make up the stent are significantly reduced. Another factor that differentiates the side effects of vascular stents from urinary stents is the fact that vascular stents tend to be endothelialised, thus ceasing to act as a foreign body, a circumstance that is not common in the urinary tract. The presence of ureteral or urethral peristalsis is perhaps one of the major pitfalls associated as a primary cause of failure in urinary metallic stents, a complication that does not occur in the vascular system, although it does in the digestive tract. This peristalsis causes a high migration rate and the appearance of urothelial hyperplasia that can become obstructive [6]. Another cause of the differences in stent deployment and success rate is the common urinary bacterial contamination, with a 100% probability of developing a biofilm on the stent surface and thus developing encrustations that can become obstructive. Although several modifications of the stent surface to reduce biofilm formation and bacterial colonization have been investigated at the moment no available biomaterials or coatings have been proven to prevent or reduce biofilm formation to a clinically relevant extent [7].

If we define biocompatibility as, the utopian state where a biomaterial presents an interface with a physiological environment without the material adversely affecting that environment or the environment adversely affecting the material. From the perspective of a biologic environment affecting the biomaterial, there are currently no biomaterials used in the urinary tract that are perfectly biocompatible. Unfortunately, urine as a liquid so saturated with salts creates a perfect storm, with a hostile environment for the implantation of biomaterials and the prolonged exposure to the urinary environment is not favourable to diminish their effects.

So, given the clinical requirement for the use of urinary stents and their clearly unacceptable adverse effects, the need to improve these medical devices and the research to do so is understandable. Firstly, a great technological development is needed to meet the needs of both patients and urologists for more effective medical devices with fewer associated side effects [8].

2   ENIUS Network

This is the main objective of this manuscript which arises from a European initiative supported by the COST Actions. It is clear that research in this area of knowledge has several limitations that have led to a slowdown in the innovation of urinary stents. Therefore, the creation of a European network dedicated to bring together different groups interested in urinary stents was the first step to break the slow trajectory of research in this medical device. ENIUS, European Network of Multidisciplinary Research to Improve the Urinary Stents, was born in 2017 with the aim of addressing the improvement of stents from a multidisciplinary point of view. We are aware that it is from this type of approach that progress can be made, since urinary stents need such different visions for their improvement as clinical urology, the industrial partners themselves, but also researchers in biomaterials or coatings, researchers in fluid dynamics, or microbiologists due to the permanent relationship between micro-organisms and stents and the urinary microbiome itself complete a plethora of researchers willing to improve stents. Therefore, bringing together so many ways of approaching the same problem can only generate knowledge. Another aspect to overcome in this field of knowledge is the great fragmentation of existing groups, which only leads to isolation. Cooperation between groups benefits everyone involved, as it allows the strengths of each group to be shared and the weaknesses of each group to be mitigated by other groups. The fact of being a multidisciplinary and cooperative network has allowed all participants to grow, to train young researchers who are aware of this important question and its social repercussions. Above all, it allows us to trust that the seed of innovation and development of new stents is in good hands, which benefits patients. It should not be forgotten that the aim of all research is to improve the lives of patients [9].

3   Conclusions

This book brings together the experience and expertise in urinary stents of the leading researchers in urinary stents. Not only because it addresses the present of urinary stents from a clinical point of view, but also because it includes the most innovative groups and future approaches.

References

1. Joshi HB, Stainthorpe A, Keeley FX Jr, MacDonagh R, Timoney AG. Indwelling ureteral stents: evaluation of quality of life to aid outcome analysis. J Endourol. 2001;15(2):151–4. https://doi.org/10.1089/089277901750134421. PMID: 11325084.

2. Zhuo D, Li M, Cheng L, Zhang J, Huang H, Yao Y. A study of diet and lifestyle and the risk of urolithiasis in 1,519 patients in Southern China. Med Sci Monit. 2019;25:4217–24. https://doi.org/10.12659/MSM.916703.
3. Lundeen CJ, Forbes CM, Wong VKF, Lange D, Chew BH. Ureteral stents: the good the bad and the ugly. Curr Opin Urol. 2020;30(2):166–70. https://doi.org/10.1097/MOU.0000000000000701.
4. Sali GM, Joshi HB. Ureteric stents: overview of current clinical applications and economic implications. Int J Urol. 2020;27(1):7–15. https://doi.org/10.1111/iju.14119.
5. Sampogna G, Grasso A, Montanari E. Expandable metallic ureteral stent: indications and results. Minerva Urol Nefrol. 2018;70(3):275–85. https://doi.org/10.23736/S0393-2249.18.03035-7.
6. Soria F, Sun F, Durán E, Sánchez FM, Usón J. Metallic ureteral stents versus endoureter-otomy as a therapeutic approach for experimental ureteral stricture. J Vasc Interv Radiol. 2005;16(4):521–9. https://doi.org/10.1097/01.RVI.0000147074.74604.35.
7. Wiesinger CG, Lee J, Herrera-Caceres JO. Future developments in ureteral stents. Curr Opin Urol. 2019;29(2):124–8. https://doi.org/10.1097/MOU.0000000000000577.
8. Abou-Hassan A, Barros A, Buchholz N, Carugo D, Clavica F, de Graaf P, de La Cruz J, Kram W, Mergulhao F, Reis RL, Skovorodkin I, Soria F, Vainio S, Zheng S. Potential strategies to prevent encrustations on urinary stents and catheters—thinking outside the box: a European network of multidisciplinary research to improve urinary stents (ENIUS) initiative. Expert Rev Med Devices. 2021;18(7):697–705. https://doi.org/10.1080/17434440.2021.1939010.
9. Domingues B, Pacheco M, de la Cruz JE, Carmagnola I, Teixeira-Santos R, Laurenti M, Can F, Bohinc K, Moutinho F, Silva JM, Aroso IM, et al. Future directions for ureteral stent technology: from bench to the market. Adv Ther. 2022;5:2100158. https://doi.org/10.1002/adtp.202100158.

Indications, Complications and Side Effects of Ureteral Stents

Daniel Pérez-Fentes, Javier Aranda-Pérez, Julia E. de la Cruz, and Federico Soria

1 Indications of Polymeric Double J Stents

Double J stents are used in a wide variety of scenarios, which we will divide into two groups of indications for didactic purposes: prophylactic and therapeutic.

1.1 Prophylactic Indications

The insertion of a double J stent can prevent the advent of perioperative complications in specific procedures involving the upper urinary tract. These interventions are mainly focused on urinary stone management, followed by reconstructive procedures.

D. Pérez-Fentes
Urology Department, Complejo Hospitalario de Santiago de Compostela, La Coruña, Spain

J. Aranda-Pérez
Urology Department, Hospital Universitario de Cáceres, Cáceres, Spain

J. E. de la Cruz
Jesús Usón Minimally Invasive Surgery Centre Foundation, Cáceres, Spain
e-mail: jecruz@ccmijesususon.com

F. Soria (✉)
Foundation, Jesús Usón Minimally Invasive Surgery Center, Cáceres, Spain
e-mail: fsoria@ccmijesususon.com

© The Author(s) 2022
F. Soria et al. (eds.), *Urinary Stents*,
https://doi.org/10.1007/978-3-031-04484-7_2

1.1.1 Stone Interventional Treatment

Stents can be placed either before or after stone treatment interventions, for different reasons. Overall, they aim at minimizing the risk of obstruction due to fragments, blood clots or edema after ureteral manipulation [1].

Prior to shock wave lithotripsy (SWL), ureteral stents try to prevent ureteral obstruction secondary to the passage of stone fragments or the formation of a steinstrasse after the treatment. Although very common in the past, it has been demonstrated that this practice doesn't increase the stone free and auxiliary treatment rates. Stenting is generally recommended for stones larger than 1.5–2 cm in diameter, since SWL in these situations will generate more fragments possibly leading to ureteral obstruction. Currently, these stone burdens are more efficiently treated by flexible ureteroscopy or miniaturized percutaneous surgery, in which a preoperative stent is not usually required. However, whenever SWL is the treatment of choice in these cases, double J stenting and its morbidity should be discussed with the patients, as well as the probable need for further lithotripsy sessions [2–6].

Prior to ureteroscopy or retrograde intrarenal surgery, the use of a double J stent aims at creating a passive dilation of the ureter that eases the insertion of the ureteroscope or the ureteral access sheath [7].

This maneuver was very common in the past due to the size of the ureteroscopes available, since not all the ureters admitted such large calibers of endoscopes or ureteral access sheaths. There are data in the literature that show that pre-stenting should lead to better stone-free rates and lessen the incidence of complications, but this finding is mainly based on retrospective studies and is therefore controversial [8–11].

Besides these data, primarily from old series, our opinion and that of the urological guidelines is that with the current armamentarium preoperative stenting should not be systematically recommended. However, placing a double J is advised when the access sheath or the ureteroscope does not go up smoothly into the ureter, in order to create a passive dilation which should allow the passage of these instruments in 1–2 weeks [12, 13].

Post ureteroscopy, be it semirigid or flexible, the use of double J is not routinely recommended, and the stenting decision must be analyzed individually. Clinicians must weigh up the risk of readmission when not leaving a stent against the morbidity of bearing it. Overall, stenting should be mandatory when there is ureteral damage, high risk of obstruction due to edema, fragments or blood clots, when an infective complication occurs or is likely to happen in the postoperative period, as well as in all doubtful cases [14–19].

Besides these recommendations, many groups place double J stents following ureteroscopy in the majority of cases, with considerable differences across countries [20]. In general, when a ureteral access sheath is used, many authors recommend leaving a double J stent at the end of the procedure, due to the considerable incidence of ureteral wall lesions found as a result of the insertion of these sheaths [21]. Therefore, it is advisable to endoscopically review the ureter after these procedures to have more information regarding the urothelium status before the decision to stent [22]. Nevertheless, there is a randomized trial showing that omitting the stent in these cases should be safe and feasible, mainly if the patient has been pre-stented [22, 23].

There are no solid data on the ideal indwelling time, but the vast majority of groups advocate for 1–2 weeks. In some situations, leaving a ureteral stent over-night or a double J on strings for 2–3 days are reasonable alternatives that can lessen the morbidity of bearing a stent for 2 weeks or longer [24–26].

Post percutaneous surgery, the use of double J has been increased in the last years due to the more frequent practice of tubeless surgeries. The decision of leaving a double J after these procedures instead of performing a totally tubeless surgery is mainly based on the surgeon's experience, the characteristics of the case and patient preferences. In this regard, some patients will opt for a percutaneous approach instead of a retrograde surgery in order not to bear a ureteral stent and its symptoms. When endoscopic combined intrarenal surgery is performed, the stenting decision follows the same principles as those previously detailed for ureteroscopic procedures [27].

1.1.2 Renal Transplantation

Ureteral stenting after renal transplantation should contribute for a watertight uretero-neocystostomy, preventing or minimizing urinary leakage that might lead to stricture [28]. A meta-analysis including five randomized controlled trials demonstrated that stented anastomoses have lower complication rates [29].

Due to the characteristics of the ureter in this indication, the length of the catheter used must be considerably shorter. Again, there is no optimal timing for stent removal after transplantation, being 2–4 weeks of indwelling time in the majority of series [30].

1.1.3 Reconstructive Surgery of the Upper Urinary Tract

Pyeloplasty, endopyelotomy, pyelolitectomy, ureteral stricture repair, ureteral trauma repair, etc.

Once more, the objective of the ureteral stent is to help in the healing process of the urinary tract, serving as a scaffold and preventing urinary leaks. In these indications, stents are traditionally removed after 4 weeks, although this dwelling time may be shortened reducing infection risk and morbidity to the patient [31, 32].

1.1.4 Non-urological Procedures Involving Ureteral Dissection

Placing a ureteral stent (either open-end straight or double J) before specific abdominal surgeries where a complex ureteral dissection is suspected makes it easier to identify the ureter during these maneuvers and may prevent accidental injuries. The pros and cons of this endoscopic intervention should be discussed with the patients. When the ureter has not been damaged during the surgery, these stents can be immediately removed or left overnight [33–35].

1.2 Therapeutic Indications

The insertion of a double J ureteral stent aims to drain an obstructed or damaged upper urinary tract.

1.2.1 Decompression of an Obstructed Collecting System

This is the most frequent indication for double J stenting, which needs to be performed in the emergency context or on a scheduled basis, depending on the severity of the case. Urinary drainage must be promptly performed in all cases of obstruction with sepsis, acute renal insufficiency or anuria due to bilateral obstruction or in solitary kidneys, as well as when there is uncontrollable pain. In some groups, percutaneous nephrostomy is preferred in infective situations, although to date there is no data to demonstrate which of these two drainage options is superior [36–38].

1.2.2 Conservative Treatment of Upper Urinary Tract Trauma

Depending on the severity of the damage, these injuries can be conservatively managed with a double J. Stenting provides canalization, reduces urinary leakage and might decrease the risk of strictures. In this scenario, bladder catheterization is advised to prevent backflow of urine through the double J ureteral stent into the upper tract [39, 40].

2 Ureteral Stents Complications

2.1 Intraoperative

2.1.1 Failure of Endoscopic Ureteral Stenting

On some occasions, it is not possible retrograde drainage of the upper urinary tract. It may be due to intrinsic cause (urothelial neoplasms) or extrinsic compression such us retroperitoneal fibrosis or tumours of the abdominopelvic area. It is necessary to treat it (especially if chemotherapy is required). Accordingly, the first treatment option is placing a retrograde ureteral stent However, the rate of stent failure is high, with a range failure rate between 12.2% and 34.6%. Guachetá-Bomba et al. found that cystoscopies result such as the bladder invasion or deformity of the trigone or the age >65 years old are negative factors when attempting an endoscopic urinary drainage [41]. Therefore, it should be considered percutaneous nephrostomy, whether retrograde drainage is not achieved, in order to maintain renal function until obstruction cause is resolved (Figs. 1, 2, 3, and 4).

Fig. 1 Ureteral orifice stricture

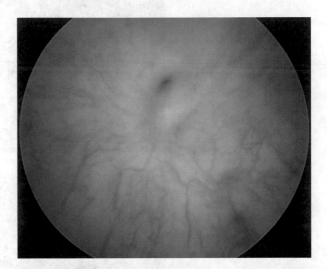

Fig. 2 Ureteral orifice balloon dilatation

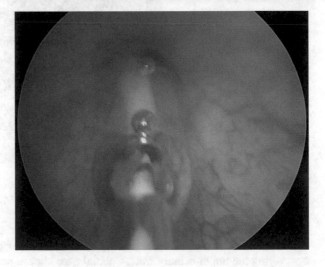

Fig. 3 Ureteral orifice involvement by urothelial carcinoma

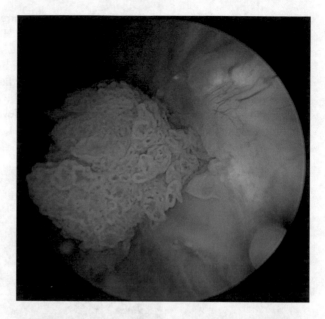

Fig. 4 Transurethral resection of bladder tumor in ureteral orifice

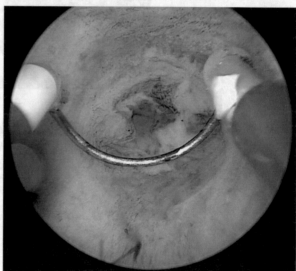

2.1.2 Ureteral Erosion or Perforation

It's a rarest complication of ureteral stent placement. The stent placement should be carefully. It is recommended to previously perform a retrograde pyelography, thus opacifying the upper urinary tract. Special care should be taken in cases of almost complete obstruction of the ureter where the passage of the stent can be complex and the ureteral wall more fragile. If observe any resistance during its progression, never use force, but observe what's happening on the fluoroscopy assessment. If find urinary leak or extravasation, it means ureteral injury. The stenting should be enough to solve the complication, allowing the ureter to heal around the stent, like an internal scaffold.

2.1.3 Stent Malposition

Malposition of a stent is defined as an incorrect position relative to initial placement [42]. A badly placed stent may be in a sub-pyelic position, if the proximal end does not reach the renal pelvis, and in a supravesical position when the distal end is can be found in the ureter. The causes of this complication are mainly due to the placement technique, both endoscopy or fluroscopy placement. This is the reason that it is so important to check the correct location of the stent after it has been placed. An appropriate length is important to avoid this complication.

2.2 Early Complications (2–4 Weeks)

2.2.1 Stent Discomfort

Pain associated with ureteral stents is one of the most common symptoms in patients, with an up to 80% rate of incidence [43]. This pain can be triggered by several reasons: vesicoureteral reflux causing an upward increase in intra-ureteral pressure, related to flank pain; ureteral spasms mainly associated with the distal ureter; and irritation of the bladder mucosa associated with the presence of a bladder foreign body [44]. However, it should be highlighted that the etiology of the pain remains unknown to date.

Mainly, it is related to two separate regions in which pain is reported by patients. Up to 60–77% of patients describe the manifestation of flank pain, which is primarily but not exclusively associated with micturition and VUR caused by the stent. The incidence of suprapubic pain, with up to 38%, is associated with adverse effects at this level related to bladder pigtail and irritation of the bladder trigone [45].

2.2.2 Vesicoureteral Reflux

The UVJ (ureterovesical junction) is a fundamental structure that protects the upper urinary tract from intermittent high pressures in the bladder. The UVJ allows, through its transient opening, the passage of urine into the bladder and prevents retrograde flow into the kidneys during the micturition. A number of factors are involved in the proper working of this anti-reflux mechanism: an appropriate length of intravesical ureter, an oblique angle of insertion of the ureter into the bladder and proper smooth muscle and extracellular matrix development, able to compress the ureteral orifice. Any abnormality in these features leads to retrograde flow of urine or VUR [46].

Vesicoureteral reflux is one of the most important drawbacks in ureteral stenting. This side effect usually appears during the voiding phase of micturition, when the pressure in the bladder increases and the stent, leaving an open communication between the bladder and the ureter, causes the urine to retrograde flow of urine [47].

Regarding the overall VUR rate in stented patients, it's 62–76%, with 80% during the voiding phase compared to 63% during the filling phase [48, 49].

In order to avoid this side effect there have been advances in stent design such as the one with anti-reflux valve, the most widely used. This stent is composed by a standard stent in which the bladder end adds a bag that encompasses the distal end of the stent. Therefore, this kind of stent just blocks the reflux that rises through the internal channel nor the one that can be produced around stent, the periprosthetic flow. Ecke et al. compare this stent with the standard ureteral stent and conclude that reduce the side effects of stents, improving quality of life, as well as being cost-effective [50]. There have been other inventions that have also incorporated a valve at the bladder end in order to prevent ureteral reflux such as McMahon et al. and Ramachandra et al. [51, 52].

2.2.3   Ureteral Smooth Muscle Spasm

A ureteral stent in the upper urinary tract, in addition to changing the dynamics of urinary flow, also has an impact on ureteral myogenic activity [53]. The increase in pressure that occurs is responded to by an increase in ureteral peristalsis during the first few hours and during this period, spasms of the smooth muscle layer of the ureter [54]. These smooth muscle spasms are triggered by the stimulation of $\alpha1$-adrenergic receptors, present at the ureteral and trigone-bladder level, which causes these contractions [55]. These contractions are more important at the level of the ureterovesical junction and distal ureter, corresponding to the higher density of nerve tissue concentrated in the adventitia and smooth muscle layer in these two regions [56].

2.2.4   Lower Urinary Tract Symptoms

Lower urinary tract symptom's (LUTS) are frequent and are clearly attributed to bladder urothelium irritation by a vesical stent end which triggers inflammation and overactivity of the bladder detrusor [57]. LUTS are classified into filling symptoms, emptying symptoms and post-mictional symptoms [58].

In a prospective analysis of the prevalence of symptoms, tolerability and complications of the ureteral stent and its impact on quality of life. Patients completed two questionnaires before stent placement, 7 days after placement, and 14 days after removal. The results concluded that 7 days after stent placement, patients experienced a significant increase symptom in terms of urinary frequency, dysuria, suprapubic pain, urgency and macroscopic hematuria, and a considerably lower quality of life. Alpha blockers, anticholinergics or beta-3 adrenergic agonists can be used to reduce the incidence of stent associated symptoms. Another strategy to achieve a decrease in associated symptoms is prevention: a smaller stent diameter and a proper stent length in order avoid distal loop crossed the bladder mid-line [59].

2.3 Late Complications (>2–4 Weeks)

2.3.1 Urinary Tract Infection (UTI)

Bacterial colonisation of the stents, with an overall rate of 42–90%, is a significant drawback, leading to biofilm formation and the development of bacteriuria and UTI [60]. European Association of Urology recommends, it is indicated prophylactic antibiotics either trimethoprim, trimethoprim-sulphamethoxazole, cephalosporin group 2 or 3 or aminopenicillin plus a beta-lactamase inhibitor, before the place-ment of a ureteral stent in order to prevent urinary tract infections, but, unfortu-nately, they are not enough [61]. It has been reported that colonisation occurs as early as 24 h after stent insertion, but it is not meant to cause infection [62]. The most common organisms isolated from stents are E. coli, Pseudomonas aeruginosa, Staphylococcus spp., and Enterococcus spp. [63]. Kris R et al. found that only about 25% of colonised ureteral stents are associated with positive urine cultures. They also demonstrated that dwell time of the stent is the strongest predictor of clinical urinary tract infection [64].

This susceptibility of stents to bacterial colonisation promotes the development of UTIs, which in some cases can trigger significant complications such as acute pyelonephritis, bacteriuria and renal failure [65]. A gender-related increased risk of stent colonisation has been observed, with a clear higher risk in women than in men, but with no gender-related risk in the appearance of UTIs [66].

To prevent biofilm formation on stents, there have been some innovations such us, coating of polyhydrogel poly (N,N-dimethylacrylamide) (PDMAA) with anti-fouling and protein repellent properties has been used by Szell et al. In vitro studies showed a five-fold decrease of bacterial load on the stent surface [67]. Unfortunately, after promising in vitro results, the human studies have not confirmed these results.

2.3.2 Stent Migration

Stent migration can occur as the ureter is a dynamic organ due to peristalsis. The precise risk factors for stent migration remain to be defined, but an appropriate selection of the stent size is not only necessary to palliate the patients' symptoms,

Fig. 5 Ureteral stent migration

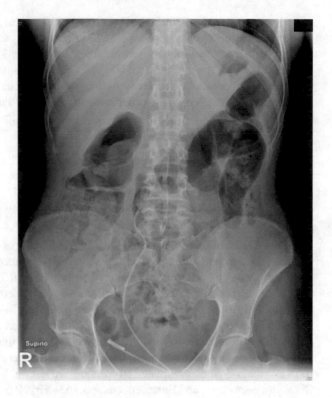

but also to avoid migration [68]. Despite the self-retentive design of the CDJ and appropriate placement, distal migration into the bladder or pelvic migration is a complication with an incidence of up to 9.5% [69] . Furthermore, biomaterials with low friction, such as silicones and hydrophilic coatings, will promote this event [52]. It has been recognised that polyurethane stents have better shape memory and can conform to the urinary tract when compared to silicone stents, decreasing the rate of ureteral stent migration [52] (Fig. 5).

2.3.3   Fragmentation and Breakage

Stent fracture is a very rare complication. It can be caused by mechanical stress, particularly through the lateral orifices, and by a decrease in tensile strength due to depolymerisation that can develop in long-term stenting. Interaction with the urine and extensive inflammatory reaction may promote fragmentation. The rate of ureteral stent fragmentation ranges between 0.3% and 10% [70]. The other factor related with stent fragmentation is stent material. Silicone stents may be more advantageous than polyethylene stents for the lower risk of fragmentation [70].

2.3.4 Forgotten Double-J Stent and Encrustation

The encrustation of forgotten stents is a serious problem due to recurrent urinary tract infections, hematuria, urinary tract obstructions, and renal failure. Similarly, to stent bacterial colonization, stent encrustation increases with stent duration. The aetiology of encrustation is multifactorial [71]: urine composition, stent material, surface properties, stent design, dwell time, urinary pH, urine flow dynamics and bacterial urease. The complexity of the encrustation process is clear, nowadays none of the biomaterials used are resistant to crystal deposition [72].

The definition of a forgotten stent is a device that remains in place for longer than the prescribed time without any medical monitoring. The reasons behind this complication can be attributed to inadequate counselling by the treating doctor and poor compliance of the patient (Figs. 6 and 7).

In a retrospective analysis for a period of 6 years by Adanaur et al., the mean indwelling time was 22.6 months (6–144 months). Of 54 patients, urolithiasis was the indication for stenting in 45 (83.3%) [73].

There have been some innovations to elude this complication such us the biodegradable ureteral stent. F Soria et al. designed a biodegradable antireflux stent that avoids vesicoureteral reflux and bladder trigone irritation as well as the forgotten

Fig. 6 X ray image.
Ureteral stent encrustation

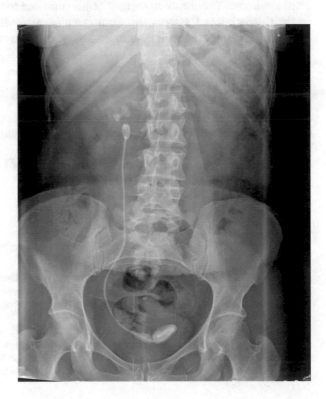

Fig. 7 Cystoscopic view. Bladder end ureteral stent encrustation. Laser Cystolithotripsy

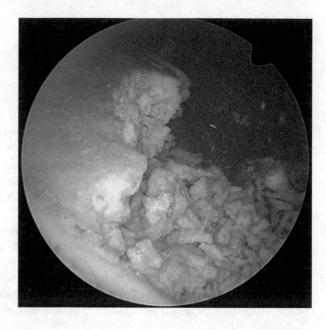

stent syndrome. There was no ureteral obstruction due to degraded stent fragments in their experimental assessment. Consequently, morbidity secondary to ureteral stents might be reduced with intraureteral biodegradable stents [74].

2.3.5 Ureteral Stent Obstruction

Obstruction increases with stent dwell time and not stent size. Causes of obstruction are due to increased debris deposition, crystals deposited on the stent surface, as well as blood clots due to haematuria. The diagnosis is usually made by deterioration of renal function, renal fossa pain or worsening of hydronephrosis. It can be solved by replacement of the stent [75].

References

1. Beysens M, Tailly TO. Ureteral stents in urolithiasis. Asian J Urol. 2018;5:274–86.
2. Al-Awadi KA, Abdul Halim H, Kehinde EO, et al. Steinstrasse: a comparison of incidence with and without J stenting and the effect of J stenting on subsequent management. BJU Int. 1999;84(6):618–21.
3. Musa AA. Use of double-J stents prior to extracorporeal shock wave lithotripsy is not beneficial: results of a prospective randomized study. Int Urol Nephrol. 2008;40:19–22.
4. Mohayuddin N, Malik HA, Hussain M, et al. The outcome of extracorporeal shockwave lithotripsy for renal pelvic stone with and without JJ stent: a comparative study. J Pak Med Assoc. 2009;59(3):143–6.

5. Shen P, Jiang M, Yang J, et al. Use of ureteral stent in extracorporeal shock wave lithotripsy for upper urinary calculi: a systematic review and meta-analysis. J Urol. 2011;186:1328–35.
6. Chandhoke PS, Barqawi AZ, Wemecke C, Chee-Away RA. A randomized outcomes trial of ureteral stents for extracorporeal shock wave lithotripsy of solitary kidney or proximal ureteral stones. J Urol. 2020;167:1981–3.
7. Hubert KC, Palmer JS. Passive dilation by ureteral stenting before ureteroscopy: eliminating the need for active dilation. J Urol. 2005;174:1079–80.
8. Ronald A, Rubenstein RA, Zhao LC, Loeb S, Shore DM, Nadler RB. Presenting improves ureteroscopic stone-free rates. J Endourol. 2007;21:1277–80.
9. Jessen JP, Breda A, Brehmer M, et al. International Collaboration in Endourology: multicenter evaluation of prestenting for ureterorenoscopy. J Endourol. 2016;30:268–73.
10. Assimos D, Crisci A, Culkin D, et al. Preoperative JJ stent placement in ureteric and renal stone treatment: results from the Clinical Research Office of Endourological Society (CROES) ureteroscopy (URS) Global Study. BJU Int. 2016;117:648–54.
11. Yang Y, Tang Y, Bai Y, Wang X, Feng D, Han P. Preoperative double-J stent placement can improve the stone-free rate for patients undergoing ureteroscopic lithotripsy: a systematic review and meta-analysis. Urolithiasis. 2018;46:493–9.
12. Mahajan PM, Padhye AS, Bhave AA, Sovani YB, Kshirsagar YB, Bapat SS. Is stenting required before retrograde intrarenal surgery with access sheath. Indian J Urol. 2009;25:326–8.
13. Ambani SN, Faerber GJ, Roberts WW, Hollingsworth JM, Wolf JR. Ureteral stents for impassable ureteroscopy. J Endourol. 2013;27:549–53.
14. Wang H, Man L, Li G, Huang G, Liu N, Wang J. Meta-analysis of stenting versus non-stenting for the treatment of ureteral stones. PLoS One. 2017;12:e0167670.
15. Nabi G, Cook J, N'Dow J, McClinton S. Outcomes of stenting after uncomplicated ureteroscopy: systematic review and meta-analysis. BMJ. 2007;334:572.
16. Assimos D, Krambeck A, Miller NL, et al. Surgical management of stones: American Urological Association/Endourological Society Guideline, PART II. J Urol. 2016;196:1161–9.
17. Türk C, Neisius A, Petrik A, et al. EAU guidelines on urolithiasis. https://uroweb.org/wp-content/uploads/EAU-Guidelines-on-Urolithiasis-2020v4-1.pdf. Accessed 20 Dec 2020.
18. Song T, Liao B, Zheng S, Wei Q. Meta-analysis of postoperatively stenting or not in patients underwent ureteroscopic lithotripsy. Urol Res. 2012;40:67–77.
19. Haleblian G, Kijvikai K, de la Rosette J, Preminger G. Ureteral stenting and urinary stone management: a systematic review. J Urol. 2008;179:424–30.
20. Muslumanoglu AY, Fuglsig S, Frattini A, et al. Risks and benefits of postoperative double-J stent placement after ureteroscopy: results from the Clinical Research Office of Endourological Society Ureteroscopy Global Study. J Endourol. 2017;31:446–51.
21. Traxer O, Thomas A. Prospective evaluation and classification of ureteral wall injuries resulting from insertion of a ureteral access sheath during retrograde intrarenal surgery. J Urol. 2013;189:580–4.
22. Sirithanaphol W, Jitpraphai S, Taweemonkongsap T, Nualyong C, Chotikawanich E. Ureteral stenting after flexible ureterorenoscopy with ureteral access sheath; is it really needed? A prospective randomized study. J Med Assoc Thail. 2017;100:174.
23. Astorza G, Catalan M, Consigliere L, Selman T, Salvadó J, Rubilar F. Is a ureteral stent required after use of ureteral access sheath in presented patients who undergo flexible ureteroscopy? Cent European J Urol. 2017;70:88–92.
24. Shigemura K, Yasufuku T, Yamanaka K, Yamahsita M, Arakawa S, Fujisawa M. How long should double J stent be kept in after ureteroscopic lithotripsy? Urol Res. 2012;40:373–6.
25. Nevo A, Mano R, Baniel J, Lifshitz DA. Ureteric stent dwelling time: a risk factor for post-ureteroscopy sepsis. BJU Int. 2017;120:117–22.
26. Komeya M, Usui K, Asai T, et al. Outcome of flexible ureteroscopy for renal stone with overnight ureteral catheterization: a propensity score-matching analysis. World J Urol. 2018;36:1871–6.

27. Garofalo M, et al. Tubeless procedure reduces hospitalization and pain after percutaneous nephrolithotomy: results of a multivariable analysis. Urolithiasis. 2013;41:347–53.
28. Wilson CH, Rix DA, Manas DM. Routine intraoperative ureteric stenting for kidney transplant recipients. Cochrane Database Syst Rev. 2013;17:CD004925.
29. Mangus RS, Haag BW. Stented versus nonstented extravesical ureteroneocystostomy in renal transplantation: a metanalysis. Am J Transplant. 2004;4:1889–96.
30. Breda A, Budde K, Figueiredo A, et al. EAU guidelines on renal transplantation. https://uroweb.org/wp-content/uploads/EAU-Guidelines-on-Renal-Transplantation-2020.pdf. Accessed 20 Dec 2020.
31. Mandhani A, Kappor R, Zaman W, et al. Is a 2-week duration sufficient for stenting in endo-pyelotomy? J Urol. 2003;169:886–9.
32. Danuser H, Germann C, Pelzer N, Rühle A, Stucki P, Mattei A. One- vs 4-week stent place-ment after laparoscopic and robot-assisted pyeloplasty: results of a prospective randomized single-centre study. BJU Int. 2014;113:931–5.
33. Chou MT, Wang CJ, Lien RC. Prophylactic ureteral catheterization in gynecologic surgery: a 12-year randomized trial in a community hospital. Int Urogynecol J Pelvic Floor Dysfunct. 2009;20:689–93.
34. Speicher PJ, Goldsmith ZG, Nussbaum DP, Turley RS, Peterson AC, Mantyh CR. Ureteral stenting in laparoscopic colorectal surgery. J Surg Res. 2014;190:98–103.
35. Coakley KM, Kasten KR, Sims SM, Prasad T, Heniford BT, Davis BR. Prophylactic ureteral catheters for colectomy: a national surgical quality improvement program-based analysis. Dis Colon Rectum. 2018;61:84–8.
36. Cepeda M, Mainez JA, de la Cruz B, Amón JH. Indications and morbidity associated with double J catheters. Arch Esp Urol. 2016;69:462–70.
37. Lynch MF, Anson KM, Patel U. Percutaneous nephrostomy and ureteric stent insertion for acute renal deobstruction: consensus based guidance. Br J Med Surg Urol. 2008;1:120–5.
38. Pearle MS, Pierce HL, Miller GL, et al. Optimal method of urgent decompression of the col-lecting system for obstruction and infection due to ureteral calculi. J Urol. 1998;160:1260–4.
39. Kitrey ND, Djakovic N, Hallscheidt P, et al. EAU guidelines on urological trauma. https://uroweb.org/wp-content/uploads/EAU-Guidelines-on-Urological-Trauma-2020.pdf. Accessed 20 Dec 2020.
40. Schwartz BF, Stoller ML. Endourologic management of urinary fistulae. Tech Urol. 2000;6:193–5.
41. Guachetá-Bomba PL, Echeverría-García F, García-Perdomo HA. Predictors for failure of endoscopic ureteric stenting in patients with malignant ureteric obstruction: systematic review and meta-analysis. BJU Int. 2021;127(3):292–9.
42. Dryer RB, Chen MY, Zagoria RJ, Regan JD, Hood CH, Kavanagh PV. Complications of ure-teral stent placement. Radiographics. 2002;22:1005–22.
43. Joshi HB, Stainthorpe A, Keeley FX, MacDonagh R, Timoney AG. Indwelling ureteral stents: evaluation of quality of life to aid outcome analysis. J Endourol. 2001;15:151–4.
44. Bonkat G, Rieken M, Müller G, Roosen A, Siegel FP, Frei R, et al. Microbial colonization and ureteral stent-associated storage lower urinary tract symptoms: the forgotten piece of the puzzle? World J Urol. 2013;31:541–6.
45. Joshi HB, Stainthorpe A, MacDonagh RP, Keeley FX, Timoney AG. Indwelling ureteral stents: evaluation of symptoms, quality of life and utility. J Urol. 2003;169:1065–9.
46. Tokhmafshan F, Brophy PD, Gbadegesin RA, Gupta IR. Vesicoureteral reflux and the extracel-lular matrix connection. Pediatr Nephrol. 2017;32:565–76.
47. Koprowski C, Kim C, Modi PK, Elsamra SE. Ureteral stent-associated pain: a review. J Endourol. 2016;30(7):744–53.
48. Yossepowitch O, Lifshitz DA, Dekel Y, Ehrlich Y, Gur U, Margel D, et al. Assessment of vesi-coureteral reflux in patients with self-retaining ureteral stents: implications for upper urinary tract instillation. J Urol. 2005;173:890–3.

49. Shao Y, Shen Z, Zhuo J, Liu H, Yu S, Xia S-J. The influence of ureteral stent on renal pelvic pressure in vivo. Urol Res. 2009;37:221–5.
50. Ecke TH, Bartel P, Hallmann S, Ruttloff J. Evaluation of symptoms and patients' comfort for JJ-ureteral stents with and without antireflux-membrane valve. Urology. 2010;75(1):212–6.
51. McMahon CW, Nief CA, Schmidt DR, Choe LJ, Aponte MG, Pelayo SL, inventor; Baylor University, assignee. Ureteral stent and method; 2017.
52. Ramachandra M, Mosayyebi A, Carugo D, Somani BK. Strategies to improve patient outcomes and QOL: current complications of the design and placements of ureteric stents. Res Rep Urol. 2020;12:303–14.
53. Janssen C, Buttyan R, Seow CY, Jäger W, Solomon D, Fazli L, et al. A role for the hedgehog effector Gli1 in mediating stent-induced ureteral smooth muscle dysfunction and aperistalsis. Urology. 2017;104:242.e1–8.
54. Johnson LJ, Davenport D, Venkatesh R. Effects of alpha-blockade on ureteral peristalsis and intrapelvic pressure in an in vivo stented porcine model. J Endourol. 2016;30:417–21.
55. Lamb AD, Vowler SL, Johnston R, Dunn N, Wiseman OJ. Meta-analysis showing the beneficial effect of α-blockers on ureteric stent discomfort. BJU Int. 2011;108:1894–902.
56. Vernez SL, Okhunov Z, Wikenheiser J, Khoyilar C, Dutta R, Osann K, et al. Precise characterization and 3-dimensional reconstruction of the autonomic nerve distribution of the human ureter. J Urol. 2017;197:723–9.
57. Park HK, Paick SH, Kim HG, Lho YS, Bae S. The impact of ureteral stent type on patient symptoms as determined by the Ureteral Stent Symptom Questionnaire: a prospective, randomized, controlled study. J Endourol. 2015;29:367–71.
58. Andersson K. Storage and voiding symptoms: pathophysiologic aspects. Urology. 2003;62:3–10.
59. Scarneciu I, Lupu S, Pricop C, Scarneciu C. Morbidity and impact on quality of life in patients with indwelling ureteral stents: a 10-year clinical experience. Pak J Med Sci. 2015;31(3):522–6.
60. Kehinde EO, Rotimi VO, Al-hunayan A, Abdul-halim H, Boland F, Al-awadi KA. Bacteriology of urinary tract infection associated with indwelling J ureteral stents. J Endourol. 2004;18:891–6.
61. Urological infections. EAU guidelines. Edn. presented at the EAU Annual Congress Amsterdam the Netherlands; 2020.
62. Cormio L, Vuopio-varkila J, Siitonen A, Talja M, Ruutu M. Bacterial adhesion and biofilm formation on various double-J stents in vivo and in vitro. Scand J Urol Nephrol. 1996;30(1):19–24.
63. Liaw A, Knudsen B. Urinary tract infections associated with ureteral stents: a review. Arch Esp Urol. 2016;69(8):479–84.
64. Klis R, Korczak-kozakiewicz E, Denys A, Sosnowski M, Rozanski W. Relationship between urinary tract infection and self-retaining double-J catheter colonization. J Endourol. 2009;23(6):1015–9.
65. Scotland KB, Lo J, Grgic T, Lange D. Ureteral stent-associated infection and sepsis: pathogenesis and prevention: a review. Biofouling. 2019;35:117–27.
66. Kehinde EO, Rotimi VO, Al-Awadi KA, Abdul-Halim H, Boland F, Al-Hunayan A, et al. Factors predisposing to urinary tract infection after J ureteral stent insertion. J Urol. 2002;167:1334–7.
67. Szell TFFD, Goelz H, Bluemel B, et al. In vitro effects of a novel coating agent on bacterial biofilm development on ureteral stents. J Endourol. 2019;33(3):225–31.
68. Slaton JW, Kropp KA. Proximal ureteral stent migration: an avoidable complication? J Urol. 1999;155:58–61.
69. Leibovici D, Cooper A, Lindner A, Ostrowsky R, Kleinmann J, Velikanov S, et al. Ureteral stents: morbidity and impact on quality of life. Isr Med Assoc J. 2005;7:491–4.
70. El-Faqih SR, Shamsuddin AB, Chakrabarti A, et al. Polyurethane internal stents in treatment of stone patients: morbidity related indwelling times. J Urol. 1991;146:1487–91.
71. Mosayyebi A, Yue QY, Somani BK, Zhang X, Manes C, Carugo D. Particle accumulation in ureteral stents is governed by fluid dynamics: in vitro study using a "stent-on-chip" model. J Endourol. 2018;32(7):639–46.

72. Lange D, Bidnur S, Hoah N, Chew BH. Ureteral stent-associated complications-where we are and where we are going. Nat Rev Urol. 2015;12:17–25.
73. Adanur S, Ozkaya F. Challenges in treatment and diagnosis of forgotten/encrusted double-J ureteral stents: the largest single-center experience. Ren Fail. 2016;38(6):920–6.
74. Soria F, Morcillo E, Serrano A, Budia A, Fernández I, Fernández-Aparicio T, Sánchez-Margallo FM. Evaluation of a new design of antireflux-biodegradable ureteral stent in animal model. Urology. 2018;115:59–64.
75. El-Faqiq SR, Shamsuddin AB, Chakrabarti A, et al. Polyurethane internal ureteral stents in treatment of stone patients: morbidity related to indwelling times. J Urol. 1991;146:1487–91.

Indications, Complications and Side Effects of Metallic Ureteral Stents

Duje Rako

1 Introduction

Even though metal might be the first material used for unblocking urinary tract, first widely used stents in the ureter were polymeric. And polymers do have their problems with longevity, compression, encrustation, irritation etc. which has led researchers to try other materials—amongst them metal alloys. First metallic stents used in ureter were made from stainless steel (Wallstent, Palmaz-Schatz) and afterwards focus was mainly on nitinol (nickel titanium oxide) as well as other alloys (tantalum, platinum, niobium, cobalt, etc.) with or without PTFE (polytetrafluoroethylene) or polymer coating. In shape/structure, they can replicate typical JJ design [1] (Passage—nitinol JJ stent, Resonance—nickel-chromium-cobalt-molybdenium JJ stent) or have coil (Memokath—nitinol coils, Allium—loose nitinol coils with polymer coating) or mesh (Uventa—nitinol mesh with PTFE coating) structure. By mechanism of deployment we can recognise baloon-expandable, self-expandable, thermo-expandable and non-expandable metallic ureteral stents.

First documented metallic stent used in ureter was vascular permanent stent (Wallstent) placed in two patients with malignant obstruction by Lugmayer in 1992 [2]. Afterwards many vascular stents were tried but high rates of complications and inability for easy removal and replacement led to their discontinuation and development of purpose-based urological metallic stents which could be more easily removed and replaced [3].

D. Rako (✉)
Croatia Polyclinic, Zagreb, Croatia

© The Author(s) 2022
F. Soria et al. (eds.), *Urinary Stents*,
https://doi.org/10.1007/978-3-031-04484-7_3

2   Indications for Metallic Ureteral Stents

For kidneys to function properly, urine produced should flow freely through ureters in order to reach bladder or substitute reservoir. Should drainage become impaired excessive intrarenal pressure will develop and can subsequently lead to kidney damage and eventually to loss of function. This blockage can come from within the ureter (internal) or outside of it (external) and by nature of cause described as malignant, benign or post radiotherapy. Two main ways of unblocking an obstructed renal unit can be considered; either internally via ureteral stent or externally by means of nephrostomy and both ways should provide uninterrupted urinary drainage.

Internal unblocking of renal unit using stent is minimally invasive and should offer long enough indwelling time with the ideal stent being easy to insert and remove, made of biocompatible and MRI-compatible material and causing no adverse host reaction (inflammation, urothelial hyperplasia, tumour ingrowth etc.) and being resistant to incrustation. Unfortunately, such stent still does not exist but some materials and designs cover many of requirements.

Even though both polymeric and metallic stents can be considered in all of benign, malignant and post-radiotherapy settings but we will usually opt for metallic stents in situations in which longer indwelling times are projected with benign conditions (resistant post inflammatory strictures), malignant obstruction (due to internal occlusion or external compression) or post-radiotherapy strictures [4].

3   Complications and Side Effects of Metallic Ureteral Stents

Even with careful and proper usage complications will inevitably arise and same is with metallic ureteral stents [5–7]. Some complications are inherent with stent design and others come from material used or applied coating. Many case reports and review papers have summarised either single stent experience or problems with specific patient population and none of them have yet discussed complications on a sufficiently large number of patients so workgroup within COST Action 16217— ENIUS (European Network of multidisciplinary research to Improve the Urinary Stents) has led literature search in order to identify, catalogue and review in a systematic way all published complications and patency rates for metallic ureteral stents used for ureteric obstructions [data prepared for publication].

In our systematic review 319 publications were identified and 111 acceptable full text papers were thoroughly examined leading to 88 being included in final analysis. That translates to database of 1749 patients with 2194 ureter units receiving 2394 stents with 1188 complications documented. It is worth noting that some of complications are due to disease itself (especially malignant) others correspond to stent type and shape or material and cation used. Even though some patients did not experience any complications or side effects, others have had multiple stent related complications but in total this translates to 68% per patient and 50% per stent risk of complication. Only 3.4% of papers (3/88) have used verified system for reporting complications (modified Clavien-Dindo classification [8]) which also poses problem in real-world data acquisition. Complication reporting in general and specifically using standardised approach is obviously not at the highest standards among academic urologic community and further actions are needed in order for that to be changed in future.

Complications related to stent placement (regardless of stent type) were low in our dataset and only 22 failures and 4 significant difficulties were documented in attempt to place 2394 stents which comes to less than 1.1% in total.

3.1   Off Label Use of Bare Metal Stents (BMS) Designed for Vascular or Gastroenterological Use in Ureteric Obstruction

First papers reporting experience with off-label use of metallic mesh stents (developed for cardiovascular use) in ureters started to emerge in 1991 with promising results initially, but as soon as 1993 reports on poor outcomes started to emerge. Review and vast personal experience published by Liatsikos et al. in 2009 started era of review papers but no comprehensive set of data reporting on complications was published as yet. Majority of data in our dataset come from experience using Wallstent™ (Schneider, Zürich, Switzerland later Boston Scientific/Microvasive, MA, USA) and other data come from use of other stents mainly Strecker (Boston Scientific, MA, USA), AccuFlex (Boston Scientific, MA, USA), Protege (Endovascular Inc., MN, USA), Luminexx (Bard GmbH, Angiomed, Karlsruhe, Germany), Sinus-Flex (Optimed, Ettingen, Germany) and Palmaz-Schatz (Johnson and Johnson, Warren, USA).

A total of 29 papers have reported on use of (mostly vascular or biliar) BMS in 345 patients (258 with malignant and 87 benign conditions) with 359 stents implanted in malignant and 98 in benign ureter units with a total of 277 complications reported which translates to 80% of patients at risk of complication or 60% per stent used. Among complications most prevalent were obstruction or occlusion in 71 (26%), tumour overgrowth or ingrowth in 59 (21%), flank or abdominal pain in 39 (14%), urothelial hyperplasia in 33 (12%). Also, four serious complications needing surgery (including two nephrectomies due to chronic pyelonephritis and two laser surgeries to remove stents) were also reported. Reported patency rates ranged from 0% to 100% with most report around 30–80% (Figs. 1, 2, and 3).

From these results we can conclude that early cardiovascular and biliary stents placed (off-label) in ureters had promising initial results but with follow up approaching 1 year they mostly suffered obstructive complications (occlusion, compression, tumour overgrowth or reactive hyperplasia) which were responsible for roughly 60% of incapacitated stents.

Fig. 1 Ureteroscopic
assessment. Metallic stent
encrustation. (Dr. F. Soria.
JUMISC. Spain)

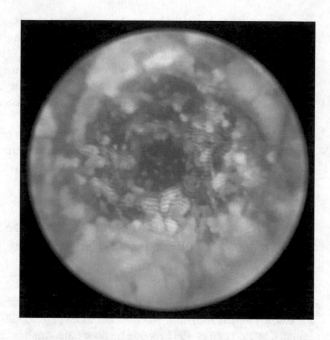

Fig. 2 Ureteroscopic
assessment. Obstructive
urothelial hyperplasia. (Dr.
F. Soria. JUMISC. Spain)

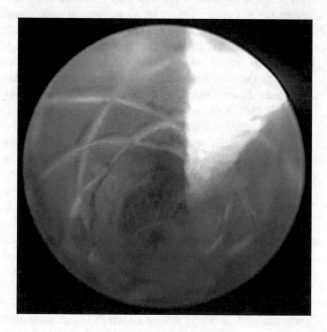

Fig. 3 Fluoroscopic view.
Ureteral metallic stent
migration. (Dr. F. Soria.
JUMISC. Spain)

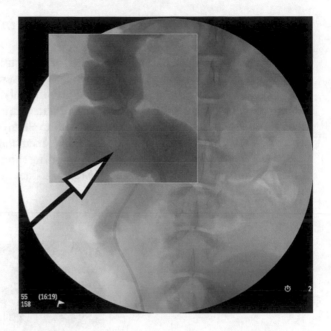

3.2 Off Label Use of Covered Metal Stents (CMS) Designed for Vascular or Gastroenterological Use in Ureteral Obstruction

Research advancements in cardiology has led to introduction of covered metal stents which were also tried in ureters and resulted in no benefit compared to off-label use of vascular/gastroenterological BMS with regards to complication rates with migrations and UTI's being most common.

Only five studies in our dataset had some data on covered metal stents including two on Passager stent (Boston Scientific Corporation, Oakland, NJ, USA), one on polyurethane tube with metal wire (Mannheim hospital, Heidelberg University, Germany), one on Dacron covered nitinol mesh stent (Stanford, Nanture, France) and one on ePTFE covered nitinol stent (Hemobahn Endoprosthesis, W. L. Gore and Associates, Inc., Flagstaff, Arizona, USA). In total they report 72 patients (49 malignant and 23 benign obstructions) with 86 ureteral units (56 and 30 respectively) with 69 complications reported namely migration/dislocation in 20 (29%), urinary tract infections (UTI) in 11 (16%), vesicoureteral reflux in 9 (13%) and reactive hyperplasia in 7 (10%) being most common. One nephrectomy was carried out due to recurrent UTI's. Patency rates reported ranged from 18.75% to 100%.

3.3 Covered Metal Stents Designed for Use in Urinary Tract

Purpose built covered metallic stents designed for use in urinary tract (Allium™ and Uventa™) could be considered as next generation of covered stents. Allium™ URS is segmental nitinol mesh stent fully covered with polymeric coating with high radial force in mid part and low radial force in outer parts. Uventa™ is segmental ureteral self-expanding metallic mesh stent with triple-layered structure consisting of nitinol mesh on outer and inner side and PTFE membrane in middle (Fig. 4).

Our search has identified only one study reporting short term outcomes with use of three Allium urethral stents (Allium™ Medical, Caesarea, Israel) in two patients resulting in one obstruction.

Fig. 4 Fluoroscopic assessment. Ureteral Uventa™ metallic stent. (Taewoong Medical, Seoul, Korea)

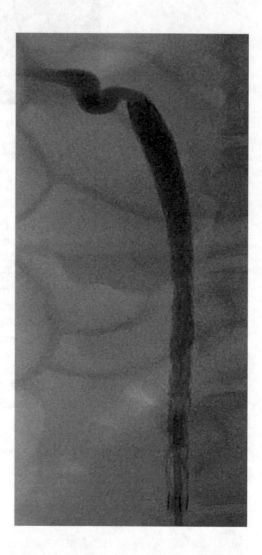

Ten reports were included on use of Uventa™ (Taewoong Medical, Seoul, Korea) stent in 202 patients (158 with malignant and 44 benign disease) across 238 ureteral units with a total of 163 complications with 16 (10%) of which were serious (7 uretero-enteric fistula, 4 uretero-arterial fistula, 2 uretero-vaginal fistula and one pseudoaneurysm, ureteral perforation and sepsis each). Other more common complications include tumour overgrowth/ingrowth in 26 (16%), flank or abdominal pain in 21 (13%) and urothelial hyperplasia in 19 (12%) of cases. Reported patency rates ranged from 30% to 100% but mainly around 65–100%.

3.4   Memokath 051™ (PNN Medical A/S, Kvistgaard, Denmark)

Memokath 051™ is a thermo-expandable, spiral-shaped (coiled) memory nickel-titanium metallic alloy segmental stent and could be considered as next generation bare metal stent with reduced complications when compared to purpose built covered metallic stents. It was more often used in benign conditions than any other stent in our review.

Data from 21 paper on use of Memokath 051™ stent report on 423 patient (188 with malignant and 235 benign condition) with 469 ureter unit (214 and 255 respectively) and 230 complications with 48% of them (111) related to migration. Obstruction, occlusion or compression is reported in further 23% of cases (52). Only one serious complication (uretero-arterial fistula post radiotherapy for colon cancer) was reported. Patency was reported anywhere between 40% and 100% with figures around 70–80% being most common especially in larger series.

3.5   Resonance™ (Cook Medical, Bloomington, IN, USA)

Resonance™ is 6 Fr double pigtail full metal (nickel-chromium-cobalt-molybdenium alloy) tight spiral stent without internal lumen and is like Memokath 051™ also considered to be next generation purpose built BMS and was most widely used stent in our review.

Twenty-eight papers in our review reported use of 1085 Resonance™ stents implanted in 707 patients (with 462 due to malignancy and 245 for benign conditions) with 944 ureter units (621 and 323 respectively) with a total of 449 complications reported with UTI being the most common with 23% (103 cases) followed by compression in 20% (91 cases) and obstruction or occlusion in further 10% (43 cases). Among eight reported significant complications three were subcapsular haematomas (all in one series), three sepsis and two surgeries due to calcification (one cystolitholapaxy and another percutaneous nephrolithotomy). With a mean follow up of 1 year reported patency rates were between 10% and 100% with larger studies usually reporting patency rates around 70–90%.

4   Conclusion and Further Recommendations

Even though metallic ureteral stents in general exhibit better patency rates than polymeric stents in comparable patient populations and provide effective long term drainage they still have high rates of complications and side effects. Metallic ureteral stents (especially segmented ones) also tend to cause less stent-related symptoms than polymeric JJ stents.

As expected, purpose-built metallic ureteric stents outperform off-label vascular and biliary stents used in past but they still have nearly 50% complication chance with 2.6% of them graded as severe. Difference among stents in predominant type of complication arise from differences inherent in stent design or material used. Despite these negative issues, metallic ureteral stents still represent most appropriate salvage options for certain groups of patients with short life expectancy or those unwilling or unable to undergo surgery.

Choice which metallic ureteral stent should be preferred over others depend on local availability, stage and localisation of disease, patient characteristics and expectations, provider (urologist, interventional radiologist) preference and experience and cost and reimbursement policy [9].

In order to have better graded recommendations there is still unmet need for multi-institutional prospective randomised trial with adequate number of patients stratified to malignant, benign and post-radiotherapy group designed as head to head superiority trial of existing metallic ureteral stents with follow up period at least 12 months in order to obtain high quality data on their patency and complication rates.

In conclusion, due to high number of complications, stent failures, side effects and stent-related symptoms, stringent follow-up of these patients is necessary.

References

1. Finney RP. Experience with new double J ureteral catheter stent. J Urol. 1978;167:1135–8, discussion 1139.
2. Lugmayr H, Pauer W. Self-expanding metal stents for palliative treatment of malignant ureteral obstruction. AJR Am J Roentgenol. 1992;159(5):1091–4.
3. Buchholz N, Hakenberg O, Masood J, Bach C, editors. Handbook of urinary stents: basic science and clinical applications. London: JP Medical Ltd; 2016.
4. Sampogna G, Grasso A, Montanari E. Expandable metallic ureteral stent: indications and results. Minerva Urol Nefrol. 2018;70(3):275–85.
5. Kallidonis P, et al. The effectiveness of ureteric metal stents in malignant ureteric obstructions: a systematic review. Arab J Urol. 2017;15(4):280–8.
6. Khoo CC, et al. Metallic ureteric stents in malignant ureteric obstruction: a systematic review. Urology. 2018;118:12–20.

7. Liatsikos EN, et al. Ureteral metal stents: 10-year experience with malignant ureteral obstruction treatment. J Urol. 2009;182(6):2613–7.
8. Dindo D, Demartines N, Clavien PA. Classification of surgical complications: a new proposal with evaluation in a cohort of a 6336 patients and results of a survey. Ann Surg. 2004;240:205–13.
9. Liatsikos E, et al. Ureteral stents: past, present and future. Expert Rev Med Devices. 2009;6(3):313–24.

Urethral Stents. Indications, Complications and Adverse Effects

Petra de Graaf, Daniel Yachia, Federico Soria, and Duje Rako

1 Introduction

Urine produced in kidneys should freely flow out through the ureters, bladder and urethra. Bladder outlet obstruction [BOO] by benign or malignant processes leads to Lower urinary tract symptoms [LUTS], reduced quality of life, and if left untreated it may damage kidneys and lead to loss of kidney function. BOO in the urethra is more prevalent in males compared to females, as the male urethra is much longer and can be caused by several conditions at different anatomical locations.

In this review we focus on the entire male urethra. Since no stents are used in female urethral obstructions, they will be excluded from this review [1].

At the prostatic urethra, the major cause for BOO is benign prostatic hyperplasia [BPH]. About 105 million men are affected globally of BPH [2]. Development of BPH typically begins after the age of 40, around half of males aged 50 and over are affected [3] with the majority [~90%] of males affected after the age of 80 [3]. Prostate cancer can also lead to BOO. More distal in the urethra, the major cause of

P. de Graaf (✉)
Department of Urology, University Medical Center Utrecht, Utrecht, The Netherlands
e-mail: p.degraaf-4@umcutrecht.nl

D. Yachia
Department of Urology, Hillel Yaffe Medical Centre, Rappaport Faculty of Medicine, Technion, Haifa, Israel
e-mail: dyachia@innoventions-med.com

F. Soria
Foundation, Jesús Usón Minimally Invasive Surgery Center, Cáceres, Spain
e-mail: fsoria@ccmijesususon.com

D. Rako
Polyclinic Croatia, Zagreb, Croatia

Zagreb University School of Medicine, Zagreb, Croatia

© The Author(s) 2022
F. Soria et al. (eds.), *Urinary Stents*,
https://doi.org/10.1007/978-3-031-04484-7_4

obstruction is strictures of the urethra. Urethral strictures due to fibrosis occur in approximately 1% of the male population over 55 years of age [4].

2 Brief History of Lower Urinary Stents

The 1980s can be seen as the decade of various stent inventions in medicine, especially for use in vascular occlusions but also for prostatic obstructions. These stents were either self expandable or balloon expandable stents [5]. The use of urethral stents starts in 1980 with the introduction of the "partial catheter"/'urological spiral' invented by Fabian [6]. This was a 21F stainless steel coil for inserting into the occluded prostatic urethra, instead of an indwelling catheter. For reducing the risk of stone formation on the stainless steel, in 1987 a group in Denmark gold-plated the 'urological spiral' and named it Prostakath [7]. Since then, a variety of metals and biostable and biodegradable polymers have been used to produce temporary or permanent stents for the management of infravesical obstructions such as benign or malignant prostatic enlargement, bladder neck stenoses, urethro-vesical anastomotic stenoses or urethral strictures. Some stents originally developed for vascular use were also adapted for use along the urethra. Examples are: The balloon expandable Palmaz Stent [only for the prostatic urethra], the self-expanding Memotherm and the Urolume which was an adaptation of the vascular Wallstent. The Wallstent was developed by Hans Wallsten as a vascular stent and later adapted to urological use under the name Urolume Wallstent [8]. The design of this stent was based on a wire braiding technology similar to the "Chinese finger trap"; an old Chinese trick in which one can insert a finger that is trapped when the finger is retracted. This braiding technology allowed the stent to self-expand and apply radial force to the surrounding tissues. The Urolume Wallstent became a very popular stent for urethral stricture. Despite the initial enthusiasm for the use of permanent stents in recurrent urethra strictures, on longer follow up they could not prove themselves as a good alternative to urethroplasty and now they are used only in selected, frail, poor surgical risk patients.

The other self-expanding stent, the Memotherm was made of a nickel titanium alloy (nitinol) wire knitted to form a tube. This thermo-sensitive stent expanded to its maximal caliber at body temperature [9]. This stent also lost its initial enthusiasm for the same Reasons as the Urolume Wallstent.

The ProstaCoil, a large caliber (24/30F), nitinol made self-expanding temporary prostatic stent was based on the UroCoil which was developed for use in frequently recurring urethral strictures [10].

Almost at the same time different polymer made stents started to appear: The polyurethane made small caliber [16F] prostatic stent named 'intra-urethral catheter—IUC' [11], a similar 16F Barnes stent [12], the larger caliber silicone made Trestle and the more recent Spanner [13].

During the same years the Biofix/SpiroFlow biodegradable prostatic coil stent made of self-reinforced polyglycolic acid [SR-PLA] was also introduced. However, it failed to support the expectations because, after losing their radial force, they crushed into the urethral lumen and caused an obstruction that had to be solved by endoscopic removal of its segments [14].

Stenting the lower urinary tract is minimally invasive approach to relieve BOO in patients unfit for surgery or in others as an alternative to surgery. What we need from a urinary stent is a patent lumen so it can support both micturition and sexual activity without serious adverse effects. The ideal urethral stent is flexible so it can support the urethral lumen in both the flaccid or erect status of the penis. In addition, the ideal stent is an off-the-shelf product, so that each patient can be treated directly.

Since their introduction in the late 1980s, stents have been studied in the urinary tract to prevent scaring contraction and re-modelling of the strictured urethral segments. Although the first reports seemed to promise excellent outcomes, longer follow-up began to cast doubts on the usefulness of urethral stenting as a primary treatment modality for urethral stricture disease [15]. Especially permanently implanted stents lead to tissue ingrowth and re-stenosis. Temporary stents prevented tissue ingrowth in their lumen but induces tissue ingrowth at their ends. Resection of this tissue or removal of the stent opened the obstructed lumen.

3   Classification of Stents

First use of a stent in the urinary tract was the permanent use of a 22F catheter for 1–4 years in a small group of 19 patients [16]. Later vascular stents were used 'off label'. The Palmaz stent, Wallstent and the Memotherm were supposed to be completely covered by urothelial tissue within a few weeks after their implantation like in the vascular tract. Less than satisfying results with these stents especially in the prostatic urethra led to development of urethral specific stents. Most of these stents had either a fixed caliber, or are self-expandable or thermo-expandable.

Differing from other tubular organs, the cross section of the prostatic urethra is rarely round. For this reason, some of the permanent stents could not become fully covered with tissue as they were supposed to become and stones could develop on the uncovered bare metal wires. Despite this drawback both the Urolume and the Memotherm are still used in selected high surgical risk patients [17]. The Palmaz stent dropped from use because its lack of radial self-expanding force.

Urethral stents can be classified in several groups. First, we can make a distinction on anatomical location. We have prostatic urethral stents—both for benign and malignant obstructions and bulbar and distal urethra stents, these are used to open the urethral lumen after traumatic pelvic bone fractures, endoscopic manipulations related and in case of recurrent infection (e.g. lichen sclerosis, gonorrhoea). An additional classification is based on the type of stent, there are permanent and removable stents, mesh stents can be either balloon expandable and self-expandable. Examples of the removable stents are among others Fabian stent/Prostacath, InStent's ProstaCoil and UroCoil, Allium's TPS, BUS and RPS. Lastly few experimental trials are reported on degradable stents.

The use of a permanent stent positioned in distal urethra may look to be an attractive treatment in the treatment of strictures. The Urolume/Wallstent and the Memotherm which are permanent stents were used as an alternative approach in such stenoses [18]. Time showed that the use of permanent stents is a contraindication in these cases because of intra-stent obstructive tissue proliferation [19, 20]. Significant complication rates were also observed when such stents were used for benign prostatic obstructions [21].

4 Aim of This Chapter

In the present chapter we provide an overview of the current literature to summarize the most common complications seen with different urethral stents for male patients with benign or malignant urethral obstruction of the urethra. Full data extraction is ongoing, this is our initial report.

5 Materials and Methods

5.1 Literature Search

Following search string: *[[[[urethra] OR urethral]] AND [[[[stent] OR endoprothesis] OR endoprosthesis] OR stents]]* was initially used both in Embase and PubMed, in February 2019 and a re-run in March 2020. Cross references were added. Figure 1 presents an outline of the literature search in a Prisma Flow Diagram [22]. Prospective, retrospective, comparative studies, case reports and case series were included.

5.2 Study Selection

Results from PubMed and the Embase were imported in Rayyan [https://rayyan. qcri.org/], where duplicates were removed. The title and abstract screen was performed by two authors independently [PdG, DR]; the full text screen was performed by the same authors, also independently of each other. Any differences in the screening results were solved by discussion. Studies were excluded when written in languages other than English, non-original papers [abstract, comment or review paper], when describing pre-clinical studies and non-human use, when studying wrong

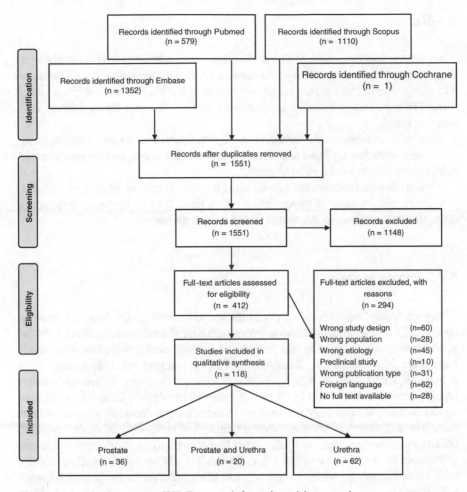

Fig. 1 Study selection process [22]. For more information, visit www.prisma-statement.org

population, e.g. wrong etiology of the urethral obstruction [mainly detrusor sphincter dyssynergia] or stenting by catheter after reconstruction surgery. The primary endpoint was cause [restricture, infection, migration and other causes for stent failure] and rate of complications and secondary endpoint was patency rate. Stent patency was calculated as number of failed stented urethra over number of total stented urethra and failed stented urethra is defined as stent not being able to do as expected so an unplanned stent removal.

6 Results

After search has been run, 1551 publications were identified and their abstracts were screened independently by two authors [PdG, DR] resulting in consensus on 412 acceptable full text papers which were thoroughly read by same authors and of those 118 were finally included in systematic review. Reasons for exclusions were listed in Fig. 1.

Over 4000 patients are described, with varying follow up. Several different stents were used, including *off label* use of covered metal stents designed for vascular use, drug eluting stents, biodegradable stents.

Papers were divided on use in anatomical location [prostate, urethra or report on both locations]. In total, 94 papers recorded on results, 24 papers on complications only. Here we summarize the results based on this division.

6.1 Prostatic Stents

Thirty-six studies report on stent use in the prostatic urethra. Of these, 34 reported on results, 2 on complications. An overview of the studies is given in Table 1. At the prostatic region the UroLume was the most used stent, used in 8 studies, other stents used were MemoKath (3), Memotherm (2), 4 reported on ProstaKath, 3 on ProstaCoil, 2 on Urospiral, 4 on Spanner and a variety of others, including 4 studies on biodegradable stents. As a full data extraction and analysis is currently performed by the authors, we can only preliminary summarize the common adverse effects, including dislocation of the stent, dysuria, retention, recurrence of obstruction and urinary incontinence. Meta-analysis cannot be performed due to different endpoints, differences in stents and most of all, differences in follow up. Overall, in studies with short follow up, success rates are much higher than in studies with longer follow up.

6.2 Stents in Both Prostatic and Urethral Region

Twenty studies reported on urethral stents both in the prostatic and the bulbar urethral region, without making clear distinction or made a combinations of results/complications in both regions. Of these, 16 reported on results, and 4 on complications. An overview of these studies is given in Table 2. Again, the Urolume was used most in this combined region (8), the other 12 studies were using a variety of stents, including a 22F catheter [16] and some titanium alloys based stents [see Table 2 for description]. Success rate in up to 50% of cases, however, short follow up may bias these results, as some complications take longer to develop.

Table 1 Data extraction prostate

Authors	Year	Report on	Number of patients	Type of stent
Van Dijk et al. [26]	2006	Results	108	Bell- shaped nitinol prostatic stent
Petas et al. [27]	1997	Results	45	Biodegradable
Laaksovirta et al. [28]	2002	Results	50	Biodegradable, self-expandable SR-PLGA copolymer stent
Talja et al. [29]	1995	Results	22	Biodegradable, self-reinforced polyglycolic acid spiral stent
Petas et al. [30]	1997	Results	72	Biodegradable, self-reinforced polyglycolic acid spiral stent
Morgentaler and DeWolf [31]	1993	Results	25	Gianturco-Z stent
Nissenkorn et al. [32]	1996	Results	15	IUC intraurethral catheter
Poulsen et al. [33]	1993	Results	30	MemoKath
Williams and White [34]	1995	Results	48	MemoKath
Kimata et al. [35]	2015	Results	37	MemoKath
Tseng et al. [36]	2007	Complications	1	Memotherm
Gesenberg and Sintermann [37]	1998	Results	123	Memotherm
Guazzoni et al. [38]	1994	Results	135	Modified Urolume
Yachia et al. [39]	1995	Results	65	ProstaCoil
Yachia and Aridogan [40]	1996	Results	27	ProstaCoil
Ovesen et al. [41]	1990	Results	1	Prostakath
Thomas et al. [42]	1993	Results	64	Prostakath
Sofer et al. [43]	1998	Complications	107	Prostakath or Urospiral
Yachia and Aridogan [44]	1996	Results	117	Prostakath vs Prostacoil
Song et al. [45]	1995	Results	13	Self-expandable metallic Z-stent
Mori et al. [46]	1995	Results	17	Shape memory alloy
Henderson et al. [47]	2002	Results	5	Spanner
Corica et al. [48]	2004	Results	30	Spanner
Tyson et al. [49]	2012	Results	20	Spanner
Goh et al. [50]	2013	Results	16	Spanner
Porpiglia et al. [51]	2018	Results	32	Temporary implantable nitinol device [TIND]
Van Dijk et al. [52]	2005	Results	35	Thermoexpandable hourglass-shaped nitinol prostatic stent
Milroy and Chapple [53]	1993	Results	54	UroLume
Williams et al. [54]	1993	Results	96	Urolume
Oesterling et al. [55]	1994	Results	126	UroLume

(continued)

Table 1 (continued)

Authors	Year	Report on	Number of patients	Type of stent
Schneider et al. [56]	1994	Results	70	UroLume
Anjum et al. [57]	1997	Results	62	Urolume
Lallas et al. [58]	2001	Results	1	UroLume
McLoughlin et al. [9]	1990	Results	19	Unclear [UroLume]
Özgür et al. [59]	1993	Results	31	Urospiral
Adam et al. [60]	1990	Results	21	Wallstent

Table 2 Data extraction prostate and urethra

Authors	year	Report on	Number of patients	Type of stent
Fair [16]	1982	Results	21	22F catheter
Perez-Marrero and Emerson [61]	1993	Results	9	Balloon expanded titanium prostatic urethral stent
Qiu et al. [62]	1994	Results	25	Chinese titanium-nickel alloy with shape memory
Choi et al. [63]	2007	Results	33	Covered nitinol stent
Boullier and Parra [64]	1991	Results	20	Expandable titanium stent
Takahashi et al. [65]	2013	Complications	4	MemoKath
Ricciotti et al. [66]	1995	Results	49	Memotherm
Egilmez et al. [67]	2006	Complications	76	Nitinol
Inoue and Misawa [68]	1997	Results	1	ProstaKath
Parra [69]	1991	Results	5	Titanium endourethral stent
Yachia and Beyar [70]	1993	Results	20	UroCoil
Corujo and Badlani [71]	1998	Complications	2	Urolume
Milroy [72]	1991	Results	45	UroLume
Oesterling [73]	1993	Results	N/A	UroLume
Sweetser et al. [74]	1993	Results	23	UroLume
Bailey et al. [75]	1998	Results	14	UroLume
Wilson et al. [76]	2002	Results	10	UroLume
Shah et al. [77]	2003	Results	465	UroLume
McNamara et al. [78]	2013	Results	45	UroLume
Chapple and Bhargava [19]	2008	Complications	14	Variety of stents

6.3   Urethral Stents

The largest set of studies was found for urethral stenting, 62 studies were selected, 44 reported on results, 18 on complications. An overview of these studies is given in Table 3. Urolume was used in 26 studies, 3 of these studies compared the stent to the Wallstent. 10 studies reported on Wallstent alone. Six studies reported on the use

Table 3 Data extraction urethra

Authors	Year	Report on	Number of patients	Type of stent
Shental et al. [79]	1998	Complications	1	Porges Urethrospiral-2 stent [as second stent, over a UroLume]
Culha et al. [80]	2014	Results	54	Allium
Silagy et al. [81]	2017	Results	15	Allium
Temeltas et al. [82]	2016	Results	28	Allium
Yachia and Beyar [83]	1991	Results	18	Biocompatible metal alloy
Isotalo et al. [84].	2002	Results	22	Biodegradable
Isotalo et al. [85]	1998	Results	22	Biodegradable
Song et al. [86]	2003	Results	12	Covered nitinol stent
Jordan et al. [87]	2013	Results	92	MemoKath
Jung et al. [88]	2013	Results	13	MemoKath
Wong et al. [89]	2014	Results	22	MemoKath
Abdallah et al. [90]	2013	Results	23	MemoKath
Barbagli et al. [91]	2017	Results	16	MemoKath
Sertcelik et al. [92]	2011	Results	47	MemoKath
Atesci et al. [93]	2014	Results	20	Memotherm
Takenaka et al. [94]	2004	Results	1	Metal
Gujral et al. [95]	1995	Results	7	Modified Z-stent, Gianturco type
Na et al. [96]	2012	Results	59	Nitinol
Eisenberg et al. [97]	2008	Complications	22	Several types
Kotsar et al. [98]	2009	Results	10	PLGA
Nissenkorn [99]	1995	Results	22	Polyurethane
Nissenkorn and Shalev [100]	1997	Results	42	Polyurethane
Kim et al. [101]	2017	Results	54	Retrievable self-expandable metallic stents
Yachia et al. [102]	1990	Results	26	Self-retaining stent
Saporta et al. [103]	1993	Results	16	UroCoil
Sikafi [104]	1996	Results	18	UroCoil
Fisher and Santucci [105]	2006	Complications	1	UroLume
Gupta and Ansari [106]	2004	Complications	1	UroLume
Paddack et al. [107]	2009	Complications	1	UroLume
Tahmaz et al. [108]	2009	Complications	1	UroLume
Cimentepe et al. [109]	2004	Results	1	UroLume
Parsons and Wright [110]	2004	Complications	3	UroLume
Rodriguez Jr. and Gelman [111]	2006	Complications	2	UroLume

(continued)

Table 3 (continued)

Authors	Year	Report on	Number of patients	Type of stent
Scarpa et al. [112]	1997	Results	2	UroLume
Gelman and Rodriguez Jr. [113]	2007	Complications	10	UroLume
Elkassaby et al. [114]	2007	Complications	13	UroLume
Milroy [115]	1993	Results	6	UroLume
Angulo et al. [116]	2018	Complications	63	Urolume
De Vocht et al. [117]	2003	Complications	15	Urolume
Hussain et al. [118]	2004	Complications	60	UroLume
Badlani et al. [119]	1995	Results	175	UroLume
Breda et al. [120]	1994	Results	82	UroLume
Donald et al. [121]	1991	Results	33	Urolume
Granieri and Peterson [122]	2014	Results	4	UroLume
Milroy and Allen [123]	1996	Results	50	UroLume
Sertcelik et al. [124]	2000	Results	60	UroLume
Shah et al. [20]	2003	Results	24	UroLume
Tillem et al. [125]	1997	Results	41	UroLume
Eisenberg et al. [126]	2007	Results	13	UroLume [11], endovascular [2]
Morgia et al. [127]	1999	Results	99	Wallstents [94], 5 other
Verhamme et al. [128]	1993	Complications	1	Wallstent
Krah et al. [129]	1992	Complications	1	Wallstent
Pansadoro et al. [130]	1994	Results	1	Wallstent
Baert et al. [131]	1993	Complications	7	Wallstent
Baert et al. [132]	1991	Results	6	Wallstent
Beier-Holgersen et al. [133]	1993	Results	10	Wallstent
Kardar and Lindstedt [134]	1998	Results	8	Wallstent/UroLume
Milroy et al. [135]	1989	Results	8	Wallstent/UroLume
Katz et al. [136]	1994	Complications	2	Wallstent/UroLume
Oosterlinck and Talja [137]	2000	Results	N/A	Various stents
Milroy et al. [138]	1989	Results	8	Various stents
Palminteri et al. [23]	2010	Complications	13	Various stents

of MemoKath, 1 on MemoTherm, 2 on UroCoil and 3 on Allium stents. The other 17 studies used other stents, described a variety of stents or the stents used were ill-defined. Reported complications included stent migration, haematuria, recurrent strictures or obstructed stents by encrustation, urinary tract infections, perineal pain and sexual dysfunction. Despite their relatively high complication rates, externally covered stents seemed more effective with fewer complications than either uncovered or internally covered stents. However, all stents intrinsically generate the risk to turn a simple stenosis into a complex stenosis requiring a staged urethroplasty, a definitive urethrostomy, or a permanent suprapubic diversion [23].

7 Discussion

In total, we analyzed 118 studies on urethral stenting, 94 on results and 24 on complications. In the studies analyzed, the UroLume was used most frequently. Full extraction of the data is in progress, we will report later on this based on this book chapter.

In modern urological practice, ureter stents and bladder catheters have become indispensable tools. The use urethral and prostate stents was introduced with optimism and hope; however, these latter stents have not shown their benefits over current procedures to treat urethral obstruction. Over the course of time, many improvements in designs and constitutive materials for urinary stents have taken place in an attempt to improve their efficacy. Nevertheless, they remain associated with several adverse effects that limit their value as tools for long-term urinary drainage. Infection, encrustation, migration, hyperplastic epithelial reaction, and patient discomfort are the most common problems [24] and, especially for urethral stricture disease, open urethral reconstruction is the treatment of choice for patients with traumatic strictures and those with previously failed urethroplasty [19]. For patients unfit for this major open surgery, research for better stents, potentially biodegradable or a combination of materials and cells will be a better option [25].

8 Limitations and Risk of Bias

The included studies used different approach on reporting complications therefore a quantitative report on the adverse effects was not possible. Publication bias is likely on the included reports, both biased on complication in the case reports, as well as bias on the outcome due to short follow up.

9 Conclusion and Future Perspectives

It is clear from papers we have analyzed that purpose-built urethral stents have outperformed off-label vascular stents, but still the ideal stent has not been identified. Despite many adverse effects, urethral stents may still be useful, in particular to the elderly unfit patient in whom a major operation is contraindicated, providing a rapid treatment that can be performed with the patient under local anesthesia. For this we need to develop better stents that can avoid the current complications and disadvantages. Cross pollination is needed between basic, translational, preclinical and clinical research, thereby combining knowledge on materials, cells, rheology, tissue, pathophysiology and pathology, with the ultimate aim better treatment options for our patients.

Acknowledgements This systematic review was part of activities from Workgroup State of art of urinary stents within COST Action 16217 ENIUS European Network of multidisciplinary research to Improve the Urinary Stents.

References

1. Agochukwu-Mmonu N, Srirangapatanam S, Cohen A, Breyer B. Female urethral strictures: review of diagnosis, etiology, and management. Curr Urol Rep. 2019;20(11):74.
2. GBD 2015 Disease and Injury Incidence and Prevalence Collaborators. Global, regional, and national incidence, prevalence, and years lived with disability for 310 diseases and injuries, 1990–2015: a systematic analysis for the Global Burden of Disease Study 2015. Lancet. 2016;388(10053):1545–602.
3. Kim EH, Larson JA, Andriole GL. Management of benign prostatic hyperplasia. Annu Rev Med. 2016;67:137–51.
4. Santucci RA, Joyce GF, Wise M. Male urethral stricture disease. J Urol. 2007;177(5):1667–74.
5. Maas D, Kropf L, Egloff L, Demierre D, Turina M, Senning A. Transluminal implantation of intravascular 'double helix' spiral prostheses; technical and biological considerations. ESAO Proc. 1982;9:252–6.
6. Fabian KM. [The intra-prostatic "partial catheter" [urological spiral] [author's transl]]. Urologe A. 1980;19[4]:236–8.
7. Mandresi A. Prostakath. Un' endoprotesi uretrale prostatica per la risoluzione della patalogia ostruttiva da cause prostatica. Riv Med Prat. 1989;288:32–4.
8. Wallsten H, Knight C, Eldin A, Milroy E. History of Wallstent. In: Yachia D, Paterson PJ, editors. Stenting the urinary tract. London: Martin Dunitz; 2004.
9. McLoughlin J, Jager R, Abel PD, Din AE, Adam A, Williams G. The use of prostatic stents in patients with urinary retention who are unfit for surgery: an interim report. Br J Urol. 1990;66(1):66–70.
10. Yachia D, Beyar M. Preservation of sexual function by insertion of 'ProstaCoil' instead of indwelling catheter in surgically unfit BPH patients. In: Proceedings of the second international congress in therapy in andrology; 1991. p. 399–402.
11. Nissenkorn I. Experience with a new self-retaining intraurethral catheter in patients with urinary retention: a preliminary report. J Urol. 1989;142(1):92–4.
12. Barnes DG, Butterworth P, Flynn JT. Combined endoscopic laser ablation of the prostate [ELAP] and temporary prostatic stenting. Minim Invasive Ther Allied Technol. 1996;5(4):333–5.
13. Corica AP, Corica F, Sagaz A. The spanner temporary prostatic stent. In: Yachia D, Paterson PJ, editors. Stenting the urinary tract. 2nd ed. London: Martin Dunitz; 2004. p. 409–18.
14. Talja M, Välimaa T, Tammela T, Petas A, Törmälä P. Bioabsorbable and biodegradable stents in urology. J Endourol. 1997;11(6):391–7.
15. Djordjevic ML. Treatment of urethral stricture disease by internal urethrotomy, dilation, or stenting. Eur Urol Suppl. 2016;15(1):7–12.

16. Fair WR. Internal urethrotomy without a catheter: use of a urethral stent. J Urol. 1982;127(4):675–6.
17. Sakamoto H, Matsuda A, Arakaki R, Yamada H. Outcome analysis of the urethral stent [Memotherm®]. Acta Urol Jpn. 2012;58(1):13–6.
18. Zivan I, Stein A. New modality for treatment of resistant anastomotic strictures after radical prostatectomy: UroLume urethral stent. J Endourol. 2001;15(8):869–71.
19. Chapple CR, Bhargava S. Management of the failure of a permanently implanted urethral stent—a therapeutic challenge. Eur Urol. 2008;54(3):665–70.
20. Shah DK, Paul EM, Badlani GH. 11-Year outcome analysis of endourethral prosthesis for the treatment of recurrent bulbar urethral stricture. J Urol. 2003;170(4):1255–8.
21. Madersbacher S. Stents for prostatic diseases: any progress after 25 years? Eur Urol. 2006;49(2):212–4.
22. Moher D, Liberati A, Tetzlaff J, Altman DG, Group P. Preferred reporting items for systematic reviews and meta-analyses: the PRISMA statement. PLoS Med. 2009;6(7):e1000097.
23. Palminteri E, Gacci M, Berdondini E, Poluzzi M, Franco G, Gentile V. Management of urethral stent failure for recurrent anterior urethral strictures. Eur Urol. 2010;57(4):615–21.
24. Dyer RB, Chen MY, Zagoria RJ, Regan JD, Hood CG, Kavanagh PV. Complications of ureteral stent placement. Radiographics. 2002;22(5):1005–22.
25. Abou-Hassan A, Barros A, Buchholz N, Carugo D, Clavica F, de Graaf P, et al. Potential strategies to prevent encrustations on urinary stents and catheters—thinking outside the box: a European network of multidisciplinary research to improve urinary stents [ENIUS] initiative. Expert Rev Med Devices. 2021;18(7):697–705.
26. Van DM, Mochtar CA, Wijkstra H, Laguna MP, Rosette DL. The bell-shaped nitinol prostatic stent in the treatment of lower urinary tract symptoms: experience in 108 patients. Eur Urol. 2006;49(2):353–9.
27. Petas A, Talja M, Tammela TLJ, Taari K, Valimaa T, Tormala P. The biodegradable self-reinforced poly-DL-lactic acid spiral stent compared with a suprapubic catheter in the treatment of post-operative urinary retention after visual laser ablation of the prostate. Br J Urol. 1997;80(3):439–43.
28. Laaksovirta S, Isotalo T, Talja M, Välimaa T, Törmälä P, Tammela TLJ. Interstitial laser coagulation and biodegradable self-expandable, self-reinforced poly-L-lactic and poly-L-glycolic copolymer spiral stent in the treatment of benign prostatic enlargement. J Endourol. 2002;16(5):311–5.
29. Talja M, Tammela T, Petas A, Valimaa T, Taari K, Viherkoski E, et al. Biodegradable self-reinforced polyglycolic acid spiral stent in prevention of postoperative urinary retention after visual laser ablation of the prostate-laser prostatectomy. J Urol. 1995;154(6):2089–92.
30. Petas A, Talja M, Tammela T, Taari K, Lehtoranta K, Valimaa T, et al. A randomized study to compare biodegradable self-reinforced polyglycolic acid spiral stents to suprapubic and indwelling catheters after visual laser ablation of the prostate. J Urol. 1997;157(1):173–6.
31. Morgentaler A, DeWolf WC. A self-expanding prostatic stent for bladder outlet obstruction in high risk patients. J Urol. 1993;150(5):1636–40.
32. Nissenkorn I, Slutzker D, Shalev M. Use of an intraurethral catheter instead of a Foley catheter after laser treatment of benign prostatic hyperplasia. Eur Urol. 1996;29(3):341–4.
33. Poulsen AL, Schou J, Ovesen H, Nordling J. MemokathR: a second generation of intraprostatic spirals. Br J Urol. 1993;72(3):331–4.
34. Williams G, White R. Experience with the Memotherm™ permanently implanted prostatic stent. Br J Urol. 1995;76(3):337–40.
35. Kimata R, Nemoto K, Tomita Y, Takahashi R, Hamasaki T, Kondo Y. Efficacy of a thermoexpandable metallic prostate stent [Memokath] in elderly patients with urethral obstruction requiring long-term management with urethral Foley catheters. Geriatr Gerontol Int. 2015;15(5):553–8.
36. Tseng KF, Tai HL, Chang CP. Case report: endoscopic removal of memotherm urethral stent with diode laser. J Endourol. 2007;21(1):100–2.

37. Gesenberg A, Sintermann R. Management of benign prostatic hyperplasia in high risk patients: long-term experience with the memotherm stent. J Urol. 1998;160(1):72–6.
38. Guazzoni G, Montorsi F, Coulange C, Milroy E, Pansadoro V, Rubben H, et al. A modified prostatic UroLume Wallstent for healthy patients with symptomatic benign prostatic hyperplasia: a European multicenter study. Urology. 1994;44(3):364–70.
39. Yachia D, Beyar M, Aridogan IA. Prostacoil [a new, large caliber, self-expanding and self-retaining temporary intraprostatic stent] in the treatment of prostatic obstructions. Ann Med Sci. 1995;4(1):25–34.
40. Yachia D, Aridogan IA. The use of a removable stent in patients with prostate cancer and obstruction. J Urol. 1996;155(6):1956–8.
41. Ovesen H, Poulsen AL, Nordling J. Differentiation between neurogenic and prostatic obstruction using the intraprostatic spiral: a case report. Scand J Urol Nephrol. 1990;24(3):179–80.
42. Thomas PJ, Britton JP, Harrison NW. The Prostakath stent: four years' experience. Br J Urol. 1993;71(4):430–2.
43. Sofer M, Chen J, Braf Z, Matzkin H. Can intraprostatic stent failure be predicted? Experience based on long-term follow-up of 107 patients. Minim Invasive Ther Allied Technol. 1998;7(4):389–93.
44. Yachia D, Aridogan IA. Comparison between first-generation [fixed-caliber] and second-generation [self-expanding, large caliber] temporary prostatic stents. Urol Int. 1996;57(3):165–9.
45. Song HY, Cho KS, Sung KB, Han YM, Kim YG, Kim CS. Self-expandable metallic stents in high-risk patients with benign prostatic hyperplasia: long-term follow-up. Radiology. 1995;195(3):655–60.
46. Mori K, Okamoto S, Akimoto M. Placement of the urethral stent made of shape memory alloy in management of benign prostatic hypertrophy for debilitated patients. J Urol. 1995;154(3):1065–8.
47. Henderson A, Laing RW, Langley SE. A Spanner in the works: the use of a new temporary urethral stent to relieve bladder outflow obstruction after prostate brachytherapy. Brachytherapy. 2002;1(4):211–8.
48. Corica AP, Larson BT, Sagaz A, Corica AG, Larson TR. A novel temporary prostatic stent for the relief of prostatic urethral obstruction. BJU Int. 2004;93(3):346–8.
49. Tyson MD, Hurd KJ, Nunez RN, Wolter CE, Humphreys MR. Temporary prostatic urethral stenting as a provocative tool to determine surgical eligibility in complex bladder outlet obstructed patients: our initial experience. Curr Urol. 2012;6(2):82–6.
50. Goh MHC, Kastner C, Khan S, Thomas P, Timoney AG. First experiences with the Spanner™ temporary prostatic stent for prostatic urethral obstruction. Urol Int. 2013;91(4):384–90.
51. Porpiglia F, Fiori C, Bertolo R, Giordano A, Checcucci E, Garrou D, et al. 3-Year follow-up of temporary implantable nitinol device implantation for the treatment of benign prostatic obstruction. BJU Int. 2018;122(1):106–12.
52. Van DM, Mochtar CA, Wijkstra H, Laguna MP, Rosette DL. Hourglass-shaped nitinol prostatic stent in treatment of patients with lower urinary tract symptoms due to bladder outlet obstruction. Urology. 2005;66(4):845–9.
53. Milroy E, Chapple CR. The urolume stent in the management of benign prostatic hyperplasia. J Urol. 1993;150(5):1630–5.
54. Williams G, Coulange C, Milroy EJG, Sarramon JP, Rubben H. The urolume, a permanently implanted prostatic stent for patients at high risk for surgery. Results from 5 collaborative centres. Br J Urol. 1993;72(3):335–40.
55. Oesterling JE, Kaplan SA, Epstein HB, Defalco AJ, Reddy PK, Chancellor MB. The North American experience with the UroLume endoprosthesis as a treatment for benign prostatic hyperplasia: long-term results. Urology. 1994;44(3):353–63.
56. Schneider HJ, De Souza JV, Palmer JH. The Urolume as a means of treating urinary outflow obstruction and its impact on waiting lists. Br J Urol. 1994;73(2):181–4.

57. Anjum MI, Chari R, Shetty A, Keen M, Palmer JH. Long-term clinical results and quality of life after insertion of a self-expanding flexible endourethral prosthesis. Br J Urol. 1997;80(6):885–8.
58. Lallas CD, Munver R, Preminger GM. Removal of a UroLume prostatic stent using the holmium laser. Urology. 2001;57(1):166–7.
59. Özgür GK, Sivrikaya A, Bilen R, Biberoĝlu K, Gümele HR. The use of intraurethral prostatic spiral in high risk patients for surgery with benign prostatic hyperplasia. Int Urol Nephrol. 1993;25(1):65–70.
60. Adam A, Jäger R, McLoughlin J, El-Din A, Machan L, Williams G, et al. Wallstent endoprostheses for the relief of prostatic urethral obstruction in high risk patients. Clin Radiol. 1990;42(4):228–32.
61. Perez-Marrero R, Emerson LE. Balloon expanded titanium prostatic urethral stent. Urology. 1993;41(1):38–42.
62. Qiu CY, Wang JM, Zhang ZX, Huang ZX, Zheng QY, Du ZQ, et al. Stent of shape-memory alloy for urethral obstruction caused by benign prostatic hyperplasia. J Endourol. 1994;8(1):65–7.
63. Choi EK, Song HY, Ji HS, Lim JO, Park H, Kim CS. Management of recurrent urethral strictures with covered retrievable expandable nitinol stents: long-term results. Am J Roentgenol. 2007;189(6):1517–22.
64. Boullier JA, Parra RO. Prostatic titanium urethral stents. A new treatment option for obstructive uropathy: early clinical results and indications. ASAIO Trans. 1991;37(3):297.
65. Takahashi R, Kimata R, Hamasaki T, Kawarasaki Y, Kondo Y. Memokath™ urethral stents induce incontinence in patients with urethral balloon catheters. J Nippon Med Sch. 2013;80(6):433–7.
66. Ricciotti G, Bozzo W, Perachino M, Pezzica C, Puppo P. Heat-expansible permanent intraurethral stents for benign prostatic hyperplasia and urethral strictures. J Endourol. 1995;9(5):417–22.
67. Egilmez T, Aridogan IA, Yachia D, Hassin D. Comparison of nitinol urethral stent infections with indwelling catheter-associated urinary-tract infections. J Endourol. 2006;20(4):272–7.
68. Inoue Y, Misawa K. Temporary spiral stent after endoscopic repair of posttraumatic stricture of prostatomembranous urethra. Urol Int. 1997;58(4):250–1.
69. Parra RO. Treatment of posterior urethral strictures with a titanium urethral stent. J Urol. 1991;146(4):997–1000.
70. Yachia D, Beyar M. New, self-expanding, self-retaining temporary coil stent for recurrent urethral strictures near the external sphincter. Br J Urol. 1993;71(3):317–21.
71. Corujo M, Badlani GH. Uncommon complications of permanent stents. J Endourol. 1998;12(4):385–8.
72. Milroy E. Permanent prostate stents. J Endourol. 1991;5(2):75–8.
73. Oesterling JE. Urologic applications of a permanent, epithelializing urethral endoprosthesis. Urology. 1993;41(1):10–8.
74. Sweetser PM, Ravalli R, Brettschneider N, Badlani G. Use of multiple Wallstents in treatment of bladder outlet obstruction. J Endourol. 1993;7(4):327–31.
75. Bailey DM, Foley SJ, McFarlane JP, O'Neil G, Parkinson MC, Shah PJR. Histological changes associated with long-term urethral stents. Br J Urol. 1998;81(5):745–9.
76. Wilson TS, Lemack GE, Dmochowski RR. UroLume stents: lessons learned. J Urol. 2002;167(6):2477–80.
77. Shah DK, Kapoor R, Badlani GH. Experience with urethral stent explantation. J Urol. 2003;169(4):1398–400.
78. McNamara ER, Webster GD, Peterson AC. The urolume stent revisited: the duke experience. Urology. 2013;82(4):933–6.
79. Shental J, Chaimowitch G, Katz Z, Rozenman J. Treatment of a recurrent bulbar urethral stricture after Urolume wallstent implantation with a second inner Urethrospiral-2 urethral stent. Urol Int. 1998;60(3):199–201.

80. Culha M, Ozkuvanci U, Ciftci S, Saribacak A, Ustuner M, Yavuz U, et al. Management of recurrent bulbar urethral stricture—a 54 patients study with Allium bulbar urethral stent [BUS]. Int J Clin Exp Med. 2014;7(10):3415–9.
81. Silagy A, Merrett C, Agarwal D. Initial experience with Allium™ stent in the management of bulbar urethral stricture. Transl Androl Urol. 2017;6:S91.
82. Temeltas G, Ucer O, Yuksel MB, Gumus B, Tatli V, Muezzinoglu T. The long-term results of temporary urethral stent placement for the treatment of recurrent bulbar urethral stricture disease? Int Braz J Urol. 2016;42(2):351–5.
83. Yachia D, Beyar M. Temporarily implanted urethral coil stent for the treatment of recurrent urethral strictures: a preliminary report. J Urol. 1991;146(4):1001–4.
84. Isotalo T, Talja M, Välimaa T, Törmälä P, Tammela TLJ. A bioabsorbable self-expandable, self-reinforced poly-L-lactic acid urethral stent for recurrent urethral strictures: long-term results. J Endourol. 2002;16(10):759–62.
85. Isotalo T, Tammela TL, Talja M, Välimaa T, Törmälä P. A bioabsorbable self-expandable, self-reinforced poly-l-lactic acid urethral stent for recurrent urethral strictures: a preliminary report. J Urol. 1998;160(6):2033–6.
86. Song HY, Park H, Suh TS, Ko GY, Kim TH, Kim ES, et al. Recurrent traumatic urethral strictures near the external sphincter: treatment with a covered, retrievable, expandable nitinol stent—initial results. Radiology. 2003;226(2):433–40.
87. Jordan GH, Wessells H, Secrest C, Squadrito JF Jr, McAninch JW, Levine L, et al. Effect of a temporary thermo-expandable stent on urethral patency after dilation or internal urethrotomy for recurrent bulbar urethral stricture: results from a 1-year randomized trial. J Urol. 2013;190(1):130–6.
88. Jung HS, Kim JW, Lee JN, Kim HT, Yoo ES, Kim BS. Early experience with a thermo-expandable stent [Memokath] for the management of recurrent urethral stricture. Korean J Urol. 2013;54(12):851–7.
89. Wong E, Tse V, Wong J. Durability of Memokath™ urethral stent for stabilisation of recurrent bulbar urethral strictures-medium-term results. BJU Int. 2014;113:35–9.
90. Abdallah MM, Selim M, Abdelbakey T. Thermo-expandable metallic urethral stents for managing recurrent bulbar urethral strictures: to use or not? Arab J Urol. 2013;11(1):85–90.
91. Barbagli G, Rimondi C, Balo S, Butnaru D, Sansalone S, Lazzeri M. Memokath stent failure in recurrent bulbar urethral strictures: results from an investigative pilot stage 2A study. Urology. 2017;107:246–50.
92. Sertcelik MN, Bozkurt IH, Yalcinkaya F, Zengin K. Long-term results of permanent urethral stent Memotherm implantation in the management of recurrent bulbar urethral stenosis. BJU Int. 2011;108(11):1839–42.
93. Atesci YZ, Karakose A, Aydogdu O. Long-term results of permanent memotherm urethral stent in the treatment of recurrent bulbar urethral strictures. Int Braz J Urol. 2014;40(1):80–5.
94. Takenaka A, Harada K, Tamada H, Fujisawa M. Re-epithelialization of a scar tract using an intraurethral metallic stent after long urethral defect. J Urol. 2004;171(3):1240–1.
95. Gujral RB, Roy S, Baijal SS, Phadke RV, Ahlawat R, Srinadh ES, et al. Treatment of recurrent posterior and bulbar urethral strictures with expandable metallic stents. J Vasc Interv Radiol. 1995;6(3):427–32.
96. Na HK, Song HY, Yeo HJ, Park JH, Kim JH, Park H, et al. Retrospective comparison of internally and externally covered retrievable stent placement for patients with benign urethral strictures caused by traumatic injury. Am J Roentgenol. 2012;198(1):W61.
97. Eisenberg ML, Elliott SP, McAninch JW. Management of restenosis after urethral stent placement. J Urol. 2008;179(3):991–5.
98. Kotsar A, Isotalo T, Juuti H, Mikkonen J, Leppiniemi J, Hänninen V, et al. Biodegradable braided poly[lactic-co-glycolic acid] urethral stent combined with dutasteride in the treatment of acute urinary retention due to benign prostatic enlargement: a pilot study. BJU Int. 2009;103(5):626–9.

99. Nissenkorn I. A simple nonmetal stent for treatment of urethral strictures: a preliminary report. J Urol. 1995;154(3):1117–8.
100. Nissenkorn I, Shalev M. Polyurethane stent for treatment of urethral strictures. J Endourol. 1997;11(6):481–3.
101. Kim MT, Kim KY, Song HY, Park JH, Tsauo J, Wang Z, et al. Recurrent benign urethral strictures treated with covered retrievable self-expandable metallic stents: long-term outcomes over an 18-year period. J Vasc Interv Radiol. 2017;28(11):1584–91.
102. Yachia D, Lask D, Rabinson S. Self-retaining intraurethral stent: an alternative to long-term indwelling catheters or surgery in the treatment of prostatism. Am J Roentgenol. 1990;154(1):111–3.
103. Saporta L, Beyar M, Yachia D. New temporary coil stent [urocoil] for treatment of recurrent urethral strictures. J Endourol. 1993;7(1):57–9.
104. Sikafi ZH. A self-expanding, self-retaining temporary urethral stent [Urocoil[TM]] in the treatment of recurrent urethral strictures: preliminary results. Br J Urol. 1996;77(5):701–4.
105. Fisher MB, Santucci RA. Extraction of UroLume endoprosthesis with one-stage urethral reconstruction using buccal mucosa. Urology. 2006;67(2):423.e10.
106. Gupta NP, Ansari MS. Holmium laser core through internal urethrotomy with explantation of UroLume stent. An ideal approach for a complicated posterior urethral stricture. Int J Urol. 2004;11(5):343–4.
107. Paddack J, Leocádio DE, Samathanam C, Nelius T, Haynes A Jr. Transitional cell carcinoma due to chronic UroLume stent irritation. Urology. 2009;73(5):995–6.
108. Tahmaz L, Cem IH, Simsek K, Zor M, Basal S, Ay H. Urethral stripping caused by stent removal and its successful treatment with hyperbaric oxygen therapy: a case report. Kaohsiung J Med Sci. 2009;25(6):334–7.
109. Cimentepe E, Unsal A, Koc A, Bayrak O, Balbay MD. Temporary urethral stenting for membranous urethral stricture helps complete healing without compromising continence. Scand J Urol Nephrol. 2004;38(6):521–2.
110. Parsons JK, Wright EJ. Extraction of UroLume endoprostheses with one-stage urethral reconstruction. Urology. 2004;64(3):582–4.
111. Rodriguez E Jr, Gelman J. Pan-urethral strictures can develop as a complication of UroLume placement for bulbar stricture disease in patients with hypospadias. Urology. 2006;67(6):1290.e12.
112. Scarpa RM, De LA, Porru D, Paulis M, Usai E. Urolume double prosthesis in the treatment of complex urethral strictures: a 5-year follow-up case report. Urology. 1997;50(3):459–61.
113. Gelman J, Rodriguez E Jr. One-stage urethral reconstruction for stricture recurrence after urethral stent placement. J Urol. 2007;177(1):188–91.
114. Elkassaby AA, Al-Kandari AM, Shokeir AA. The surgical management of obstructive stents used for urethral strictures. J Urol. 2007;178(1):204–7.
115. Milroy E. Treatment of sphincter strictures using permanent UroLume stent. J Urol. 1993;150(5):1729–33.
116. Angulo JC, Kulkarni S, Pankaj J, Nikolavsky D, Suarez P, Belinky J, et al. Urethroplasty after urethral Urolume stent: an international multicenter experience. Urology. 2018;118:213–9.
117. De VT, Van VG, Boon TA. Self-expanding stent insertion for urethral strictures: a 10-year follow-up. BJU Int. 2003;91(7):627–30.
118. Hussain M, Greenwell TJ, Shah J, Mundy A. Long-term results of a self-expanding wallstent in the treatment of urethral stricture. BJU Int. 2004;94(7):1037–9.
119. Badlani GH, Press SM, Defalco A, Oesterling JE, Smith AD. Urolume endourethral prosthesis for the treatment of urethral stricture disease: long-term results of the North American Multicenter Urolume trial. Urology. 1995;45(5):846–56.
120. Breda G, Xausa D, Puppo P, Ricciotti G, Zanollo A, Guadaloni P, et al. Urolume in urethral stenosis: Italian club of minimally invasive urology experience. J Endourol. 1994;8(4):305–9.
121. Donald JJ, Rickards D, Milroy EJ. Stricture disease: radiology of urethral stents. Radiology. 1991;180(2):447–50.

122. Granieri MA, Peterson AC. The management of bulbar urethral stricture disease before referral for definitive repair: have practice patterns changed? Urology. 2014;84(4):946–9.
123. Milroy E, Allen A. Long-term results of urolume urethral stent for recurrent urethral strictures. J Urol. 1996;155(3):904–8.
124. Sertcelik N, Sagnak L, Imamoglu A, Temel M, Tuygun C. The use of self-expanding metallic urethral stents in the treatment of recurrent bulbar urethral strictures: long-term results. BJU Int. 2000;86(6):686–9.
125. Tillem SM, Press SM, Badlani GH. Use of multiple urolume endourethral prostheses in complex bulbar urethral strictures. J Urol. 1997;157(5):1665–8.
126. Eisenberg ML, Elliott SP, McAninch JW. Preservation of lower urinary tract function in posterior urethral stenosis: selection of appropriate patients for urethral stents. J Urol. 2007;178(6):2456–61.
127. Morgia G, Saita A, Morana F, Macaluso CP, Serretta V, Lanza P, et al. Endoprosthesis implantation in the treatment of recurrent urethral stricture: a multicenter study. J Endourol. 1999;13(8):587–90.
128. Verhamme L, Van Poppel H, Voorde VD, Baert L. Total fibrotic obliteration of urethral stent. Br J Urol. 1993;72(3):389–90.
129. Krah H, Djamilian M, Seabert J, Allhoff EP, Stief C, Jonas U. Significant obliteration of the urethral lumen after Wallstent implantation. J Urol. 1992;148(6):1901–2.
130. Pansadoro V, Scarpone P, Emiliozzi P. Treatment of a recurrent penobulbar urethral stricture after Wallstent implantation with a second inner Wallstent. Urology. 1994;43(2):248–50.
131. Baert L, Verhamme L, Van Poppel H, Vandeursen H, Baert J. Long-term consequences of urethral stents. J Urol. 1993;150(3):853–5.
132. Baert L, Van PH, Werbrouck P. Implantation of the urethral stent for treatment of complex urethral strictures. Evaluation of the functional and radiological results. Urol Int. 1991;47(1):35–9.
133. Beier-Holgersen R, Brasso K, Nordling J, Andersen JT. The 'Wallstent': a new stent for the treatment of urethral strictures. Scand J Urol Nephrol. 1993;27(2):247–50.
134. Kardar AH, Lindstedt E. Role of Wallstent® in urethral stricture. Ann Saudi Med. 1998;18(5):463–5.
135. Milroy EJG, Chapple C, Eldin A, Wallsten H. A new treatment for urethral strictures: a permanently implanted urethral stent. J Urol. 1989;141(5):1120–2.
136. Katz G, Shapiro A, Pode D. Obstruction of urethral stents by mucosal overgrowth. J Endourol. 1994;8(1):73–4.
137. Oosterlinck W, Talja M. Endoscopic urethroplasty with a free graft on a biodegradable polyglycolic acid spiral stent. A new technique. Eur Urol. 2000;37(1):112–5.
138. Milroy EJG, Chapple CR, Eldin A, Wallsten H. A new stent for the treatment of urethral strictures. Preliminary report. Br J Urol. 1989;63(4):392–6.

Ureteral Stents. Impact on Patient's Quality of Life

M. Bargues-Balanzá, G. Ordaz-Jurado, A. Budía-Alba, and F. Boronat-Tormo

1 Introduction

The ureteral stent is a tubular device with multiple lateral holes that is placed inside the ureter to prevent or treat an obstruction in order to ensure the permeability of the urinary tract. In 1967, Zimskind et al. [1] described the endoscopic placement of the first permanent ureteral stents. Subsequently, Finney et al. [2] improved the shape of the device by describing the double J stent (DJS).

Its main indications are unblocking the upper urinary tract of both extrinsic and intrinsic causes, allowing healing after a urinary anastomosis or ureteral trauma and as prevention of obstruction after endourological techniques or iatrogenic ureteral injury [3, 4].

With the endourological techniques increase, their routine use has raised. Its placement prior to ureterorenoscopy (URS) is not generally necessary, although some studies report a better stone-free rate and fewer intraoperative complications [5, 6]. Randomized prospective trials have found that routine stenting after uncomplicated URS (complete stone removal) is not necessary; stenting might be associated with higher post-operative morbidity and costs [7–10].

Although in the first published scientific literature, no side effects associated with its use were described, Pollard and Macfarlane [11] in 1988 presented the first series that describes the morbidity associated with ureteral stents, with a decrease in quality of life in 80% of patients and 90% of urinary symptoms associated with the

M. Bargues-Balanzá · G. Ordaz-Jurado · A. Budía-Alba (✉) · F. Boronat-Tormo
Lithotripsy and Endourology Unit. Urology Department, La Fe University and Polytechnic Hospital, Valencia, Spain
e-mail: bargues_marbal@gva.es; ordaz_dom@gva.es; boronat_fra@gva.es

© The Author(s) 2022
F. Soria et al. (eds.), *Urinary Stents*,
https://doi.org/10.1007/978-3-031-04484-7_5

stent (SRS). Subsequent studies confirmed similar morbidity rates [12, 13], confirming the side effects associated with its use.

The objective of this chapter is to evaluate the impact on the quality of life of patients with ureteral stents.

2 Symptoms Related to Ureteral Stents

The main symptoms related to urinary stents are:

2.1 Lower Urinary Tract

Storage symptoms of the lower urinary tract are the most prevalent ones in patients with ureteral stents and that cause the greatest loss of quality of life. They are related to the bladder mucosa irritation, produced by mechanical scratching of the stent and, it has been related to the spasmodic contractions of the ureter produced by the presence of an inner foreign body. There are also factors related to the type of stent selected:

Ureteral stent length: A published randomized clinical trial [14] confirmed that urgency and dysuria were common with longer stents and negatively affected the patients' quality of life. Along the same lines, Taguchi et al. [15] and Al-kandari [16] also found greater urgency, dysuria, as well as a worse quality of life in patients with ureteral stents that crossed the bladder midline. The gold standard for measuring the required stent length remains the insertion of a graduated ureteral catheter, measuring the distance between ureteropelvic junction (UPJ) and ureterovesical junction (UVJ) [17]. Lee at al [18] correlated the length of the stent with the height of the patient. On the other hand, Ho et al. [19] proposed a mathematical formula (length = 0.125 × body height + 0.5 cm) to calculate the length of the stent.

Calibre of urinary stents: Another aspect evaluated, is whether the thickness of the ureteral stent can influence the worsening of symptoms and the deterioration of the patient's quality of life. Candela et al. [20] compared stent diameter and composition with patient symptoms occurring from stent placed for a variety of reasons. They did not find a difference in terms of patient tolerance. Erturk et al. [21] performed a study comparing pain and storage urinary symptoms in patients undergoing stent positioning of different sizes after ureteroscopy. They showed no differences between the studied groups. Similarly Chandhoke et al. [22] in a study conducted with patients having shock wave lithotripsy (SWL) noted no significant differences in terms of pain and irritation using stents of two different diameters. Along the same lines, Damiano et al. [23] found no differences between stents of different diameters, but they did reflect a higher frequency of migration in those with a smaller diameter.

Distal coil shape: As the distal coil of the stent is hypothesized to be in part responsible for SRS, several design alterations have been proposed to reduce SRS. A loop, a tail and a simple suture in several trials have replaced the conventional distal coil [24].

Stent composition: The stent composition can influence symptoms depending on its biocompatibility and the tissue reaction. Currently used biomaterials for stent construction are synthetic polymers or (proprietary) copolymers such as silicone, polyethylene, polyurethane, C-Flex®, Silitek®, Pellethane®, Vertex® and Percuflex™ [24]. The most biocompatible material is silicone, but its high coefficient of friction can make stent insertion difficult [25]. Scarneciu et al. [26] used the Flanagan life scale (QOLS) as a tool for evaluating quality of life with different stent materials (40.98% aliphatic polyurethane, hydrophilic polyurethane coating (20.72%), carbothane (17.82%).), silicon (20.46%). None of the materials proved to be superior in terms of symptomatology.

2.2 Pain

Pain is one of the symptoms that occurs in up to 80% of patients, predominantly in the lower back associated with urination. Intravesical pressure increases with detrusor contraction and this pressure increase can be transmitted by reflux to the renal unit, triggering flank pain [27]. Suprapubic pain can result from local bladder irritation by the distal coil or as a secondary sign of associated complication such as encrustation or infection [14]. Different stents have been designed with anti-reflux mechanisms to reduce the pain associated with reflux; at the distal end of the stent, a valve mechanism allows drainage of the kidney but closes with increasing intravesical pressure [28]. Ritter et al. [29] compared the antireflux stent with a conventional stent, without finding significant differences, probably due to a small sample size (29 patients). However, Ecke et al. [30] reached a significantly lower complication rate and higher acceptance rate with an antirefluxive stent. Although many promising designs have been developed, these have not entered routine clinical practice yet [24] (Fig. 1).

Fig. 1 Encrustations on stent

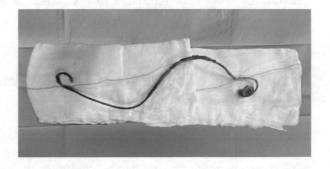

2.3   Urinary Tract Infection

Patients with ureteral stents are prone to urinary tract infection. Therefore, antibiotics should be administered prophylactically before stent placement and removal [31]. The ureteral stent acts as a foreign body and therefore bacteria often colonize them, usually within the first 2 weeks after stent placement.

Colonization rates of the ureteral stent are 100% in patients with permanent stents and 69.3% in patients with temporary stents [32, 33]. However, long-term therapy does not provide benefit in patients with asymptomatic bacteriuria. Additionally, diabetes mellitus, chronic renal failure and pregnancy were associated with a higher risk of stent related bacteriuria [34]. Biofilm formation on the stent surface has been implicated as an important step in the process of stent associated UTI, stent encrustation and SRS. The impact of biofilms on stent morbidity has been discussed controversially [35]. Within this biofilm, microorganisms are protected from host defences and antibiotics, which may lead to an accelerated development of antibiotic resistance.

Coatings have been proven to prevent or reduce biofilm formation to a clinically relevant extent [36]. The associated symptoms of long-lasting DJS and the influence of biofilm formation have also been evaluated. Biofilm formation on ureteral stents does not seem to be the relevant driver of symptoms. Long-term Double-J stenting provides a valuable treatment option, if stent-associated symptoms are low during the initial indwelling period. Thus, symptoms remain stable over the long-term course and the majority of patients are satisfied with the treatment [37].

The indwelling time is the most important risk factor for encrustation [24], that can make it difficult or impossible to remove it. The encrustation and cellular adherence, which, in turn, promotes urinary tract infection, can induce impaired healing in case of ureteral damage [38]. Cadieux et al. [39] show that although triclosan-eluting stents did not show a clinical benefit in terms of urine and stent cultures or overall case symptoms compared with controls, it resulted in decreased antibiotic prescription and significantly fewer symptomatic infections. Urine pH and supersaturation also play a very important role, the incidence of embedded stent could be minimized by acidifying the urine and increasing urinary crystallization inhibitors. Torrecilla et al. [40] describe a significant decrease in encrustation in the group that received treatment with L-methionine and phytate compared to the control group. Removal of embedded ureteral stents requires careful planning to avoid fragmentation.

3   Assessment of the Quality of Life of Patients with Urinary Stents

According to the World Health Organization (WHO), QoL is described as the individual's perception of their life positions under the perspective of the culture and value system in which they are inserted, including individual goals, expectations, standards and priorities [41]. Different tools have been designed to determine the quality of life in different settings.

The most widely used tool to assess the impact on quality of life in patients with ureteral stents is the Ureteral Stent Symptom Questionnaire (USSQ) specifically designed to obtain a psychometrically valid measure to evaluate symptoms and impact on quality of life of ureteral stents. It was developed and published by Joshi et al. [42] in 2003 as a valid instrument to evaluate the impact and compare different types of stent in six health domains: three specific to the stent (voiding symptoms, pain, additional problems) and three general aspects (general health status, work environment and sexual life) in 38 items.

Another widely used tool has been the International Prostate Symptom Score (IPSS), which is the most widely used questionnaire to quantify the symptoms derived from benign prostatic hyperplasia. It is not a specific to evaluate the impact of the stent. However, it has been widely used for this purpose, especially prior to the publication of the USSQ. It consists of eight questions: three filling symptoms questions, four emptying symptoms questions, and one quality of life question.

Other questionnaires to assess health-related quality of life (HRQoL) in the general population are the SF-36 health questionnaire, EuroQoL 5D, and the Flanagan's Quality of Life Scale. The SF-36 [43] is made up of 36 items that assesses eight scales: Physical function, physical role, bodily pain, general health, vitality, social function, emotional role, and mental health. As a limitation of the questionnaire, it does not include some important health aspects such as sleep disorders, cognitive function, family function and sexual function. Another frequently used questionnaire, the EuroQoL-5D (EQ-5D) [44] assesses five dimensions of health status: mobility, personal care, daily activities, pain/discomfort and anxiety/depression and includes the visual analog pain scale (VAS).

The use of these tools has made it possible to quantify the impact on quality of life produced by urinary stents.

3.1 Impact on Quality of Life in Patients of Ureteral Stent

Ureteral stent placement has a variable degree of impact across all general health domains. Many patients report fatigue, dependence to perform daily activities, and even reduce their social life while presenting symptoms associated with the stent. The stent can also lead to a worsening in the quality of sleep and the appearance of anxiety [45].

Studies that have used the USSQ questionnaire have shown that patients with ureteral stents present an increase in LUTS with a significantly reduced quality of life on the scales of body pain, perception of general health, mental health, social functioning and physical functioning.

There is some controversy regarding stent tolerance based on the age of the patient. Irani et al. observed that stents are less well tolerated by younger patients [46]. However, Joshi et al. [12] did not observe any correlation between urinary symptoms and the age of the patients [47].

The fall in the sexual sphere has an important impact on the quality of life. The use of DJS can produce various symptoms within the sexual sphere such as pain during sexual intercourse, dyspareunia, ejaculodynia, erectile dysfunction or decreased libido among others. The study by Joshi et al. [12] revealed that 35% of sexually active patients had pain during sexual intercourse. Sexual health, although affected by stents, might have been perceived as a lesser problem. It seems not a major problem with short stent indwelling time (week 1) but it becomes important as the stent endures. The impact of stents was not only related to the pain during sexual activity, but also appeared to be affecting overall sexual satisfaction.

Other studies such as that of Leibovici et al. [48], described that 62.6% of sexually active patients had pain during intercourse (32% men), ejaculodynia (46%), dyspareunia (62%), erectile dysfunction (20%), decreased libido (38% men and 66% women) and fear that intercourse would be harmful to the DJS (54% women). Globally, women presented more problems than men did. A meta-analysis carried out by Lu et al. [49] in which five prospective studies were included, to analyse sexual health after an endourological procedure or stent, showed that in patients without a double-J stent, the change in sexual function after endourological procedures was not significant in men nor women. However, in patients with indwelling double-J stent, sexual function scores significantly declined after the procedure in both men and women. One study reported that sexual deterioration in women recovered 1 month after stent removal [50]. In another study, the IIEF score remained unchanged on the tenth day after stent removal when compared with the preoperative baseline value [51]. These results suggest that sexual function was impaired after employing a stent but recovered soon following stent removal.

On the other hand, Zhu et al. [52] and Giannarini et al. [53] showed impairment in sexual health in patients compared to that in healthy individuals at 4 weeks after stent placement. By contrast, some studies showed no significant difference when comparing sexual health at the fourth week after placement with the fourth week after removal [54]. A slight improvement of symptoms after stent removal may account for these results.

The described symptoms related to the ureteral stent can be the cause of sick leave, depending on the type of work activity, with a significant impact on the productivity of the active population [13].

Joshi et al. [12] found that 26% of patients who wore DJS for 4 weeks spent more than 2 days in bed (range 3–14 days) and 42% had to reduce activities by more than 3 half days or more (4–28 half days). Similarly, the presence of the stent resulted in a reduction in the quality of work.

Along the same lines, Leibovici et al. [48] found that 45% of patients lost some days of work during the first 2 weeks after stent placement. At 30 and 45 days after placement, 30% and 32% respectively also lost days of work due to sick leave. All days off were attributed to DJS-related symptoms. Although there seems to be a progressive tolerance over time with less loss of workdays due to work leave [13].

4 Innovations for the Improvement of Stented Patients Quality of Life

Informing the patient about the symptoms and the impact on quality of life prior to the placement of a stent can help to understand the symptoms and improve their perception, as described by Abt et al. [55]. However, the influence of information on the incidence and extent of symptoms appears limited.

Management should be focused on the prevention and management of symptoms. In this sense, research has focused on new materials and stent designs that would be more compatible to the physiologic properties of the urinary tract and medications that can ameliorate the sensitivity and motor response of the bladder. All research efforts are focused on approaching the ideal conditions that a stent should meet. The ideal stent would provide adequate urinary drainage, resist migration, encrustation and bacterial colonization. It should be easy to insert and remove, minimize stent-related morbidity, and low cost. Resistant to compression, biodurable and biocompatible.

The stent design aims to improve patient comfort, stent handling and reduce the incidence of urinary tract infections and encrustations. Modern science still offers many alternatives in order to invent the "ideal stent". Thermo-expandable stents are increasingly being studied, thermo-expandable shape memory stents, stents made of biodegradable or bioabsorbable materials, coated stents with various substances as heparin, various enzymes, hydrogel, antibiotics and antifungal medication or anti-inflammatory medication [26].

References

1. Zimskind PD, Fetter TR, Wilkerson JL. Clinical use of long-term indwelling silicone rubber ureteral splints inserted cystoscopically. J Urol. 1967;97(5):840–4.
2. Finney RP. Experience with new double J ureteral catheter stent. J Urol. 1978;120(6):678–81.
3. Damiano R, Oliva A, Esposito C, De Sio M, Autorino R, D'Armiento M. Early and late complications of double pigtail ureteral stent. Urol Int. 2002;69(2):136–40.
4. Ringel A, Richter S, Shalev M, Nissenkorn I. Late complications of ureteral stents. Eur Urol. 2000;38(1):41–4.
5. Jessen JP, Breda A, Brehmer M, Liatsikos EN, Millan Rodriguez F, Osther PJS, et al. International Collaboration in Endourology: multicenter evaluation of prestenting for ureterorenoscopy. J Endourol. 2016;30(3):268–73.
6. Assimos D, Crisci A, Culkin D, Xue W, Roelofs A, Duvdevani M, et al. Preoperative JJ stent placement in ureteric and renal stone treatment: results from the Clinical Research Office of Endourological Society (CROES) ureteroscopy (URS) Global Study. BJU Int. 2016;117(4):648–54.
7. Song T, Liao B, Zheng S, Wei Q. Meta-analysis of postoperatively stenting or not in patients underwent ureteroscopic lithotripsy. Urol Res. 2012;40(1):67–77.
8. Haleblian G, Kijvikai K, de la Rosette J, Preminger G. Ureteral stenting and urinary stone management: a systematic review. J Urol. 2008;179(2):424–30.

9. Nabi G, Cook J, N'Dow J, McClinton S. Outcomes of stenting after uncomplicated ureteroscopy: systematic review and meta-analysis. BMJ. 2007;334(7593):572.
10. Moon TD. Ureteral stenting—an obsolete procedure? J Urol. 2002;167(5):1984.
11. Pollard SG, Macfarlane R. Symptoms arising from double-J ureteral stents. J Urol. 1988;139(1):37–8.
12. Joshi HB, Stainthorpe A, MacDonagh RP, Keeley FX, Timoney AG, Barry MJ. Indwelling ureteral stents: evaluation of symptoms, quality of life and utility. J Urol. 2003;169(3):1065–9; discussion 1069.
13. Ordaz-Jurado G, Budía-Alba A, Bahilo-Mateu P, López-Acón JD, Trassierra-Villa M, Boronat-Tormo F. [Impact in the quality of life of the patients with double J catheter]. Arch Esp Urol. 2016;69(8):471–8.
14. Miyaoka R, Monga M. Ureteral stent discomfort: etiology and management. Indian J Urol. 2009;25(4):455–60.
15. Taguchi M, Yoshida K, Sugi M, Matsuda T, Kinoshita H. A ureteral stent crossing the bladder midline leads to worse urinary symptoms. Cent Eur J Urol. 2017;70(4):412–7.
16. Al-Kandari AM, Al-Shaiji TF, Shaaban H, Ibrahim HM, Elshebiny YH, Shokeir AA. Effects of proximal and distal ends of double-J ureteral stent position on postprocedural symptoms and quality of life: a randomized clinical trial. J Endourol. 2007;21(7):698–702.
17. Barrett K, Ghiculete D, Sowerby RJ, Farcas M, Pace KT, Honey RJD. Intraoperative radiographic determination of ureteral length as a method of determining ideal stent length. J Endourol. 2017;31(S1):S-101.
18. Lee C, Kuskowski M, Premoli J, Skemp N, Monga M. Randomized evaluation of Ureteral Stents using validated Symptom Questionnaire. J Endourol. 2005;19(8):990–3.
19. Ho C-H, Chen S-C, Chung S-D, Lee Y-J, Chen J, Yu H-J, et al. Determining the appropriate length of a double-pigtail ureteral stent by both stent configurations and related symptoms. J Endourol. 2008;22(7):1427–31.
20. Candela JV, Bellman GC. Ureteral stents: impact of diameter and composition on patient symptoms. J Endourol. 1997;11(1):45–7.
21. Erturk E, Sessions A, Joseph JV. Impact of ureteral stent diameter on symptoms and tolerability. J Endourol. 2003;17(2):59–62.
22. Chandhoke PS, Barqawi AZ, Wernecke C, Chee-Awai RA. A randomized outcomes trial of ureteral stents for extracorporeal shock wave lithotripsy of solitary kidney or proximal ureteral stones. J Urol. 2002;167(5):1981–3.
23. Damiano R, Autorino R, De Sio M, Cantiello F, Quarto G, Perdonà S, et al. Does the size of ureteral stent impact urinary symptoms and quality of life? A prospective randomized study. Eur Urol. 2005;48(4):673–8.
24. Beysens M, Tailly TO. Ureteral stents in urolithiasis. Asian J Urol. 2018;5(4):274–86.
25. Denstedt JD, Wollin TA, Reid G. Biomaterials used in urology: current issues of biocompatibility, infection, and encrustation. J Endourol. 1998;12(6):493–500.
26. Scarneciu I, Lupu S, Pricop C, Scarneciu C. Morbidity and impact on quality of life in patients with indwelling ureteral stents: a 10-year clinical experience. Pak J Med Sci. 2015;31(3):522–6.
27. Koprowski C, Kim C, Modi PK, Elsamra SE. Ureteral stent-associated pain: a review. J Endourol. 2016;30(7):744–53.
28. Kim HW, Park C-J, Seo S, Park Y, Lee JZ, Shin DG, et al. Evaluation of a polymeric flap valve-attached ureteral stent for preventing vesicoureteral reflux in elevated intravesical pressure conditions: a pilot study using a porcine model. J Endourol. 2016;30(4):428–32.
29. Ritter M, Krombach P, Knoll T, Michel MS, Haecker A. Initial experience with a newly developed antirefluxive ureter stent. Urol Res. 2012;40(4):349–53.
30. Ecke TH, Bartel P, Hallmann S, Ruttloff J. Evaluation of symptoms and patients' comfort for JJ-ureteral stents with and without antireflux-membrane valve. Urology. 2010;75(1):212–6.

31. Wolf JS, Bennett CJ, Dmochowski RR, Hollenbeck BK, Pearle MS, Schaeffer AJ, et al. Best practice policy statement on urologic surgery antimicrobial prophylaxis. J Urol. 2008;179(4):1379–90.

32. Riedl CR, Plas E, Hübner WA, Zimmerl H, Ulrich W, Pflüger H. Bacterial colonization of ureteral stents. Eur Urol. 1999;36(1):53–9.

33. Kehinde EO, Rotimi VO, Al-Hunayan A, Abdul-Halim H, Boland F, Al-Awadi KA. Bacteriology of urinary tract infection associated with indwelling J ureteral stents. J Endourol. 2004;18(9):891–6.

34. Akay AF, Aflay U, Gedik A, Sahin H, Bircan MK. Risk factors for lower urinary tract infection and bacterial stent colonization in patients with a double J ureteral stent. Int Urol Nephrol. 2007;39(1):95–8.

35. Betschart P, Zumstein V, Buhmann MT, Albrich WC, Nolte O, Güsewell S, et al. Influence of biofilms on morbidity associated with short-term indwelling ureteral stents: a prospective observational study. World J Urol. 2019;37(8):1703–11.

36. Stewart PS. Mechanisms of antibiotic resistance in bacterial biofilms. Int J Med Microbiol. 2002;292(2):107–13.

37. Betschart P, Zumstein V, Buhmann MT, Altenried S, Babst C, Müllhaupt G, et al. Symptoms associated with long-term double-J ureteral stenting and influence of biofilms. Urology. 2019;134:72–8.

38. Kram W, Buchholz N, Hakenberg OW. Ureteral stent encrustation. Pathophysiology. Arch Esp Urol. 2016;69(8):485–93.

39. Cadieux PA, Chew BH, Nott L, Seney S, Elwood CN, Wignall GR, et al. Use of triclosan-eluting ureteral stents in patients with long-term stents. J Endourol. 2009;23(7):1187–94.

40. Torrecilla C, Fernández-Concha J, Cansino JR, Mainez JA, Amón JH, Costas S, et al. Reduction of ureteral stent encrustation by modulating the urine pH and inhibiting the crystal film with a new oral composition: a multicenter, placebo controlled, double blind, randomized clinical trial. BMC Urol. 2020;20(1):65.

41. WHOQOL—Measuring Quality of Life| The World Health Organization [Internet]. [citado 10 de diciembre de 2020]. https://www.who.int/toolkits/whoqol.

42. Joshi HB, Newns N, Stainthorpe A, MacDonagh RP, Keeley FX Jr, Timoney AG. Ureteral stent symptom questionnaire: development and validation of a multidimensional quality of life measure. J Urol. 2003;169(3):1060–4.

43. Ware JE, Sherbourne CD. The MOS 36-item short-form health survey (SF-36). I. Conceptual framework and item selection. Med Care. 1992;30(6):473–83.

44. Brooks R. EuroQol: the current state of play. Health Policy. 1996;37(1):53–72.

45. Vega Vega A, García Alonso D, García Alonso CJ. Evaluación de clínica y calidad de vida con catéteres ureterales de tipo doble pig-tail. Actas Urol Esp. 2007;31(7):738–42.

46. Irani J, Siquier J, Pirès C, Lefebvre O, Doré B, Aubert J. Symptom characteristics and the development of tolerance with time in patients with indwelling double-pigtail ureteric stents. BJU Int. 1999;84(3):276–9.

47. Ucuzal M, Serçe P. Ureteral stents: impact on quality of life. Holist Nurs Pract. 2017;31(2):126–32.

48. Leibovici D, Cooper A, Lindner A, Ostrowsky R, Kleinmann J, Velikanov S, et al. Ureteral stents: morbidity and impact on quality of life. Isr Med Assoc J. 2005;7(8):491–4.

49. Lu J, Lu Y, Xun Y, Chen F, Wang S, Cao S. Impact of endourological procedures with or without double-J stent on sexual function: a systematic review and meta-analysis. BMC Urol. 2020;20(1):13.

50. Eryildirim B, Tuncer M, Kuyumcuoglu U, Faydaci G, Tarhan F, Ozgül A. Do ureteral catheterisation procedures affect sexual functions? A controlled prospective study. Andrologia. 2012;44(Suppl 1):419–23.

51. Mosharafa A, Hamid MAE, Tawfik M, Rzzak OAE. Effect of endourological procedures on erectile function: a prospective cohort study. Int Urol Nephrol. 2016;48(7):1055–9.
52. Zhu C, Qu J, Yang L, Feng X. The Chinese linguistic validation of the Ureteral Stent Symptom Questionnaire. Urol Int. 2019;102(2):194–8.
53. Giannarini G, Keeley FX, Valent F, Manassero F, Mogorovich A, Autorino R, et al. Predictors of morbidity in patients with indwelling ureteric stents: results of a prospective study using the validated Ureteric Stent Symptoms Questionnaire. BJU Int. 2011;107(4):648–54.
54. Tanidir Y, Mangir N, Sahan A, Sulukaya M. Turkish version of the Ureteral Stent Symptoms Questionnaire: linguistic and psychometric validation. World J Urol. 2017;35(7):1149–54.
55. Abt D, Warzinek E, Schmid H-P, Haile SR, Engeler DS. Influence of patient education on morbidity caused by ureteral stents. Int J Urol. 2015;22(7):679–83.

Strategies to Improve the Quality of Life of Stented Patients

E. Emiliani, A. K. Kanashiro, I. Girón-Nanne, and O. Angerri-Feu

1 Introduction

Since its introduction in 1967, double-J stents have been an essential tool for urologists worldwide playing a major role in urinary drainage for a wide range of scenarios. However, they present a significant drawback, since up to 80% of patients present bothersome symptoms that negatively affect quality of life [1]. The aim to create innocuous stents is an ongoing challenge and strategies to prevent side-effects have yet to be achieved. In this chapter we will consider different approaches to reduce stented patient's morbidity without the use of drugs. These strategies include proper stenting indication, stent composition and length selection, and correct placement technique, which will be discussed below.

2 Indications of Double-J Stenting

As double J stents are related to high rates of bothersome and distress, the best way to improve quality of life of patients is to avoid stenting altogether. Consequently, as they are often necessary it is imperative to correctly indicate a stent placement, following conscious and evidence-based criteria. Unfortunately, despite the well-known morbidity and economic burden that stents involve, these are thought to be overused in contemporary practice [2].

E. Emiliani (✉) · A. K. Kanashiro · I. Girón-Nanne · O. Angerri-Feu
Department of Urology, Fundación Puigvert, Autonomous University of Barcelona,
Barcelona, Spain
e-mail: akanashiro@fundacio-puigvert.es; oangerri@fundacio-puigvert.es

© The Author(s) 2022
F. Soria et al. (eds.), *Urinary Stents*,
https://doi.org/10.1007/978-3-031-04484-7_6

2.1   Urgent Indications

In case of obstructive acute pyelonephritis, anuria or sepsis, urgent decompression is needed, where placement of a ureteral stent is an option [3]. Other absolute indications include intolerable acute renal colic, renal failure, or solitary kidney [4]. Relative indications are steinstrasse, pregnancy, long-standing impacted stone and recent history of sepsis or urinary tract infection (UTI) [4].

3   Non-urgent Indications

3.1   Shockwave Lithotripsy (SWL)

Traditionally, pre-SWL stenting for renal stones, especially in larger stones, was thought to help reduce obstructive and infective complications. However, in recent years the need of ureteral stents has been questioned. Several systematic reviews and meta-analysis reveal no difference in terms of stone-free rate, fever or need of auxiliary treatments between stented on non-stented groups; but rather the stent-group demonstrated more retreatment and stent-related symptoms [5–7]. Some authors suggest that stenting may reduce formation of steinstrasse, but specifically in SWL of stones >20 mm, which currently is not standard clinical practice [3]. From an economic point of view, pre-stenting significantly raises healthcare costs, without presenting a clinical benefit and affecting quality of life [5]. Thus, stenting before SWL is not recommended [3, 5]. However, stenting may be considered in cases of ongoing pain, and when SWL cannot be done in a timely manner [5].

3.2   Ureterrenoscopy (URS) and Retrograde Intra-renal
Surgery (RIRS)

Thanks to technological advancements and development of new miniaturized endoscopes, ureteroscopy has become a widely used technique for ureteral and renal stone treatment. Regarding double-J stents in the perioperative scenario, several issues arise: if they are advantageous when placed before a surgery, and if they are necessary after every procedure.

3.3 Pre-operative Stenting

The routine ureteral stenting before surgery remains controversial. A double-J stent will cause a passive ureteral dilatation, and therefore facilitating instrument insertions and possibly reducing complications. This is especially relevant for ureteral access sheath (UAS) insertion, which allow multiple and easier access to the collecting system and decreases renal pressure, but UAS can cause severe ureteral injury. In 2013 Traxer et al. [8], stated that pre-stenting decreases by sevenfold the risk of severe access sheath related injuries. Several groups have discussed the need of stenting before URS/RIRS, with dissenting results and conclusions. Several studies report better stone free rates (SFRs) and decreased complications in pre-stented patients, specifically for renal stones [9–12]. However, these improved outcomes come at a price, with a higher care cost and negatively impacting quality of life of patients. Moreover, an additional procedure may not be available in every centre. Other groups advocate ureteroscopy without prior stenting, arguing that in most cases, RIRS can be successfully accomplished in a single surgery, without differences in intraoperative complications, whilst avoiding the bothersome symptoms associated to stents and with less costs [6, 13].

EAU guidelines conclude that pre-stenting is not necessary prior to URS, but may facilitate and improve outcomes, especially for renal stones [3]. AUA guidelines do not recommend routine stenting prior to every URS, since they consider the added medical cost and comorbidity associated to stents overweight the potential benefit of presenting in outcomes [14]. Therefore, if feasible, pre-stenting may be an option for elective renal surgery, especially when UAS is likely to be used during surgery (10–15 mm renal stones). Nonetheless, additional randomized controlled trials are still needed to corroborate findings.

3.4 Post-operative Stenting

Typically, many urologists routinely place a double-J stent after URS, based on the idea that the stent will reduce the incidence of postoperative complications and promote passage of residual stones. However, in recent years, the need of standardized postoperative stent has been questioned. Several randomized trials and meta-analysis have shown similar stone free rate and stricture formation outcomes between stenting and non-stenting groups after uncomplicated URS. Moreover, non-stented patients presented less urinary tract symptoms, as well as decreasing healthcare costs [15–17]. EAU and AUA recommend that

Table 1 Recommendations for postoperative stenting

• Ureteric injury/perforation during URS
• Balloon dilatation during surgery
• Ureteral stricture or anatomical anomalies that will difficult stone passage
• Ureteral wall edema
• Large stone burden (>15 mm) or long operation time
• Anatomical or functional solitary kidney
• Previous history of renal failure
• Recent or recurrent UTI or sepsis
• Pregnancy
• Bilateral URS
• Long-standing impacted stone
• If second look surgery is planned

stenting is not necessary after uncomplicated URS [3]. It is important to correctly identify patients where postoperative stenting is recommended [4, 14, 18] (Table 1).

4 Stent Timing

The ideal duration of stenting is unknown, but a single straightforward maxim can be applied in every situation: as little time as possible [2]. This is based on the logical premise that a lesser indwelling time will shorten patient symptoms and side-effects associated to stents [19].

In general, after obstructive pyelonephritis, definite stone removal should be delayed until the infection is cleared with antimicrobial therapy, approximately 2–3 weeks [3]. In most cases, urologists prefer stenting for 1–2 weeks after surgery [3].

In patients with high risk of stent encrustation (cystinuria, sarcoidosis or brushite stones) a quick removal should be prioritized.

In conclusion, minimizing stent indwelling time is crucial, as it is a significant cause of stent encrustation and negatively impacting patient quality of life [19].

5 Stent Materials and Symptoms

5.1 Soft Vs. Hard Stents

Since its description in 1967, many efforts have been made towards the development of the ideal stent, modifying material, shape, length, and coating. Regarding, stent composition, its chemical and physical properties determine its hardness, flexibility, tensile strength, which in turn can have a different effect on patient symptoms. Scientists and engineers have focused on optimizing catheter hardness and flexibility to strive to improve stent tolerability and therefore improve quality of life.

Hardness is a physical property of biomaterials such as stents that can be measured using a durometer. This device measures the resistance of materials under pre-established conditions according to the American Society for Testing and Materials (ASTM) [20]. There are many types of durometers, although for soft materials such as stents the durometer called "A" is used. The hardness for biomaterials is measured in an arbitrary scale and varies between 40 A and 90 A (that includes the letter "A" from the durometer used for guidance) [21, 22]. The arbitrary division of hardness classifies materials it into soft if scores less than 64 A and hard if scores from 65 to 90 A, for example, the Percuflex Plus® stent is classified as hard for having more than 65 A, while the Contour® stent belongs to the soft group for having less than 64 A according to the manufacturer's data [23].

Further, the tensile force (the stretching forces of the stent) is an important factor for maintaining the patency of the stent, but it can affect patient's comfort, because is related to hardness in a directly proportional way. The higher the tensile force the hardest and more rigid the stent is. This hardness or rigidity is considered by some authors as the cause of increased hematuria and urgency due to bladder irritation [24, 25].

The application of thermoplastic elastomers has facilitated the development of soft stents that show more flexibility. In recent years, the use of proprietary polymer stents, such as C-flex®, Percuflex®, Silitek®, Dual Durometer®, Sof-Flex®, and poly-urethane has increased [23].

Currently, numerous polymeric materials are now available and at the disposal of urologists, from relatively stiff (polyurethane) to relatively soft (silicone). A softer biomaterial "intuitively" should cause fewer symptoms in the patient with a stent, compared to a harder biomaterial, however there is still controversy whether stent material has a major impact in patient discomfort. Bregg and Riehle [25] found no association between the degree of symptoms and the composition, shape or length of the stent in a study with 50 patients. In the same way, Pryor et al. [26] reported no differences in the incidence and severity of lower tract symptoms between four types of stents (74 patients) with different hardness, but both studies were done without a standard measure of symptoms caused by stent.

Lennon et al. [27] conducted a randomized controlled trial with 155 patients comparing polyurethane and Sof-Flex® stents, both from the same manufacturer (Cook Medical, IN, US), finding a significantly higher incidence of dysuria, renal and supra-pubic pain in the group of hard stents, but without differences in reflux pain, urgency, frequency, hematuria, tolerance, encrustation or stent placement. The symptom assessment was performed by the endoscopist who removed the stent using a simple, non-validated questionnaire. Normal activity and return to work were quicker in patients with softer stents (67% vs 45%).

In a prospective randomized trial, Joshi et al. [22]. Compared in 130 patient's hard stents (Percuflex® (6 Fr)) Boston Scientific, MA, USA, versus soft stents (Contour® (6 Fr), (Boston Scientific, MA, USA) founding no significant differences in the USSQ (The quality of life and stents symptoms score) between the two groups in 1–4 weeks after insertion of the stent.

Dual hardness stents such as the Sof-Curl® (ACMI, MA, USA) and the Polaris® (Boston Scientific, MA, USA) incorporate a smooth transition of hard biomaterials from the proximal (renal) end to a softer biomaterial for the distal (bladder) end to minimize the "hypothetical" bladder discomfort caused by irritation from a hard material. Two randomized controlled trials [28, 29] evaluated these devices with the USSQ without demonstrating a significant benefit for the Polaris® compared with the Percuflex® or the InLay® (Bard Medical, GA, USA).

Some stent biomaterials also soften by 50% at body temperature with better tolerance according to Lee et al. [30] although Park et al. [31] identified some advantages in terms of pain, physical activities, work, and antibiotic use in favor of a softer catheter end.

Silicone stents have the property of being highly biocompatible with human tissues, as well as being soft compounds. Recent studies place them as a great alternative to reduce the adverse effects caused by double J ureteral stents [32, 33]. Hendlin et al. investigated 12 commercial stents to test the effect of composition material on mechanical strength after exposure to artificial urine. The Black Silicone® stent and C-Flex stent exhibited strong coil strength with and without exposure to urine [34].

With the current evidence, the composition of stents, specifically its stiffness, seems to influence patient stent-related symptoms. Current tendencies advocate the use of softer stents, which appear to have a better tolerance profile for patients. However, certain controversy remains, and stent composition is not the only factor to take into consideration in the design of the ideal stent.

6   Ureteral Stent Position and Its Relation to Symptoms

As previously mentioned, stents involve significant morbidity that negatively affects quality of life. Several aspects to help mitigate symptoms have been examined, such as stent indication, duration, and biomaterial composition. In addition, a correlation between the position of a ureteral stent and stent-related symptom is also postulated [35–37]. Proper positioning of pigtails of the stent can help decrease patient discomfort [35]. This depends on accurate stent length selection and proper placement technique, which are discussed below. These straightforward approaches can considerably improve quality of life, and therefore it is important for the urologist to take into consideration and apply to daily clinical practice.

6.1 Ureteral Stent Placement Techniques

Many studies have compared the tolerance of different types of ureteral stents, regarding stent composition, but there are few papers analysing predictive factors related to placement technique [38].

Bladder irritation causing urinary frequency and urgency, even suprapubic pain is very common with ureteral stents. The cause of this discomfort is probably secondary to the irritation caused by a foreign body so close to the bladder neck, leading to trigone irritation by the distal end of the stent which has proven to be worse if the stent length is large, it makes sense to think that less foreign material inside bladder generates less irritation and less symptoms [39].

The ideal stent placement should avoid that the bladder coil crosses the mid pelvis (referenced by the symphysis pubis) on an x-ray line to mitigate symptoms (Fig. 1). Moreover, the best scenario is when only the distal coil is in the bladder, just coming out the ureteral orifice meaning less foreign body inside the bladder and therefore less symptoms [38, 39].

Rane et al. [37] showed that stents crossing the midline of the bladder or having incomplete loops at the lower end highly increased the morbidity of the stent.

Stents crossing the midline of the bladder resulted in significantly more patients experiencing bothersome symptoms that those with the coil not crossing the midline (77% vs. 33% respectively $P \leq 0.01$). So, proper stent length and an appropriate placement based on the patient's ureteral length is necessary to improve comfort.

Dysuria is usually experienced near the end of voiding. Again, this event presumably is attributable to trigonal irritation by the distal end of the stent, which is worse

Fig. 1 Proper Double J placement where the distal coil does not pass the midline

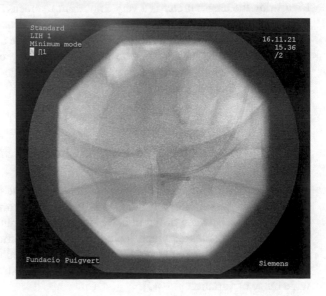

even the bladder is empty. This pain can be transmitted into the urethra, giving rise to the typical burning sensation. It is important to achieve a well-formed bladder coil with the stent because incomplete (straight) loops, that point ad pokes the trigone may increase symptoms [38].

Considerable evidence demonstrates the impact of distal coil placement, but limited literature exists regarding proximal end positioning. El-Nahas et al. concluded that caliceal position of the upper coil is a significant factor affecting discomfort, with an estimated relative risk of discomfort of four times for caliceal position [35]. On the other hand, Liatsikos et al. performed a randomized prospective study comparing symptomatology associated placement of the upper coil in the upper pole versus renal pelvis. The group that placement of stent in the upper pole appears to be better tolerated, regarding urgency, dysuria, and quality of life [36]. The possible pathophysiological explanation of proximal coil positioning in worsening symptoms is still unknown, and to date, a clinically relevant impact of pyelic or caliceal placement remains controversial.

7   Ureteral Length Measurement

One of the most important aspects for an adequate stent placement is a prior selection of an appropriate stent length. Different lengths are available, from 24 to 30 cm and can be individualized depending on patient's anatomy [40]. It is very important for patients to have their stent length measured. There is substantial evidence that excessively long stents that cross the bladder midline cause greater morbidity. Measuring the length ureter is a very important manoeuvre for urologists to implement correctly to reduce the symptoms associated with ureteral stents.

However, as simple as it sounds, the prediction of the ureteral length has always been a challenge for urologists who want to accurately choose the double J stent size to reduce symptoms on patients. Nowadays a wide variety of methods have been used for this purpose.

7.1   Ureteral Length Measurement by Body Shape

The predictions and methods may vary widely due to the different body shapes but also due to the presence of any anomalies as dilated or tortuous ureters [41].

Correlations between different body shapes and heights have been widely used for ureteral length measurements including anthropometric measures over the body surface [42]. Although the ureteral length has been linked to the patients height [40, 43, 44] the ureteral length has not been reliably demonstrated as this method has a wide range of variation [45–47].

7.2 Ureteral Length Measurement by Computed Tomography and Intravenous Urography

Measurements using diverse lengths such as the uretero-vesical length (with adjustments) [48, 49], the height of lumbar vertebrae (L1-L5) or calculations of the computed tomography (CT) axial images [50] have been used for ureteral length measure with high correlations [51], and with higher equivalence than measuring patients height [42].

Predictive models assessing the ureteral length with CT and intravenous urography have been described using age, sex, side and pyelo-vesical length as evaluation values. Although these reports have shown good correlation compared to endoscopic measurements [52] this has also been revoked in recent analysis of predictive formulas [53].

7.3 Endoscopic Ureteral Length Measurement

One of the most reliable methods to determine the ureteral length is by placing a ruled 5–6 French open-ended catheter it into the renal pelvis over a guidewire and measuring the length by using the references in the catheter as a referral [54, 55]. This method also has been used as the standard for comparison with new techniques.

As discussed, an accurate ureteral length measurement is a difficult task. Using body height as a reference to approximately calculate the ureteral length does not always give a proper correlation [56] and the best way to decide stent length is the direct endoscopic measurement [56]. From our clinical point of view, it is mandatory to perform a retrograde pyelography during stent placements for many reasons being the most important the accurate evaluation of the upper urinary tract's anatomy, including calices, infundibulum's and the renal pelvis. When you introduce an open ended catheter to perform a retrograde pyelography it is very easy to measure the ureteral length and select the proper stent by using the references in the catheter as a referral [54, 55]. Once the pyelography is done, the decision of where to place the proximal coil is taken (the pelvis or any of the calyces) and then measure of the distance until the ureteral orifice by references in the catheter is performed. It's important to know that after positioning, the stent could move from the original position and migrate downwards depending on the kidney's anatomy, so more pigtail segment may lie in the bladder than the one left.

8 Conclusions

Stents have become an indispensable tool for urologists; unfortunately there is still no idyllic symptom-free stent. It is the urologist's responsibility to try to minimize morbidity as much as possible. Throughout this chapter, we have focused on

Table 2 Strategies to improve the quality of life of stented patients

Avoid stenting when clinically possible. Thoroughly evaluate the necessity of stent placement, reserving its indication in imperative cases or after careful and evidence-based criteria
Minimize stenting time as much as possible. When there is a high risk of stent encrustation, a quick removal should be prioritized
Make individualized stent material selection. Become familiar with the stent repertoire available to you, and choose the variety depending on purpose, stenting time, previous patient experience, and risk of encrustation. Consider a softer biomaterial to reduce symptoms specially when long-term catheterization is warranted
Measure ureteral length and choose stent length accordingly. If possible, perform a direct endoscopic measurement. To do this, perform a retrograde pyelography before stent placement and measure in situ the ureteral length utilizing the open-ended catheter's marks as a reference
Ensure a proper stent positioning. The ideal position of a stent occurs when both coils are correctly formed, the proximal end in the upper pole (somewhat controversial) and the distal end should avoid crossing the mid pelvis of the bladder

different issues that urologist should take into consideration regarding stent indication, selection, and placement. Table 2 summarizes different approaches proposed to implement in daily practice to help reduce adverse effects and complications in catheterized patients.

References

1. Joshi HB, Stainthorpe A, Keeley FX Jr, MacDonagh R, Timoney AG. Indwelling ureteral stents: evaluation of quality of life to aid outcome analysis. J Endourol. 2001;15:151–4.
2. Betschart P, Zumstein V, Piller A, Schmid HP, Abt D. Prevention and treatment of symptoms associated with indwelling ureteral stents: a systematic review. Int J Urol. 2017;24(4):250–9.
3. Türk C, et al. EAU guidelines on urolithiasis. Edn. presented at the EAU Annual Congress Amsterdam 2020. ISBN 978-94-92671-07-3.
4. Miyaoka R, Monga M. Ureteral stent discomfort: etiology and management. Indian J Urol. 2009;25(4):455–60.
5. National Institute for Health and Care Excellence. Renal and ureteric stones: assessment and management Stents before surgery (NICE guideline NG118); 2019. https://www.nice.org.uk/guidance/ng118.
6. Wang H, Man L, Li G, Liu N, Wang H. Meta-analysis of stenting versus non-stenting for the treatment of ureteral stones. PLoS One. 2017;12(1):e0167670.
7. Shen P, et al. Use of ureteral stent in extracorporeal shock wave lithotripsy for upper urinary calculi: a systematic review and meta-analysis. J Urol. 2011;186(4):1328–35.
8. Traxer O, Thomas A. Prospective evaluation and classification of ureteral wall injuries resulting from insertion of a ureteral access sheath during retrograde intrarenal surgery. J Urol. 2013;189(2):580–4.
9. Assimos D, et al. Preoperative JJ stent placement in ureteric and renal stone treatment: results from the Clinical Research Office of Endourological Society (CROES) Ureteroscopy (URS) Global Study. BJU Int. 2016;117:648.

10. Jessen JP, et al. International Collaboration in Endourology: multicenter evaluation of prestenting for ureterorenoscopy. J Endourol. 2016;30:268.
11. Rubenstein RA, Zhao LC, Loeb S, et al. Prestenting improves ureteroscopic stone-free rates. J Endourol. 2007;21:1277.
12. Netsch C, Knipper S, Bach T, et al. Impact of preoperative ureteral stenting on stone-free rates of ureteroscopy for nephroureterolithiasis: a matched-paired analysis of 286 patients. Urology. 2012;80:1214.
13. Mahajan PM, Padhye AS, Bhave AA, Sovani YB, Kshirsagar YB, Bapat SS. Is stenting required before retrograde intrarenal surgery with access sheath. Indian J Urol. 2009;25(3):326–8.
14. Assimos, et al. Surgical management of stones: AUA Endourological Society Guideline. 2016 American Urological Association Education and Research.
15. Song T, et al. Meta-analysis of postoperatively stenting or not in patients underwent ureteroscopic lithotripsy. Urol Res. 2012;40:67.
16. Ibrahim HM, Al-Kandari AM, Shaaban HS, et al. Role for ureteral stenting after uncomplicated ureteroscopy for distal ureteral stones: a randomized controlled trial. J Urol. 2008;180:961.
17. Seklehner S, et al. A cost analysis of stenting in uncomplicated semirigid ureteroscopic stone removal. Int Urol Nephrol. 2017;49:753.
18. Schwartzmann I, Gaya JM, Breda A. Cateterización tras ureteroscopia, ¿Siempre, nunca cuándo? Arch Esp Urol. 2016;69(8):565–70.
19. Bibby LM, Wiseman OJ. Double JJ ureteral stenting: encrustation and tolerability. Eur Urol Focus. 2020;7(1):7–8. https://doi.org/10.1016/j.euf.2020.08.014.
20. Beysens M, Tailly TO. Ureteral stents in urolithiasis. Asian J Urol. 2018;5(4):274–86. https://doi.org/10.1016/j.ajur.2018.07.002. Epub 2018 Jul 25. PMID: 30364608; PMCID: PMC6197553.
21. Mardis HK, Kroeger RM, Morton JJ, Donovan JM. Comparative evaluation of materials used for internal ureteral stents. J Endourol. 1993;7(2):105–15. https://doi.org/10.1089/end.1993.7.105. PMID: 8518822.
22. Joshi HB, Chitale SV, Nagarajan M, Irving SO, Browning AJ, Biyani CS, Burgess NA. A prospective randomized single-blind comparison of ureteral stents composed of firm and soft polymer. J Urol. 2005;174(6):2303–6. https://doi.org/10.1097/01.ju.0000181815.63998.5f. PMID: 16280829.
23. Tschada RK, Henkel TO, Jünemann KP, Rassweiler J, Alken P. Spiral-reinforced ureteral stent: an alternative for internal urinary diversion. J Endourol. 1994;8(2):119–23. https://doi.org/10.1089/end.1994.8.119. PMID: 8061668.
24. Mardis HK, Kroeger RM, Hepperlen TW, Mazer MJ, Kammandel H. Polyethylene double-pigtail ureteral stents. Urol Clin North Am. 1982;9(1):95–101. PMID: 7080301.
25. Bregg K, Riehle RA Jr. Morbidity associated with indwelling internal ureteral stents after shock wave lithotripsy. J Urol. 1989;141(3):510–2. https://doi.org/10.1016/s0022-5347(17)40875-5. PMID: 2918584.
26. Pryor JL, Langley MJ, Jenkins AD. Comparison of symptom characteristics of indwelling ureteral catheters. J Urol. 1991;145(4):719–22. https://doi.org/10.1016/s0022-5347(17)38433-1. PMID: 2005686.
27. Lennon GM, Thornhill JA, Sweeney PA, Grainger R, McDermott TE, Butler MR. 'Firm' versus 'soft' double pigtail ureteric stents: a randomised blind comparative trial. Eur Urol. 1995;28(1):1–5. https://doi.org/10.1159/000475010. PMID: 8521886.
28. Davenport K, Kumar V, Collins J, Melotti R, Timoney AG, Keeley FX Jr. New ureteral stent design does not improve patient quality of life: a randomized, controlled trial. J Urol. 2011;185(1):175–8. https://doi.org/10.1016/j.juro.2010.08.089. Epub 2010 Nov 13. PMID: 21074809.
29. Wiseman O, Ventimiglia E, Doizi S, Kleinclauss F, Letendre J, Cloutier J, Traxer O. Effects of silicone hydrocoated double loop ureteral stent on symptoms and quality of life in patients undergoing flexible ureteroscopy for kidney stone: a randomized multicenter clinical study. J

Urol. 2020;204(4):769–77. https://doi.org/10.1097/JU.0000000000001098. Epub 2020 May 5. PMID: 32364838.

30. Lee C, Kuskowski M, Premoli J, Skemp N, Monga M. Randomized evaluation of Ureteral Stents using validated Symptom Questionnaire. J Endourol. 2005;19(8):990–3. https://doi.org/10.1089/end.2005.19.990. PMID: 16253066.

31. Park HK, Paick SH, Kim HG, Lho YS, Bae S. The impact of ureteral stent type on patient symptoms as determined by the ureteral stent symptom questionnaire: a prospective, randomized, controlled study. J Endourol. 2015;29(3):367–71. https://doi.org/10.1089/end.2014.0294. Epub 2014 Oct 9. PMID: 25153249.

32. Gadzhiev N, Gorelov D, Malkhasyan V, Akopyan G, Harchelava R, Mazurenko D, Kosmala C, Okhunov Z, Petrov S. Comparison of silicone versus polyurethane ureteral stents: a prospective controlled study. BMC Urol. 2020;20(1):10. https://doi.org/10.1186/s12894-020-0577-y. PMID: 32013936; PMCID: PMC6998278.

33. Hendlin K, Dockendorf K, Horn C, Pshon N, Lund B, Monga M. Ureteral stents: coil strength and durometer. Urology. 2006;68(1):42–5. https://doi.org/10.1016/j.urology.2006.01.062. PMID: 16844448.

34. Ho CH, et al. Predictive factors for ureteral double-J-stent-related symptoms: a prospective, multivariate analysis. J Formos Med Assoc. 2010;109(11):848–56.

35. Liatsikos EN, Gershbaum D, Kapoor R, et al. Comparison of symptoms related to positioning of double-pigtail stent in upper pole versus renal pelvis. J Endourol. 2001;15:299–302.

36. Ahmed MA, et al. Effects of proximal and distal ends of double-J ureteral stent position on postprocedural symptoms and quality of life: a randomized clinical trial. J Endourol. 2007;21(7):698–702.

37. Rane A, Saleemi A, Cahill D, et al. Have stent-related symptoms anything to do with placement technique? J Endourol. 2001;7:741–5.

38. Duvdevani M, Chew BH, Denstedt JD, et al. Minimizing symptoms in patients with ureteric stents. Curr Opin Urol. 2006;16:77–82.

39. Ramachandra M, Mosayyebi A, Somani BK, et al. Strategies to improve patient outcomes and QOL: current complications of the design and placements of ureteric stents. Res Rep Urol. 2020;12:303–14.

40. Pilcher JM, Patel U. Choosing the correct length of ureteric stent: a formula based on the patient's height compared with direct ureteric measurement. Clin Radiol. 2002;57(1):59–62.

41. Hruby GW, Ames CD, Yan Y, Monga M, Landman J. Correlation of ureteric length with anthropometric variables of surface body habitus. BJU Int. 2007;99(5):1119–22.

42. Paick SH, Park HK, Byun SS, Oh SJ, Kim HH. Direct ureteric length measurement from intravenous pyelography: does height represent ureteric length? Urol Res. 2005;33:199–202.

43. Lee BK, Paick SH, Park HK, Kim HG, Lho YS. Is a 22 cm ureteric stent appropriate for Korean patients smaller than 175 cm in height? Korean J Urol. 2010;51:642–6.

44. Shah J, Kulkarni RP. Height does not predict ureteric length. Clin Radiol. 2005;60:812–4.

45. Ho CH, Huang KH, Chen SC, Pu YS, Liu SP, Yu HJ. Choosing the ideal length of a double-pigtail ureteral stent according to body height: study based on a Chinese population. Urol Int. 2009;83:70–4.

46. Jeon SS, Choi YS, Hong JH. Determination of ideal stent length for endourologic surgery. J Endourol. 2007;21(8):906–10.

47. Shrewsberry AB, Al-Qassab U, Goodman M, Petros JA, Sullivan JW, Ritenour CW, Issa MM. A +20% adjustment in the computed tomography measured ureteral length is an accurate predictor of true ureteral length before ureteral stent placement. J Endourol. 2013;27(8):1041–5.

48. Jung SI, Park HS, Yu MH, Kim YJ, Lee H, Choi WS, Park HK, Kim HG, Paick SH. Korean ureter length: a computed tomography-based study. Investig Clin Urol. 2020;61(3):291–6.

49. Kawahara T, Ito H, Terao H, Yoshida M, Ogawa T, Uemura H, Kubota Y, Matsuzaki J. Which is the best method to estimate the actual ureteral length in patients undergoing ureteral stent placement? Int J Urol. 2012;19(7):634–8.

50. Barrett K, Foell K, Lantz A, Ordon M, Lee JY, Pace KT, Honey RJ. Best stent length predicted by simple CT measurement rather than patient height. J Endourol. 2016;30(9):1029–32.
51. Kawahara T, Sakamaki K, Ito H, Kuroda S, Terao H, Makiyama K, Uemura H, Yao M, Miyamoto H, Matsuzaki J. Developing a preoperative predictive model for ureteral length for ureteral stent insertion. BMC Urol. 2016;16(1):70.
52. Kuo J, Rabley A, Domino P, Otto B, Moy ML, Bird VG. Evaluation of patient factors that influence predictive formulas for determining ureteral stent length when compared to direct measurement. J Endourol. 2020;34(8):805–10.
53. Kawahara T, Ito H, Terao H, et al. Choosing an appropriate length of loop type ureteral stent using direct ureteral length measurement. Urol Int. 2012;88:48–53.
54. Leslie SW, Sajjad H. Double J placement methods comparative analysis. In: StatPearls [Internet]. Treasure Island (FL): StatPearls Publishing; 2020. PMID: 29494060.
55. Shah J, Kilkami RP. Height does not predict ureteric length. Clin Radiol. 2005;60:812–4.
56. Pilcher JM, Patel U. Choosing the correct length of ureteric stents: a formula based on the patient's height compared with direct ureteric measurement. Clin Radiol. 2002;57:59–62.

Use of Drugs to Reduce the Morbidity of Ureteral Stents

Milap Shah, B. M. Zeeshan Hameed, Amelia Pietropaolo, and Bhaskar K. Somani

1 Introduction

Double 'J' (DJ) ureteral stenting is amongst the commonest procedures performed in urology as an adjunct since its first inception in 1978 by Finney [1]. However, there are complications (SRS) such as infection, and encrustation associated with its use, together with uncomfortable lower urinary tract symptoms (LUTS). The latter are known as stent related symptoms (SRS) and are commonly reported in the literature. SRS mentioned in literature are urgency, frequency, dysuria, haematuria, pain in the suprapubic and flank region. These can result in decreased sexual activity, reduced work performance, as well as decreased quality of life (QoL) in more than two-third of the patients [2]. Advancements have been made in stent design in order to try to reduce the irritation and discomfort using different biomaterials and coatings. Despite this, drugs still hold the key in reducing the morbidity related to the ureteral stents. In this chapter we attempt to throw light on the pharmacotherapy used to reduce ureteral stent related morbidity.

M. Shah (✉)
Department of Urology, Kasturba Medical College Manipal, Manipal Academy of Higher Education, Manipal, India

B. M. Z. Hameed
Department of Urology, Father Muller Medical College, Mangalore, India

A. Pietropaolo · B. K. Somani
Department of Urology, University Hospital Southampton, Southampton, UK

© The Author(s) 2022
F. Soria et al. (eds.), *Urinary Stents*,
https://doi.org/10.1007/978-3-031-04484-7_7

73

2   Reasons for Stent Related Symptoms (SRS)

Discomfort caused by the ureteral stents is one of the most common problems associated with DJ stenting. In order to better identify the gravity of the problem and
quantify the level of discomfort, Ureteral Stent Symptom Questionnaire (USSQ)
was developed and validated by Joshi et al. [2]. USSQ paved the way for multiple
studies that tried to identify the cause of stent related discomfort. One study from
Al-Kandari et al., reported that the distal end of stent crossing midline was one of
the major causes of stent related discomfort [3]. Another randomised control trial
(RCT) by Chew et al., showed that excess length of stent in the bladder caused
severe urgency and dysuria in patients [4]. As described by Ramsay and Venkatesh
et al., stent related reflux of urine during micturition was reported to cause ipsilateral renal pain [5, 6]. Also movement of stent occurs has been described during
daily routine activities and it moves up to 2 cm in both in kidney and bladder sides,
adding to irritation and inflammation of the urothelium [7, 8]. Significant progresses
have been made in stent design keeping these factors in mind, to reduce the irritation
and discomfort using suitable biomaterials to improve the biocompatibility, however the stent's movement is unavoidable. One of the intriguing effects of stent
placement is the activation of "hyperperistalsis" during which the ureter contracts
trying to expel the stent. This mechanism continues until the ureteric peristaltic
activity stops and reaches a state of "aperistalsis" [9, 10]. This was proposed as one
of the theories to understand the cause of ipsilateral pain and hydronephrosis and
was explained by Rajpathy et al. as a consequence of the slow drainage of urine
from the kidneys caused by the aperistalsis. Many authors have shown that selective
alpha blockers such as Tamsulosin and Alfuzosin, have the effect of decreasing stent
related pain and discomfort by reducing the peak ureteral contraction pressure and
the global contractility [11–17]. The mechanisms of action of these drugs that have
the effect of minimising SRS, is still under study. Several studies have suggested
that both these mechanisms may be possible, either decreasing the peristalsis or
relaxing the hyperperistaltic obstructed segment of ureter thereby restoring normal
peristaltic movement. The latter mechanism if true, may also reduce the hydronephrosis caused by the aperistalsis after stent insertion [11–17].

2.1   Role of Alpha-1 Blockers/Antagonists

The alpha-adrenoreceptors, when activates, result in the contraction of the smooth
muscles. They are present in the distal ureteric mucosa, trigone of bladder and in the
prostatic urethra. The ureteral stents cause stimulation of these regions which lead
to irritation, contraction and spasms, thereby causing LUTS. Pain in the flank region
caused by urinary reflux through the stents has also been documented [13, 18–21].
The earliest mention of alpha-1 blockers for the treatment of (LUTS) was reported
in 1900 by Michel et al. [22]. Alpha-blocker inhibits the above mentioned contraction and thereby relaxes the smooth muscles which in turn prevents spasms and

decreases the resistance of bladder outlet. This mechanism also reduces intra-vesical pressure during voiding which indirectly decreases the urinary reflux to the kidneys [23, 24].

2.1.1 Silodosin

Silodosin is a highly selective alpha-1a blocker with 160 and 55 times affinity towards alpha-1a subtype and 1b and 1d receptors respectively. In 1995, it was initially introduced as KMD-3213 and since then its role in medical management of Benign Prostatic Enlargement (BPE) has been established [24–27]. Silodosin has high affinity towards the alpha-1a receptor subtype, which are densely located in the smooth muscles of lower urinary tract. Owing to this highly selective action, it has lower adverse cardiovascular effects such as postural or orthostatic hypotension [24]. This implies that Silodosin has higher safety index than other alpha-1 blockers for patients with SRS especially those affected by cardiovascular disease, frailty, postural instability and low blood pressure.

2.1.2 Tamsulosin

Tamsulosin is a selective alpha 1a and 1d-adrenoreceptor blocker [28]. The dosage is once daily and causes less postural/orthostatic hypotension as compared to other non-selective drugs of the same class [29]. The mechanism of action in relieving SRS has been described by Lamb et al. and it is similar to the other drugs of the same category [30].

2.1.3 Alfuzosin

Also Alfuzosin effectively inhibits Alpha-1 adrenoreceptor-mediated contraction of bladder, prostate and proximal urethral smooth muscle with a favourable side effect profile [31–36]. Alfuzosin also has once-a-day dosage which has resulted in better patient compliance [33]. The two most commonly reported side effects are headache and dizziness. However their intensity is mild and does not require alteration of dosage or stoppage of medication [34].

2.1.4 Naftopidil

Naftopidil is found to have very high affinity towards alpha 1D subtype of adrenergic receptors as compared to others (3 times higher than alpha 1a; 17 times higher than alpha 1b) [36]. Hence, theoretically naftopidil may be more beneficial in treating SRS [37]. However not enough literature is available regarding their use in alleviating SRS.

2.2 Role of Antimuscarinics/Anticholinergics

2.2.1 Solifenacin and Tolterodine

Detrusor muscle incorporates a high density of muscarinic receptors. Tolterodine and Solifenacin are competitive antagonists of the muscarinic receptors, thereby; they modify the contractility of the detrusor muscle. They are available in immediate, modified or extended release formulations. Firstly, as SRS may be due to the detrusor overactivity (OAB/DOA) caused by the bladder wall irritation, these are inhibited by antimuscarinics. Secondly, subclinical OAB/DOA may be highlighted by SRS and can also be managed by this group of drugs [38, 39]. Adverse effects associated with antimuscarinics are headache, blurred vision, orthostatic hypotension, dry mouth, constipation, and urinary retention [38, 39]. This can influence the patient's quality of life and reduce the compliance to the medication.

2.3 Post Ganglionic Blockers

2.3.1 Oxybutynin

Oxybutynin has anti-cholinergic action at the post ganglion level of the smooth muscles, thereby providing an antispasmodic effect. Similarly to Solifenacin and Tolterodine, Oxybutynin is also available in immediate and extended release formulations [40]. One major drawback of its extended use is that, Oxybutynin can cross the blood-brain barrier and cause cognitive impairment in patients >65 years of age [40].

2.3.2 Trospium Chloride

Trospium chloride has a parasympatholytic effect by opposing the action of acetylcholine on muscarinic receptors in bladder. It therefore relaxes the bladder smooth muscle. This has proved to be effective in relieving SRS related to bladder muscle spasms due irritation by the stent [41]. This drug is also better tolerated in older age groups due to fewer incidences of central nervous system (CNS) adverse reactions thanks to its reduced ability to cross the blood-brain barrier.

2.4 Beta-3 Agonists

2.4.1 Mirabegron

The role of Mirabegron is already established in overactive bladder by reducing the detrusor overactivity. Hence, it was postulated to also be able to reduce the overactivity caused by the ureteral stent in the bladder, thereby decreasing SRS. Mirabegron belongs to the family of Beta-3 agonist's drugs and its mechanism of actions seems reducing SRS similarly to antimuscarinics. In view to its reduced side effects, its role in SRS treatment is currently being reconsidered [42–44].

2.5   Nonsteroidal Anti-inflammatory Drugs (NSAIDs)

Cyclooxygenase receptors are present in tunica muscularis of urothelium, ureters as well as in tunica media of blood vessels. By targeting these receptors in the ureters, NSAIDs can contribute to manage stent related pain. They inhibit the prostaglandin synthesis causing ureteral relaxation which indirectly decreases intrarenal and intra-ureteral pressure [45, 46]. Thus their use in alleviating stent related pain and discomfort is justified.

2.6   Phosphodiesterase 5-Inhibitors (PDE5I)

2.6.1   Tadalafil

Smooth muscle relaxation is mediated by an intracellular increase of cAMP and cGMP. The role of PDE5-I is already established in medical expulsion therapy (MET) for ureteral stones and decreasing LUTS in benign enlargement of prostate [47–49]. This led to the idea of their usage in alleviating stent related symptoms. Although the studies are in a preliminary stage, the results have suggested PDE5I to be a better option in patients with sexual dysfunction related to ureteral stents [49].

3   Miscellaneous

3.1   Botulinum Toxin

Botulinum toxin type A (BotoxA) injection has an established role in management of overactive bladder (OAB) based on its mechanism of inhibition of presynaptic acetylcholine release. Based on this, it was hypothesized that stent related discomfort caused by overactivity due to ureteral irritation could be managed by the same mechanism. Gupta et al. administered Periureteral BotoxA injection (10 U/mL) at three locations. The results suggested that after these injections, the analgesic requirement reduced significantly. Their role is still experimental as the exact pain-relieving mechanism is not known. It is postulated that this works inhibiting the release of various neuromodulators such as substance P, calcitonin gene-related protein (CGRP) as well as glutamate. The associated risks mentioned are urinary retention due to muscle paralysis, bleeding from the periureteral injection sites and vesicoureteral reflux [50–53].

3.2 Pregabalin

Pregabalin is a gamma-aminobutyric acid (GABA) agent and it has been FDA approved for neuropathic pain, central pain and chronic pain. Recent interest has developed in the use of this drug to treat LUTS [54, 55]. Pregabalin works by reducing the neuronal excitability by decreasing the synaptic neurotransmitter release which in turn inhibits afferent C nerve fiber evoked responses for inflammation [55]. It also centrally inhibits the dorsal horn neuron which results in reduced sensation of pain caused by inflammation. Despite there is no clear evidence in the literature supporting the use of pregabalin in reducing SRS, few authors have hypothesized it can play this role based on its combined peripheral and central mechanisms of action [55].

3.3 Calcium Channel Blockers (CCB)

There is no strong evidence to support the role of CCB in relief of stent related symptoms. Recently, Lee et al. hypothesized that ureteral relaxation can be improved with local administration of vasodilators such as CCB [56]. The authors found that CCB (nifedipine) significantly relaxed the human ureteral smooth muscle cells with reduced ureteral contraction amplitude and frequency by 90% and 50%, respectively [56]. Hence, their use in conditions such as ureteric calculus and stent related symptoms cannot be ignored.

4 Evidence Regarding Combination Therapy

4.1 Alpha-Blocker and Anti-muscarinics/ Anticholinergics Combination

Various studies including more than 700 patients, have described the role of combination therapy to be better than placebo across all domains of USSQ such as general health, urinary symptoms, work performance, sexual health and pain score as well as significantly decreased IPPS and QoL scores [55, 57–62].

Studies have been carried out comparing combination therapy versus monotherapy.

Alpha blockers monotherapy have been compared with combination therapy and antimuscarinics single treatment with combination therapy. The comparative studies [55, 57–62] included more than 500 and 700 patients respectively. The analysis clearly showed greater benefit with combination therapy in terms of USSQ domain scores, reduction of International prostate symptom score (IPSS) and improvement in QoL score. The values across all domains were statistically significant in favour of combination therapy as compared to either monotherapy [55, 57–62].

5 Complementary and Alternative Medications (CAM)

CAM is aimed to prevent or treat a condition but is not considered a part of the conventional medicine approach [63]. There are no published reports or evidences directly pointing to the benefits of alternative plant based or herbal medications in preventing ureteral stent related symptoms. However the results from few reports indicate their effect in reducing bladder over activity.

5.1 Chinese Herbal Medicines

Chinese herbal medications namely Hachi-mi-jio-gan and Gosha-jinki-gan contain multiple herbs which activate the spinal kappa opioid receptors and cause reduction in the bladder sensation and contractility. Their benefits on IPSS, overactive bladder symptom score (OABSS) and QoL scores have been demonstrated in various studies [64–67].

5.2 Capsaicin

Capsaicin belongs to the genus Capsicum. It has a similar action to the previously mentioned Chinese herbs desensitizing C-afferent neurons and thereby decreasing bladder contractility and sensations. However, no many human studies have been performed using this ingredient to date [68].

5.3 Pumpkin Seed Extract

Pumpkin seed oil extracts have been used to treat LUTS. Several studies have demonstrated their beneficial effects in reducing storage symptoms and improving OAB symptoms [67–69].

5.4 Homeopathic Options

Natrum miraticum, causticum, sepia, paeira, zincum and pulsatilla are some of the homeopathic medications used to treat LUTS such as increased urinary frequency or urinary retention due to bladder paralysis especially in the post- operative period [70, 71]. There have not been any human clinical trials assessing the efficacy of these medications with ureteric stents.

6 Conclusions

In terms of monotherapy, Alpha blockers as well as Antimuscarinics are effective in reducing SRS. Role of Mirabegron in the field is currently gaining importance. However, combination therapy reaches better outcomes than monotherapy alone while in cases with sexual dysfunction along with stent related symptoms, PDE5-I are better than other options. The role of complementary therapy for SRS with natural remedies is promising but needs to be assessed further. More randomised studies and laboratory trials are necessary to analyse possible alternative treatments for SRS that can heavily affects patients' quality of life.

References

1. Finney RP. Experience with new double J ureteral catheter stent. J Urol. 2002;167(2):1135–8.
2. Joshi HB, Stainthorpe A, MacDonagh RP, Keeley FX, Timoney AG. Indwelling ureteral stents: evaluation of symptoms, quality of life and utility. J Urol. 2003;169(3):1065–9.
3. Al-Kandari AM, Al-Shaiji TF, Shaaban H, Ibrahim HM, Elshebiny YH, Shokeir AA. Rapid communication: effects of proximal and distal ends of double-J ureteral stent position on postprocedural symptoms and quality of life: a randomized clinical trial. J Endourol. 2007;21(7):698–702.
4. Chew BH, Knudsen BE, Nott L, Pautler SE, Razvi H, Amann J, Denstedt JD. Pilot study of ureteral movement in stented patients: first step in understanding dynamic ureteral anatomy to improve stent comfort. J Endourol. 2007;21(9):1069–76.
5. Ramsay JW, Payne SR, Gosling PT, Whitfield HN, Wickham JE, Levison DA. The effects of double J stenting on unobstructed ureters. An experimental and clinical study. Br J Urol. 1985;57(6):630–4.
6. Venkatesh R, Landman J, Minor SD, Lee DI, Rehman J, Vanlangendonck R, Ragab M, Morrissey K, Sundaram CP, Clayman RV. Impact of a double-pigtail stent on ureteral peristalsis in the porcine model: initial studies using a novel implantable magnetic sensor. J Endourol. 2005;19(2):170–6.
7. Kinn AC, Lykkeskov-Andersen H. Impact on ureteral peristalsis in a stented ureter. An experimental study in the pig. Urol Res. 2002;30(4):213–8.
8. Dunn CJ, Matheson A, Faulds DM. Tamsulosin: a review of its pharmacology and therapeutic efficacy in the management of lower urinary tract symptoms. Drugs Aging. 2002;19:135–16.
9. Davenport K, Timoney AG, Keeley FX. A comparative in vitro study to determine the beneficial effect of calcium-channel and α1-adrenoceptor antagonism on human ureteric activity. BJU Int. 2006;98(3):651–5.
10. Rajpathy J, Aswathaman K, Sinha M, Subramani S, Gopalakrishnan G, Kekre N. An in vitro study on human ureteric smooth muscle with the a1-adrenoceptor subtype blocker, tamsulosin. BJU Int. 2008;102(11):1743.
11. Damiano R, Autorino R, De Sio M, Giacobbe A, Palumbo IM, D'Armiento M. Effect of tamsulosin in preventing ureteral stent-related morbidity: a prospective study. J Endourol. 2008;22(4):651–6.

12. Wang CJ, Huang SW, Chang CH. Effects of specific α-1A/1D blocker on lower urinary tract symptoms due to double-J stent: a prospectively randomized study. Urol Res. 2009;37(3):147–52.
13. Beddingfield R, Pedro RN, Hinck B, Kreidberg C, Feia K, Monga M. Alfuzosin to relieve ureteral stent discomfort: a prospective, randomized, placebo controlled study. J Urol. 2009;181:170–6.
14. Deliveliotis C, Chrisofos M, Gougousis E, Papatsoris A, Dellis A, Varkarakis IM. Is there a role for alpha1-blockers in treating double-J stent-related symptoms? Urology. 2006;67(1):35–9.
15. Damiano R, Autorino R, De Sio M, Cantiello F, Quarto G, Perdonà S, Sacco R, D'Armiento M. Does the size of ureteral stent impact urinary symptoms and quality of life? A prospective randomized study. Eur Urol. 2005;48(4):673–8.
16. Erturk E, Sessions A, Joseph JV. Impact of ureteral stent diameter on symptoms and tolerability. J Endourol. 2003;17(2):59–62.
17. Pryor J, Carey P, Lippert M. Migration of silicone ureteral catheters. J Endourol. 1988;2(3):283–6.
18. Thomas RA. Indwelling ureteral stents: impact of material and shape on patient comfort. J Endourol. 1993;7(2):137–40.
19. Duvdevani M, Chew BH, Denstedt JD. Minimizing symptoms in patients with ureteric stents. Curr Opin Urol. 2006;16(2):77–82.
20. Mokhtari G, Shakiba M, Ghodsi S, Farzan A, Nejad SH, Esmaeili S. Effect of terazosin on lower urinary tract symptoms and pain due to double-J stent: a double-blind placebo-controlled randomized clinical trial. Urol Int. 2011;87(1):19–22.
21. Clifford GM, Farmer RD. Medical therapy for benign prostatic hyperplasia: a review of the literature. Eur Urol. 2000;38(1):2–19.
22. Michel MC. The pharmacological profile of the α1A-adrenoceptor antagonist silodosin. Eur Urol Suppl. 2010;9(4):486–90.
23. Roehrborn CG, Schwinn DA. α1-Adrenergic receptors and their inhibitors in lower urinary tract symptoms and benign prostatic hyperplasia. J Urol. 2004;171(3):1029–35.
24. Yoshida M, Kudoh J, Homma Y, Kawabe K. New clinical evidence of silodosin, an α1A selective adrenoceptor antagonist, in the treatment for lower urinary tract symptoms. Int J Urol. 2012;19(4):306–16.
25. Shibata K, Foglar R, Horie K, Obika K, Sakamoto A, Ogawa S, Tsujimoto G. KMD-3213, a novel, potent, alpha 1a-adrenoceptor-selective antagonist: characterization using recombinant human alpha 1-adrenoceptors and native tissues. Mol Pharmacol. 1995;48(2):250–8.
26. Richter S, Ringel A, Shalev M, Nissenkorn I. The indwelling ureteric stent: a 'friendly' procedure with unfriendly high morbidity. BJU Int. 2000;85(4):408–11.
27. Tolley D. Ureteric stents, far from ideal. Lancet. 2000;356(9233):872–3.
28. Navanimitkul N, Lojanapiwat B. Efficacy of tamsulosin 0.4 mg/day in relieving double-J stent-related symptoms: a randomized controlled study. J Int Med Res. 2010;38(4):1436–41.
29. Wang CJ, Huang SW, Chang CH. Effects of tamsulosin on lower urinary tract symptoms due to double-J stent: a prospective study. Urol Int. 2009;83(1):66–9.
30. Lamb AD, Vowler SL, Johnston R, Dunn N, Wiseman OJ. Meta-analysis showing the beneficial effect of alpha-blockers on ureteric stent discomfort. Database of Abstracts of Reviews of Effects (DARE): Quality-assessed reviews [Internet]. 2011.
31. Wilde MI, Fitton A, McTavish D. Alfuzosin. Drugs. 1993;45(3):410–29.
32. Mehik A, Alas P, Nickel JC, Sarpola A, Helström PJ. Alfuzosin treatment for chronic prostatitis/chronic pelvic pain syndrome: a prospective, randomized, double-blind, placebo-controlled, pilot study. Urology. 2003;62(3):425–9.
33. Höfner K, Jonas U. Alfuzosin: a clinically uroselective α 1-blocker. World J Urol. 2002;19(6):405–12.

34. Karadeniz A, Pişkin İ, Eşsiz D, Altintaş L. Relaxation responses of trigonal smooth muscle from rabbit by alpha 1-adrenoceptor antagonists alfuzosin, doxazosin and tamsulosin. Acta Vet Brno. 2008;77(1):81–8.

35. Van Moorselaar RJ, Hartung R, Emberton M, Harving N, Matzkin H, Elhilali M, Alcaraz A, Vallancien G, ALF-ONE Study Group. Alfuzosin 10 mg once daily improves sexual function in men with lower urinary tract symptoms and concomitant sexual dysfunction. BJU Int. 2005;95(4):603–8.

36. Takei RI, Ikegaki I, Shibata K, Tsujimoto G, Asano T. Naftopidil, a novel α1-adrenoceptor antagonist, displays selective inhibition of canine prostatic pressure and high affinity binding to cloned human α1-adrenoceptors. Jpn J Pharmacol. 1999;79(4):447–54.

37. Kohjimoto Y, Hagino K, Ogawa T, Inagaki T, Kitamura S, Nishihata M, Iba A, Matsumura N, Hara I. Naftopidil versus flopropione as medical expulsive therapy for distal ureteral stones: results of a randomized, multicenter, double-blind, controlled trial. World J Urol. 2015;33(12):2125–9.

38. Shalaby E, Ahmed AF, Maarouf A, Yahia I, Ali M, Ghobish A. Randomized controlled trial to compare the safety and efficacy of tamsulosin, solifenacin, and combination of both in treatment of double-J stent-related lower urinary symptoms. Adv Urol. 2013;752382.

39. Lee YJ, Huang KH, Yang HJ, Chang HC, Chen J, Yang TK. Solifenacin improves double-J stent-related symptoms in both genders following uncomplicated ureteroscopic lithotripsy. Urolithiasis. 2013;41(3):247–52.

40. Lexi-Drugs. Lexicomp Online(R) Hudson, Ohio: LexiComp, Inc.; 2015. www.crlonline.com/lco/action/home.

41. Abdelhamid MH, Zayed AS, Ghoneima WE, Elmarakbi AA, El Sheemy MS, Aref A, et al. Randomized, double-blind, placebo-controlled trial to compare solifenacin versus trospium chloride in the relief of double-J stent-related symptoms. World J Urol. 2017;35(8):1261–8.

42. Cui Y, Zong H, Yang C, Yan H, Zhang Y. The efficacy and safety of mirabegron in treating OAB: a systematic review and meta-analysis of phase III trials. Int Urol Nephrol. 2014;46(1):275–84.

43. Warren K, Burden H, Abrams P. Mirabegron in overactive bladder patients: efficacy review and update on drug safety. Ther Adv Drug Saf. 2016;7:204–16.

44. Betschart P, Zumstein V, Piller A, Schmid HP, Abt D. Prevention and treatment of symptoms associated with indwelling ureteral stents: a systematic review. Int J Urol. 2017;24(4):250–9.

45. Chaignat V, Danuser H, Stoffel MH, Z'Brun S, Studer UE, Mevissen M. Effects of a non-selective COX inhibitor and selective COX-2 inhibitors on contractility of human and porcine ureters in vitro and in vivo. Br J Pharmacol. 2008;154(6):1297–307.

46. Tadros NN, Bland L, Legg E, Olyaei A, Conlin MJ. A single dose of a non-steroidal anti-inflammatory drug (NSAID) prevents severe pain after ureteric stent removal: a prospective, randomised, double-blind, placebo-controlled trial. BJU Int. 2012;111(1):101–5.

47. Kyriazis I, Kallidonis P, Georgiopoulos I, Al-Aown A, Sakellaropoulos G, Stolzenburg JU, Liatsikos E. In vitro evaluation of ureteral contractility: a comparative assessment of human, porcine and sheep ureteral response to vardenafil. Urol Int. 2015;94(2):234–9.

48. Bayraktar Z, Albayrak S. Sexual intercourse as a new option in the medical expulsive therapy of distal ureteral stones in males: a prospective, randomized, controlled study. Int Urol Nephrol. 2017;49(11):1941–6.

49. Sharma G, Sharma AP, Mavuduru RS, Devana SK, Bora GS, Singh SK, Mandal AK. Role of phosphodiesterase inhibitors in stent-related symptoms: a systematic review and meta-analysis. World J Urol. 2020;38(4):929–38.

50. Cui M, Khanijou S, Rubino J, Aoki KR. Subcutaneous administration of botulinum toxin A reduces formalin-induced pain. Pain. 2004;107(1–2):125–33.

51. Ishikawa H, Mitsui Y, Yoshitomi T, Mashimo K, Aoki S, Mukuno K, Shimizu K. Presynaptic effects of botulinum toxin type A on the neuronally evoked response of albino and pigmented rabbit iris sphincter and dilator muscles. Jpn J Ophthalmol. 2000;44(2):106–9.

52. Durham PL, Cady R, Cady R. Regulation of calcitonin gene-related peptide secretion from trigeminal nerve cells by botulinum toxin type A: implications for migraine therapy. Headache. 2004;44(1):35–43.
53. Gupta M, Patel T, Xavier K, Maruffo F, Lehman D, Walsh R, Landman J. Prospective randomized evaluation of periureteral botulinum toxin type A injection for ureteral stent pain reduction. J Urol. 2010;183(2):598–602.
54. Falahatkar S, Beigzadeh M, Mokhtari G, Esmaeili S, Kazemnezhad E, Amin A, Herfeh NR, Falahatkar R. The effects of pregabalin, solifenacin and their combination therapy on ureteral double-J stent-related symptoms: a randomized controlled clinical trial. Int Braz J Urol. 2021;47:596–609.
55. Ragab M, Soliman MG, Tawfik A, Raheem AA, El-Tatawy H, Farha MA, Magdy M, Elashry O. The role of pregabalin in relieving ureteral stent-related symptoms: a randomized controlled clinical trial. Int Urol Nephrol. 2017;49(6):961–6.
56. Lee CX, Cheah JH, Soule CK, Ding H, Whittaker CA, Karhohs K, Burds AA, Subramanyam KS, Carpenter AE, Eisner BH, Cima MJ. Identification and local delivery of vasodilators for the reduction of ureteral contractions. Nat Biomed Eng. 2020;4(1):28–39.
57. Bhattar R, Tomar V, Yadav SS, Dhakad DS. Comparison of safety and efficacy of silodosin, solifenacin, tadalafil and their combinations in the treatment of double-J stent-related lower urinary system symptoms: a prospective randomized trial. Turk J Urol. 2018;44(3):228.
58. Tehranchi A, Rezaei Y, Khalkhali H, Rezaei M. Effects of terazosin and tolterodine on ureteral stent related symptoms: a double-blind placebo-controlled randomized clinical trial. Int Braz J Urol. 2013;39:832–40.
59. Dellis AE, Keeley FX Jr, Manolas V, Skolarikos AA. Role of α-blockers in the treatment of stent-related symptoms: a prospective randomized control study. Urology. 2014;83(1): 56–62.
60. Park J, Yoo C, Han DH, Shin DW. A critical assessment of the effects of tamsulosin and solifenacin as monotherapies and as a combination therapy for the treatment of ureteral stent-related symptoms: a 2× 2 factorial randomized trial. World J Urol. 2015;33(11):1833–40.
61. Abdelaal AM, Al-Adl AM, Abdelbaki SA, Al Azab MM, Al Gamal KA. Efficacy and safety of tamsulosin oral-controlled absorption system, solifenacin, and combined therapy for the management of ureteric stent-related symptoms. Arab J Urol. 2016;14(2):115–22.
62. Maldonado-Avila M, Garduño-Arteaga L, Jungfermann-Guzman R, Manzanilla-Garcia HA, Rosas-Nava E, Procuna-Hernandez N, Vela-Mollinedo A, Almazan-Treviño L, Guzman-Esquivel J. Efficacy of tamsulosin, oxybutynin, and their combination in the control of double-J stent-related lower urinary tract symptoms. Int Braz J Urol. 2016;42:487–93.
63. Rees AM, editor. The complementary and alternative medicine information source book. ABC-CLIO; 2001.
64. Gotoh A, Goto K, Sengoku A, Shirakawa T, Akao Y, Fujisawa M, Okada H, Arakawa S, Sasaki H, Kamidono S. Inhibition of urinary bladder motility by a spinal action of U-50488H in rats. J Pharm Pharmacol. 2002;54(12):1645–50.
65. Yoshimura K, Terai A, Arai Y. Two-week administration of low-dose Hachimi-jio-gan (Ba-Wei Di-Huang-Wan) for patients with benign prostatic hyperplasia. Hinyokika kiyo. 2003;49(9):509–14.
66. Chancellor MB, de Groat WC. Intravesical capsaicin and resiniferatoxin therapy: spicing up the ways to treat the overactive bladder. J Urol. 1999;162(1):3–11.
67. Ojiako OA, Igwe CU. Short communication nutritional and anti-nutritional compositions of Cleome rutidosperma, Lagenaria siceraria, and Cucurbita maxima seeds from Nigeria. J Med Food. 2007;10(4):735–8.
68. Friederich M, Theurer C, Schiebel-Schlosser G. Prosta Fink Forte capsules in the treatment of benign prostatic hyperplasia. Multicentric surveillance study in 2245 patients. Forsch Komplementarmed Klass Naturheilkd. 2000;7(4):200–4.

69. Nishimura M, Ohkawara T, Sato H, Takeda H, Nishihira J. Pumpkin seed oil extracted from Cucurbita maxima improves urinary disorder in human overactive bladder. J Tradit Complement Med. 2014;4(1):72–4.
70. Chernin D. The complete homeopathic resource for common illnesses. North Atlantic Books; 2006.
71. Gollmann W. The homoeopathic guide in all diseases of the urinary and sexual organs. 1855.

Ureteral Stent Designs to Reduce Stent-Related Symptoms and Improve Patient Quality of Life

Julia E. de la Cruz, Francisco M. Sánchez-Margallo, and Federico Soria

1 Introduction

Considering the impact on the quality of life of patients caused by double-J stents (DJS), different stent designs have been developed focusing mainly on the decrease or suppression of vesicoureteral reflux (VUR) and the reduction of bladder trigone irritation, for the improvement of patient comfort [1–4]. Many of these designs are based on changes at the distal end, such as the attachment of antireflux membranes and valves, their replacement by less voluminous designs or the complete removal of this section to create intraureteral stents [5–10].

2 Antireflux Membranes and Valves

Antireflux membranes and valves are devices incorporated to the distal end of a standard DJS design, with the purpose of preventing intraluminal reflux through the internal channel of the stent. There are two variants, the antireflux-membrane valve and the polymeric flap valve [5, 6, 11].

The antireflux membrane valve consists of a transparent silicone membrane in the shape of a pouch, that is attached at the vesical end of a DJS, wrapped around the outlet of the internal channel and the lateral orifices [5, 11, 12] (Fig. 1). This design is currently available for clinical use and its antireflux mechanism works as a one-way valve, automatically collapses as the bladder pressure increases thus

J. E. de la Cruz (✉) · F. M. Sánchez-Margallo · F. Soria
Foundation, Jesús Usón Minimally Invasive Surgery Center, Cáceres, Spain
e-mail: msanchez@ccmijesususon.com; fsoria@ccmijesususon.com

© The Author(s) 2022
F. Soria et al. (eds.), *Urinary Stents*,
https://doi.org/10.1007/978-3-031-04484-7_8

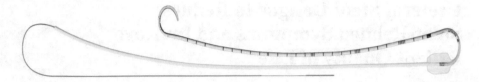

Fig. 1 Double-J ureteral stent with the antireflux-membrane valve. Reprinted from: Ecke et al. [5], with per-mission from Elsevier and T. H. Ecke as right holders of the image

preventing intraluminal VUR [12]. This membrane valve allows only antegrade urine movement with minimal impact on pressure and flow resistance but has the limitation of preventing antegrade insertion of the stent [5, 12].

In terms of its clinical evaluation, a significant decrease in VUR and suprapubic and flank pain during urination were observed, as well as a reduction in hydrone-phrosis degree and rate of stent exchange [5]. A significant improvement in patient comfort, compared to current DJS, is described, suggesting that it may be due to less damage to the bladder urothelium provided by the antireflux-membrane valve [5, 13]. Nevertheless, Ritter et al. [14], by means of the Ureteral Stent Symptom Questionnaire (USSQ), do not show significant differences against a DJS, in the symptoms or in the quality of life of the patients, although it does deliver a signifi-cant reduction of the VUR. Thus, although this antireflux membrane has shown a significant reduction in VUR, a direct relationship between this trend and the improvement of patient symptomatology cannot be made.

The polymeric flap valve, developed by Park et al. [15], consists of a polymeric device that attaches to the vesical edge of the DJS, shaped as two lip-like mem-branes and an inner cavity [15]. Manufactured by 3D printing, flexible Tango-Plus FLX980 is used as the material of this flap valve [15]. The mechanism of this device is based on the difference between ureteral and bladder pressures. When the intra-vesical pressure rises, the valve occludes, preventing the retrograde flow of urine [15]. The efficacy of the valve was analysed *in vivo* by Kim et al. [6] in the porcine model. By means of a simulated voiding cystourethrography, the study revealed significant lower grades of VUR. However, low grade VUR was still present with a rate of 18% since this flap valve does not prevent extraluminal VUR either. This is a 24 h acute study, therefore potential long-term complications, such as possible valve obstruction due to encrustation remain uncertain [16, 17].

In the end, these designs block urine reflux through the internal channel of the DJS, but fail to prevent VUR in its entirety. In stented ureters, VUR occurs both through the lumen of the stent and around it. The extraluminal reflux will prevail as long as there is a stent reaching the ureterovesical junction (UVJ) through the ure-teral orifice [18].

3   Distal End Modifications

Changes in the stents' distal ends pursue a common objective, the reduction of material at the level of the UVJ and bladder trigone in order to mitigate the discomfort in stented patients [7, 8, 10, 11].

The modification of the distal end of the Tail Stent (Boston Scientific® Corporation, USA) consists of a progressive narrowing of its diameter, from 7 to 3 Fr, in a distal direction [7]. Unlike a standard DJS, this vesical end is not a pigtail, but straight, with the aim of reducing the volume of the stent at the ureteral orifices and bladder [7]. Regarding its assessment in the clinical setting, it causes 21% less lower urinary tract symptoms (LUTS) than a DJS, but provides no significant improvement in stent-related pain and urothelial inflammation [7].

On the other hand, the Buoy stent (Cook® Medical, USA), a stent with the features of a tail stent, except for its proximal largest diameter of 10 Fr, was analysed in the porcine model [19]. This Buoy stent provides effective urine drainage, adequate ureteral healing after endoureterotomy and causes less histologic damage of the UVJ, when compared to a standard 7 Fr CDJ and to a Endopyelotomy stent (Cook® Medical, USA) [19]. Nevertheless, the potential of this design to improve patient comfort remains unknown.

The Polaris™ Loop® design, developed by Boston Scientific® (Boston Scientific® Corporation, USA), consists of a 6 Fr single pigtail stent with a double loop at its distal end, whose diameter is equal or inferior to 3 Fr, reducing almost 70% of material at the distal level, with regard to a standard DJS [10] (Fig. 2). Thus the interaction of the stent with the bladder urothelium and the intramural ureter is restricted, reducing discomfort of patients [10]. Most of the clinical improvements induced by this design are not significant compared to DJS's commercial designs [10, 20]. Many comparative studies with standard DJS show that despite there is a reduction in pain, filling symptoms, and analgesic consumption provided by the Polaris™ Loop®, these results are not significant [10, 20].

Fig. 2   Distal end of the Polaris™ Loop® ureteral stent, Boston Scientific (Boston Scientific Corporation, USA)

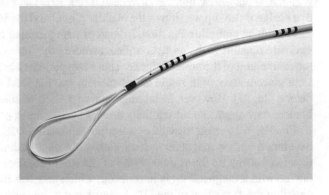

Another upgrade of ureteral stent designs is the suture stent, a single pigtail stent whose distal end has been replaced by one or two suture threads [8, 11]. A preliminary version of this design was firstly described in 1993 by Hübner et al. [21], although the most representative devices with this design are JFil® and MiniJFil®, developed by Vogt et al. [8, 22–25]. They claim that the intact areas of the ureter do not require the urinary drainage provided by a DJS and therefore, in proximal ureteral obstructions, the material of distal sections of the DJS can be replaced by a narrower component, such as a suture thread [8]. The JFil® is constituted by 50% of polymeric DJS, arranged in a proximal position and the remaining 50% composed by two suture threads, whereas the MiniJFil® has only the proximal pigtail, to which the suture threads have been attached. In both cases, the suture is double, made of 5-0 polypropylene, presenting a total diameter of 0.6 Fr [8]. Clinical studies evidenced an effective urinary drainage capacity, as well as a significant reduction in urinary pain and symptoms [8]. Besides, MiniJFil® has demonstrated its clinical safety and efficacy used after ESWL and ureteroscopic lithotripsy [22]. Nevertheless, this design is not exempt from complications, since up to 20% migration is detected, which in the case of being proximal, represents an endourological challenge, in addition to the potential risk of disrupting urine drainage [8].

As for the significant reduction of urinary symptoms and pain provided by these designs, the authors suggest its potential to limit the occurrence of VUR [8]. However, VUR incidence has not been analysed in patients and, similarly to the aforementioned antireflux designs, the presence of the suture crossing the ureteral orifice could again prevent the complete eradication of this adverse effect [8, 22]. All these designs have in common, that the potential inhibition of VUR may be partial. Regardless of calibre, the stent in all cases traverses the ureteral orifice preventing its closure when intravesical pressure rises and therefore perpetuating the incompetence of the antireflux mechanism of the UVJ.

With regard to further modifications of DJS's distal end, recently B. Vogt has published two clinical cases presenting the treatment of malignant ureteral obstructions with a new polymeric ureteral stent design [26, 27]. The main feature of this innovative design is the suppression of the bladder pigtail and the incorporation of a silicone piece with an antireflux function. Instead of being located on the bladder, this distal structure remains at the ureteral orifice, avoiding the interaction of the material with the urothelium of the vesical trigone. These two patients have proven the feasibility of stent placement both in single and in tandem and the safety and effectiveness of the device [26, 27]. However, distal migration of a stent with such characteristics in the bladder may aggravate substantially urinary symptoms in patients [27].

Finally, in an effort to avoid cystoscopic removal of DJS, a ureteral stent has been developed with a magnetic system consisting of a cylinder shaped magnet fixed through a string on the vesical pigtail of the stent [28]. For its extraction, a retrieval device with a magnetic tip is introduced; which attaches to the magnet of the stent, enabling the extraction of the DJS by pulling out the catheter [28]. Clinical evaluations of the Black-Star® stent (Urotech®, Germany) using USSQ and visual analogue scales have revealed a lower incidence of pain and discomfort during removal with the use of this system, especially in men [28, 29]. On the other hand, the likelihood of the onset of encrustations on urinary stents should be considered, since it might disable the magnetic extraction system of this device [29].

4   Intraureteral Stents

Provided that a device at the UVJ disrupts its antireflux mechanism and triggers urinary symptoms and pain, the next step appeared to be to develop ureteral stents that spare the whole distal end, becoming intraureteral stents. Under this rationale, Soria et al. have developed an antireflux intraureteral ureteral stent registered as BraidStent® [9]. This intraureteral stent is a self-retaining design comprising a proximal pigtail, a central braided body of 3 Fr lacking internal channel, and a double helix as the distal end [9] (Fig. 3). The development of this intraureteral design is based on the principle that the way to prevent both intraluminal and extraluminal reflux is to preserve the UVJ intact [18, 30].

The validation of the BraidStent® by Soria et al. [9] in the swine model showed that this design meets the requirements of a DJS for passive ureteral dilation, completely avoiding VUR and significantly decreasing macroscopic and histologic damage in UVJ, which will probably reduce discomfort in stented patients [31, 32]. In addition, the effect of the stent on ureteral healing has been evaluated experimentally, showing that selective intubation of the affected area provides surgical success rates of over 85%, suggesting ureteral surgery as one of the indications that may benefit from this intraureteral design [33]. However, since the endoscopic removal of an intraureteral stents involves certain difficulty, a biodegradable BraidStent® has been developed and has undergone experimental assessment, showing a safe, controlled and predictable degradation rate [34, 35]. The biodegradable BraidStent® and its counterpart coated with heparin, the BraidStent®-H, maintain the characteristics proven in previous studies that tested the biostable BraidStent® [9, 32, 36–38].

The benefits arisen from the suppression of stent material at the UVJ on patients' quality of life are substantiated in the randomized study by Yoshida et al. [39]. In which the insertion of an intraureteral stent after ureteroscopic lithotripsy causes significantly less pain and urinary symptoms, as well as an also significant reduction in the consumption of analgesic drugs [39]. However, despite being designated as an

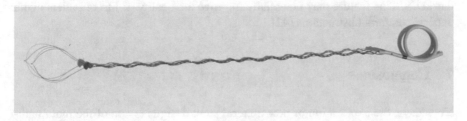

Fig. 3 BraidStent®, self-retaining, antireflux ureteral stent developed by Soria et al.

intraureteral stent, a thread attached to the stent reaches the bladder to enable cysto-scopic removal, supporting the idea that an intraureteral device would benefit from biodegradable properties. Once more, it is uncertain whether this vesical thread may interfere on the onset of VUR, since the study did not assess this parameter [39].

It is of note that indications for any intraureteral stent are going to be more lim-ited than those of a standard DJS. Circumstances requiring the dilatation of the UVJ will not be amenable to treatment with intraureteral designs, but with rather other stent catheterizing the ureteral orifice. Such designs will therefore offer the possibil-ity of avoiding the adverse effects related to the distal end of DJS to a certain pro-portion of patients requiring stenting, excluding those with distal ureteral lesions close to the UVJ, those who require prestenting for ureteroscopic treatment, or with lithiasic fragments after lithotripsy [9, 33, 34].

5   Modifications of the Core Architecture of a DJS

With different features to those presented above, the Percuflex™ Helical ureteral stent (Boston Scientific® Corporation, USA), is a spiral cut flexible ureteral stent, which maintains the morphology of a standard DJS at the distal ends. This device is com-mercially available, whose spiral conformation has been developed to adapt to the shape of the ureter and to better accommodate patient movement [40, 41]. This design, under experimental conditions, drains urine in a comparable way to a DJS Percuflex™ Plus (Boston Scientific® Corporation, USA) [40]. In a comparative clinical study, an improvement in patient comfort is described by a significant reduction of the need for analgesics, although it does not report a significant decrease in pain intensity [41].

6   Dual-Lumen Ureteral Stents

Dual-lumen ureteral stent (Gyrus ACMI Corporation, USA) is a device that has been designed to improve urine drainage in extrinsic compressions. This design consists of two DJS attached to each other to provide two internal drainage path-ways. In its *ex vivo* evaluation, this prototype provides significantly more extra and intraluminal drainage under extrinsic compression conditions, compared to a stan-dard DJS. This feature may potentially improve the quality of life of patients with extrinsic ureteral obstructions [42].

7   Conclusions

Nowadays, the exploration of new ureteral stent designs is one of the main path-ways, along with the development of materials and coatings, to improve the per-formance of current DJS. So far, it seems that these new designs mainly tend to modify the standard double pigtail design by progressively reducing and eliminating the presence of stent material at the level of the UVJ. In the context of suture stents and intraureteral stents, they have shown promising results in terms of improving patients' quality of life. However, indications of these devices differ from those of standard DJS, not being suitable for all patients that require ureteral stenting. The shortcoming of stents with modified distal ends is that in the event of complications or proximal migrations, their removal is technically more challenging than the removal of a DJS which may involve a potential risk for the patient.

Ultimately, design improvements aim at diversification, towards the development of more specific devices to adapt to different circumstances, so that the adverse effects resulting from the generalized use of standard DJS can be avoided. For the development of new designs, it is desirable that simultaneous modifications are made to the materials to enhance their performance, being of particular interest the ability to degrade safely.

References

1. Beysens M, Tailly TO. Ureteral stents in urolithiasis. Asian J Urol. 2018;5:274–86.
2. Chew BH, Lange D. Advances in ureteral stent development. Curr Opin Urol. 2016;26:277–82.
3. Mosayyebi A, Manes C, Carugo D, Somani BK. Advances in ureteral stent design and materials. Curr Urol Rep. 2018;19(35):1–9.
4. Forbes C, Scotland KB, Lange D, Chew BH. Innovations in ureteral stent technology. Urol Clin North Am. 2019;46:245–55.
5. Ecke TH, Bartel P, Hallmann S, Ruttloff J. Evaluation of symptoms and patients' comfort for JJ-ureteral stents with and without antireflux-membrane valve. Urology. 2010;75:212–6.
6. Kim HW, Park C-J, Seo S, Park Y, Lee JZ, Shin DG, et al. Evaluation of a polymeric flap valve-attached ureteral stent for preventing vesicoureteral reflux in elevated intravesical pressure conditions: a pilot study using a porcine model. J Endourol. 2016;30:428–32.
7. Dunn MD, Portis AJ, Kahn SA, Yan Y, Shalhav AL, Elbahnasy AM, et al. Clinical effectiveness of new stent design: randomized single-blind comparison of tail and double-pigtail stents. J Endourol. 2000;14:195–202.
8. Vogt B, Desgrippes A, Desfemmes F-N. Changing the double-pigtail stent by a new suture stent to improve patient's quality of life: a prospective study. World J Urol. 2015;33:1061–8.
9. Soria F, Morcillo E, Serrano A, Rioja J, Budía A, Sánchez-Margallo FM. Preliminary assessment of a new antireflux ureteral stent design in swine model. Urology. 2015;86:417–22.
10. Lingeman JE, Preminger GM, Goldfischer ER, Krambeck AE. Assessing the impact of ureteral stent design on patient comfort. J Urol. 2009;181:2581–7.
11. Soria F, de la Cruz JE, Morcillo E, Rioja J, Sánchez-Margallo FM. Catéteres ureterales antirreflujo. Arch Esp Urol. 2016;69:544–52.
12. Yamaguchi O, Yoshimura Y, Irisawa C, Shiraiwa Y. Prototype of a reflux-preventing ureteral stent and its clinical use. Urology. 1992;40:326–9.
13. Ahmadzadeh M. Flap valve ureteral stent with an antireflux function: a review of 46 cases. Urol Int. 1992;48:466–8.
14. Ritter M, Krombach P, Knoll T, Michel MS, Haecker A. Initial experience with a newly developed antirefluxive ureter stent. Urol Res. 2012;40:349–53.
15. Park C-J, Kim H-W, Jeong S, Seo S, Park Y, Moon HS, et al. Anti-reflux ureteral stent with polymeric flap valve using three-dimensional printing: an in vitro study. J Endourol. 2015;29:933–8.

16. Sighinolfi MC, Sighinolfi GP, Galli E, Micali S, Ferrari N, Mofferdin A, et al. Chemical and mineralogical analysis of ureteral stent encrustation and associated risk factors. Urology. 2015;86:703–6.
17. Bithelis G, Bouropoulos N, Liatsikos EN, Perimenis P, Koutsoukos PG, Barbalias GA. Assessment of encrustations on polyurethane ureteral stents. J Endourol. 2004;18:550–6.
18. Mosli HA, Farsi HM, Al-Zimaity MF, Saleh TR, Al-Zamzami MM. Vesicoureteral reflux in patients with double pigtail stents. J Urol. 1991;146:966–9.
19. Krebs A, Deane LA, Borin JF, Edwards RA, Sala LG, Khan F, et al. The "buoy" stent: evaluation of a prototype indwelling ureteric stent in a porcine model. BJU Int. 2009;104:88–92.
20. Lee JN, Kim BS. Comparison of efficacy and bladder irritation symptoms among three different ureteral stents: a double-blind, prospective, randomized controlled trial. Scand J Urol. 2015;49:237–41.
21. Hübner WA, Plas EG, Trigo-Rocha F, Tanagho EA. Drainage and reflux characteristics of antireflux ureteral double-J stents. J Endourol. 1993;7:497–9.
22. Vogt B, Desfemmes F-N, Desgrippes A, Ponsot Y. MiniJFil®: a new safe and effective stent for well-tolerated repeated extracorporeal shockwave lithotripsy or ureteroscopy for medium-to-large kidney stones? Nephrourol Mon. 2016;8:e40788.
23. Vogt B, Desgrippes A, Desfemmes F-N. Sondes JFil et MiniJFil: Progrès décisifs dans la tolérance des sondes urétérales et propriétés inattendues du fil urétéral. Prog Urol. 2014;24:441–50.
24. Vogt B, Desgrippes A, Desfemmes F. Sonde JFil et MiniJFil: analyse des données de 280 patients et applications pratiques de la dilatation urétérale. Prog Urol. 2014;24:795–6.
25. Vogt B, Desgrippes A, Desfemmes F. Sondes JFil et MiniJFil. Stratégie dans le traitement de gros calculs rénaux et utilisation d'un urétéroscope souple 11F avec Lithoclast. Prog Urol. 2014;24:896.
26. Vogt B. Ureteral stent obstruction and stent's discomfort are not irreparable damages. Urol Case Rep. 2018;20:100–1.
27. Vogt B. Challenges to attenuate ureteric stent-related symptoms: reflections on the need to fashion a new dynamic stent design consequent upon a case report. Res Rep Urol. 2019;11:277–81.
28. Rassweiler M-C, Michel M-S, Ritter M, Honeck P. Magnetic ureteral stent removal without cystoscopy: a randomized controlled trial. J Endourol. 2017;31:762–6. https://doi.org/10.1089/end.2017.0051.
29. Sevcenco S, Eredics K, Lusuardi L, Klingler HC. Evaluation of pain perception associated with use of the magnetic-end ureteric double-J stent for short-term ureteric stenting. World J Urol. 2018;36:475–9.
30. Janssen C, Buttyan R, Seow CY, Jäger W, Solomon D, Fazli L, et al. A role for the hedgehog effector Gli1 in mediating stent-induced ureteral smooth muscle dysfunction and aperistalsis. Urology. 2017;104:242.e1–8.
31. Joshi HB, Newns N, Stainthorpe A, MacDonagh RP, Keeley FX, Timoney AG, et al. Ureteral stent symptom questionnaire: development and validation of a multidimensional quality of life measure. J Urol. 2003;169:1060–4.
32. Joshi HB, Okeke A, Newns N, Keeley FXJ, Timoney AG. Characterization of urinary symptoms in patients with ureteral stents. Urology. 2002;59:511–6.
33. Soria F, Morcillo E, de la Cruz JE, Serrano A, Estébanez J, Sanz JL, et al. Antireflux ureteral stent proof of concept assessment after minimally invasive treatment of obstructive uropathy in animal model. Arch Esp Urol. 2018;71:607–13.
34. Soria F, Morcillo E, Serrano A, Budía A, Fernandez I, Fernández-Aparicio T, et al. Evaluation of a new design of antireflux-biodegradable ureteral stent in animal model. Urology. 2018;115:59–64.
35. Soria F, de la Cruz JE, Budía A, Serrano A, Galán-Llopis JA, Sánchez-Margallo FM. Experimental assessment of new generation of ureteral stents: biodegradable and antireflux properties. J Endourol. 2020;34:359–65.

36. Soria F, de la Cruz JE, Fernandez T, Budia A, Serrano Á, Sanchez-Margallo FM. Heparin coating in biodegradable ureteral stents does not decrease bacterial colonization-assessment in ureteral stricture endourological treatment in animal model. Transl Androl Urol. 2021;10(4):1700–10.
37. Soria F, de La Cruz JE, Budia A, Cepeda M, Álvarez S, Serrano Á, et al. Iatrogenic ureteral injury treatment with biodegradable antireflux heparin-coated ureteral stent—animal model comparative study. J Endourol. 2021;35(8):1244–9.
38. Soria F, de La Cruz JE, Caballero-Romeu JP, Pamplona M, Pérez-Fentes D, Resel-Folskerma L, et al. Comparative assessment of biodegradable-antireflux heparine coated ureteral stent: animal model study. BMC Urol. 2021;21(1):1–8. https://doi.org/10.1186/s12894-021-00802-x.
39. Yoshida T, Inoue T, Taguchi M, Matsuzaki T, Murota T, Kinoshita H, et al. Efficacy and safety of complete intraureteral stent placement versus conventional stent placement in relieving ureteral stent related symptoms: a randomized, prospective, single blind, multicenter clinical trial. J Urol. 2019;202:164–70.
40. Mucksavage P, Pick D, Haydel D, Etafy M, Kerbl DC, Lee JY, et al. An in vivo evaluation of a novel spiral cut flexible ureteral stent. Urology. 2012;79:733–7.
41. Chew BH, Rebullar KA, Harriman D, McDougall E, Paterson RF, Lange D. Percuflex helical ureteral stents significantly reduce patient analgesic requirements compared to control stents. J Endourol. 2017;31:1321–5.
42. Hafron J, Ost MC, Tan BJ, Fogarty JD, Hoenig DM, Lee BR, et al. Novel dual-lumen ureteral stents provide better ureteral flow than single ureteral stent in ex vivo porcine kidney model of extrinsic ureteral obstruction. Urology. 2006;68(4):911–5.

Encrustation in Urinary Stents

Wolfgang Kram, Noor Buchholz, and O. W. Hakenberg

1 Introduction

Insertion of a ureteral stent is an acute measure to restore the urinary flow from the kidney to the bladder in cases of acute or chronic obstruction or a functional disturbance of ureteral peristalsis. In cases with chronic obstruction and poor prognosis due to surgical or anesthetic inoperability or sometimes patient preference, ureteral stenting may be used as a permanent treatment. In such cases, regular exchange of the ureteral stent at specified intervals is necessary and constitutes a minimally invasive endourological procedure.

With long-standing ureteral stenting, the problems of stent encrustation, biofilm formation, and bacterial colonization become important. Excessive stent encrustation to stent blockage and, consequently, pain, fever, renal infection, impairment of renal function and even renal failure.

Encrustations of urinary stents are due to the crystallization of soluble minerals in urine, predominantly calcium oxalate salts [1]. The quantification of this process is highly individualized. Patients with a high excretion of crystal-forming ions in the urine tend to have fast and excessive formation of encrustations on any stent.

This process can occur without significant bacterial contamination but facilitates the adherence, persistence and multiplication of bacteria in biofilms.

Uropathogenic microorganisms (usually enterobacteria) are either introduced into the bladder when a catheter is inserted, or they migrate into the bladder along a transurethral catheter over time. From the bladder, bacteria ascend through the ureter and especially along a ureteral stent into the kidneys. This

W. Kram (✉) · O. W. Hakenberg
Department of Urology, University Medical Center Rostock, Rostock, Germany
e-mail: wolfgang.kram@med.uni-rostock.de; oliver.hakenberg@med.uni-rostock.de

N. Buchholz
Scientific Office, U-merge Ltd., London-Athens-Dubai, London, UK

© The Author(s) 2022
F. Soria et al. (eds.), *Urinary Stents*,
https://doi.org/10.1007/978-3-031-04484-7_9

Table 1 Natural defense mechanisms of the urinary tract

Commensal flora
Urinary flow (ureteral peristalsis)
Skin and mucous membrane
Bladder mucosa: Mucin production
Tamm-Horsefall glycoprotein
Local immune responses

Implants are exempted from those and therefore prone to encrustations

catheter-associated urinary tract infection (CAUTI) is associated with the long-term use of indwelling transurethral bladder catheters [2]. With an indwelling bladder catheter, bacterial colonization will occur within a few days. This problem is clinically highly relevant since ureteral stenting and the use of indwelling bladder catheters are often necessary and combined after urological surgical procedures. This inevitably leads to a high rate of contamination and, consequently, bacteriuria. Bacteria will usually spread throughout the urinary tract but with an unimpeded urinary flow and normal ureteral and bladder function this usually does not lead to clinical problems.

However, with the formation of biofilms on urological implants there will be bacterial colonization. Bacteria are protected from the natural local defense mechanisms of the urinary tract in those biofilms (Table 1). Not only will this lead to more clinically relevant urinary tract infections, but antibiotics are also less effective because they cannot adequately reach bacteria in biofilms. Furthermore, bacteria incorporated in biofilms have a reduced metabolic rate which further reduces the efficacy of most antibiotics. As a result, bacteria in biofilm develop antibiotic resistance more quickly [3, 4].

1.1 Bacteria and Biofilm Formation

Biofilms develop when microorganisms settle in the area between two different phases and are immobilized in a matrix of extracellular polymeric substances (EPS) [5]. These cannot be effectively cleared neither by humoral and cellular immune defense mechanisms nor by antibiotics. Biofilm development can be separated into four such phases (Fig. 1):

1. Reversible aggregation of proteins, polysaccharides and macrolide molecules.

    The binding of proteins to the catheter surface depends on the catheter material (surface energy, mechanical properties and morphology), electrostatic interactions and the composition of the surrounding medium [4]. Within minutes, a dense formation, the *conditioning film*, develops on the substrate [6, 7].

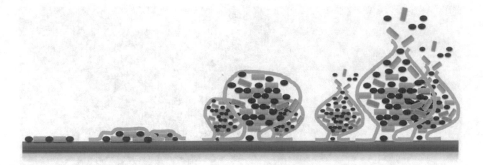

Fig. 1 Biofilm development in four phases

2. Irreversible apposition of proteins and bacteria.

   Bacteria reach the substrate through electrostatic interactions [8, 9]. The production of extracellular polymeric substances (EPS) is influenced in the now closed system by *quorum sensing*, a regulatory system which requires a certain cell density of the same species of bacteria [10].

3. Development of a mature biofilm.

   With further growth, the three-dimensional macro-colonies accumulate to form a bacterial layer. Bacterial immobilization is highest in the close vicinity of the material surface [11].

4. Biofilm spread through degradation of matrix polymers.

   With increasing maturation of the biofilm, cells or clusters of cells can separate and slough from the biofilm. Through the release of enzymes, bacteria can actively leave the biofilm and migrate [12, 13].

1.2 Physicochemical Aspects of Urinary Stents Encrustation and Stone Formation

Multiple influences on the composition of the bacterial mix in a biofilm lead to a heterogeneous biofilm development. Although bacteria are predominant, pathological crystallization may develop and lead to encrustations on catheter materials even without significant microbial presence.

Regarding the crystallization process (formation of urinary stones) there are different theories:

- Oversaturation of the urine with crystal forming ions (nucleation),
- formation of stone matrix with secondary crystallization of complex macromolecules on the surface,

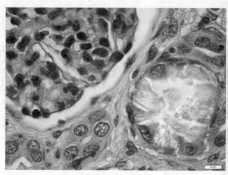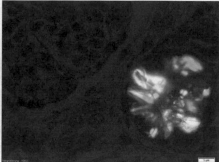

Fig. 2 Histology showing renal kidney injury in a porcine model. Induction of calcium oxalate crystallization (hydroxy-L-proline). No encrustations were seen on the indwelling ureteral stent over 6 weeks. Left: hematoxylin-eosine, 40×; right: polarized light, 40×. BX43 lens UPLSAPO 2 40×/0,95, BX-POL and U-GAN, Olympus

- formation of Randall plaques,
- relative lack of inhibitors or oversupply of promoters of crystallization,
- idiopathic crystallization of calcium oxalate.

Crystallization is influenced by many exogenous and endogenous factors in a multifactorial way. It is thus the result of a complex interaction of many physicochemical and biochemical processes. For the development of urinary stones, the initiating mechanism could be the formation of poly-crystalline in the distal tubules of nephrons. However, crystaluria does not necessarily imply the development of urinary stones. Microscopic crystals are commonly excreted in the urine by healthy individuals with urinary oversaturation (Fig. 2).

The essential factor is the balance between lithogenic and inhibitory substances in the urine. If this equilibrium is disturbed, urinary oversaturation with lithogenic substances will result in spontaneous homogeneous nucleation. Crystals with the same structure will bind to initial aggregates and finally stones. If catheter material or crystals are present in urine, macromolecular urinary compounds will lead to heterogeneous nucleation depending on the degree of oversaturation (metastable oversaturation).

Calcium oxalate, calcium phosphate, magnesium phosphate and uric acid are the minerals that most commonly crystallize in urine [14] (Table 2).

Urinary compounds can modulate the process of crystal nucleation, aggregation and encrustation on urinary stents. These comprise compounds normally present in urine such as the Tamm-Horsefall proteins, glycosaminoglycanes and pyrophosphates [17]. Some of these may have inhibitory as well as promotive effects on nucleation and aggregation. This is discussed with some controversy in the literature [18–21]. Low molecular weight substances such as zinc, magnesium, sulfate

Table 2 Composition of urinary stones [15, 16]

Stone type	Chemical composition	Mineral	Population (%)
Calcium oxalate	Calcium oxalate-monohydrate	Whewellite	70–80
	Calcium oxalate-dihydrate	Weddellite	42
Calcium phosphate	Calcium phosphate	Apatite	30
	Calcium hydrogen phosphate-dihydrate	Brushite	1
	Tricalcium phosphate	Whitlockite	<0.1
	Carbonate apatite	Dahllite	1
Magnesium-ammonium-phosphate	Magnesium-ammonium-phosphate-hexahydrate	Struvite	6
	Magnesium hydrogen-phosphate-trihydrate	Newberyite	<0.1
Uric acid and urate	Uric acid	Uricite	10
	Uric acid-monohydrate	Uricite (mono)	0.1
	Uric acid-dihydrate	Uricite (ortho)	6
	Ammonium hydrogenurate		0.5
Genetically determined	Cystine	Uricite (hexa)	0.4
	Xanthine		<0.1
	2,8-dihydroxyadenine		<0.1

and pyrophosphate bind to calcium and form soluble complexes and do therefore have an inhibitory influence on crystallization.

2 Risks Factors and Complications

2.1 Risks Factors and Complications of Urinary Stone Formation

A polygenetic defect in combination with other facilitating factors (e.g. dietary and climatic conditions) can lead to urolithiasis [22]. Important cofactors are hypercalciuria, hyperoxaluria, hypocitraturia, and hyperuricosuria as well as a lack of inhibitory substances [23]. Idiopathic hypercalciuria is the most common etiological factor for calcium stones. In addition, some physiological conditions such as pregnancy influence the urine composition [24]. Pathological conditions such as renal diseases, especially glomerular changes, or disturbances of urine transportation can lead to urinary stone formation. The latter can result from upper or lower urinary tract obstruction, renal dystopia (nephroptosis, pelvic kidney), other malformations such as horse-shoe kidney, ureteroceles, vesico-ureteral reflux, neurogenic bladder dysfunction, or immobilization (e.g. after a fracture).

2.2 Risk Factors and Complications of Encrustations on Stents and Catheters

Pathophysiology of urolithiasis and catheter encrustation are closely related. Studies have shown that the indwelling time of a catheter is the most important risk factor for oxalate-dependent encrustations. However, there is no significant correlation between the volume of encrustation and catheter-associated symptoms [25]. Yet, studies looked at the quantification of encrustations depending on the indwelling time, the differentiation of bacterial colonization, and risk factors associated with these processes [26–29]. Roupret et al. found for ureteral stents with a mean indwelling time of 55.5 days a correlation between stone composition and catheter encrustation of over 70% [30].

Catheter encrustations occur faster in the presence of infection than oxalate-dependent encrustations, and are also associated with risk factors. An important risk factors is residual bladder urine (incomplete bladder emptying) in the presence of an implant, leading to infections. Other risk factors are inflammatory urinary tract obstruction, neurogenic bladder dysfunctions, and urinary diversions using intestinal loops, such as an ileal conduit [31]. This may be further aggravated by additional renal conditions such as distal tubular acidosis, hyperphosphaturia, or medullary sponge kidneys [32].

One important mechanism of biofilm formation is the infection with urease-producing bacteria. Broomfield et al. [33] investigated the capacity of urease-positive bacteria to induce encrustations on ureteral implants. They found that Proteus mirabilis, Proteus vulgaris und Providencia rettgeri have the highest urease activity and induce the highest rate of encrustations. Urease leads to production of ammonia through hydrolysis of urea, with an increase in urinary pH. The alkaline milieu leads to increased crystallization of magnesium-ammonium-phosphate (struvite) as well as calcium-hydroxyapatite (apatite) [34]. Due to improved urological diagnostics, the relative proportion of infectious stones (struvite) has been lowered to 6% of all urinary stones (Table 2). In urological guidelines, there is consensus that in view of the danger of life-threatening infections and/or renal damage as well as the high rate of recurrence, infectious stones and the associated implants should be completely removed [35–38].

In studies of biofilm quantification, Ganderton et al. found that there is no clear relationship between indwelling time and biofilm mass [39]. Presumably there is a relationship with the colonizing ability of the primary bacterial species that settles on the biofilm. Also, catheter design may have important implications for urinary flow through and around the catheter, affecting encrustation formation [40].

An important point would be the contamination-free ureteral stent extraction [41]. Transurethral extraction lead to bacterial contamination from the distal urethra. In addition, catheter encrustations might be dislodged. This is in line with studies that have shown that the rate of bacterial colonization with ureteral stents as well as urethral catheters is higher than the rate of urinary infections [42, 43]. Thus, routine urine cultures are not predictive of catheter cultures.

3 Preventive Strategy of Encrustations and Biofilm Formation

The surface characteristics of a biomaterial (e.g. smoothness of surface, electric charge) as well as the virulence factors of microorganisms, and the presence of adhesins all determine the time course and characteristics of biofilm formation. Most urinary stents are made of polymer mixtures with characteristics that are intended to reduce encrustations [44]. These mixtures are often proprietary, but are usually based on polyurethane (Silhouette®, Bardex® and Tecoflex®). There are also other polymer combinations that can be used such as hydrogel with urethane, silicone, polyvinyl chloride (Aquavene®), styrole, ethylene-butylene, styrole-block copolymers (C-Flex®) and polyester (Silitek®) [45]. Currently used biocompatible polymers, e.g. Elastollan, Styroflex and Greenflex have good mechanical stability and flexibility, with antiadhesive properties and can be used for thin-walled catheters with good urine drainage [46].

Additional compounds need to be added to these basic materials to provide for x-ray opacity. This usually reduces the mechanical flexibility. Usually, 25–30% barium sulfate, a biocompatible salt with high electron density is used for this purpose.

Another way to reduce the degree of encrustation and bacterial adhesions is to coat the catheter surface with different materials. For urinary stents, surface coatings with covalently bound heparin, polytetrafluoroethylene (PTFE), hydrogels, plasma-bound carbon (DLC—diamond-like carbon), or urease-inhibitors can be used [47]. Strategies to reduce microbial adhesions, to induce bactericidal properties (contact killing), to impede the 'quorum sensing' of microbes, and generally to interfere with the initial adhesion process include the formation of a surface film or the release of a bactericidal compound including antibiotics, bacteriophages, metal oxide nanoparticles, other meta ions, and carbon compounds, ionic polymers, as well as polymers and biofilms with non-pathogenic bacteria. Studies with silver nanoparticles and with hydrophilic poly(p-xylene) (PPX-N) coated catheters found a reduced rate of biofilm formation and reduced bacterial adhesions [48, 49]. Watterson et al. Reported that the coating of urinary stents with enzymes metabolizing oxalate significantly reduced encrustations [50].

Whilst urinary stents impregnated with and releasing e.g. silver ions, hydrogel or antibiotics significantly delayed bacterial adherence in the first days, they did not reduce the rate of significant infections and had no clinical benefit in long-term indwelling catheters. Furthermore, the long-term antibiotic release from stent material might lead to bacterial resistance which can have serious clinical consequences.

Concerning long-term indwelling catheters, surface coatings with covalent bindings seem to hold some promise. Surfaces with double-ion polymers such as phosphorylcholine [51] and covalently bound heparin have been tested [52]. Another class of materials are antibacterial cationic polymers. The contact-active covalently bound coating absorbs proteins and bacteria with a negatively charged cell membrane or cell wall and develops antimicrobial activity through high hydrophilicity with high ionic charges [53].

4 Current Methods for Reducing Encrustation and Biofilm Formation

As an alternative to conventional implants, biodegradable ureteral stents (BUS) may avoid the procedure of transurethral catheter removal. Another theoretical advantage is the constantly changing material surface which impairs the development of a conditioning biofilm and thus reduces the interaction of the material with microbes. Biodegradable implants consist of several natural and synthetic polymers, whereby the most important biological degrading process is hydrolysis. Barros et al. developed the HydrUStent®. This ureteral stent is completely dissolved after 10 days in urine. X-ray opacity is however given during the first 24 h only [54]. The BraidStent®, a heparin-coated polyurethane ureteral stent has an in-dwelling time of up to 6 weeks in animal tests. The heparin coating allows for an early reduction in bacterial colonization. However, this effect is limited in the long term [55].

Champagne et al. examined the degradation of zinc compounds in artificial urine to try to circumvent the limitations of alloys based on iron and magnesium regarding biocompatibility and controlled degradation under physiological conditions. Zinc alloys are degraded more slowly than magnesium alloys and might be an ideal biomaterial to reduce bacterial adhesions and encrustations on stents [56].

Currently, systems on the basis of computer-based fluid analysis and microfluid models (stent-on-chip, microfluidic chips) are being developed to examine and simulate the flow of urine in a stented ureter. These models are also intended to examine the flow in the presence of additional obstruction, i.e. through encrustation. With changes in the thickness of the stent wall and the design of the side holes significant reductions in particle formation could be achieved [57–59]. Future simulation systems will take a variety of pathological reactions of the stented and the obstructed ureter into account [60].

5 Current Methods for the Examination of Encrustation and Biofilm on Urinary Stents

Elwood et al. observed that conditioning biofilms on urinary stents contain calcium-binding proteins, among them uromodulin, and that these can serve as a nidus for further crystalline growth and encrustation. These proteins were the same on different stent materials and in different patients. This seems to indicate that the physical properties of the stent surface and not the interaction between bacterial adhesins and urinary proteins are the main determinants for bacterial interactions with stent material [61].

Rebl et al. examined the relationship between physical properties of polymer surfaces and their ability to withstand encrustations. The important parameters to characterize the surfaces were:

- contact angle,
- zeta potential,
- morphology.

The contact angle between a fluid drop and a plane surface is a measure for hydrophilicity. Synthetic urine with a pH of 6.5 was used. The zeta potential describes a specific surface charge which develops between in a watery solute on the interface between a solid material and the watery solution. The comparative analyses in the screening model did show that the negative surface charge of about −60 mV and the hydrophilicity of the polymer (<85°) correlated with a reduced amount of encrustations. The main components of infection stones are struvite with a surface charge of −17.5 mV and carbonate apatite with −16 mV surface charge at a pH of 8.0 [62].

Morphological examinations of stent encrustations are preferably carried out by means of scanning electron microscopy (SEM), energy dispersive X-ray spectroscopy (EDX), and Fourier-transform infrared spectroscopy (FTIR) and show the

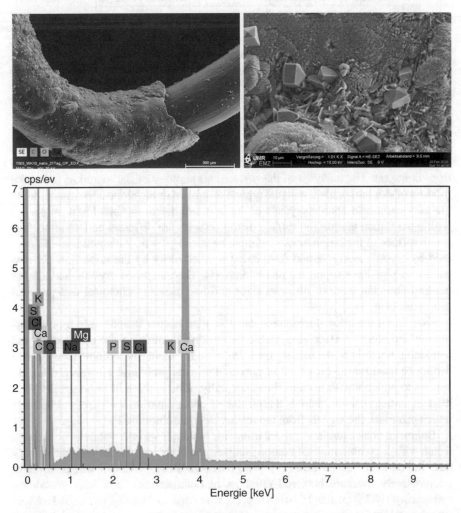

Fig. 3 EDX analysis of encrustations on a ureteral stent (rat). Top left, the mapping shows the elements Ca, C, and O, which are calcium-containing crystals. Top right, SEM image shows a rough surface with calcium oxalate crystals. Bacterias find good conditions here. Bottom: the line spectrum shows the Ca- and P-containing matrix of calcium oxalate and a small proportion of calcium phosphate. FE-SEM Merlin VP compact (Zeiss) with EDX detector XFlash 6/30 (Bruker)

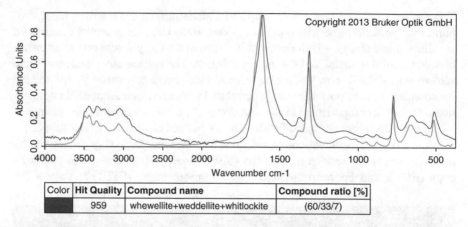

Fig. 4 FTIR analysis of encrustations on a ureteral stent (Fig. 3) in a rat model. Measured absorption spectra of the mineral deposits in red. Absorption spectra of the OPUS reference library are shown in blue. The encrustation consists of calcium oxalate monohydrate (whewellite), calcium oxalate dihydrate (weddellite) and tricalcium phosphate (whitlockite) 60/33/7. ALPHA FTIR spectrometer, OPUS™ library, Bruker

characteristic interactions of the catheter surface with the surrounding urine in clinical studies. Figures 3 and 4 show the morphological examination of stent encrustations in the rat. The analyses of the surface morphology of the materials showed a mixture of calcium oxalate with the typical dumbbell or envelope appearance, some granular carbonate apatite crystals of some micrometers in size. Fluid properties within the lumen and on the surface of the catheter are different and variable. The rough surface of the polymer can facilitate bacterial growth. Adherent bacteria covered by crystals are protected from being washed away by the urine flow. *In vivo* studies in pigs have supported this hypothesis. The examined crystals had similar compositions but were of different sizes and had differing chemical and physical properties (Fig. 5).

Examining the urine microbiome can also give further insights into biofilm formation and catheter-associated problems through identifying the commensal and residential bacteria of the urinary tract. Individual patient microbiome analysis can further be used for the prognosis of potential clinical problems. However, this only applies to patients with bacteriuria as normally urine is thought to be sterile. With bladder catheterization, there is a high risk of contamination with urethral bacteria which can mask the signals from the residential microbiota [62].

Buhmann et al. examined several urine microbiota from encrustations on ureteral stents with a combination of complementary methods in patients without urinary tract infections or bacteriuria [63]. With real time PCR (qPCR) it was possible to quantitatively estimate bacterial numbers in encrustations, and next generation sequencing (NGS) of the 16S-rRNA gene was used to identify bacterial DNA. It was shown that the insertion of a ureteral stent for up to 6 weeks was associated with a lower bacterial colonization of the encrustations. In patients without clinically

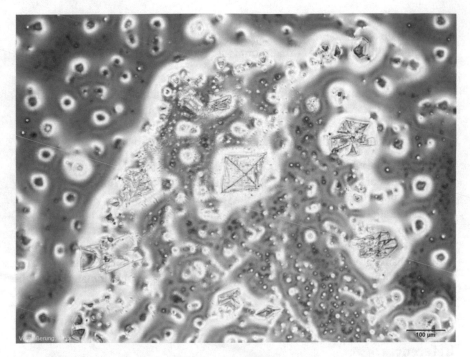

Fig. 5 Induced crystal formation in the pig model: precipitates of calcium oxalate in urine. The crystals have different sizes as well as different chemical and physical properties. Calcium dihydrate (weddellite), calcium monohydrate (whewellite): small crystals with dumbbell shape or envelope shape. BX43—phase contrast lens UPLSAPO 2 40x/0.95, Olympus

relevant urinary tract infections facultative pathogenic bacteria seem to be predominant.

The identification of bacteria with MALDI-ToF MS (matrix-assisted laser desorption ionization-time-of-flight mass spectrometry) is currently used in combination with other technologies to increase the scope of relevant analyses. MALDI-ToF MS can be used for the fast identification of bacteria in encrustations without prior culture or subculture [64]. However, for the identification of bacteria in urine microbiological culture and selective identification of bacteria are still required [65].

6 Conclusions

Crystallization processes in urine, bacterial adherence and encrustation of biomaterials in the urinary tract are usually the result of a multifactorial process with an interplay between many physicochemical and biochemical processes. While all non-infectious urinary stones and encrustations develop on the basis of metabolic, endocrine or renal disturbances, the presence of bacteria in the urinary tract, especially of those producing urease and their enzymatic activity, increases the urinary pH. This changes the solubility product of calcium and magnesium salts which, in turn, facilitates encrustations.

Taken together, the use of urinary implants is characterized by three interrelated problems:

a tendency for encrustations through the deposition of urinary crystal-forming ions, facilitation of bacterial colonization and persistence despite antibiotic prophylaxis/ treatment, and mechanical irritation with resulting reaction of the ureteral tissues.

Coated catheters which potentially could minimize the risk of a complicated urinary tract infection and could allow for longer indwelling times without complications are to date not recommended by urological guidelines [66, 67].

Work is underway for new concepts to develop biomaterials with reduced encrustation propensity and biofilm formation. Promising candidates are coated materials with anti-adhesive properties through covalent binding, high hydrophilicity, and good mechanical properties allowing for adequate patient comfort. For urinary tract catheters with an in-dwelling time under 6 weeks, self-absorbing biomaterials might be a good solution.

References

1. Grases F, Sohnel O, Costa-Bauza A, Ramis M, Wang Z. Study on concretions developed around urinary catheters and mechanisms of renal calculi development. Nephron. 2001;88(4):320–8.
2. Tenke P, Kovacs B, Jackel M, Nagy E. The role of biofilm infection in urology. World J Urol. 2006;24(1):13–20.
3. Jain A, Gupta Y, Agrawal R, Khare P, Jain SK. Biofilms—a microbial life perspective: a critical review. Crit Rev Ther Drug Carrier Syst. 2007;24(5):393–443.
4. Choong S, Whitfield H. Biofilms and their role in infections in urology. BJU Int. 2000;86(8):935–41.
5. Flemming HC, Wingender J. Relevance of microbial extracellular polymeric substances (EPSs)—part I: structural and ecological aspects. Water Sci Technol. 2001;43(6):1–8.
6. Denstedt JD, Wollin TA, Reid G. Biomaterials used in urology: current issues of biocompatibility, infection, and encrustation. J Endourol. 1998;12(6):493–500.
7. van Loosdrecht MC, Lyklema J, Norde W, Zehnder AJ. Influence of interfaces on microbial activity. Microbiol Rev. 1990;54(1):75–87.
8. Donlan RM, Costerton JW. Biofilms: survival mechanisms of clinically relevant microorganisms. Clin Microbiol Rev. 2002;15(2):167–93.
9. Mikkelsen H, Sivaneson M, Filloux A. Key two-component regulatory systems that control biofilm formation in Pseudomonas aeruginosa. Environ Microbiol. 2011;13(7):1666–81.
10. Senturk S, Ulusoy S, Bosgelmez-Tinaz G, Yagci A. Quorum sensing and virulence of Pseudomonas aeruginosa during urinary tract infections. J Infect Dev Ctries. 2012;6(6):501–7.
11. O'Toole G, Kaplan HB, Kolter R. Biofilm formation as microbial development. Annu Rev Microbiol. 2000;54:49–79.
12. Costerton JW, Stewart PS, Greenberg EP. Bacterial biofilms: a common cause of persistent infections. Science (New York, NY). 1999;284(5418):1318–22.

13. Verstraeten N, Braeken K, Debkumari B, Fauvart M, Fransaer J, Vermant J, et al. Living on a surface: swarming and biofilm formation. Trends Microbiol. 2008;16(10):496–506.
14. Wang Z, Zhang Y, Zhang J, Deng Q, Liang H. Recent advances on the mechanisms of kidney stone formation (review). Int J Mol Med. 2021;48(2):149.
15. Cloutier J, Villa L, Traxer O, Daudon M. Kidney stone analysis: "Give me your stone, I will tell you who you are!". World J Urol. 2015;33(2):157–69.
16. Schubert G. Stone analysis. Urol Res. 2006;34(2):146–50.
17. Khan SR, Kok DJ. Modulators of urinary stone formation. Front Biosci. 2004;9:1450–82.
18. Aggarwal KP, Narula S, Kakkar M, Tandon C. Nephrolithiasis: molecular mechanism of renal stone formation and the critical role played by modulators. Biomed Res Int. 2013;2013:292953.
19. Ratkalkar VN, Kleinman JG. Mechanisms of stone formation. Clin Rev Bone Miner Metab. 2011;9(3–4):187–97.
20. Ryall RL. Urinary inhibitors of calcium oxalate crystallization and their potential role in stone formation. World J Urol. 1997;15(3):155–64.
21. Baumann JM, Affolter B. The paradoxical role of urinary macromolecules in the aggregation of calcium oxalate: a further plea to increase diuresis in stone metaphylaxis. Urolithiasis. 2016;44(4):311–7.
22. Sakhaee K, Maalouf NM, Sinnott B. Clinical review. Kidney stones 2012: pathogenesis, diagnosis, and management. J Clin Endocrinol Metab. 2012;97(6):1847–60.
23. Sofer M, Denstedt JD. Encrustation of biomaterials in the urinary tract. Curr Opin Urol. 2000;10(6):563–9.
24. Semins MJ, Matlaga BR. Management of stone disease in pregnancy. Curr Opin Urol. 2010;20(2):174–7.
25. Joshi HB, Newns N, Stainthorpe A, MacDonagh RP, Keeley FX Jr, Timoney AG. Ureteral stent symptom questionnaire: development and validation of a multidimensional quality of life measure. J Urol. 2003;169(3):1060–4.
26. Sighinolfi MC, Sighinolfi GP, Galli E, Micali S, Ferrari N, Mofferdin A, et al. Chemical and mineralogical analysis of ureteral stent encrustation and associated risk factors. Urology. 2015;86(4):703–6.
27. Torrecilla C, Fernandez-Concha J, Cansino JR, Mainez JA, Amon JH, Costas S, et al. Reduction of ureteral stent encrustation by modulating the urine pH and inhibiting the crystal film with a new oral composition: a multicenter, placebo controlled, double blind, randomized clinical trial. BMC Urol. 2020;20(1):65.
28. Betschart P, Zumstein V, Buhmann MT, Albrich WC, Nolte O, Güsewell S, et al. Influence of biofilms on morbidity associated with short-term indwelling ureteral stents: a prospective observational study. World J Urol. 2019;37(8):1703–11.
29. Betschart P, Zumstein V, Buhmann MT, Altenried S, Babst C, Müllhaupt G, et al. Symptoms associated with long-term double-J ureteral stenting and influence of biofilms. Urology. 2019;134:72–8.
30. Roupret M, Daudon M, Hupertan V, Gattegno B, Thibault P, Traxer O. Can ureteral stent encrustation analysis predict urinary stone composition? Urology. 2005;66(2):246–51.
31. Rieu P. [Infective lithiasis]. Ann Urol. 2005;39(1):16–29.
32. Bichler KH, Eipper E, Naber K, Braun V, Zimmermann R, Lahme S. Urinary infection stones. Int J Antimicrob Agents. 2002;19(6):488–98.
33. Broomfield RJ, Morgan SD, Khan A, Stickler DJ. Crystalline bacterial biofilm formation on urinary catheters by urease-producing urinary tract pathogens: a simple method of control. J Med Microbiol. 2009;58(Pt 10):1367–75.
34. Stickler DJ. Clinical complications of urinary catheters caused by crystalline biofilms: something needs to be done. J Intern Med. 2014;276(2):120–9.
35. Espinosa-Ortiz EJ, Eisner BH, Lange D, Gerlach R. Current insights into the mechanisms and management of infection stones. Nat Rev Urol. 2019;16(1):35–53.

36. Jiang P, Xie L, Arada R, Patel RM, Landman J, Clayman RV. Qualitative review of clinical guidelines for medical and surgical management of urolithiasis: consensus and controversy 2020. J Urol. 2021;205(4):999–1008.
37. Seitz C, Bach T, Bader M, Berg W, Knoll T, Neisius A, et al. [Update of the 2Sk guidelines on the diagnostics, treatment and metaphylaxis of urolithiasis (AWMF register number 043-025) : What is new?]. Der Urologe Ausg A. 2019;58(11):1304–12.
38. Türk C, Petřík A, Sarica K, Seitz C, Skolarikos A, Straub M, et al. EAU guidelines on diagnosis and conservative management of urolithiasis. Eur Urol. 2016;69(3):468–74.
39. Ganderton L, Chawla J, Winters C, Wimpenny J, Stickler D. Scanning electron microscopy of bacterial biofilms on indwelling bladder catheters. Eur J Clin Microbiol Infect Dis. 1992;11(9):789–96.
40. Waters SL, Heaton K, Siggers JH, Bayston R, Bishop M, Cummings LJ, et al. Ureteric stents: investigating flow and encrustation. Proc Inst Mech Eng H J Eng Med. 2008;222(4):551–61.
41. Buhmann MT, Abt D, Altenried S, Rupper P, Betschart P, Zumstein V, et al. Extraction of biofilms from ureteral stents for quantification and cultivation-dependent and -independent analyses. Front Microbiol. 2018;9:1470.
42. Gunardi WD, Karuniawati A, Umbas R, Bardosono S, Lydia A, Soebandrio A, et al. Biofilm-producing bacteria and risk factors (gender and duration of catheterization) characterized as catheter-associated biofilm formation. Int J Microbiol. 2021;2021:8869275.
43. Klis R, Szymkowiak S, Madej A, Blewniewski M, Krzeslak A, Forma E, et al. Rate of positive urine culture and double-J catheters colonization on the basis of microorganism DNA analysis. Cent European J Urol. 2014;67(1):81–5.
44. Forbes C, Scotland KB, Lange D, Chew BH. Innovations in ureteral stent technology. Urol Clin North Am. 2019;46(2):245–55.
45. Venkatesan N, Shroff S, Jayachandran K, Doble M. Polymers as ureteral stents. J Endourol. 2010;24(2):191–8.
46. Rebl H, Renner J, Kram W, Springer A, Fritsch N, Hansmann H, et al. Prevention of encrustation on ureteral stents: which surface parameters provide guidance for the development of novel stent materials? Polymers. 2020;12(3):558.
47. Morris NS, Stickler DJ. The effect of urease inhibitors on the encrustation of urethral catheters. Urol Res. 1998;26(4):275–9.
48. Heidari Zare H, Juhart V, Vass A, Franz G, Jocham D. Efficacy of silver/hydrophilic poly(p-xylylene) on preventing bacterial growth and biofilm formation in urinary catheters. Biointerphases. 2017;12(1):011001.
49. Zhu Z, Wang Z, Li S, Yuan X. Antimicrobial strategies for urinary catheters. J Biomed Mater Res A. 2019;107(2):445–67.
50. Watterson JD, Cadieux PA, Beiko DT, Cook AJ, Burton JP, Harbottle RR, et al. Oxalate-degrading enzymes from Oxalobacter formigenes: a novel device coating to reduce urinary tract biomaterial-related encrustation. J Endourol. 2003;17(5):269–74.
51. Diaz Blanco C, Ortner A, Dimitrov R, Navarro A, Mendoza E, Tzanov T. Building an anti-fouling zwitterionic coating on urinary catheters using an enzymatically triggered bottom-up approach. ACS Appl Mater Interfaces. 2014;6(14):11385–93.
52. Cauda F, Cauda V, Fiori C, Onida B, Garrone E. Heparin coating on ureteral double J stents prevents encrustations: an in vivo case study. J Endourol. 2008;22(3):465–72.
53. Zhou C, Wu Y, Thappeta KRV, Subramanian JTL, Pranantyo D, Kang ET, et al. In vivo anti-biofilm and anti-bacterial non-leachable coating thermally polymerized on cylindrical catheter. ACS Appl Mater Interfaces. 2017;9(41):36269–80.
54. Barros AA, Oliveira C, Ribeiro AJ, Autorino R, Reis RL, Duarte ARC, et al. In vivo assessment of a novel biodegradable ureteral stent. World J Urol. 2018;36(2):277–83.
55. Soria F, de La Cruz JE, Caballero-Romeu JP, Pamplona M, Pérez-Fentes D, Resel-Folskerma L, et al. Comparative assessment of biodegradable-antireflux heparine coated ureteral stent: animal model study. BMC Urol. 2021;21(1):32.

56. Champagne S, Mostaed E, Safizadeh F, Ghali E, Vedani M, Hermawan H. In vitro degradation of absorbable zinc alloys in artificial urine. Materials (Basel). 2019;12(2):295.
57. Mosayyebi A, Yue QY, Somani BK, Zhang X, Manes C, Carugo D. Particle accumulation in ureteral stents is governed by fluid dynamics: in vitro study using a "stent-on-chip" model. J Endourol. 2018;32(7):639–46.
58. De Grazia A, LuTheryn G, Meghdadi A, Mosayyebi A, Espinosa-Ortiz EJ, Gerlach R, et al. A microfluidic-based investigation of bacterial attachment in ureteral stents. Micromachines. 2020;11(4):408.
59. Amitay-Rosen T, Nissan A, Shilo Y, Dror I, Berkowitz B. Failure of ureteral stents subject to extrinsic ureteral obstruction and stent occlusions. Int Urol Nephrol. 2021;53(8):1535–41.
60. Kram W, Buchholz N. Letter to the editor, international urology and nephrology-in silico-in vitro-in vivo: can numerical simulations based on computational fluid dynamics (CFD) replace studies of the urinary tract? Int Urol Nephrol. 2021;53(9):1835–6.
61. Elwood CN, Lo J, Chou E, Crowe A, Arsovska O, Adomat H, et al. Understanding urinary conditioning film components on ureteral stents: profiling protein components and evaluating their role in bacterial colonization. Biofouling. 2013;29(9):1115–22.
62. Salter SJ, Cox MJ, Turek EM, Calus ST, Cookson WO, Moffatt MF, et al. Reagent and laboratory contamination can critically impact sequence-based microbiome analyses. BMC Biol. 2014;12:87.
63. Buhmann MT, Abt D, Nolte O, Neu TR, Strempel S, Albrich WC, et al. Encrustations on ureteral stents from patients without urinary tract infection reveal distinct urotypes and a low bacterial load. Microbiome. 2019;7(1):60.
64. Tsuchida S, Umemura H, Nakayama T. Current status of matrix-assisted laser desorption/ionization-time-of-flight mass spectrometry (MALDI-TOF MS) in clinical diagnostic microbiology. Molecules (Basel). 2020;25(20):4775.
65. Li Y, Wang T, Wu J. Capture and detection of urine bacteria using a microchannel silicon nanowire microfluidic chip coupled with MALDI-TOF MS. Analyst. 2021;146(4):1151–6.
66. Lam TB, Omar MI, Fisher E, Gillies K, MacLennan S. Types of indwelling urethral catheters for short-term catheterisation in hospitalised adults. Cochrane Database Syst Rev. 2014;9(9):Cd004013.
67. Jahn P, Beutner K, Langer G. Types of indwelling urinary catheters for long-term bladder drainage in adults. Cochrane Database Syst Rev. 2012;10:Cd004997.

Forgotten Ureteral Stent Syndrome

Cristina de la Encarnación Castellano, Àngela Canós Nebot, Juan Pablo Caballero Romeu, Federico Soria, and Juan Antonio Galán Llopis

1 Introduction

Ureteral stents are one of the most widely employed tools in urology and have been in use for more than four decades. Their indications have widened over the years, making the management of their complications an essential role in the urologist's practice. In this regard, the "retained or forgotten ureteral stent" syndrome remains a challenge. This syndrome is defined as the group of signs and symptoms produced by a JJ stent that has not been removed 2 or more weeks after the end of its maximum life [1].

Data on the frequency of forgotten ureteral stents vary widely between series, ranging from 3% to 51% of stents that are placed [1, 2]. Identification of the forgotten stent occurs on average 29 months after placement, with a range of 7–180 months [3].

2 Risk Factors for Forgotten Ureteral Stent Syndrome

The main risk factor for the development of forgotten ureteral stent syndrome is the time since placement of the stent [4]. However, the time to onset of the syndrome will depend on the chemical characteristics of the urine, its hydrodynamics, the catheter material itself and other factors related to the patient and the care provided.

C. de la Encarnación Castellano · À. Canós Nebot
Urology Department, Alicante University General Hospital, Alicante, Spain

J. P. Caballero Romeu (✉) · J. A. Galán Llopis
Urology Department, Alicante University General Hospital, Alicante, Spain

Alicante Institute for Health and Biomedical Research (ISABIAL), Alicante, Spain

F. Soria
Foundation, Jesús Usón Minimally Invasive Surgery Center, Cáceres, Spain
e-mail: fsoria@ccmijesususon.com

© The Author(s) 2022
F. Soria et al. (eds.), *Urinary Stents*,
https://doi.org/10.1007/978-3-031-04484-7_10

Table 1 Conditions that promote the development of forgotten ureteral stent syndrome

Factors modifying the chemical characteristics of urine	Factors affecting urine dynamics	Stent related factors	Patient-related factors
Personal history of lithiasis (9,10) Hyperuricosuria Hypercalciuria Hyperoxaluria Hypocitraturia Metabolopathies (10) Urinary pH alterations Renal failure Dehydration Urinary sepsis Chemotherapy (10) Pregnancy (9)	Intrinsic and extrinsic obstructive uropathy Congenital urinary malformations (10) Functional pathology of the lower urinary tract	Time since placement (4.9) Internal diameter Stent manufacturing material (10) Stent replacement by cystoscopy (1) Double-loop stents (11)	Low sociocultural level (1,3,12) Lack of health system or health insurance protection Good tolerance to the catheter Low adherence to treatment and follow-up (6,10) Poor doctor-patient communication (3) Age >60 years (1) Cognitive impairment History of urological, abdominal or pelvic surgery (13)

Matthew F et al. found that 75.5% of ureteral stents were encrusted within 6 months, 42.8% were encrusted within 4 months and 14.3% within 2 months. The time of highest incidence was between the fourth and fifth month (36.7%). Furthermore, in those patients who had experienced previous stents encrustation, the time to encrustation of the second was shorter, 3.3 months, than that of the first, 6 months, [5, 6].

Although it is not possible to estimate an incidence of encrustation, these data suggest that stents should be changed at least within 4 months of placement and preferably every 2 months. In patients with a previous history of encrustation, it is recommended that the dwell time of the stent be shortened to the minimum necessary, every 6 weeks [5, 6].

Other factors that favour the development of forgotten ureteral stent syndrome (FUSS) are detailed below [7–9] (Table 1).

3 Pathophysiology of the Forgotten Ureteral Stent

The forgotten ureteral stent syndrome depends on several factors. First of all, we will pay attention to the factors that favour encrustation, both of the internal channel of the stents and their external surface.

On the one hand, the surface of ureteral stents can become damaged, especially in their bend parts, making these areas more susceptible to crystal deposition. In addition, ureteral catheters can cause mechanical irritation of the urothelium, which favours colonisation by bacteria. These uropathogenic bacteria can be carried during stenting into the upper urinary tract.

Under the right conditions, crystals will be deposited both inside the ureteral stent and on the outside. The deposited material consists mainly of calcium oxalate mono- and dihydrate. It may also be associated with the deposition of phosphate crystals, uric acid and/or struvite and/or cystine. In addition to crystals, protein material such as Tamm-Horsfall or alpha 1-microglobulin may be deposited.

Crystal deposition can occur in the absence of bacteria, but when bacteria are present, and maintain high enzyme activity, the adhesion, persistence and proliferation of fouling sites increases. In addition, bacteria cause a change in urinary pH that causes the solubility of calcium and magnesium in urine to be altered, creating a vicious circle. Up to 90% of ureteral stents are colonised by microorganisms and according to published patient series a frequency of recurrent UTIs between 27% and 73.6% is reported [3, 10].

The biofilm development is often essential in the encrustation of ureteral stents [11] and is closely associated with the presence of urease-positive bacteria. Biofilms have a very complex formation and development process that is divided into four phases: (1) reversible agglomeration of proteins, polysaccharides and macromolecules; (2) irreversible deposition of proteins and bacteria; (3) maturation of the biofilm; and (4) spreading of the biofilm.

Singh et al. [12] found a higher percentage of encrustation in the proximal tip of the JJ stent, with the proximal segment of the ureter being the second most frequently affected area. In that study, encrustation of the bladder tip was rare.

Encrustation or mucoprotein deposits affect up to 68% of JJ stents, but only 4% of these patients show clinical signs of obstruction [13]. Furthermore, it appears that extraluminal obstruction reduces urinary flow to a greater degree than intraluminal obstruction [14]. Legrand et al. [15] have demonstrated a higher rate of encrustation in stents placed for lithiasis indication (8% before 4 months, almost 17% after), than in those patients with non-lithiasis indication (e.g. malignancy) with encrustation rates of 1.3% at 4 months and 5.2% at 6 months.

4 Symptoms and Complications Associated with the Forgotten Ureteral Stent

Patients with ureteral stents can present with a number of symptoms that make up the "ureteral stent syndrome" [2, 5, 6, 10, 16, 17] (Table 2).

Although the pathophysiology of the development of these signs and symptoms is not fully understood, the irritation produced by the distal end of the stent on the

Table 2 Symptoms of ureteral stent syndrome

Filling symptoms
Dysuria
Haematuria
Hypogastric or suprapubic abdominal pain
Ipsilateral renal fossa pain

bladder mucosa (mainly the bladder trigone), as well as the presence of vesicoureteral reflux seem to be related to the described symptoms. The use of catheters made of harder materials has also been associated with a higher incidence of symptoms such as dysuria, hypogastric or renal fossa pain [18].

Some patients may be unaware of a history of ureteral stent placement during the anamnesis, but the presence of these symptoms in a patient with a surgical history should lead us to believe that he or she may have a stent [2]. Furthermore, it is not uncommon for forgotten ureteral catheters to be asymptomatic and to be an incidental finding when they are incidentally found in an abdominopelvic imaging test [9].

The previously described symptoms, in addition to being present in patients with a ureteral stent who are aware of this condition, may also be present in FUSS. In this scenario, the symptoms depend on the complications generated by the time elapsed and the risk factors described above.

From compliance with the maximum ureteral stent dwell time to the occurrence of complications related to excess stent placement time is considered to take on average between 3 and 24 months [19].

Although most authors consider that the longer the stent placement time, the retrospective study by Lin TF et al. [1] found no significant differences in this regard. However, in this study, patients with a forgotten JJ stent placement accounted for 3.8% (18 patients) of the 479 patients analysed. Thus, only three of the patients with forgotten catheter placement developed complications. The sample size might be insufficient to draw conclusions [1].

4.1   Flank Pain

Pain may be due to vesicoureteral reflux or hydronephrosis. During micturition, the increased bladder pressure is transmitted through the stent placement and retrograde to the renal pelvis. The stent placement overrides the anti-reflux mechanism of the distal ureter causing a sudden increase in intra-pelvic pressure.

Hydronephrosis may be due to lithiasis formation, displacement or migration of the catheter placement, fragmentation or obstruction, among other causes.

On the one hand, the frequency of ureteral JJ stent migration ranges between 3% and 10% of the stents that are placed. It should be specified that migration can be proximal or distal; the latter being up to three times more frequent [20]. Factors involved in intra-ureteral stent movements include length, diameter and stent material. In general, stents made of softer, hydrophilic materials have a greater trend towards dislodgement [21]. Although stent length is usually chosen based on the patient's height, some studies suggest radiographic measurement of the distance between the pyeloureteral junction and the uretero-vesical junction as a strategy to further adjust the stent to the patient [21]. Also to prevent migration, double-J retention systems for stents were designed. Even so, sometimes even the proximal J-end can descend from the renal pelvis into the ureter or even the bladder, leading to urinary obstruction [7, 10].

Finally, the risk of catheter fragmentation is particularly high 14 weeks after stenting. Long-term exposure of stents to urine components produce the degeneration of the polymers. Thus, in cases of urinary tract infection and/or urothelial inflammation, the rate of degradation is higher. Stents composed of polyethylene polymers are the most easily degraded and are more prone to fragmentation. It is noted that the fragmentation lines usually coincide with the stent placement holes, so reducing the number of these holes could reduce the risk and/or the number of stent fragments [6, 18, 22].

4.2 Urinary Tract Infections

The stenting duration time also increases the likelihood of persistent UTI, since the longer the stent placement time, the higher the level of colonisation (up to 75% of stents that have been in place for more than 90 days are colonised).

As we have already indicated, bacteriuria is almost a constant in these patients, and up to 27–73.6% of cases develop UTIs that are likely to be recurrent and multi-resistant to antibiotics. This is because microorganisms remain in biofilms [3, 10, 23]. Biofilms hinder antimicrobial penetration and, in their matrix, microorganisms tend to express antimicrobial resistance genes and remain metabolically dormant, making antimicrobials even less effective [24]. Other factors that may favors the persistence of UTIs include the high prevalence of diabetes or renal failure in these patients.

The severity of infections generated by a forgotten ureteral stent varies widely: from simple cystitis [24] to severe acute pyelonephritis and septic shock of urinary origin [1, 2].

In renal transplant recipients, the most common presentation is recurrent UTIs and deterioration of renal function [25, 26]. In these patients the most common composition of the deposited material is struvite. Immunosuppression in transplant recipients favours colonisation of the urinary tract by urease-positive bacteria. In contrast to non-transplanted patients, patients with a renal graft do not have episodes of renal colic due to denervation of the graft [25].

4.3 Problems in Removal of Ureteral Stent

As mentioned above, the percentage of stent with surface encrustations increases with the stenting duration, with up to 75.5% of stents being found to be encrusted to a lesser or greater extent 6 months after placement [2, 6, 9, 15, 19, 27].

Extensive encrustation can lead to difficulties or impossibility in retrieval of the ureteral stent. This is why each case must be assessed individually to propose the method of stent removal depending on the degree of encrustation. Ureteral stents can be removed under local anaesthesia and using the flexible cystoscope in uncomplicated cases with low risk of encrustation. In patients with extensive stent encrustation rate, the removal should be performed under general anaesthesia, using fluoroscopy to monitor the procedure.

4.4 Irritation and Tissue Injury

Long-term stents can alter ureteral tissue vascularisation and cause tissue injury, potentially leading to urinary fistulae and even uretero-arterial fistulae [28]. It should be highlighted that although polyurethane stents combine the flexibility of silicone and the rigidity of polyethylene, they appear to be the least biocompatible devices and are associated with the highest degree of urothelial injury and erosion in animal models. In contrast, silicone stents have been associated with the least ureteral tissue reactions in animal models [18].

4.5 Renal Failure

Recurrent infections, vesicoureteral reflux and encrustation, fragmentation or migration of the ureteral stents are conditions that may finally lead to deterioration of renal function. In some clinical series, up to 18.4% of patients with forgotten stents have been found to have chronic kidney disease at different stages, and up to 5.2% of patients eventually require renal replacement therapy [3].

5 Diagnosis of Forgotten/Encrusted Ureteral Stent

In patients with the signs and symptoms described above, an X-ray of the urinary tract, blood tests and urine culture should be considered initially [29]. Urinary tract X-rays can not only confirm the existence of the stent but also show whether it is encrustated. The degree of encrustation can be more precisely defined by performing an abdominopelvic CT scan without iodine contrast. Grades of stent encrustation are listed in the FECal Ureteral Grading System classification [2, 29]:

- Grade 1: minimal linear encrustation at one of the two J-ends of the stent.
- Grade 2: Circular encrustation totally encompassing one of the two J-ends of the stent.

– Grade 3: Circular encrustation totally encompassing either of the two J-ends together with linear encrustation in some segments of the ureteral section of the stent.
– Grade 4: circular encrustation completely encompassing both J-ends of the catheter placement.
– Grade 5: extensive encrustation encompassing both J-ends and the entire ureteral segment of the catheter placement.

This classification makes it possible to standardise the assessment of the extent of encrustation of stents and can guide decision-making on the treatment required [1].

Ultrasonography of the urinary tract is of interest to assess the existence or not of hydronephrosis, which may suggest obstruction and/or encrustation of the stent [29]. Assessment of the proximal end should be done with an empty bladder to avoid artefact due to excessive bladder distension.

Other anatomical-functional studies such as intravenous urography or CT urography can complete the evaluation of patients with forgotten ureteral stents. If the loss of renal function is severe, these studies may not be performed. For the assessment of the degree of functionality of both renal units, the isotopic renogram is of interest, mainly for individualised therapeutic options [12] (Figs. 1, 2, 3 and 4).

Fig. 1 Urinary tract X ray. Patient with 5 level FeCal score

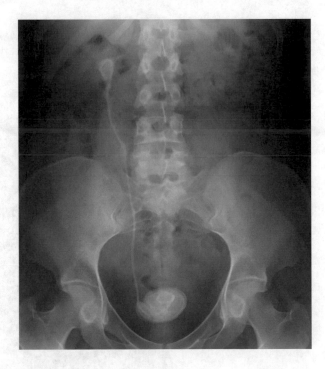

Fig. 2 Urinary tract CT. Patient with 5 level FeCal score

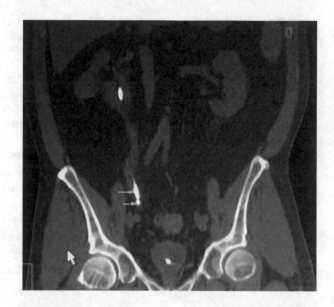

Fig. 3 Excretory urography. Ureteral stent encrustation

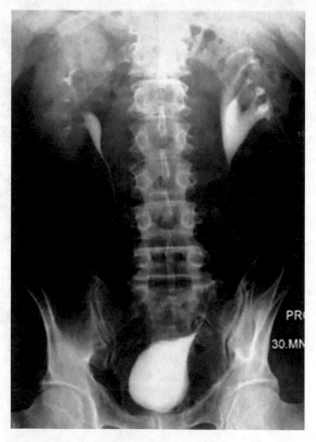

Fig. 4 CT Urography.
Ureteral stent encrustation

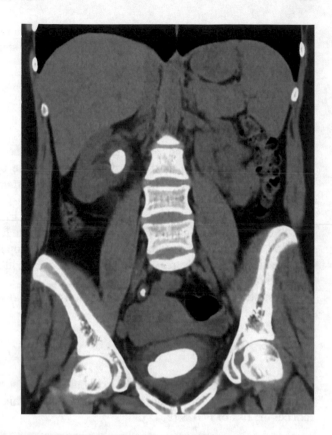

6 Preventive Strategies for Forgotten Ureteral Stent

The development of protocols to reduce unnecessary JJ ureteral stent placement and minimise dwell time is the first step in preventing the occurrence of FUSS.

Additional strategies in the same direction include patient follow-up and education as well as the development of new materials that may prevent or delay the development of complications.

6.1 Health Education

Healthcare professionals are responsible for establishing the follow-up of patients with ureteral stents, and for determining the length of time placement according to the type of stent. Before discharge from hospital, the patient should be adequately educated about his or her condition [19, 27].

It is essential to inform and convey the importance of stent placement time to the patient so that he/she is involved in the removal planning process [16].

Patients who move between regions or countries are a major concern and should be informed of the implications of not withdrawing the stent placement in a timely manner [10].

6.2 Surveillance and Monitoring Systems

Its purpose is to remove the catheter placement within the required timeframe.

Notebooks and paper card recording, in which the operator records patient details on paper. It has proven to be an unreliable system, with a failure rate of 22.4% [25].

Computerised tracking: Several computerised registries have been developed and implemented showing significant improvement in the follow-up of patients with ureteral catheters. The computerised tracking system proposed by Ather et al. demonstrated a significant decrease in the incidence of forgotten catheters from 12.5% to 1.2% after the first year of its application [25].

Registration using new software applications is developed below.

6.3 Simple Removal System

In uncomplicated cases, stents can be externalised by attaching them to the bladder catheter after procedures such as ureterorenoscopy. This facilitates removal and reduces the risk of FUUS [9, 19].

6.4 Innovation in Stents

Development of biodegradable stents, which dissolve after a predictable time (14–28 days from insertion), leaving no fragments that could cause obstruction (polyglycolic acid and glycomer 631). This would eliminate the need for stent withdrawal [9, 25, 30, 31]. However, there is currently non-evidence on their use as results are only available from animal studies [18].

6.4.1 Use of Stents with Coatings of Different Materials

- Glycosaminoglycans, heparin or silver reduce or prevent stent biofilm formation [9, 18, 25].
- PDMMA (dimethylacrylamide) polyhydrogel, triclosan, polyacrylonitrile or antiseptics such as chlorhexidine: reduce biofilm formation and catheter-associated UTIs [9].

6.4.2 Anti-reflux Stents [17, 30, 32]

- Stent with a very thin distal end, thinner than the rest of the stent. This allows minimal interference at the ureterovesical junction.
- Traditional ureteral stent placement with a valve attached to the distal end, which functions as an anti-reflux valve.
- Intraureteral stent placement that does not cross the ureteral orifice and therefore does not generate vesicoureteral reflux.
- Stents in which the distal pigtail is replaced by a 0.3Fr thread suture.

6.4.3 Use of New Technologies in the Prevention of Forgotten Ureteral Stent Syndrome

The main drawback of traditional ureteral catheter patient follow-up strategies (paper card registry, electronic registry) is that the information is only available at the centre where the registration takes place. In addition, this register requires infrastructure and personnel to perform enrolment and follow-up [33].

To overcome this shortcoming, the Ureteral Stent Tracker™ (UST) has been developed (P Visible Health, Inc., in partnership with Boston Scientific). It is a mobile application to track patients with ureteral catheters [34].

A unique profile with name and registration number is created for each patient. Within the profile, the date of insertion, laterality, expected removal date, and confirmed date of removal are included. Care plans are visually coded to allow easy identification of patients with catheters that have exceeded their planned removal date. This information is also sent as a weekly email reminder to all involved healthcare professionals [34].

Comparing the effectiveness and usefulness of the app with the classical card-based appointment system to prevent FUSS, it was concluded that patients followed up via the mobile app had fewer delays and losses to follow-up [35].

Unlike paper-based systems, computer tracking has improved data entry, rapid search capability, and access from multiple sites [34].

7 Conclusions

The growing importance of the use of double j ureteral stents for several indications makes the FUSS a complication with a not insignificant frequency. The properties of urine and the presence of bacteria can promote catheter encrustation. This can result in a highly variable range of signs and symptoms. Patients may have no clinical presentation or may have severe urinary tract infections and/or renal failure.

New biomaterials for stent manufacture and coatings should reduce the main complications associated with this syndrome are currently under development. New technologies aimed at planning and remembering stent removal or replacement could dramatically reduce the incidence of this syndrome.

References

1. Lin TF, Lin WR, Chen M, Yang TY, Hsu JM, Chiu AW. The risk factors and complications of forgotten double-J stents: a single-center experience. J Chin Med Assoc. 2019;82(10):767–71.
2. Ulker V, Celik O. Endoscopic, single-session management of encrusted, forgotten ureteral stents. Medicina (Kaunas). 2019;55(3):58.
3. Murtaza B, Alvi S. Forgotten ureteral stents: an avoidable morbidity. J Coll Physicians Surg Pak. 2016;26(3):208–12.
4. El-Faqih AB, Shamsuddin A, Chakrabarti R, Atassi AH, Kardar MK, Osman IH. Polyurethane internal ureteral stents in treatment of stone patients: morbidity related to indwelling times. J Urol. 1991;146(6):1487–91.
5. Bultitude MF, Tiptaft RC, Glass JM, Dasgupta P. Management of encrusted ureteral stents impacted in upper tract. Urology. 2003;62(4):622–6.
6. Goel H, Kundu A, Maji T, Pal D. Retained fragmented double J ureteric stent: a report of four cases with review of the literature. Saudi J Kidney Dis Transpl. 2015;26(4):747.
7. Kawahara T, Ito H, Terao H, Yoshida M, Matsuzaki J. Ureteral stent encrustation, incrustation, and coloring: morbidity related to indwelling times. J Endourol. 2012;26(2):178–82.
8. Kawahara T, Ishida H, Kubota Y, Matsuzaki J. Ureteroscopic removal of forgotten ureteral stent. BMJ Case Rep. 2012;1:2–4.
9. Vanderbrink BA, Rastinehad AR, Ost MC, Smith AD. Encrusted urinary stents: evaluation and endourologic management. J Endourol. 2008;22(5):905–12.
10. Lawrentschuk N, Russell JM. Ureteric stenting 25 years on: routine or risky? ANZ J Surg. 2004;74(4):243–7.
11. Kram W, Buchholz NNP, Hakenberg OW. Ureteral stent encrustation. Pathophysiology. Arch Esp Urol. 2016;69(8):485–93.
12. Singh I, Gupta NP, Hemal AK, Aron M, Seth A, Dogra PN. Severely encrusted polyurethane ureteral stents: management and analysis of potential risk factors. Urology. 2001;58(4):526–31.
13. Thomas R. Indwelling ureteral stents: impact of material and shape on patient comfort. J Endourol. 1993;7(2):137–40.
14. Burgos Revilla FJ, Sáez Garrido JC, Vallejo Herrador J, Lovaco Castellano F, del Hoyo Campos J. Comportamiento hidrodinámico de los catéteres endourológicos. Arch Esp Urol. 1995:627–36.
15. Legrand F, Saussez T, Ruffion A, Celia A, Djouhri F, Musi G, Kalakech S, Desriac I, Roumeguère T. Double loop ureteral stent encrustation according to indwelling time: results of a European Multicentric Study. J Endourol. 2021;35(1):84–90.
16. Murtaza B, Niaz WA, Akmal M, Ahmad H, Mahmood A. A rare complication of forgotten ureteral stent. J Coll Physicians Surg Pak. 2011;21(3):190–2.
17. Fishman JR, Presto AJ. The forgotten ureteral stent. West J Med. 1994;160(6):569–70.
18. Beysens M, Tailly TO. Ureteral stents in urolithiasis. Asian J Urol. 2018;5(4):274–86. https://doi.org/10.1016/j.ajur.2018.07.002.
19. Neto ACL. Forgotten double-J ureteral stent. Int Braz J Urol. 2019;45(6):1087–9.
20. Garrido Abad P, Fernández Arjona M, Fernández González I, Santos Arrontes D, Pereira Sanz I. Migración proximal de catéter doble J: presentación de un caso y revisión de la literatura. Arch Esp Urol. 2008;3:428–31.
21. Lange D, Bidnur S, Hoag N, Chew BH. Ureteral stent-associated complications-where we are and where we are going. Nat Rev Urol. 2015;12(1):17–25. https://doi.org/10.1038/nrurol.2014.340.

22. Mahmood SN, Toffeq HM, Hussen M, Karim A, Jamal C, Said AA, et al. Endourologic management of a 15-year-old neglected, fragmented, and encrusted ureteral stent. J Endourol Case Rep. 2018;4(1):201–4.
23. De Grazia A, Somani BK, Soria F, Carugo D, Mosayyebi A. Latest advancements in ureteral stent technology. Transl Androl Urol. 2019;8(1):S436–41.
24. Brotherhood H, Lange D, Chew BH. Advances in ureteral stents. Transl Androl Urol. 2014;3(3):314–9.
25. Veltman Y, Shields JM, Ciancio G, Bird VG. Percutaneous nephrolithotomy and cystolithalapaxy for a "forgotten" stent in a transplant kidney: case report and literature review. Clin Transpl. 2010;24(1):112–7.
26. Lasaponara F, Dalmasso E, Santià S, Sedigh O, Bosio A, Pasquale G, et al. A 8-year-forgotten ureteral stent after kidney transplantation: treatment and long-term follow-up. Urologia. 2013;80(1):80–2.
27. Adanur S, Ozkaya F. Challenges in treatment and diagnosis of forgotten/encrusted double-J ureteral stents: the largest single-center experience. Ren Fail. 2016;38(6):920–6.
28. Moghul M, Almpanis S. Stent cards: a simple solution for forgotten stents? BMJ Open Qual. 2019;8(2):2018–9.
29. Barreiro DM, Losada JB, Montiel FC, Lafos N. Urinary incontinence and urosepsis due to forgotten ureteral stent. Urol Case Rep. 2016;8:63–5. https://doi.org/10.1016/j.eucr.2016.07.004.
30. Soria F, De La Cruz JE, Morcillo E, Rioja J, Sánchez-Margallo FM. Catéteres ureterales antirreflujo. Arch Esp Urol. 2016;69(8):544–52.
31. Chew BH, Paterson RF, Clinkscales KW, Levine BS, Shalaby SW, Lange D. In vivo evaluation of the third generation biodegradable stent: a novel approach to avoiding the forgotten stent syndrome. J Urol. 2013;189(2):719–25. https://doi.org/10.1016/j.juro.2012.08.202.
32. Vogt B, Desfemmes FN, Desgrippes A, Ponsot Y. MiniJFil®: a new safe and effective stent for well-tolerated repeated extracorporeal shockwave lithotripsy or ureteroscopy for medium-to-large kidney stones? Nephrourol Mon. 2016;8(5):4–10.
33. Ziemba JB, Ludwig WW, Ruiz L, Carvalhal E, Matlaga BR. Preventing the forgotten ureteral stent by using a mobile point-of-care application. J Endourol. 2017;31(7):719–24.
34. Lynch MF, Ghani KR, Frost I, Anson KM. Preventing the forgotten ureteral stent: implementation of a web-based stent registry with automatic recall application. Urology. 2007;70(3):423–6.
35. Ulker V, Atalay HA, Cakmak O, Yucel C, Celik O, Kozacioglu Z. Smartphone-based stent tracking application for prevention of forgotten ureteral double-J stents: a prospective study. Int Braz J Urol. 2019;45(2):376–83.

Endourological Management of Encrusted Ureteral Stents

Patrick Jones, Amelia Pietropaolo, and Bhaskar K. Somani

1 Introduction

Ureteral stents are a minimally invasive method to secure urinary drainage from the upper urinary tract(s). Since the first description of the double 'pigtail' stent in 1978 by Finney et al., they have become established as a fundamental part of the endourologist's toolkit [1]. Indeed, valuation for the global stent market is estimated to exceed $560 million by 2026 [2]. Despite an evolution in stent technology which has seen a plethora of developments related to material, design and surface coating, a number of limitations persist [3]. This includes complications such as bleeding, pain and bothersome urinary symptoms. Up to 80% of patients experience negative effect on their quality of life [4]. Stent encrustation (SE) is a further possible adverse sequela, which occurs as a result of crystal deposition (Fig. 1) [5, 6]. These crystals form due a change in the pH of the urine due to bacterial activity e.g. *Proteus mirabilis*. The latter are associated with urease production and therefore accumulation of ammonia resulting in a pH rise accordingly [7, 8]. A degree of SE is reported to occur in up to 47% of patients according to some studies [9, 10]. In severe cases, SE renders standard cystoscopic removal impossible. Management of such cases can be a complex problem, which requires a step wise approach to ensure safe removal and secure the best possible outcome for the patient [11].

P. Jones · A. Pietropaolo · B. K. Somani (✉)
Department of Urology, University Hospital Southampton NHS Foundation Trust,
Southampton, UK
e-mail: b.k.somani@soton.ac.uk

Fig. 1 Encrusted stent
removed from patient

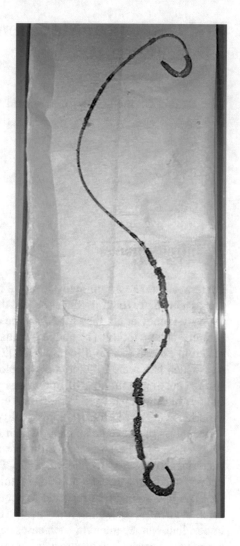

Left undiagnosed and or untreated, SE that occurs both intra and extra luminally, can lead to a host of serious complications including infection (and potentially life-threatening sepsis), stent fracture (Fig. 2), obstruction and deterioration in renal function [12].

Furthermore, over 50% of lawsuits arising from endourological surgery are stent related e.g. lost to follow up or forgotten stents [13]. Given the rise in the prevalence of kidney stone disease (KSD) and the worldwide trend for minimally invasive interventions which often employ ureteral stent insertion, the volume of stent encrustations may also be set to rise [14]. Awareness and understanding of the endourological management is therefore of paramount importance.

Fig. 2 Plain radiograph showing fractured stent at lower end

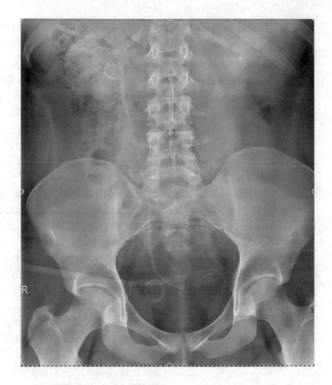

2 Risk Factors

The temporal relationship between stent indwelling time and morbidity is now well recognised [15]. Moreover, stent duration is generally considered the greatest risk factor for SE [5]. The relevance of this is now arguably greater than ever before given the near universal delays in operating as a result of the Covod-19 global pandemic [16, 17]. Many cases of SE may be related to a 'forgotten' stent which Molina et al. found to take place in up to 12% of stent placements. This can be a result of poor patient compliance [18]. Previous studies have revealed the correlation between forgotten stents and socio-economic background as well as lack of health insurance [19]. A history of prior and concurrent KSD predispose the patient to a higher chance of SE. Risk of SE is also heightened further in the context of pregnancy due to metabolic changes such as reduced secretion of parathyroid hormone and the rise in filtered calcium associated with the rise in glomerular filtration rate during pregnancy [2]. Kavoussi et al. found that pregnant women with nephrostomy tubes in situ required exchange as often as every 2 weeks in selected cases due to SE [20]. Malabsorptive states and malignant processes are also catalysts for pro-encrustation. As well as patient factors, the properties of the stent e.g. material and caliber will also play a role. Kawahara et al. found the rate of SE to be significantly lower when ≥7 Fr stents were used [9]. Unfortunately, even newer modifications such as metallic stents are not exempt from SE.

3   Clinical Assessment and Treatment Planning

While the clinical history can highlight the group of patients with greater likelihood of SE, an important pre-operative step is imaging. The first line modality is plain X-Ray (Fig. 3), but a low threshold should be maintained for expediting a computed tomography (CT) scan with a stone protocol applied. This may be selected in the first instance if the person has a history of uric acid stones. Although it holds the advantage of no radiation exposure, the role of ultrasound in the assessment of SE is very limited and is not routinely practiced in most centres.

Imaging can be complemented through use of grading system for SE. The two most commonly used nomograms are Kidney, Ureter, Bladder (KUB) and the Forgotten encrusted, calcified (FECal) Double J classification [12, 21]. These validated tools allow the surgeon to better predict those cases which will warrant multiple procedures, a multi-modal intervention plan e.g. combined endourological approach and those cases with long operative time (e.g. >3 h). It further helps to counsel the patient and manage expectations. More recently, the Visual Grading for Ureteral Encrusted Stent (V-GUES) has been developed [22]. If a patient attends for routine removal of ureteral stent under local anaesthetic (LA) and resistance is encountered, it should be abandoned and an up-to-date imaging organised. Understanding the impact on quality of life caused by the stent is also a valuable

Fig. 3 Plain radiograph showing encrustation at distal coil

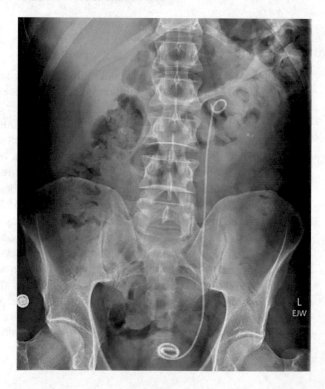

step and this can be assessed using a patient reported outcome measure (PROM) such as the ureteral stent symptom questionnaire (USSQ) [23].

If the CT scan reveals poor condition of the renal parenchyma, consideration for nuclear renal scan should be given. Should this reveal less than 15–20% renal function, a simple nephrectomy may represent an alternate treatment option for that patient [12]. However, if both the parenchymal appearances and renal function are satisfactory, a more minimally invasive treatment can be selected for removal of encrusted stent. It is now standard practice among many endourology centres to have regular stone multidisciplinary team (MDT) to discuss such complex cases. This not only allows for a shared treatment plan to be established but it also facilitates assessment by dietician and referral to metabolic clinic after the initial treatment [24].

Careful review of the patients imaging will allow to determine the severity of SE as well as whether it occupies both the proximal and distal ends of the ureteral stent or the whole length of the stent. Minimal linear encrustation at one end of the ureteral stent could permit standard removal of the stent by cystoscopy. However, if encrustations found are more than this then formal treatment of SE is warranted. Any planned procedure should be accompanied by collection of urine culture and antibiotic sensitivities prior to treatment. It is a further possibility that SE may only be discovered intra-operatively.

Retrospective and prospective studies have described different surgical approaches of stent retrieval related to the location and volume of encrustation.

In some cases, stent encrustation is an unexpected intraoperative finding and the surgeon has no choice than to abandon the procedure and repeat the treatment in after further planning. This allows strategic planning of staged stent removal with appropriate equipment and staff preventing further complications.

Mapping of SE can be done pre-operatively with imaging or can be described by the surgeon intra-operatively. The absence of standardisation in describing the location of encrustation(s) can make management planning and comparison of outcomes very difficult. It therefore highlights the need for dissemination and adoption of classifications systems in order to facilitate surgical planning. Use of a tool to grade severity of SE will also help guide a clinician as to whether they have the necessary expertise for the proposed treatment or whether onward referral to a specialist centre is warranted.

4 Minimally Invasive Approaches

Before the advancements in modern technologies, open surgery remained a go to option for difficult cases. Indeed, its role serves a purpose in less developed countries [5]. However, such is the expanded application of ureteroscopy and percutaneous nephrolithotomy (PCNL), that even highly complex cases of SE can be handled using these minimally invasive interventions. The surgeon must bear in mind the option of using a combined modality approach. At time of patient counselling, it should also be explained that multiple sessions can be warranted.

5   Cystolithotripsy and Cystolitholapaxy

In cases of encrustation to the distal or bladder portion of the stent, cystolithola-paxy using stone punch can be an effective method for fragmentation. If SE is limited to this site only, then it can be sufficient for then grasping and removing the stent. In certain cases, when the encrustation bulk around the distal coil of the stent is too large to be released with the stone punch, an alternative and less inva-sive method is laser cystolithotripsy (Fig. 4). This is particularly effective in cases where the calcification has formed a large bladder stone surrounding the stent. The focused effect of the Holmium laser is able to gradually fragment and dust the encrustation preserving the stent integrity. The technique can be accomplished with 550 μm laser fiber, high energy settings (1–2 J). Use of resectoscope rather than rigid cystoscope can help maintain low pressure bladder irrigation. When all encrustations are released, the stent can be finally removed with normal grasper and all the fragments evacuated with bladder washout. The disadvantages of these methods e.g. cystolithotripsy, is the requirement for general anaesthesia and laser training. Lam et al. carried out an institutional review of their cases and reported that on average 2.7 procedures (range 1–4) are required to clear heavily encrusted stents [25].

Fig. 4 Endoscopic view of encrusted distal coil at time of cystolithotripsy

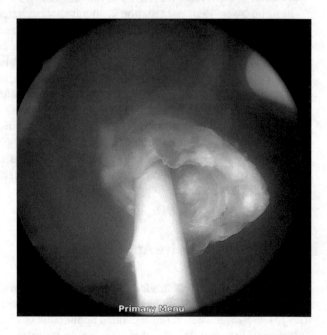

Primary Menu

6 Shockwave Lithotripsy (SWL)

SWL represents a minimally invasive intervention in endourology. While its clinical application for treatment of KSD is far reaching, in the setting of SE, it is more limited. Its role for SE is largely restricted to cases of low volume encrustations. Its application favours cases where the area of encrustation is localised to the proximal, intra-renal portion of the stent [26]. Use of SWL for this scenario is more suitable if in the setting of high volume centre with a fixed lithotripter. It can also be implemented before planned stent removal with grasper. SWL is a preferred modality in those patients with a high anaesthetic risk.

7 Ureteroscopy

Ureteroscopy can allow for use of laser to remove encrustations (recommended fragmentation settings 0.4–0.6 J, 5–20 Hz). This should be performed in standard lithotomy procedure under a general anaesthetic. Intravenous antibiotic prophylaxis should be administered at induction. After placement of a cystoscopically guided safety wire (0.035 in.), the semi-rigid ureteroscope can be inserted parallel to the stent. Holmium laser treatment of encrustation can allow gradual release of the encrustations around the stents in order to create space and proceed retrogradely towards the kidney. In many cases series, rigid and flexible ureteroscopy are described as the definitive treatment to completely remove encrustation with the aid of Holmium laser.

When this is not possible, because of heavy encrustation encasing the stent, it can be divided using the laser and 'piecemeal strategy' of retrograde removal of the stent can be carried out [27]. Cutting the distal portion of the stent with laser allows for creation of more space (recommended cutting settings 1–1.5 J, 5–10 Hz).

Although fluoroless endourological surgery has gained increased attention in the modern era, use of fluoroscopy is still advocated in these complex cases [28]. However, the principle of 'as low as reasonably achievable' (ALARA) should still be upheld [29]. Once sufficient space has been established, the scope can be advanced and a further section of the stent can be cut and removed using grasper or basket in a step wise fashion. This method has also been termed 'coil resection'. In cases where an additional operative session is determined to be required or where no initial entry with the semi rigid ureteroscope is possible, a small calibre stent (e.g. 4.8 Fr) can be inserted in parallel to allow passive dilatation of the ureter and the patient is booked to return at a later date. SWL can also be considered in these cases during the interval period. A smaller sized ureteroscope can also be used where there is limited space to

Fig. 5 Fluoroscopic view
of flexible ureteroscope
and cut proximal loop of
stent

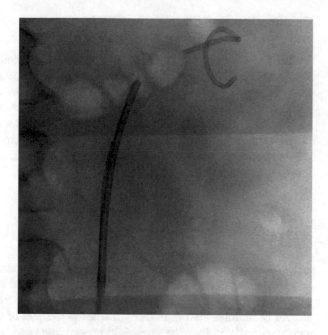

accommodate an instrument alongside the encrusted stent. Where the distal portion of
the stent can be safely withdrawn to the urethral meatus, it can be secured (clamp or
stitch) in order to fix its position and provide gentle traction.

Where proximal encrustation exists, treatment can be carried out using flexible
ureteroscopy. Placement of ureteral access sheath (UAS) can facilitate this process.
The cut proximal loop can then be removed via the UAS and hence reduce trauma
on exit (Fig. 5). Once clearance has been achieved, a new ureteric stent should be
temporarily inserted with a fixed date for removal supplied to the patient before
discharge. Thomas et al. successfully treated over 90% of cases (n = 51) at their
institution with use of ureteroscopy (semi-rigid and/or flexible) alone [30]. The
advantages of newer generations of lasers e.g. high powered 100 W machine lend
themselves well to these cases of heavy encrustation [31]. The introduction of the
Holmium YAG (Ho:YAG) laser has heightened the reach of what can be achieved.
High precision is enabled with reduced tissue trauma as a result [32, 33].

Smaller hospitals should consider a centralised process and onward referral of
these cases for treatment in a high volume centre [34]. Furthermore, patients may
require post-operative admission to high dependency unit (HDU) or intensive care
units (ICU) given potential for septic shower and serious morbidity which could
occur especially in multiple comorbidities [35].

8   Percutaneous Nephrolithotomy (PCNL)

In cases of heavy encrustation within the kidney, a percutaneous approach may be
necessitated. This will allow for antegrade nephroscopy and fragmentation to be
undertaken from above. Due to high stone burden of the renal encrustation around

the proximal coil of the stent, up to 20% of cases warrant PCNL and anterograde approach. Although universal consensus does not exist in regard to the optimal approach when there exists both distal and proximal SE, it is the opinion of the authors as well as most published reports, that the distal portion should be handled and released of SE first [5]. Patients should also be consented for proceeding to a combined antegrade approach at the same anaesthetic if retrograde surgery alone is not sufficient. The procedure can be indeed performed with combined retrograde and anterograde approach in the presence of the correct equipment, positioning and staff in order to grant the best expertise and outcome but also keeping in mind patients' preference and safety.

9 Open Approach

The majority of severely encrusted stents described in the literature can be removed with one endourological procedures or a combination of them. However, when these minimally invasive techniques fail to achieve a full stent clearance, open pyelolithotomy still serves as an option. Nephrectomy with removal of the encrusted stent is considered the last resort, especially in patients where the kidney function has been compromised from prolonged obstruction [5].

10 Encrusted Nephrostomy Tube

This represents another potential clinical scenario. The intra-renal portion can become heavily encrusted or a prolonged period in situ can lead to tissue bridges forming. The same principles of planning and treatment apply for this situation. As well lithotripsy down the established track and ureteroscopic treatment from below, another consideration is to establish an additional percutaneous calyx puncture to treat the large encrustation burden if it is present via a PCNL procedure.

11 Prevention

Patient and surgeon education are arguably the most effective treatment tool [36, 37].

Careful counselling and an ethos of shared responsibility between patient and surgeon is of paramount importance. Implementation of strategies such as stent registries and more recent adjuncts such as novel use of mobile based reminder systems are possible remedies for this widespread problem [38, 39]. Ather et al. implemented a modern software tracking system and this significantly reduced the incidence of overdue stents from 12.5% to 1.2% [40].

Preventative medical management and metabolic treatment can still play a role in encrustation treatment and prevention. Torrecilla et al. performed a randomised trial between urine acidifier and crystallization inhibitor capsules vs placebo in patients with encrusted stents [41]. The outcomes showed decrease of overall encrustation in the experimental arm compared to placebo. It also delivered shorter removal time and higher success rate of stent removal at first attempt, which did not require additional surgical procedures. Medical management can especially be useful for SE related to prior treatment of uric acid stones and acidic urine, where the patients can have urinary alkalinization to dissolve the encrustations [37].

12 Conclusion

The development of SE is multifactorial, and a vigilant approach is required in order to help prevent it and this should be mirrored when treating this clinical problem as well. The evolution of minimally invasive endourology allows for virtually all cases to now be managed successfully without the need for open surgery. A tailored management strategy should be formulated and use of an algorithm such as FECal or V-GUES system is recommended as part of this work up. The need for a multi-modal treatment plan should be considered. Patients should be carefully counselled of additional procedures and made aware that multiple sittings may be warranted.

Conflict of Interests No relevant disclosures.

References

1. Finney RP. Experience with new double J ureteral catheter stent. 1978. J Urol. 2002;167(2 Pt 2):1135–8; discussion 1139. https://doi.org/10.1016/s0022-5347(02)80361-5. PMID: 11905888.
2. Tomer N, Garden E, Small A, Palese M. Ureteral stent encrustation: epidemiology, pathophysiology, management, and current technology. J Urol. 2021;205(1):68–77. https://doi.org/10.1097/JU.0000000000001343.
3. Mosayyebi A, Manes C, Carugo D, Somani BK. Advances in ureteral stent design and materials. Curr Urol Rep. 2018;19(5):35. https://doi.org/10.1007/s11934-018-0779-y. PMID: 29637309; PMCID: PMC5893657.
4. Lingeman JE, Preminger GM, Goldfischer ER, Krambeck AE. Assessing the impact of ureteral stent design on patient comfort. J Urol. 2009;181(6):2581–7. https://doi.org/10.1016/j.juro.2009.02.019.
5. Vanderbrink BA, Rastinehad AR, Ost MC, Smith AD. Encrusted urinary stents: evaluation and endourologic management. J Endourol. 2008;22(5):905–12. https://doi.org/10.1089/end.2006.0382.
6. Aravantionos E, Gravas S, Karatzas AD, Tzortzis V, Melekos M. Forgotten, encrusted ureteral stents: a challenging problem with an endourologic solution. J Endourol. 2006;20:1045–9.

7. Wilks SA, Fader MJ, Keevil CW. Novel insights into the Proteus mirabilis crystalline biofilm using real-time imaging. PLoS One. 2015;10(10):e0141711. https://doi.org/10.1371/journal.pone.0141711.

8. Mosayyebi A, Vijayakumar A, Yue QY, Bres-Niewada E, Manes C, Carugo D, et al. Engineering solutions to ureteral stents: material, coating and design. Cent European J Urol. 2017;70(3):270–4. https://doi.org/10.5173/ceju.2017.1520. Epub 2017 Aug 28. PMID: 29104790; PMCID: PMC5656375.

9. Kawahara T, Ito T, Terao H, Yoshida M, Matsuzaki J. Ureteral stent encrustation, and colouring: morbidity related to indwelling times. J Endourol. 2012;26:178–82.

10. Al-Aown A, Kyriazis I, Kallidonis P. Ureteral stents: new ideas, new designs. Ther Adv Urol. 2010;2(2):85–92.

11. Rana AM, Sabooh A. Management strategies and results for severely encrusted retained ureteral stents. J Endourol. 2007;21(6):628–32. https://doi.org/10.1089/end.2006.0250.

12. Acosta-Miranda AM, Milner J, Turk TM. The FECal double-J: a simplified approach in the management of encrusted and retained ureteral stents. J Endourol. 2009;23:409–15.

13. Duty B, Okhunov Z, Okeke Z, Smith A. Medical malpractice in endourology: analysis of closed cases from the state of New York. J Urol. 2012;187(2):528–32. https://doi.org/10.1016/j.juro.2011.10.045.

14. Geraghty RM, Jones P, Somani BK. Worldwide trends of urinary stone disease treatment over the last two decades: a systematic review. J Endourol. 2017;31(6):547–56. https://doi.org/10.1089/end.2016.0895.

15. Legrand F, Saussez T, Ruffion A, Celia A, Djouhri F, Musi G, et al. Double loop ureteral stent encrustation according to indwelling time: results of a European Multicentric Study. J Endourol. 2021;35(1):84–90. https://doi.org/10.1089/end.2020.0254. Epub 2020 Nov 6. PMID: 32799700.

16. Proietti S, Gaboardi F, Giusti G. Endourological stone management in the era of the COVID-19. Eur Urol. 2020;78(2):131–3. https://doi.org/10.1016/j.eururo.2020.03.042. Epub 2020 Apr 14. PMID: 32303384; PMCID: PMC7195508.

17. Ho HC, Hughes T, Bozlu M, Kadıoğlu A, Somani BK. What do urologists need to know: diagnosis, treatment, and follow-up during COVID-19 pandemic. Turk J Urol. 2020;46(3):169–77. https://doi.org/10.5152/tud.2020.20119. PMID: 32301692; PMCID: PMC7219975.

18. Molina WR, Pessoa R, Donalisio da Silva R, Kenny MC, Gustafson D, Nogueira L, et al. A new patient safety smartphone application for prevention of "forgotten" ureteral stents: results from a clinical pilot study in 194 patients. Patient Saf Surg. 2017;11:10. https://doi.org/10.1186/s13037-017-0123-3. PMID: 28396695; PMCID: PMC5381069.

19. Divakaruni N, Palmer CJ, Tek P, Bjurlin MA, Gage MK, Robinson J, et al. Forgotten ureteral stents: who's at risk? J Endourol. 2013;27(8):1051–4. https://doi.org/10.1089/end.2012.0754. Epub 2013 Jul 13. PMID: 23590526.

20. Kavoussi LR, Albala DM, Basler JW, Apte S, Clayman RV. Percutaneous management of urolithiasis during pregnancy. J Urol. 1992;148(3 Pt 2):1069–71. https://doi.org/10.1016/s0022-5347(17)36820-9.

21. Arenas JL, Shen JK, Keheila M, Abourbih SR, Lee A, Stokes PK, et al. Kidney, ureter, and bladder (KUB): a novel grading system for encrusted ureteral stents. Urology. 2016;97:51–5. https://doi.org/10.1016/j.urology.2016.06.050. Epub 2016 Jul 12. PMID: 27421780.

22. Manzo BO, Alarcon P, Lozada E, Ojeda J, Morales C, Gökce MI, et al. A novel visual grading for ureteral encrusted stent classification to help decide the endourologic treatment. J Endourol. 2021;35(9):1314–9. https://doi.org/10.1089/end.2020.1225. Epub 2021 Aug 13. PMID: 33730863.

23. Mehmi A, Jones P, Somani BK. Current status and role of patient-reported outcome measures (PROMs) in endourology. Urology. 2021;148:26–31. https://doi.org/10.1016/j.urology.2020.09.022. Epub 2020 Sep 28. PMID: 32991909.

24. Hughes T, Pietropaolo A, Archer M, Davis T, Tear L, Somani BK. Lessons learnt (clinical outcomes and cost savings) from virtual stone clinic and their application in the era post-COVID-19: prospective outcomes over a 6-year period from a university teaching hospital. J Endourol. 2021;35(2):200–5. https://doi.org/10.1089/end.2020.0708. Epub 2020 Aug 14. PMID: 32731751.
25. Lam JS, Gupta M. Tips and tricks for the management of retained ureteral stents. J Endourol. 2002;16(10):733–41. https://doi.org/10.1089/08927790260472881. PMID: 12542876.
26. Bultitude MF, Tiptaft RC, Glass JM, Dasgupta P. Management of encrusted ureteral stents impacted in upper tract. Urology. 2003;62(4):622–6. https://doi.org/10.1016/s0090-4295(03)00506-5. PMID: 14550429.
27. Pietropaolo A, Whitehurst L, Somani BK. Piecemeal retrograde removal of encrusted and encased stuck ureteral stent: video tips and tricks. Videourology. 2020; https://doi.org/10.1089/vid.2019.0057.
28. Emiliani E, Kanashiro A, Chi T, Pérez-Fentes DA, Manzo BO, Angerri O, et al. Fluoroless endourological surgery for stone disease: a review of the literature-tips and tricks. Curr Urol Rep. 2020;21(7):27. https://doi.org/10.1007/s11934-020-00979-y. PMID: 32444987.
29. Cabrera F, Preminger GM, Lipkin ME. As low as reasonably achievable: methods for reducing radiation exposure during the management of renal and ureteral stones. Indian J Urol. 2014;30(1):55–9. https://doi.org/10.4103/0970-1591.124208. PMID: 24497684; PMCID: PMC3897055.
30. Thomas A, Cloutier J, Villa L, Letendre J, Ploumidis A, Traxer O. Prospective analysis of a complete retrograde ureteroscopic technique with holmium laser stent cutting for management of encrusted ureteral stents. J Endourol. 2017;31:476–81.
31. Pietropaolo A, Jones P, Whitehurst L, Somani BK. Role of 'dusting and pop-dusting' using a high-powered (100 W) laser machine in the treatment of large stones (≥ 15 mm): prospective outcomes over 16 months. Urolithiasis. 2019;47(4):391–4. https://doi.org/10.1007/s00240-018-1076-4. Epub 2018 Aug 21. PMID: 30132276; PMCID: PMC6647176.
32. Kronenberg P, Somani B. Advances in lasers for the treatment of stones-a systematic review. Curr Urol Rep. 2018;19(6):45. https://doi.org/10.1007/s11934-018-0807-y. PMID: 29774438; PMCID: PMC5958148.
33. Bhanot R, Jones P, Somani B. Minimally invasive surgery for the treatment of ureteric stones—state-of-the-art review. Res Rep Urol. 2021;13:227–36. https://doi.org/10.2147/RRU.S311010. PMID: 33987110; PMCID: PMC8110280.
34. Vajpeyi V, Chipde S, Khan FA, Parashar S. Forgotten double-J stent: experience of a tertiary care center. Urol Ann. 2020;12(2):138–43. https://doi.org/10.4103/UA.UA_73_19.
35. Whitehurst L, Jones P, Somani BK. Mortality from kidney stone disease (KSD) as reported in the literature over the last two decades: a systematic review. World J Urol. 2019;37(5):759–76. https://doi.org/10.1007/s00345-018-2424-2.
36. Ramachandra M, Mosayyebi A, Carugo D, Somani BK. Strategies to improve patient outcomes and QOL: current complications of the design and placements of ureteric stents. Res Rep Urol. 2020;12:303–14. https://doi.org/10.2147/RRU.S233981. PMID: 32802807; PMCID: PMC7403435.
37. De Grazia A, Somani BK, Soria F, Carugo D, Mosayyebi A. Latest advancements in ureteral stent technology. Transl Androl Urol. 2019;8(Suppl 4):S436–41. https://doi.org/10.21037/tau.2019.08.16. PMID: 31656749; PMCID: PMC6790420.
38. Chen MY, Skewes J, Woodruff MA, Rukin NJ. Using bespoke 3D-printed models to improve patient understanding of an encrusted ureteric stent. J Clin Urol. 2019;14(2):137–9. https://doi.org/10.1177/2051415819876514.
39. Tang VC, Gillooly J, Lee EW, Charig CR. Ureteric stent card register—a 5-year retrospective analysis. Ann R Coll Surg Engl. 2008;90(2):156–9. https://doi.org/10.1308/003588408X242123. PMID: 18325220; PMCID: PMC2443315.

40. Ather MH, Talati J, Biyabani R. Physician responsibility for removal of implants: the case for a computerized program for tracking overdue double-J stents. Tech Urol. 2000;6(3):189–92. PMID: 10963484.
41. Torrecilla C, Fernández-Concha J, Cansino JR, Mainez JA, Amón JH, Costas S, et al. Reduction of ureteral stent encrustation by modulating the urine pH and inhibiting the crystal film with a new oral composition: a multicenter, placebo controlled, double blind, randomized clinical trial. BMC Urol. 2020;20(1):65. https://doi.org/10.1186/s12894-020-00633-2. PMID: 32503502; PMCID: PMC7275439.

Pediatric Ureteral Stents

Tariq Abbas, Tarek Ibrahim, Mohamed AbdelKareem, and Mansour Ali

1 Introduction

Ureteral stents are considered of the significant revaluations in endourological practice and have become an integral part of the contemporary urologic practice. The widespread utilization of ureteric stents in children has lagged behind that in adults because of difficulties encountered for design and sizes optimization manufacturing. However, ureteral stents are considered essential tools in the management of several pediatric urological conditions ranging from, but not limited to, ureteropelvic junction obstruction (UPJO), calculi, and ureteric obstruction [1].

2 Classification of Stents

There are different indications for ureteral stents insertion, and accordingly, there is no one ideal stent. Efforts are made to provide the highest stents quality and reduce potential complications (Table 1).

T. Abbas (✉)
Urology Division, Surgery Department, Sidra Medicine, Doha, Qatar

College of Medicine, Qatar University, Doha, Qatar

Weill Cornell Medical College-Qatar, Doha, Qatar

T. Ibrahim · M. AbdelKareem
Department of Urology, Hamad Medical Corporation, Doha, Qatar
e-mail: Mabdelkareem@hamad.qa

M. Ali
Urology Division, Surgery Department, Sidra Medicine, Doha, Qatar
e-mail: Mali2@sidra.org

© The Author(s) 2022
F. Soria et al. (eds.), *Urinary Stents*,
https://doi.org/10.1007/978-3-031-04484-7_12

Table 1 Characteristics of the ideal urinary stent

- Stiff to be inserted easily, flexible with tapering to avoid injury during insertion
- Maintaining coil strength to reduce migration
- Maintaining patency and urine flow
- Softer after insertion, when exposed to urine or kept within body temperature
- Tolerated well by the patients without causing irritation or discomfort
- Causes the least mucosal irritation by being inert, having a smooth surface and a surface coating with the least coefficient of friction
- Coated by a substance that prevents encrustation and reduces the possibility of infection
- Cost efficient
- Matching the durability according to the indication and easily removed or dissolvable

Table 2 Different design patterns, materials, and features of ureteric stents

	Type of stent	Advantage	Further readings
Upper coil design	Open end	Standard open end for maximal drainage	
	Closed end	Less reflux and pain	
	Flexible coil length	No need for length calculation	
Lower coil design	Tail stents	Thin strips instead of bladder loop to reduce bladder friction and cause less bladder irritation	No significant difference [2]
	Dual Durometer	Easy insertion due to the proximal part and softer bladder coil to cause less bladder irritation	No significant difference [2]
	Magnetic tip	Easier stent removal [3]	
Shaft	Rounded smooth	Standard. Used routinely in most cases	
	Grooved	Enhance passage of stone fragments	
	Spiral	Maintain patency with external compression [4]	In vivo study, no significant difference [5]
	Self-expandable Mesh stent	To increase flow, reduce reflux	The animal study did not show a significant difference [6]
	Endopyelotomy stent	Smooth transition from 14 Fr at the renal coil to 7 Fr taper at the bladder coil	
Material	Metallic	Resist blockage by external compression	[7]
	Polyurethane	Easy insertion, better drainage	
	Silicone	Less bladder irritation, resist encrustation	
Coating	PTFE	Easy insertion, low friction reduces bacterial colonization	
	PC/PVP	Hydrophilic ease insertion, less encrustation and bacterial biofilm formation	
	Antibiotic/ triclosan/silver	Reduces bacterial colonization and growth	
	Heparin	Less encrustation and bacterial biofilm formation	

The ureteral stents design comprises three significant parts; renal coil, shaft, and bladder coil (Table 2). A string may be attached to the lower end to facilitate stent removal without an additional procedure. The stent circumference ranges, and the

Table 3 Different indications of ureteral stents insertion

• Intraluminal ureteral obstruction (e.g., stones, clots, tumor)
• Intramural obstruction (e.g., UPJO)
• Extramural obstruction (e.g., tumor, aberrant artery causing UPJO, retrocaval ureter)
• Post endoscopic surgery in ureteral orifice edema
• Ureteral or renal pelvis iatrogenic injury, and residual stones
• Post ureteral anastomosis and re-implantation
• Prior to extensive pelvic procedures to avoid ureteral injury
• Prior to external shockwave lithotripsy to avoid steinstrasse
• Prior to retrograde intrarenal surgery, if a tight ureter
• Ureteral and renal pelvicalyceal injury

length varies. Stents function by allowing urine flow within the stent lumen and alongside the ureteral lumen. Some different materials and designs will be discussed later in this chapter.

3 Indications of Upper Tract Drainage

The indications for stent usage in the pediatric age group are almost similar to that in adults, including relieve of obstruction that might be intrinsic or extrinsic causes, following ureteroscopy, especially complicated one, post reconstructive procedure for both upper and lower urinary tract and before shockwave lithotripsy. The most common encounters for insertion of ureteric stents in children are UPJO, calculi, and ureteric obstruction (Table 3). The double-J ureteric stent has been described to permit for efficient, reversible internalized drainage of children with primary non-refluxing megaureter (PNRM) [8].

4 Techniques of Ureteral Stenting

4.1 Insertion Approach

Ureteral stents can be inserted either retrogradely through the urethra or antegradely through a percutaneous tract. In children, retrograde double-J stenting seems more reliable and safer than antegrade stenting [9, 10] with greater success and lower complication rates [11, 12].

4.2 Retrograde Stenting

It is performed in a lithotomy position. Initially, starting by cystoscopy and localizing the ureteric orifice, which is then cannulated with a guidewire and open-ended ureteral catheter. A retrograde pyelogram can be obtained to examine the pelvicalyceal system and the stone. Replacement of a stiff bodied wired guidewire through the ureteral catheter and removal of the catheter. The self-retaining stent is then slide over the guidewire through the ureter under vision via a cystoscope sheath and fluoroscopy. Marks guide this along the stent that demarcates the ureteral length.

4.3   Antegrade Stenting

The guidewire is passed from the kidney through the ureter to the bladder under fluoroscopic guidance through the pre-formed percutaneous nephrostomy tract. Then, the stent is slide over the guidewire and checked its position by fluoroscopy.

5   Calculation of Stent Length

The selection of stent length is of high importance as it is needed to balance the risk between stent migration in case of using short stent versus stent irritation and stent-related pain that occurs with longer stents [13]. There are different methods to choose the most optimum length. This has been attempted by measuring the ureteral length from the UPJ to the ureteral orifice using a scaled ureteral catheter while performing pyelography [14]. Similarly, this has been tackled by measuring the length between two points; (from the center of the renal pelvis to the symphysis pubis in IVU or KUB X-ray [15]. CT scan can be utilized for the measurement by multiplying the number of slices by the interval cut the thickness of slices in the area between the renal veins to the vesicoureteric junction. A formula (stent length = age in years +10) has been introduced as a reproducible manner to predict JJ stent length irrespective of laterality or gender.

Concerning the management of ureteral stent implantation, antibiotic therapy appears to be essential to prevent infection [16], which can have rates as high as 28%.

6   The Current Problems and Limitations

The indwelling nature of ureteric stents is complicated by several unwanted effects including a feeling of pain, irritative voiding symptoms, and/or urinary tract infection (UTI). There are several potential complications in the currently utilized urinary catheters in general and ureteric stents in particular (Table 4).

Table 4 Potential early and late complications of ureteral stents insertion

Complications of the procedure	Potential post-procedural complications
• Infection	• Pain; renal, suprapubic, or groin
• Renal pelvis, ureteral, and bladder injury ranging from mucosal erosion, submucosal false passage to perforation	• Urinary symptoms; dysuria, hematuria, increased urinary frequency, nocturia, urgency, incontinence, sense of incomplete bladder emptying
• Extravasation of contrast	• Stent migration
• Stent dislodgment	• Stent encrustation
• Failure to insert the stent	• Stent fracture
	• Stent occlusion externally by tumor compression or internally by blood clots or encrustation
	• Forgotten stents

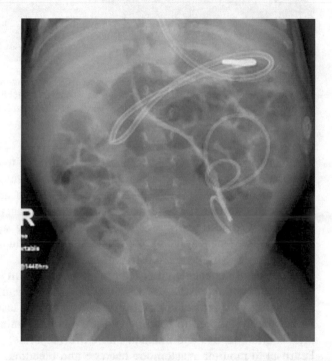

Fig. 1 Abdominal X-ray of 3 months old infant with migrated left JJ stent inserted post left open pyeloplasty

The straight catheters are used to migrate downwards towards the bladder or upwards towards the kidneys. Finney was the first to introduce indwelling ureteral stents with a double J pigtail design, each pigtail coils at one end of the stent [17]. This design reduced migration and is still used nowadays. Complications encountered include upward migration in 3.3%, slipping in 4.2% (Fig. 1). High urinary tract infection with the presence of stents and catheters as considered being foreign bodies.

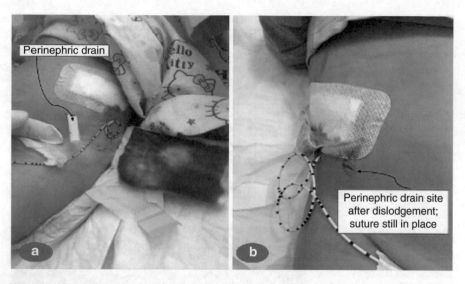

Fig. 2 (**a**) Showing the gauze on top of the perinephric drain soaked with urine and blood with no accurate measurement and bothering both the baby and the parents. (**b**) Dislodegement of the perinephric drain with the first 24 h of surgery while the stitch is still in place

Complications encountered include febrile urinary tract infections in 10.8%, bacteriuria in 27.7% [18]. A recent prospective, randomized, controlled was conducted to investigate the effectiveness of continuous antibiotic prophylaxis in patients with JJ stent. The incidence of febrile urinary tract infections with CAP was significantly reduced [3.8% vs. 19% (p 0.015)]. A long stent with an extra length within the bladder cavity causes more irritation [19]. Stent irritation symptoms were found to be more if the stent crossed the midline [20].

A frequently encountered problem is the unreliability of post-operative contrast studies in the presence of the stent. This often occurs because of the inability to selectively control contrast opacification in the urinary tract that needs to be accurately tailored to each patient's situation. Drainage of the perinephric area is often needed and mandates an extra (separate) perinephric drain (e.g., Penrose) to monitor anastomotic leakage and bleeding. This has the drawback of extra wounds and scar and discomfort at the time of removal, which is the bedside (Fig. 2).

Traditional perinephric drains lack the efficacy draining of localized or small perinephric collections and are vulnerable to dislodgement. We have introduced a double-lumen externalized ureteral stent that can drain both the urinary tract and the perinephric space and better control the area of interest during contrast studies [21] (Fig. 3).

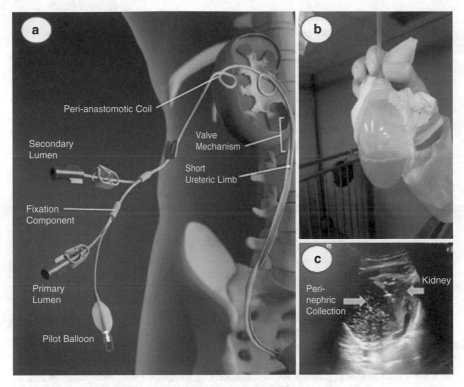

Fig. 3 (**a**) The stent is implanted in situ in a human. (**b**) Fluid collection. (**c**) US with perinephric collection demonstrated. (With permission (CC-BY) from [21])

7   Future Directions

Ureteral stents are encountering technological advancements to overcome the problems faced upon placement. Attempts to modify the traditional tube design have included changing the shape of the stent's ends even further to inhibit migration. Moreover, integrating an antibacterial component will ultimately decrease the associated high risk of acquired urinary tract infections.

Other attempts have involved replacing the bladder end of the stent with highly flexible strands or loops to reduce the stent's size in the bladder end to decrease the discomfort felt by a patient. In these designs, the stent may resemble a traditional tubular stent starting at the renal end and progressing for a significant distance, e.g., about 12 cm, or such a distance to start the flexible strands or loops about the iliac vessels of the patient. This significant distance was employed to prevent the migration of the stent further. Stents of this type suffer from the problem that stents of multiple sizes must be created, and then a physician must select what size stent to use based on approximations of the patient's physiology. In addition, even with the reduced size of the strands or loops, significant patient discomfort may result [22]. Efforts are undergoing to reduce current problems related to ureteral stents placement. Specifically, for the pediatric population, an additional procedure is needed to remove the stent under general anesthesia. Magnetic tip stents were introduced to facilitate the removal without the need for another anesthesia [23, 24].

Recently, biodegradable stents are being evaluated that would typically degrade from 15 to 30 days [25]. A mixture of materials was tried to gain maximum efficiency and the least complications. The mixture allowed the stent's gradual degradation so that the stents would dissolve from inside out and the body followed by the pigtails. This guarantees better stent stability without migration and keeps integrity till full resorption [26]. A novel design was recently introduced with an antireflux mechanism [27]. Likewise, coating materials would further improve the characteristics of stents and drug-eluting coating of biodegradable stents would widen the range of usage and reduce complications [28]. Antibacterial and anti-inflammatory coatings would reduce stents infection and irritation.

References

1. Dyer RB, Chen MY, Zagoria RJ, Regan JD, Hood CG, Kavanagh PV. Complications of ureteral stent placement. Radiographics. 2002;22:1005–22. https://doi.org/10.1148/radiographics.22.5 .g02se081005.
2. Davenport K, Kumar V, Collins J, Melotti R, Timoney AG, Keeley FX. New ureteral stent design does not improve patient quality of life: a randomized, controlled trial. J Urol. 2011;185:175–8. https://doi.org/10.1016/j.juro.2010.08.089.
3. Taylor WN, McDougall IT. Minimally invasive ureteral stent retrieval. J Urol. 2002;168:2020–3. https://doi.org/10.1097/01.ju.0000033964.15384.e2.
4. Stoller ML, Schwartz BF, Frigstad JR, Norris L, Park JB, Magliochetti MJ. An in vitro assessment of the flow characteristics of spiral-ridged and smooth-walled JJ ureteric stents. BJU Int. 2000;85:628–31. https://doi.org/10.1046/j.1464-410x.2000.00489.x.
5. Mucksavage P, Pick D, Haydel D, Etafy M, Kerbl DC, Lee JY, et al. An in vivo evaluation of a novel spiral cut flexible ureteral stent. Urology. 2012;79:733–7. https://doi.org/10.1016/j. urology.2011.10.062.
6. Olweny EO, Portis AJ, Sundaram CP, Afane JS, Humphrey PA, Ewers R, et al. Evaluation of a chronic indwelling prototype mesh ureteral stent in a porcine model. Urology. 2000;56:857–62. https://doi.org/10.1016/s0090-4295(00)00734-2.
7. Wah TM, Irving HC, Cartledge J. Initial experience with the resonance metallic stent for antegrade ureteric stenting. Cardiovasc Intervent Radiol. 2007;30:705–10. https://doi.org/10.1007/ s00270-007-9043-4.
8. Castagnetti M, Cimador M, Sergio M, De Grazia E. Double-J stent insertion across vesicoureteral junction—is it a valuable initial approach in neonates and infants with severe primary nonrefluxing megaureter? Urology. 2006;68:870–5. https://doi.org/10.1016/j.urology.2006.05.052.

9. Resorlu B, Sancak EB, Resorlu M, Gulpinar MT, Adam G, Akbas A, et al. Retrograde intrarenal surgery in pediatric patients. World J Nephrol. 2014;3:193–7. https://doi.org/10.5527/wjn.v3.i4.193.

10. Babu R, Arora A, Raj N. Stenting antegrade via veress needle during laparoscopic PyeloplastY ("SAVVY" Technique). J Indian Assoc Pediatr Surg. 2019;24:117–9. https://doi.org/10.4103/jiaps.JIAPS_38_18.

11. Chandrasekharam VVSS. Is retrograde stenting more reliable than antegrade stenting for pyeloplasty in infants and children? Urology. 2005;66:1301–4. https://doi.org/10.1016/j.urology.2005.06.132.

12. Sertic M, Amaral J, Parra D, Temple M, Connolly B. Image-guided pediatric ureteric stent insertions: an 11-year experience. J Vasc Interv Radiol. 2014;25:1265–71. https://doi.org/10.1016/j.jvir.2014.03.028.

13. Slaton JW, Kropp KA. Proximal ureteral stent migration: an avoidable complication? J Urol. 1996;155:58–61.

14. Pollack HM, Banner MP. Percutaneous nephrostomy and related pyeloureteral manipulative techniques. Urol Radiol. 1981;2:147–54. https://doi.org/10.1007/BF02926716.

15. Wills MI, Gilbert HW, Chadwick DJ, Harrison SC. Which ureteric stent length? Br J Urol. 1991;68:440. https://doi.org/10.1111/j.1464-410x.1991.tb15375.x.

16. El-Faqih SR, Hussain I. Urolithiasis in the middle east: epidemiology and pathogenesis. In The management of lithiasis. Dordrecht: Springer; 1997. p. 35–41. https://doi.org/10.1007/978-94-011-5396-6_4.

17. Finney RP. Experience with new double J ureteral catheter stent. J Urol. 1978;120:678–81. https://doi.org/10.1016/s0022-5347(17)57326-7.

18. Al-Marhoon MS, Shareef O, Venkiteswaran KP. Complications and outcomes of JJ stenting of the ureter in urological practice: a single-centre experience. Arab J Urol. 2012;10:372–7. https://doi.org/10.1016/j.aju.2012.08.004.

19. Rane A, Saleemi A, Cahill D, Sriprasad S, Shrotri N, Tiptaft R. Have stent-related symptoms anything to do with placement technique? J Endourol. 2001;15:741–5. https://doi.org/10.1089/08927790152596352.

20. Al-Kandari AM, Al-Shaiji TF, Shaaban H, Ibrahim HM, Elshebiny YH, Shokeir AA. Effects of proximal and distal ends of double-J ureteral stent position on postprocedural symptoms and quality of life: a randomized clinical trial. J Endourol. 2007;21:698–702. https://doi.org/10.1089/end.2007.9949.

21. Abbas TO, Ali M, Moog R. "Double-Lumen Valve-Controlled Intra-Operative Pyeloplasty Stent (VIPs)": a new technology for post-pyeloplasty stenting—proof of concept study in a preclinical large animal model. Res Rep Urol. 2020;12:61–74. https://doi.org/10.2147/RRU.S238572.

22. Steven YC. Ureteral Stent Patent US8192500B2. 2019.

23. Mykulak DJ, Herskowitz M, Glassberg KI. Use of magnetic internal ureteral stents in pediatric urology: retrieval without routine requirement for cystoscopy and general anesthesia. J Urol. 1994;152:976–7. https://doi.org/10.1016/s0022-5347(17)32634-4.

24. Mitchell A, Bolduc S, Moore K, Cook A, Fermin C, Weber B. Use of a magnetic double J stent in pediatric patients: a case–control study at two Canadian pediatric centers. J Pediatr Surg. 2020;55:486–9. https://doi.org/10.1016/J.JPEDSURG.2019.03.014.

25. Zhang MQ, Zou T, Huang YC, Shang YF, Yang GG, Wang WZ, et al. Braided thin-walled biodegradable ureteral stent: preliminary evaluation in a canine model. Int J Urol. 2014;21:401–7. https://doi.org/10.1111/iju.12297.

26. Liu X, Li F, Ding Y, Zou T, Wang L, Hao K. Intelligent optimization of the film-to-fiber ratio of a degradable braided bicomponent ureteral stent. Materials (Basel, Switzerland). 2015;8:7563–77. https://doi.org/10.3390/ma8115397.

27. Soria F, de la Cruz JE, Budia A, Serrano A, Galan-Llopis JA, Sanchez-Margallo FM. Experimental assessment of new generation of ureteral stents: biodegradable and antireflux properties. J Endourol. 2020;34:359–65. https://doi.org/10.1089/end.2019.0493.
28. Yang L, Whiteside S, Cadieux PA, Denstedt JD. Ureteral stent technology: drug-eluting stents and stent coatings. Asian J Urol. 2015;2:194–201. https://doi.org/10.1016/J.AJUR.2015.08.006.

Flow Dynamics in Stented Ureter

Shaokai Zheng, Dario Carugo, Francesco Clavica, Ali Mosayyebi, and Sarah Waters

1 Introduction

Urinary flow is governed by the principles of fluid mechanics. Urodynamic investigations are frequently employed to diagnose lower urinary tract symptoms [1, 2], and many recent studies have focused on the fundamental flow dynamics of the ureter using fluid mechanical modelling methods, both theoretical and experimental [3]. Such studies have revealed the fundamental kinematics and dynamics of urinary flow in various physiological and pathological conditions, which are cornerstones for future development of diagnostic knowledge and innovative devices.

In a nutshell, there are three primary approaches to study the fluid mechanical characteristics of urinary flow: reduced order, computational, and experimental methods. Reduced-order methods exploit the disparate length scales inherent in the system to reveal the key dominant physics. Computational models can simulate

S. Zheng (✉) · F. Clavica
ARTORG Center for Biomedical Engineering Research, Faculty of Medicine, University of Bern, Bern, Switzerland
e-mail: shaokai.zheng@unibe.ch; francesco.clavica@unibe.ch

D. Carugo
Department of Pharmaceutics, UCL School of Pharmacy, University College London, London, United Kingdom
e-mail: d.carugo@ucl.ac.uk

A. Mosayyebi
Bioengineering Sciences, Faculty of Engineering and Physical Sciences, University of Southampton, Southampton, United Kingdom
e-mail: a.mosayyebi@soton.ac.uk

S. Waters
Oxford Centre for Industrial and Applied Mathematics, Mathematical Institute, University of Oxford, Oxford, United Kingdom
e-mail: sarah.waters@maths.ox.ac.uk

© The Author(s) 2022
F. Soria et al. (eds.), *Urinary Stents*,
https://doi.org/10.1007/978-3-031-04484-7_13

fully three-dimensional, time-dependent flows in physiologically-inspired anatomical domains. Finally, experimental models provide an excellent counterpart to reduced and computational models by providing physical tests under various physiological and pathological conditions.

2 Fundamental Characteristics of the Stented Ureter for Modelling Purposes

The key components of the human urinary system are illustrated in Fig. 1. The base flow is established by urine transport from the kidneys to the bladder. The generated urinary flow rates are in the order of 1 mL/min for each kidney [3], but can be higher or lower based on fluid intake or pathological conditions such as polyuria and diabetes mellitus.

For most fluid mechanical studies, the kidneys and bladder are treated as boundaries of the ureteric domain where pressure conditions are prescribed. The intraluminal renal pelvic pressure averages 12–15 cmH$_2$O [4, 5], and is generally considered to be below 20 cmH$_2$O for healthy individuals. The intraluminal renal pelvic pressure is often imposed as the inlet pressure boundary condition (BC) for ureteric flow models.

The bladder pressure is usually defined as the detrusor pressure, which is clinically measured by subtracting the intra-abdominal pressure from the intravesical pressure. The detrusor pressure remains small (roughly 2–5 cmH$_2$O) during the filling phase, but rises in the voiding phase, especially in men as a result of the extra resistance caused by the prostate. In a retrospective study of 976 healthy

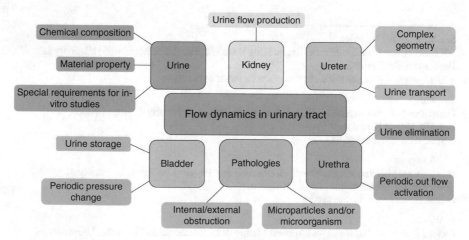

Fig. 1 Illustration of the key components of human urinary system and the primary considerations in designing a physiological model. For multi-organ models, connections between components need to be carefully addressed as well

individuals, the detrusor pressure at maximum flow rate during voiding was reported as 38.3 ± 11.5 cmH$_2$O for males and 32 ± 10.6 cmH$_2$O for females [6]. The voiding time of a normal bladder (capacity of approximately 500 mL) is around 40 s for healthy individuals [6]. The magnitude and duration of the pressures during filling and voiding can be used to specify the outlet condition of the ureteric domain, in contrast to explicitly including the bladder and urethra in the model.

The ureter is usually described as a tube of approximately 22–30 cm in length [7], and 1–6 mm in diameter [8]. The diameter is smaller at the ureteropelvic junction (UPJ), ureterovesical junction (UVJ), and where the ureters turn medially and cross the common iliac vessels. The ureter is typically modelled as either a straight or an undulated tube [9, 10].

Finally, to complete a model setup, characteristics of the stent need to be prescribed. This is straightforward for in-vitro studies at the macroscopic level, where commercially available stents can be directly used in the model ureter. For research into the fundamental physics, design parameters such as stent length, diameter (outer/inner), side hole arrangements (e.g. diameter, spacing, vertex angle), and material properties can be investigated at different scales (e.g. local behaviour in vicinity of side holes of varying geometries).

3   Reduced Models

Reduced-order methods are often employed to develop theoretical models of the flow dynamics within a (stented) ureter. Here we highlight the approaches adopted, and refer the interested reader to the review paper by Zheng et al. [3] for discussion of the details of the mathematical equations.

Lubrication theory was used to derive some of the earliest reduced models for the ureter [11–13], motivated by the small aspect ratio of the ureter (i.e. ratio of radius to length is small or R/L $\ll 1$) and the small reduced Reynolds number of ureteric flow (Re ~ 1). In the lubrication regime, the full Navier–Stokes equation was simplified to derive the urine flux and pressure distribution within a ureter subject to prescribed displacement of the ureter walls [11] to model the effects of peristalsis. The insertion of a catheter (or stent) was shown not to affect the pressure distribution within the ureter, providing confidence that urological pressure measurements made with a catheter are trustworthy [12].

Major limitations of the earliest models include the neglect of kidney and bladder activities, and the treatment of the catheter or stent as a solid tube without side holes, so that the permeability of the walls of the catheter or stent was neglected. This was ameliorated by Cummings et al. [14], where the kidney and bladder were treated with dynamic pressure BCs and the stent walls were assumed to be permeable. The ureter was considered to be a passive linearly-elastic tube that deformed in response to the transmural pressure across it. Their results indicate that during voiding the bladder pressure rises significantly and reflux can occur. Stents with higher permeability cause less total reflux than those with smaller permeability, which suggests that more side holes can help reduce urine reflux. The model was further developed to incorporate more physiological descriptions of bladder pressure variation [15] (i.e. during voiding or spasms), a nonlinear elastic ureter wall law [15, 16], and the urine production from kidneys [16]. The authors argued that reflux exacerbates stent encrustation (primarily caused by the crystalline deposits of salts from urine) by returning bladder urine and bacteria to the ureter and renal pelvis. Increased duration of bladder spasm pulse and higher peak pressure during voiding were both shown to increase the total reflux, suggesting that patients should not squeeze hard during voiding, and the stent design should be optimized to reduce bladder irritations.

We note that peristalsis of the ureter wall can be strongly affected by the presence of an implanted ureteral stent, even ceasing completely, as concluded from several experiments using porcine models [17, 18] and a human patient study with indwelling double-J stent [19]. It is therefore common to neglect peristalsis in stented ureter models, especially for in-vitro investigations.

Finally, there have been models dealing with micro-particle laden (e.g. stone fragments or crystalline particles) urine flows. In this context, urine is modeled as a multiphase medium with solid particles [20–22]. In these models, the coupling is one way: the particles do not affect the flow dynamics, but the fluid flow governs the transport of the particles. The ureter is modeled as a two-dimensional channel with solid boundaries under peristaltic waves, and the fluid phase is solved by the Navier–Stokes equations. The effect of the fluid flow on particle transport is then determined by solution of the Basset–Boussinesq–Oseen equation. These methods are largely used to study particle trajectories and sedimentation under ureteric peristaltic waves. The exact results from these studies are therefore less relevant in the case of a stented ureter, since the peristaltic movement is largely impeded by the indwelling stent.

4   Computational Methods

While reduced models are useful to probe the underlying physics of the urinary system with minimal requirements for computational power, full computational models are able to simulate multiple configurations in clinically realistic settings by systematically varying physiological and stent-related parameters. Two solution techniques exist to solve full computational models. The conventional Computational Fluid Dynamic (CFD) approach solves only for the fluid domain and treats all solid components as prescribed BCs, whereas the Fluid–Structure Interaction (FSI) approach solves the governing equations for both the fluid and solid domains, coupled via conditions at the fluid–solid interface [23, 24].

CFD has been widely used to study design parameters of stents, such as number of side holes [9, 10, 25–27], inter-hole distance [10, 26, 27] and angular positions [10, 25–27] in various ureter shapes [10, 26] with different levels of ureteral obstructions [10, 25, 27, 28]. Results from straight ureter models showed that most of the side holes are inactive (no through flow) in the absence of blockages [25], except perhaps the ones nearest to the UPJ or UVJ [10, 25]. With a local blockage present, the side holes in the vicinity of the blockage become increasingly active as the degree of blockage increases [25, 28]. Increasing the number of side holes (consequently decreasing the side hole interval) was shown to promote total flow rates [26, 27, 29], but the angular arrangement of side holes showed no impact on the total flow rate [27]. In the case of curved ureter models, the total flow rate was smaller compared to straight ureters [10], and the side holes were found to be active even in the absence of obstruction [26]. The stent wall thickness and the vertex angle of side holes were also studied in a CFD model of a microfluidic chip that replicated only a segment of the stented ureter [30]. Based on the local wall shear stress level, reducing stent wall thickness and adopting a 45° vertex angle for the side hole edges were proposed as strategies to reduce encrustation rates in inactive side holes.

The peristaltic movement of ureter wall is often omitted in CFD studies. In a few exceptions, a periodic wave of the ureter wall was prescribed and the effect of obstruction level was investigated [31, 32]. Nonetheless, the FSI method is more suitable for this type of study, where the ureter wall is modeled as a solid with appropriate constitutive equations capturing its material properties (e.g. elasticity). Previous FSI studies mainly focused on the characteristics of peristaltic waves such as maximum height, wave speed, and number of waves per ureter length [33, 34]. The proximal segment of the ureter was shown to suffer from a higher level of wall shear stress associated with a back flow at the beginning of peristalsis [33–35]. When an obstruction was introduced, higher shear stresses and pressure gradients were observed near the obstruction [36, 37]. Notably, a comparison between a full axisymmetric 3D ureter model and its corresponding 2D case showed negligible differences in shear stress and pressure gradient levels along the entire ureter length [36], and suggested that the simpler 2D axisymmetric model should be always considered first. Finally, in a study of a stented ureter [38], strains and stresses over the ureter obtained from a FSI study suggested a rigid-body behavior. The authors therefore recommended CFD as a cost efficient, but equally accurate option, for similar cases, where peristalsis is not considered.

5 Experimental Methods

In addition to providing physical insights, experimental models are also essential for the generation of data to calibrate and validate theoretical and computational models. Once validated by detailed comparison of theoretical model predictions with experimental data, theoretical and computational models can go beyond the experimental results by simulating more complex geometries and boundary conditions. Specifically, for the upper urinary tract (UUT), experimental studies have focused on the following aspects: (1) bacterial growth, (2) drainage capabilities of stents, and (3) the interplay between fluid mechanics and encrustation.

5.1   Bacterial Growth

Studies on bacterial growth in ureters aim to investigate encrustation and biofilm formation from a chemical and biological point of view. In the earliest studies [39, 40] on UUT, stents were not considered and the bladder was modelled as a static flask with periodic emptying cycles to simulate micturition. Volume capacity, residual volume and frequency of micturition were taken into account to study the bacterial susceptibility to antibiotics. It was demonstrated that the amount of bacteria in the urinary tract can be reduced with frequent micturition [39].

After stents were introduced in the clinical setting, several studies focused on investigating encrustation and biofilm growth in stented ureters. In general, different types of results can be achieved when static or dynamic models are used. Static models [41] were normally characterized by big reservoirs filled with artificial urine in which stents were immersed for a defined time interval. The results of these studies showed that 60% of the surface was covered by encrustation (mainly characterised by hydroxyapatite and struvite crystals) within 2 weeks, and that encrustation reached 100% coverage after 10 weeks.

Dynamic models were later introduced to overcome the main limitations of the static models and mimic more closely the physiological conditions. For example, filling and emptying cycles were introduced to model micturition which was not possible with static models. To this end, Chong et al. [42] introduced a syphon at the bladder outlet to automatically empty the bladder, when bladder volume reached a defined value (this volume could be controlled by changing the height of the syphon).

To facilitate comparison of stent designs, multi-testing platforms were introduced to enable simultaneous testing of several stent samples [43–45]. These experimental models were normally closed loops and constant urine flow was enforced by means of volumetric pumps (periodic bladder filling/emptying was not considered). Encrustation in dynamic models was found to be significantly lower than in static models, demonstrating the pivotal role of the flow on biofilm and encrustation growth.

5.2   Drainage Capabilities

Quantification of the drainage behaviour of ureteral stents is essential for assessing/ comparing stent performance. Hofmann and Hartung [46] used a reservoir to model the kidney and a 9-F (3 mm) polyvinyl tube with a stent inside (placed below the kidney) to model a stented ureter. To quantify the intraluminal drainage of stents, threads were tied around the polyvinyl tube to simulate obstructions. A similar approach was followed by Lange et al. [47] who used casted spheres to model ureteral obstructions. By keeping the head pressure constant, the performance of different stents were compared in terms of total flow rates [47]. A pressure driven flow setup was also adopted by Kim et al. [48]. In their experiments, stents of different diameters were inserted in silicone ureters. These ureter models closely mimicked the architecture of real human ureters as their geometry was based on computed tomographic (CT) scans from patients. Curved ureters were compared with simplified straight ureters in their study. These experiments showed that higher hydraulic resistance is associated with bigger stents (i.e., stents with higher diameters) and curved ureters [48].

In contrast to the pressure-driven flows highlighted above, Olweny et al. [49] adopted a flow-driven approach to quantify the drainage properties of ureteral stents: constant flow was enforced and the pressure difference across the stent samples was measured. The hydraulic resistance of each stent sample was calculated using Poiseuille's law. Their in-vitro results, however, did not match the associated in-vivo data, probably because of the morphological changes induced in the ureters by the presence of the indwelling stents.

In order to reproduce more physiologically realistic conditions, Graw and Engelhardt [50] provided an experimental setup to mimic ureteral peristalsis using 24 inflatable cuffs surrounding an inner tube which modelled the ureter (a thin-walled tube with four lobes). The peristaltic wave, causing the bolus propagation, was reproduced by periodically activating the pressure in each cuff. Their investigations allowed to measure the pressure waveform associated to the bolus propagation; few suggestions were also provided to help the selection of catheters for intraluminal pressure measurements in ureters. Moreover, a bladder model reproducing the physiological pressure–volume curves was introduced by Kim et al. [51]. In their model, micturition was achieved using an outlet valve which opened at target pressure values. Measured peak bladder pressure, in this model, was found in the physiological range 20–80 cmH$_2$O (during micturition).

5.3 Interplay Between Fluid Mechanics and Encrustation

Flow-particle models investigate the interplay between fluid mechanics and encrustation/biofilm development in stented ureters (in addition to drainage capabilities of stents). Clavica et al. [52] and Carugo et al. [53] developed an in-vitro transparent model of the ureter based on measurements in porcine ureters. They quantified the relation between renal pressure and parameters including urine viscosity, urine flow rate, and level of obstruction. Notably, using fluorescent particles flowing in the transparent model, they were the first to provide flow visualisation in stented ureters and to observe the presence of laminar vortices near stent side-holes. It was hypothesised that these vortices can be anchoring sites for crystal and bacterial deposits [52, 53]. Following these findings, microfluidic 'stent-on-chip' models were developed by Mosayyebi et al. [54] to investigate intraluminal and extraluminal flows in stented ureters at the microscale level. In this study, flow streamlines at selected locations were obtained using fluorescent tracers and comparisons with computational equivalents were provided. An inverse correlation between particle accumulation and wall shear stress was identified. In further studies, the same research group investigated: (1) a novel side hole [30] with an optimised 'streamlined architecture' which led to lower particle deposition and (2) the influence of wall shear stress on bacterial adhesion [55]. Similarly to particle accumulation, it was found that low wall shear stress are associated with higher bacterial coverage.

6 Conclusion

In summary, this chapter has highlighted the various approaches established to study the flow dynamics in stented ureter. While the interdisciplinary approaches to date have provided a wealth of insight into the fluid mechanical properties of the stented ureter, the next challenge is to develop new theoretical, computational and experimental models to capture the complex interplay between the fluid dynamics in stented ureters and biofilm/encrustation growth. Such studies will (1) enable identification of clinically relevant scenarios to improve patients' treatment, and (2) provide physical guidelines for next-generation stent design.

References

1. Abrams P. Urodynamics. 3rd ed. London: Springer; 2006.
2. Griffiths D. Urodynamics: the mechanics and hydrodynamics of the lower urinary tract. Bristol: Adam Hilger in Collaboration with the Hospital Physicists Association; 1980.
3. Zheng S, Carugo D, Mosayyebi A, Turney B, Burkhard F, Lange D, et al. Fluid mechanical modeling of the upper urinary tract. WIREs Mech Dis. 2021;13:e01523.
4. Rattner William H, Fink S, Murphy JJ. Pressure studies in the human ureter and renal pelvis. J Urol. 1957;78(4):359–62.
5. Walzak MP, Paquin AJ. Renal pelvic pressure levels in management of nephrostomy. J Urol. 1961;85(5):697–702.
6. Alloussi SH, Lang C, Eichel R, Ziegler M, Stenzl A, Alloussi S. Urodynamical benchmarks: a retrospective analyses of 976 combined urodynamics with no pathological findings to evaluate standard values. Eur Urol Suppl. 2010;9(2):227.
7. Hickling DR, Sun T-T, Wu X-R. Anatomy and physiology of the urinary tract: relation to host defense and microbial infection. Microbiol Spectr. 2015;3(4):2012.
8. Zelenko N, Coll D, Rosenfeld AT, Smith RC. Normal ureter size on unenhanced helical CT. Am J Roentgenol. 2004;182(4):1039–41.
9. Kim K-W, Kim H-H, Choi YH, Lee SB, Baba Y, Suh S-H. Arrangement of side holes in a double J stent for high urine flow in a stented ureter. J Mech Sci Technol. 2020;34:949–54.
10. Kim H-H, Choi YH, Lee SB, Baba Y, Kim K-W, Suh S-H. Numerical analysis of the urine flow in a stented ureter with no peristalsis. Biomed Mater Eng. 2015;26(s1):S215–S23.
11. Lykoudis PS, Roos R. The fluid mechanics of the ureter from a lubrication theory point of view. J Fluid Mech. 1970;43(4):661–74.
12. Roos R, Lykoudis PS. The fluid mechanics of the ureter with an inserted catheter. J Fluid Mech. 1971;46(4):625–30.
13. Kiil F. Urinary flow and ureteral peristalsis. In: Lutzeyer W, Melchior H, editors. Urodynamics: upper and lower urinary tract. Berlin: Springer; 1973. p. 57–70.
14. Cummings LJ, Waters SL, Wattis JAD, Graham SJ. The effect of ureteric stents on urine flow: reflux. J Math Biol. 2004;49(1):56–82.
15. Waters S, Heaton K, Siggers J, Bayston R, Bishop M, Cummings L, et al. Ureteric stents: investigating flow and encrustation. Proc Inst Mech Eng Part H J Eng Med. 2008;222(4):551–61.
16. Siggers JH, Waters S, Wattis J, Cummings L. Flow dynamics in a stented ureter. Math Med Biol. 2009;26(1):1–24.
17. Kinn AC, Lykkeskov-Andersen H. Impact on ureteral peristalsis in a stented ureter. An experimental study in the pig. Urol Res. 2002;30(4):213–8.
18. Venkatesh R, Landman J, Minor SD, Lee DI, Rehman J, Vanlangendonck R, et al. Impact of a double-pigtail stent on ureteral peristalsis in the porcine model: initial studies using a novel implantable magnetic sensor. J Endourol. 2005;19(2):170–6.

19. Mosli Hisham A, Farsi Hasan MA, Al-Zimaity Mohammed F, Saleh Tarik R, Al-Zamzami MM. Vesicoureteral reflux in patients with double pigtail stents. J Urol. 1991;146(4):966–9.
20. Jiménez-Lozano J, Sen M, Corona E. Analysis of peristaltic two-phase flow with application to ureteral biomechanics. Acta Mech. 2011;219(1–2):91–109.
21. Rath H, Reese G. Peristaltic flow of non-Newtonian fluids containing small spherical particles. Arch Mech. 1984;36(2):263–77.
22. Riaz A, Sadiq MA. Particle–fluid suspension of a non-Newtonian fluid through a curved passage: an application of urinary tract infections. Front Phys. 2020;8:109.
23. Hirt CW, Amsden AA, Cook JL. An arbitrary Lagrangian–Eulerian computing method for all flow speeds. J Comput Phys. 1974;14(3):227–53.
24. Benra F-K, Dohmen HJ, Pei J, Schuster S, Wan B. A comparison of one-way and two-way coupling methods for numerical analysis of fluid–structure interactions. J Appl Math. 2011;2011:16.
25. Tong JCK, Sparrow EM, Abraham JP. Numerical simulation of the urine flow in a stented ureter. J Biomech Eng. 2006;129(2):187–92.
26. Kim KW, Choi YH, Lee SB, Baba Y, Kim HH, Suh SH. Numerical analysis of the effect of side holes of a double J stent on flow rate and pattern. Biomed Mater Eng. 2015;26:S319–S27.
27. Kim H-H, Choi YH, Lee SB, Baba Y, Kim K-W, Suh S-H. Numerical analysis of urine flow through the side holes of a double J stent in a ureteral stenosis. Technol Health Care. 2017;25(S1):63–72.
28. Carugo D, Zhang X, Drake JM, Clavica F, editors. Formation and characteristics of laminar vortices in microscale environments within an obstructed and stented ureter: a computational study. In Proceedings of the 18th International Conference on Miniaturized Systems for Chemistry and Life Sciences, MicroTAS; October 26–30, 2014; San Antonio, TX, USA. The Chemical and Biological Microsystems Society; 2014.
29. Kim KW, Choi YH, Lee SB, Baba Y, Kim HH, Suh SH. Analysis of urine flow in three different ureter models. Comput Math Methods Med. 2017;2017:5172641.
30. Mosayyebi A, Lange D, Yann Yue Q, Somani BK, Zhang X, Manes C, et al. Reducing deposition of encrustation in ureteric stents by changing the stent architecture: a microfluidic-based investigation. Biomicrofluidics. 2019;13(1):014101.
31. Najafi Z, Gautam P, Schwartz BF, Chandy AJ, Mahajan AM. Three-dimensional numerical simulations of peristaltic contractions in obstructed ureter flows. J Biomech Eng. 2016;138(10):101002.
32. Najafi Z, Schwartz BF, Chandy AJ, Mahajan AM. A two-dimensional numerical study of peristaltic contractions in obstructed ureter flows. Comput Methods Biomech Biomed Eng. 2018;21(1):22–32.
33. Vahidi B, Fatouraee N, Imanparast A, Moghadam AN. A mathematical simulation of the ureter: effects of the model parameters on ureteral pressure/flow relations. J Biomech Eng. 2011;133(3):031004–9.
34. Vahidi B, Fatouraee N. A biomechanical simulation of ureteral flow during peristalsis using intraluminal morphometric data. J Theor Biol. 2012;298:42–50.
35. Hosseini G, Ji C, Xu D, Rezaienia MA, Avital E, Munjiza A, et al. A computational model of ureteral peristalsis and an investigation into ureteral reflux. Biomed Eng Lett. 2018;8(1):117–25.
36. Takaddus AT, Chandy AJ. A three-dimensional (3D) two-way coupled fluid–structure interaction (FSI) study of peristaltic flow in obstructed ureters. Int J Numer Methods Biomed Eng. 2018;34(10):e3122.
37. Takaddus AT, Gautam P, Chandy AJ. A fluid–structure interaction (FSI)-based numerical investigation of peristalsis in an obstructed human ureter. Int J Numer Methods Biomed Eng. 2018;34(9):e3104.
38. Gómez-Blanco JC, Martínez-Reina FJ, Cruz D, Pagador JB, Sánchez-Margallo FM, Soria F. Fluid structural analysis of urine flow in a stented ureter. Comput Math Methods Med. 2016;2016:5710798.
39. O'Grady F, Pennington JH. Bacterial growth in an in vitro system simulating conditions in the urinary bladder. Br J Exp Pathol. 1966;47(2):152–7.
40. Greenwood D, O'Grady F. An in vitro model of the urinary bladder. J Antimicrob Chemother. 1978;4(2):113–20.

41. Tunney MM, Bonner MC, Keane PF, Gorman SP. Development of a model for assessment of biomaterial encrustation in the upper urinary tract. Biomaterials. 1996;17(10):1025–9.
42. Choong SKS, Wood S, Whitfield HN. A model to quantify encrustation on ureteric stents, urethral catheters and polymers intended for urological use. BJU Int. 2000;86(4):414–21.
43. Cauda V, Chiodoni A, Laurenti M, Canavese G, Tommasi T. Ureteral double-J stents performances toward encrustation after long-term indwelling in a dynamic in vitro model. J Biomed Mater Res Part B Appl Biomater. 2017;105(8):2244–53.
44. Gorman SP, Garvin CP, Quigley F, Jones DS. Design and validation of a dynamic flow model simulating encrustation of biomaterials in the urinary tract. J Pharm Pharmacol. 2003;55(4):461–8.
45. Hobbs T, Schultz LN, Lauchnor EG, Gerlach R, Lange D. Evaluation of biofilm induced urinary infection stone formation in a novel laboratory model system. J Urol. 2018;199(1):178–85.
46. Hofmann R, Hartung R. Ureteral stents—materials and new forms. World J Urol. 1989;7(3):154–7.
47. Lange D, Hoag NA, Poh BK, Chew BH. Drainage characteristics of the 3F MicroStent using a novel film occlusion anchoring mechanism. J Endourol. 2011;25(6):1051–6.
48. Kim K-W, Kim H-H, Choi YH, Lee SB, Baba Y. Urine flow analysis using double J stents of various sizes in in vitro ureter models. Int J Numer Methods Biomed Eng. 2020;3:e3294.
49. Olweny EO, Portis AJ, Afane JS, Brewer AV, Shalhav AL, Luszczynski K, et al. Flow characteristics of 3 unique ureteral stents: investigation of a Poiseuille flow pattern. J Urol. 2000;164(6):2099–103.
50. Graw M, Engelhardt H. Simulation of physiological ureteral peristalsis. Urol Int. 1986;41(1):1–8.
51. Kim J, Lee MK, Choi B. A study on the fluid mechanical urinary bladder simulator and reproduction of human urodynamics. Int J Precis Eng Manuf. 2011;12(4):679–85.
52. Clavica F, Zhao X, ElMahdy M, Drake MJ, Zhang X, Carugo D. Investigating the flow dynamics in the obstructed and stented ureter by means of a biomimetic artificial model. PLoS One. 2014;9(2):e87433.
53. Carugo D, Elmahdy M, Zhao X, Drake M, Zhang X, Clavica F, editors. An artificial model for studying fluid dynamics in the obstructed and stented ureter. In 35th Annual International Conference of the IEEE Engineering in Medicine and Biology Society (EMBC); July 3–7 2013; Osaka, Japan. IEEE; 2013. p. 5335–8.
54. Mosayyebi A, Yue QY, Somani BK, Zhang X, Manes C, Carugo D. Particle accumulation in ureteral stents is governed by fluid dynamics: in vitro study using a "stent-on-chip" model. J Endourol. 2018;32(7):639–46.
55. De Grazia A, LuTheryn G, Meghdadi A, Mosayyebi A, Espinosa-Ortiz JE, Gerlach R, et al. A microfluidic-based investigation of bacterial attachment in ureteral stents. Micromachines. 2020;11(4):408.

Methodology for the Development and Validation of New Stent Designs: *In Vitro* and *In Vivo* Models

Wolfgang Kram, Julia E. de la Cruz, Owen Humphreys, Noor Buchholz, and Federico Soria

1 *In-Vitro* Encrustation Models: A Critical Review

Implantation of biomaterials into the urinary tract is hampered by crystal formation, bacterial adherence and, ultimately, encrustation through biofilm formation resulting from a multifactorial disturbance of the delicate balance between numerous physico-chemical and biochemical processes. Non-infectious stone formation and encrustation usually result from metabolic imbalances, often on the tubular level. In contrast, infectious stone formation and biofilm-induced encrustation are linked to the enzymatic activity of bacteria. Best known are urease-producing species such as *Proteus mirabilis*, which increase the pH of the urine. This alkalization, in turn, decreases the solubility of urinary calcium and magnesium salts and thus facilitates encrustation.

Consequently, the use of urinary implants is complicated by several factors stent surface encrustation through deposition of crystal-forming urinary ions, bacterial colonization and biofilm formation despite antibiotic treatment and prophylaxis, mechanical irritation of the urothelium by encrustation, and alterations of urine flow in and around the stent due to encrustation [1].

W. Kram
Department of Urology, University Medical Center Rostock, Rostock, Germany
e-mail: wolfgang.kram@med.uni-rostock.de

J. E. de la Cruz (✉) · F. Soria
Foundation, Jesús Usón Minimally Invasive Surgery Center, Cáceres, Spain
e-mail: jecruz@ccmijesususon.com; fsoria@ccmijesususon.com

O. Humphreys
UCD Centre for Biomedical Engineering, University College Dublin, Dublin, Ireland
e-mail: owen.humphreys@ucdconnect.ie

N. Buchholz
Scientific Office, U-merge Ltd., London-Athens-Dubai, Athens, Greece

© The Author(s) 2022
F. Soria et al. (eds.), *Urinary Stents*,
https://doi.org/10.1007/978-3-031-04484-7_14

The development of *in vitro* models to simulate bacterial infections and biofilm formation started after the initial observation of sessile bacteria and their role in chronic infections in humans. Biofilms form an irregular network matrix. They protect the bacteria from physical, chemical and biological stresses. Shear stress caused by the flow of the fluid medium is hereby one of the main factors impacting on the formation of a stable biofilm.

Early approaches focused on the use of continuous flow systems, such as the chemostat model, which had the advantage of a regular supply of fresh fluid medium whilst maintaining a constant volume [2]. Many *in vitro* models designed to mimic encrustation on urological devices have been derived from classical microbiological approaches, and often do not reflect important physiological factors such as the complex and variable physico-chemical urinary environment *in vivo,* or infection with mixed species.

In 1973, Finlayson and Dubois described a dynamic flow *in vitro* encrustation model which used both, a constant flow of artificial urine and a magnetic stirrer [3]. A number of adaptations to this model have been devised over time to enable the study of urinary encrustations utilizing both, human and artificial urine [4]. Depending on particular research questions, two groups of *open* systems were designed: The Continuous Flow Stirred Tank Reactor (CFSTR) and the Plug Flow Reactor (PFR). The Modified Robbins Device (MRD) was designed to monitor biofilm formation with different flow speeds in an axial direction, and in a completely mixed reactor using diffusion. This PFR-system consists of a pipe with multiple threaded holes containing coupons. The biofilm reactor of the Center for Disease Control (CDC) is a current, commercially available flow-based CFSTR-system. A vessel with a polyethylene lid bears independent rods housing removable coupons. Inside the reactor, there is a rotating magnetic stirrer exerting a constant high shear force on the coupons. The number of revolutions can be varied and is independent of the feed speed. The system allows for a perfect mixing and operates at a steady state. With this system, structure and physiology of biofilm formation can be monitored by confocal laser scanning microscopy (CLSM) in a non-invasive fashion [5]. The CDC biofilm reactor is indispensable for prototype testing, but less suitable for screening testing. Another disadvantage of the semi-open design of the CDC reactor is its susceptibility to contamination.

This led to the development of high-throughput static biofilm models. Microtiter plate (MTP)-based static systems are the perhaps most commonly used biofilm model systems. They are an important tool to study especially the early stages of biofilm formation. In these systems, biofilms are typically grown on either the bottom or the sidewalls of a MTP. MTP-based systems are *closed* systems without in- or outflow from the reactor. Consequently, during an experiment the composition of the environment inside the well of an MTP changes. Nutrients are depleted whilst signaling molecules accumulate. It has been suggested that a part of the accumulated biomass may not result from biofilm formation, but rather from cell sedimentation and subsequent entrapment of cell sediments within the matrix of extracellular polymeric substances (EPS).

The Calgary Biofilm Device (CBD) represents a modification of the MTP-based systems, where biofilms are formed on lids with rods that fit into the bacteria-containing wells of the MTP. A newer system to study biofilm formation and encrustation on implants uses this CBD as a commercially available high-throughput screening assay. However, the lid is configured in such a way that materials are held in a matrix. The bottom is a welled plate into which the implant materials to be tested can be inserted. The matrix in combination with the high-throughput capability of the assay allow the study of several encrustation parameters. The use of MTP-based assays offers many of advantages. MTP are cheap and they provide the opportunity for multiplexing, as multiple organisms and treatments can be incorporated in a single experimental run [6].

Both, MTP/CBD-based and flow-based systems share some limitations. One common pitfall in designing *in vitro* biofilm models is the use of bacterial strains with a low virulence which, in turn, results in a low translation rate from *in vitro* to *in vivo* studies.

Most *in vitro* encrustation models use synthetic urine, based on urease reactions or urease-producing bacteria. However, in real life most urinary tract infections are caused by *E. coli*. These are acid-producing, and, consequently the urinary pH does not increase. Whilst models using urease-related alkalization are relatively easy to design, the multifactorial physiological conditions in stone- and encrustation formation are not properly represented. In fact, 80% of all urinary stones and probably most urinary implant encrustations consist to a large part of calcium and oxalate. Only 10% of urinary stones contain uric acid crystals, and struvite as a typical infectious stone is clinically found in less than 10% of urinary stones, typically in alkaline urine with a pH > 7. Yet, alkalization models do focus on this group of stones.

In clinical practice, guidelines mandate that urinary catheters and stents with such infectious stone encrustations must always be removed due to the presence of inactive bacteria protected by the biofilm [7]. Using these models seems therefore non-relevant for the development of new stents for a large target population of patients.

The above-mentioned encrustation models could be complimented by *in vitro* calcium oxalate crystallization methods from urolithiasis research. There are different options to choose from. These vary from simple experiments in defined inorganic solutions to whole human urine experiments replicating urine flow dynamics [8]. Currently, models are being developed that combine the advantages of continuous flow and static models. One such system is the *stent-on-chip* microfluidic model (SOC). SOC tries to simulate the hydrodynamic areas of a stented ureter under physiological conditions, including drainage holes and the cavity formed by a ureteral obstruction. Encrustation formation over time is monitored and measured by optical microscopy [9].

For the future, examination of the urinary microbiome may provide promising insight into the underlying mechanisms of biofilm formation and encrustation on urinary implants. It has been suggested that the urinary tract is not, contrary to earlier assumptions, a perfectly sterile environment and that commensal bacteria may play a role in patient susceptibility to infection and in the composition of the urinary microbiome associated with stent complications [10].

OMICs (genomics, transcriptomics, proteomics and metabolomics) have improved our understanding of microbial interactions in the urinary tract. It is now possible to identify all microbial species that colonize the urinary tract. Combining results from OMICs studies with *in vitro* biofilm research has the potential of making a real impact in clinical practice in the future.

2 Preclinical *In Vivo* Evaluation of Urinary Stents

Experimental *in vivo* trials represent the final step in the preclinical validation of a medical device. These *in vivo* evaluations should be preceded by the corresponding *in silico* simulations, *in vitro* and *ex vivo* studies of the newly developed device. The urinary tract constitutes a complex dynamic environment with a high variability, where *in vitro* and *ex vivo* models often fail to reflect certain factors that are decisive for the safety and effectiveness of a urinary stent. These factors include urodynamic behavior of the urinary tract, the changing physico-chemical conditions and the multifactorial nature of urinary tract infections, biofilm and encrustations. Besides, ureteral peristalsis and the potential presence of vesicoureteral reflux may play a crucial role in the success of new designs of ureteral stents [1, 11, 12].

Prior to its translation into a clinical setting, the safety and performance of a urinary stent requires to be tested in a whole organism, provided currently by animal models. Animal models overcome the aforementioned limitations of reproducibility in laboratory setting and also allow the evaluation of the systemic effect of a new device on the host, including its potential systemic toxicity [13]. The rational sequence of the preclinical assessment of a new stent design or innovation should follow the order from in silico, *in vitro* and *ex vivo* studies, to finally *in vivo* trials. This thus allows the reduction of the number of animal models used to a minimum that provides adequate statistical power, increasing the likelihood of success of these experimental trials and preserving animal welfare [14, 15].

Concerning animal welfare in experimental studies, ethical evaluation of projects involving animal testing is mandatory in the EU since January 2013, through the Directive 2010/63/EU of the European Parliament and of the Council [16]. Establishing the basic rules applicable to the protection of animals used in experimentation and other scientific purposes [15, 16]. In order to ensure moral standards, scientific validity, and public trust, all projects must be evaluated and approved by an ethical committee prior to development. The use of animals for research should be justified by carefully evaluating each procedure, as to the scientific validity, usefulness and relevance of the expected result of that use. The potential harm to the animal will be balanced against the expected benefits of the project [15, 17].

With regard to the translational perspective of animal research, the choice of the species should be based on the similarity of the conditions studied with those of the human being. Ideally, we should seek for the model that provides anatomic, urodynamic, pathophysiological, histological and biochemical levels as identical as possible to that of humans. Non-human primates represent the closest model in this regard, except for two anatomic variations, they possess unipapillary kidneys and the left kidney lies lower in the abdomen, as opposed to human kidneys [18]. Nevertheless, the scientific literature has not reported the assessment of urinary stents in primates, which may be due to ethical, legal, economic and logistical considerations [16, 19].

2.1   Porcine Model

The porcine species are the animal models most frequently used for the assessment of urinary stent designs. The anatomy of the human and porcine urinary tracts are highly similar, rendering this model ideal for analyzing the behavior of the urinary tract in the presence of new devices [20] (Fig. 1). Pigs have multipapillary kidneys, with 8–12 papillae compared to humans, which usually have 4–18 [21]. Porcine ureters tend to be longer and more tortuous than those of humans [20, 22, 23]. Moreover, porcine renal physiology parallels that of humans with respect to

Fig. 1 Corrosion endocast shows pelvicalyceal system and renal vessels. Dorsal view

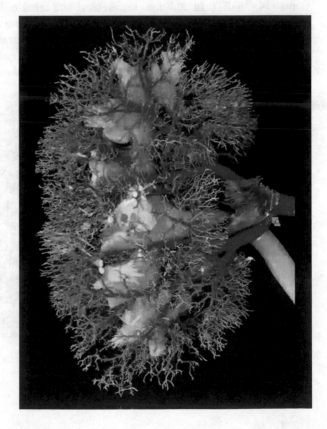

maximal urine concentration, glomerular filtration rate and total renal blood flow [24]. Since the male porcine urethra prevents retrograde approach due to its sigmoid morphology, research involving endourologic procedures is performed on females. Ideally, interventions should be carried out on 35–40 kg models, as the dimensions of their urinary tract at that weight are comparable to a human adult [25, 26].

The devices assessed in the porcine model are mainly ureteral stents, including polymeric stents, antireflux, biodegradable, drug-eluting and metallic stents [24–29]. This animal enables the transurethral retrograde insertion of the devices, although antegrade and cystostomy approaches have also been described [24, 29–32]. The evaluation of the performance *in vivo* of the urinary devices involves blood and urinalysis, urine culture and imaging tests that include the ultrasonographic assessment of the hydronephrosis degrees [33] (Fig. 2). Radiologic tests comprising excretory urography and retrograde ureteropyelography, provide valuable information on urinary patency, stent migration, radiopacity and fashion of degradation of biodegradable devices [12, 34, 35] (Fig. 3). As a limitation, this animal model prevents the assessment of vesicoureteral reflux by means of a voiding cystourethrography; which can be examined via a simulated voiding cystourethrography [27, 36] (Fig. 4). Histological analysis may be performed for the analysis of biocompatibility, tissue damage and more specifically, of the ureteral healing provided with the stents [34, 36, 37]. In addition, intravesical and renal pressures in stented ureters have also been measured, as well as ureteral peristalsis and contractility [29, 38, 39]. Research on urinary stents in the porcine species is generally performed on healthy intact models. However, pigs may undergo the surgical and pharmacological induction of pathologic features such as ureteral strictures and urolithiasis [31, 35, 40].

Fig. 2 Ultrasonographic assessment of the hydronephrosis degrees in a porcine model of obstructive uropathy

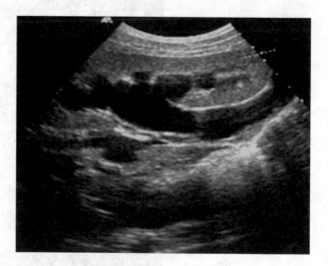

Fig. 3 Retrograde ureteropyelography of the proximal ureter, renal pelvis and calyxes of a healthy porcine model. The use of radiologic catheters with radiopaque marks enables the measurement of upper urinary tract dimensions and perform a follow-up of their development

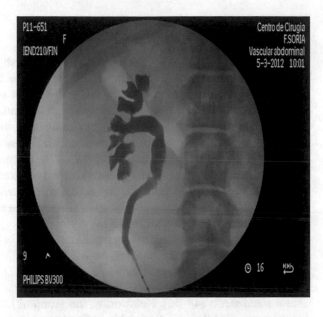

Fig. 4 Simulated voiding cystourethrography in a porcine model stented with a double-j ureteral stent. *Vesicoureteral reflux reaches the lumbar ureter

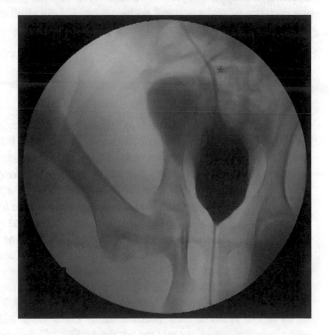

2.2   Canine Model

The validation of urethral and prostatic stents is generally not performed on pigs, given the particularities of male porcine urethra and the anatomical differences of the accessory sex glands [22]. The dog has proven to be an adequate model for the study of prostate diseases, as it develops benign prostatic hyperplasia (BPH) and prostate cancer both spontaneously and experimentally induced [41, 42]. Metallic, covered, drug-eluting and biodegradable urethral stents have been assessed in healthy and in BPH induced canine models, via transurethral insertion [43–45]. Urethral diameter is measured by means of a retrograde urethrography, which enables the monitoring of position, expansion, patency and migration of the stents [44–46]. Besides, histological evaluation is also included for the follow-up of stent-related urethral damage and urothelial hyperplasia [44, 47]. Nevertheless, the use of urodynamic studies for testing the therapeutic response in BPH canine models does not seem reliable as, unlike humans, canine hyperplastic prostate produces rectal obstruction rather than lower urinary tract symptoms [42].

The canine model has occasionally been chosen for the evaluation of biodegradable ureteral stents [48–50]. Noteworthy, the group of Lumiaho et al., tested their first prototypes of their biodegradable ureteral stent in dogs, placing them with an open surgical approach [49, 50]. The analysis of renal function, ureteral patency and the presence of vesicoureteral reflux are carried out similarly to the methodology in pigs, in addition to renograms [48–50].

2.3   Rat Model

Smaller laboratory animals, such as rabbits and rats, provide the advantages of easier handling, are more cost effective and require less infrastructure and logistics [40]. Unlike porcine and canine models, whose dimensions and anatomy allow the evaluation of the urinary stents that will be tested in future clinical trials, the devices inserted on rabbits and rats may differ from the definitive prototype under development. Small laboratory animals are therefore of great use for the assessment of stent upgrades including biomaterials, coatings and the release of substances [51, 52].

As for the rat model, it enables the analysis of the antimicrobial and anti-encrustation potential of new stents, since urolithiasis and urinary tract infection (UTI) can be experimentally induced in a controlled manner [40, 52]. UTI models are performed by the intravesical instillation of bacterial suspensions, being the most common *S. aureus*, *E. faecalis* and *P. aeruginosa* [52–54]. The induction of urolithiasis in rats to promote stent encrustation is carried out with dietary manipulations, gastrointestinal resections and the administration of lithogenic agents [40]. These animals are often chosen for the validation of both urethral and ureteral stents. Ureteral stents are inserted through a cystotomy in either the bladder or the ureter [51, 55, 56]. Besides the evaluation of the device's performance, when placed in the ureter, uretero-ureteral anastomosis may also be performed for the histological analysis of ureteral healing and scarring processes [13, 55, 56]. Urethral stents are tested in the bladder and the urethra, and depending on stent size and characteristics, transurethral placement may be feasible [57–59]. The rat's urethra allows the detection, as well as the histological analysis, of injuries during stent placement and the development of urethral strictures secondary to fibrotic and hyperplastic tissue formation [59].

2.4 Rabbit Model

The rabbit has been used for biocompatibility studies of stent materials. To this end, stent samples can be inserted in the muscle by blunt dissection, preferably the dorsal muscle to prevent the animal from self-mutilation [60]. The scientific literature regarding urinary stent validation in this animal model is scarce, probably due to the significant differences between rabbit's and human's urine composition [61]. The potential of biomaterials and drug-release against stent-related urinary tract infections has been assessed by transurethral intravesical placement of ureteral stent samples, for the performance of microbiological cultures and histological analysis [62, 63]. The rabbit's urethra enables the evaluation of urethral and prostatic stents, including placement, degradation of materials, therapeutic success and histology in both healthy and urethral stricture models [64, 65].

3 Guidelines for Animal Research

Finally, for reporting animal research, it is recommended to follow the ARRIVE guidelines [66]. These guidelines have been developed to ensure that studies involving live animals follow methodological rigour, are reported in enough detail and enable reproducibility. This tool is primarily aimed for the writing and revision of scientific publications. However, they are also valuable for study planning and conducting, as they help researchers to design rigorous and reliable *in vivo* experiments, minimize bias and to record important information about study methods. Besides, ethical review boards, funders, institutions and learned societies may rely on them to help promote best practice and ensure rigorous design and transparent reporting of *in vivo* preclinical research [66].

References

1. Kram W, Buchholz N, Hakenberg OW. Ureteral stent encrustation. Pathophysiology. Arch Esp Urol. 2016;69(8):485–93.
2. Novick A, Szilard L. Description of the chemostat. Science. 1950;112(2920):715–6.
3. Finlayson B, Dubois L. Kinetics of calcium oxalate deposition in vitro. Investig Urol. 1973;10(6):429–33.
4. Gilmore BF, et al. Models for the assessment of biofilm and encrustation formation on urological materials. In Biomaterials and tissue engineering in urology. Sawston: Woodhead Publishing; 2009. p. 59–81.

5. Gilmore BF, et al. Validation of the CDC biofilm reactor as a dynamic model for assessment of encrustation formation on urological device materials. J Biomed Mater Res Part B Appl Biomater. 2010;93(1):128–40.
6. Azeredo J, et al. Critical review on biofilm methods. Crit Rev Microbiol. 2017;43(3):313–51.
7. Hesse A, et al. Study on the prevalence and incidence of urolithiasis in Germany comparing the years 1979 vs. 2000. Eur Urol. 2003;44(6):709–13.
8. Chow K, et al. A stone farm: development of a method for simultaneous production of multiple calcium oxalate stones in vitro. Urol Res. 2004;32(1):55–60.
9. Mosayyebi A, et al. Reducing deposition of encrustation in ureteric stents by changing the stent architecture: a microfluidic-based investigation. Biomicrofluidics. 2019;13(1):014101.
10. Buhmann MT, et al. Encrustations on ureteral stents from patients without urinary tract infection reveal distinct urotypes and a low bacterial load. Microbiome. 2019;7(1):60.
11. Lumiaho J, Heino A, Pietilainen T, Ala-Opas M, Talja M, Valimaa T, et al. The morphological, in situ effects of a self-reinforced bioabsorbable polylactide (SR-PLA 96) ureteric stent; an experimental study. J Urol. 2000;164:1360–3.
12. Barros AA, Oliveira C, Ribeiro AJ, Autorino R, Reis RL, Duarte ARC, et al. In vivo assessment of a novel biodegradable ureteral stent. World J Urol. 2018;36:277–83.
13. Kram W, Rebl H, Wyrwa R, Laube T, Zimpfer A, Maruschke M, et al. Paclitaxel-coated stents to prevent hyperplastic proliferation of ureteral tissue: from in vitro to in vivo. Urolithiasis. 2020;48(1):47–56.
14. De Angelis I, Ricceri L, Vitale A. The 3R principle: 60 years taken well. Preface. Annali dell'Istituto superiore di sanita. 2019;55:398–9.
15. Tjärnström E, Weber EM, Hultgren J, Röcklinsberg H. Emotions and ethical decision-making in animal ethics committees. Animals. 2018;8(10):1–19.
16. European Commission. Directive 2010/63/EU of the European Parliament and of the Council of 22 September 2010 on the protection of animals used for scientific purposes. Brussels: European Union; 2010.
17. Hansen LA, Goodman JR, Chandna A. Analysis of animal research ethics committee membership at American institutions. Animals. 2012;2(1):68–75.
18. Roberts J. The urinary system. In: Fiennes RN, editor. Pathology of simian primates part I: general pathology. London: Karger; 1972. p. 821–40.
19. Crisóstomo Ayala V, Maynar Moliner M, Sun F, Usón Gargallo J, Sánchez Margallo FM. Ultrasonographic histological study on the evolution of a canine model of hormone-induced benign prostatic hyperplasia. Actas Urol Esp. 2009;33(8):895–901.
20. Pereira-Sampaio MA, Favorito LA, Sampaio FJB. Pig kidney: anatomical relationships between the intrarenal arteries and the kidney collecting system. Applied study for urological research and surgical training. J Urol. 2004;172:2077–81.
21. Cullen-McEwen L, Sutherland MR, Black MJ. The human kidney: parallels in structure, spatial development, and timing of nephrogenesis. In Kidney development, disease, repair and regeneration. Amsterdam: Elsevier Inc.; 2015. p. 27–40.
22. Swindle M, Smith AC. Comparative anatomy and physiology of the pig. Scand J Lab Anim Sci. 1998;23:1–10.
23. Sampaio FJ, Pereira-Sampaio MA, Favorito LA. The pig kidney as an endourologic model: anatomic contribution. J Endourol. 1998;12:45–50.
24. Sachs DH. The pig as a potential xenograft donor. Vet Immunol Immunopathol. 1994;43(1–3):185–91.
25. Tunc L, Resorlu B, Unsal A, Oguz U, Diri A, Gozen AS, et al. In vivo porcine model for practicing retrograde intrarenal surgery. Urol Int. 2014;92(1):64–7.
26. Soria F, Rioja LA, Blas M, Durán E, Usón J. Evaluation of the duration of ureteral stenting following endopyelotomy: animal study. Int J Urol. 2006;13:1333–8.

27. Lumiaho J, Heino A, Aaltomaa S, Vålimaa T, Talja M. A short biodegradable helical spiral ureteric stent provides better antireflux and drainage properties than a double-J stent. Scand J Urol Nephrol. 2011;45:129–33.
28. Liatsikos EN, Karnabatidis D, Kagadis GC, Katsakiori PF, Stolzenburg J-U, Nikiforidis GC, et al. Metal stents in the urinary tract. EAU-EBU Update Ser. 2007;5(2):77–88. https://doi.org/10.1016/j.eeus.2006.11.003.
29. Venkatesh R, Landman J, Minor SD, Lee DI, Rehman J, Vanlangendonck R, et al. Impact of a double-pigtail stent on ureteral peristalsis in the porcine model: initial studies using a novel implantable magnetic sensor. J Endourol. 2005;19:170–6.
30. Seitz C, Liatsikos E, Porpiglia F, Tiselius H-G, Zwergel U. Medical therapy to facilitate the passage of stones: what is the evidence? Eur Urol. 2009;56:455–71.
31. Soria F, Morcillo E, Serrano A, Budía A, Fernandez I, Fernández-Aparicio T, et al. Evaluation of a new design of antireflux-biodegradable ureteral stent in animal model. Urology. 2018;115:59–64.
32. Soria F, Morcillo E, Pamplona M, Uson J, Sanchez-Margallo FM. Evaluation in an animal model of a hybrid covered metallic ureteral stent: a new design. Urology. 2013;81:458–63.
33. Soria F, de La Cruz JE, Fernandez T, Budia A, Serrano Á, Sanchez-Margallo FM. Heparin coating in biodegradable ureteral stents does not decrease bacterial colonization-assessment in ureteral stricture endourological treatment in animal model. Transl Androl Urol. 2021;10(4):1700–10.
34. Chew BH, Paterson RF, Clinkscales KW, Levine BS, Shalaby SW, Lange D. In vivo evaluation of the third generation biodegradable stent: a novel approach to avoiding the forgotten stent syndrome. J Urol. 2013;189:719–25.
35. Soria F, de La Cruz JE, Budia A, Cepeda M, Álvarez S, Serrano Á, et al. Iatrogenic ureteral injury treatment with biodegradable antireflux heparin-coated ureteral stent—animal model comparative study. J Endourol. 2021;35(8):1244–9.
36. Soria F, de la Cruz JE, Budía A, Serrano A, Galán-Llopis JA, Sánchez-Margallo FM. Experimental assessment of new generation of ureteral stents: biodegradable and antireflux properties. J Endourol. 2020;34:359–65.
37. Soria F, Delgado MI, Rioja LA, Blas M, Pamplona M, Durán E, et al. Ureteral double-J wire stent effectiveness after endopyelotomy: an animal model study. Urol Int. 2010;85:314–9.
38. Janssen C, Buttyan R, Seow CY, Jäger W, Solomon D, Fazli L, et al. A role for the hedgehog effector Gli1 in mediating stent-induced ureteral smooth muscle dysfunction and aperistalsis. Urology. 2017;104:242.e1–8.
39. Johnson LJ, Davenport D, Venkatesh R. Effects of alpha-blockade on ureteral peristalsis and intrapelvic pressure in an in vivo stented porcine model. J Endourol. 2016;30:417–21.
40. Tzou DT, Taguchi K, Chi T, Stoller ML. Animal models of urinary stone disease. Int J Surg. 2016;36:596–606. https://doi.org/10.1016/j.ijsu.2016.11.018.
41. Sun F, Báez-Díaz C, Sánchez-Margallo FM. Canine prostate models in preclinical studies of minimally invasive interventions: Part I, canine prostate anatomy and prostate cancer models. Transl Androl Urol. 2017;6(3):538–46.
42. Sun F, Báez-Díaz C, Sánchez-Margallo FM. Canine prostate models in preclinical studies of minimally invasive interventions: Part II, benign prostatic hyperplasia models. Transl Androl Urol. 2017;6(3):547–55.
43. Yoon CJ, Song H-Y, Kim JH, Park HG, Kang HS, Ro J-Y, et al. Temporary placement of a covered, retrievable, barbed stent for the treatment of hormone-induced benign prostatic hyperplasia: technical feasibility and histologic changes in canine prostates. J Vasc Interv Radiol. 2010;21(9):1429–35.
44. Han K, Park J-H, Yang S-G, Lee DH, Tsauo J, Kim KY, et al. EW-7197 eluting nano-fiber covered self-expandable metallic stent to prevent granulation tissue formation in a canine urethral model. PLoS One. 2018;13(2):e0192430.

45. Park J-H, Song H-Y, Shin JH, Kim JH, Jun EJ, Cho YC, et al. Polydioxanone biodegradable stent placement in a canine urethral model: analysis of inflammatory reaction and biodegradation. J Vasc Interv Radiol. 2014;25(8):1257–64.
46. Lee JH, Kim SW, Il YB, Ha U-S, Sohn DW, Cho Y-H. Factors that affect nosocomial catheter-associated urinary tract infection in intensive care units: 2-year experience at a single center. Korean J Urol. 2013;54(1):59–65.
47. Wang C-J, Huang S-W, Chang C-H. Effects of specific alpha-1A/1D blocker on lower urinary tract symptoms due to double-J stent: a prospectively randomized study. Urol Res. 2009;37:147–52.
48. Li G, Wang Z-X, Fu W-J, Hong B-F, Wang X-X, Cao L, et al. Introduction to biodegradable polylactic acid ureteral stent application for treatment of ureteral war injury. BJU Int. 2011;108:901–6.
49. Lumiaho J, Heino A, Tunninen V, Ala-Opas M, Talja M, Valimaa T, et al. New bioabsorbable polylactide ureteral utent in the treatment of ureteral lesions: an experimental study. J Endourol. 1999;13:107–12.
50. Lumiaho J, Heino A, Kauppinen T, Talja M, Alhava E, Valimaa T, et al. Drainage and anti-reflux characteristics of a biodegradable self-reinforced, self-expanding X-ray-positive poly-L,D-lactide spiral partial ureteral stent: an experimental study. J Endourol. 2007;21:1559–64.
51. Hildebrandt P, Sayyad M, Rzany A, Schaldach M, Seiter H. Prevention of surface encrustation of urological implants by coating with inhibitors. Biomaterials. 2001;22(5):503–7.
52. Wang X, Cai Y, Xing H, Wu W, Wang G, Li L, et al. Increased therapeutic efficacy of combination of azithromycin and ceftazidime on Pseudomonas aeruginosa biofilm in an animal model of ureteral stent infection. BMC Microbiol. 2016;16(1):124. https://doi.org/10.1186/s12866-016-0744-1.
53. Cirioni O, Silvestri C, Ghiselli R, Kamysz W, Minardi D, Castelli P, et al. In vitro and in vivo effects of sub-MICs of pexiganan and imipenem on Pseudomonas aeruginosa adhesion and biofilm development. Le Infez Med. 2013;21(4):287–95.
54. Minardi D, Cirioni O, Ghiselli R, Silvestri C, Mocchegiani F, Gabrielli E, et al. Efficacy of tigecycline and rifampin alone and in combination against enterococcus faecalis biofilm infection in a rat model of ureteral stent. J Surg Res. 2012;176:1–6.
55. Maruschke M, Kram W, Nebe JB, Vollmar B, Zimpfer A, Hakenberg OW. Development of a rat model for investigation of experimental splinted uretero-ureterostomy, ureteral stenting and stenosis. In Vivo. 2013;27(2):245–9.
56. Wang T, Yu Z, Chen C, Song Y, Zeng X, Su Y, et al. Ureteral anastomosis with a polyimide stent in rat kidney transplantation. Ren Fail. 2020;42:193–9.
57. Lim KS, Jeong MH, Bae IH, Park JK, Park DS, Kim JM, et al. Effect of polymer-free TiO$_2$ stent coated with abciximab or alpha lipoic acid in porcine coronary restenosis model. J Cardiol. 2014;64(5):409–18. https://doi.org/10.1016/j.jjcc.2014.02.015.
58. Park J-H, Kim T-H, Cho YC, Bakheet N, Lee SO, Kim S-H, et al. Balloon-expandable biodegradable stents versus self-expandable metallic stents: a comparison study of stent-induced tissue hyperplasia in the rat urethra. Cardiovasc Interv Radiol. 2019;42(9):1343–51.
59. Kim KY, Park J-H, Kim DH, Tsauo J, Kim MT, Son W-C, et al. Sirolimus-eluting biodegradable poly-l-lactic acid stent to suppress granulation tissue formation in the rat urethra. Radiology. 2018;286(1):140–8.
60. Wang X, Zhang L, Chen Q, Hou Y, Hao Y, Wang C, et al. A nanostructured degradable ureteral stent fabricated by electrospinning for upper urinary tract reconstruction. J Nanosci Nanotechnol. 2015;15:9899–904.
61. Block WD, Hubbard RW. Amino acid content of rabbit urine and plasma. Arch Biochem Biophys. 1962;96:557–61.
62. Fung LCT, Mittelman MW, Thorner PS, Khoury AE. A novel rabbit model for the evaluation of biomaterial associated urinary tract infection. Can J Urol. 2003;10(5):2007–12.

63. Cadieux PA, Chew BH, Knudsen BE, DeJong K, Rowe E, Reid G, et al. Triclosan loaded ureteral stents decrease *Proteus mirabilis* 296 infection in a rabbit urinary tract infection model.
J Urol. 2006;175:2331–5.
64. Fu W-J, Zhang B-H, Gao J-P, Hong B-F, Zhang L, Yang Y, et al. Biodegradable urethral stent
in the treatment of post-traumatic urethral strictures in a war wound rabbit urethral model.
Biomed Mater. 2007;2(4):263–8. https://doi.org/10.1088/1748-6041/2/4/009.
65. Kotsar A, Isotalo T, Mikkonen J, Juuti H, Martikainen PM, Talja M, et al. A new biodegradable
braided self-expandable PLGA prostatic stent: an experimental study in the rabbit. J Endourol.
2008;22(5):1065–9.
66. du Sert NP, Hurst V, Ahluwalia A, Alam S, Avey MT, Baker M, et al. The arrive guidelines 2.0:
updated guidelines for reporting animal research. PLoS Biol. 2020;18(7):1–12.

Methodology on Clinical Evaluation of Urinary Stents

Maja Sofronievska Glavinov, Sotir Stavridis, Senad Bajramovic, and Stefan Arsov

1 Introduction

In the framework of COST CA16217 "European Network of multidisciplinary research to improve the Urinary Stents (ENIUS)", WG3 group worked on the validation of protocols for new stent designs. In this chapter, we address a methodology on clinical evaluation of urinary stents as well as the importance of clinical data and patients' feedback regarding urinary stents.

This methodology is meant to provide guidance on clinical aspects of urinary stent development, thus assisting all stakeholders in innovation and improvement of new stents designs during clinical investigation in both, pre- and post-market evaluation.

In addition, as part of the methodology for urinary stents development, we were also focused to effective determination of any undesirable side effects that can appear in stented patients. That is the reason we performed analysis of all tools developed in order to obtain and deliver such information from the patients who underwent urinary stent placement and suggest a newer approach in obtaining this feedback through The Urinary Stent Related Health (UriSteRH) questionnaire (Table 1).

M. Sofronievska Glavinov (✉)
University Surgical Clinic "St.Naum Ohridski", Skopje, Republic of North Macedonia

S. Stavridis
University Clinic of Urology, Clinical Complex "Mother Theresa",
Skopje, Republic of North Macedonia

S. Bajramovic
Clinical Center University of Sarajevo, Sarajevo, Bosnia and Herzegovina

S. Arsov
Center for Public Health, Skopje, Republic of North Macedonia

© The Author(s) 2022   173
F. Soria et al. (eds.), *Urinary Stents*,
https://doi.org/10.1007/978-3-031-04484-7_15

Table 1 The Urinary Stent Related Health (UriSteRH) questionnaire

COST Action CA 16
ID

ENIUS (European Network of Multidisciplinary Reaserch to Imrove the Urinary stents

Urinary Stent Related Health (UriSteRH)

* 1. Age

☐ <20   ☐ 20-29   ☐ 30-39   ☐ 40-49   ☐ 50-59   ☐ > 60

☐ Other (please specify)

* 2. Gender

☐ Male   ☐ Female

* 3. Type of urinary stent

☐ J-J polymer

☐ J-J silicone

☐ Metallic ureter stent

☐ Folley catheter - latex

☐ Folley catheter - silicone

☐ Thieman catheter - latex

☐ Thieman catheter - silicone

☐ Metallic prostate stent

☐ Other (please specify)

*4. Time after stent implantation

☐ 24 hours   ☐ 1 week   ☐ 1 month   ☐ 3 months   ☐ Other (please specify)____

*5. Rate pain (suprapubic or flank) after stent placement.

No pain, excellent	Mild, bothersome	Moderate, tolerable	Severe, bad	Extreme, intolerable
1	2	3	4	5

Table 1 (continued)

*6. Rate pain during voiding after stent placement

No pain, excellent	Mild, bothersome	Moderate, tolerable	Severe, bad	Extreme, intolerable
1	2	3	4	5

*7. Rate your Social life (cinema,theatre,shopping etc) after stent placement

Excellent	Good	Tolerable	Bad	Unsatisfactory
1	2	3	4	5

*8. Rate mood and sleep disturbances (depression, anxiety, insomnia)

No disturbances, Excellent	Mild, bothersome	Moderate, tolerable	Severe, bad	Extreme, intolerable
1	2	3	4	5

*9. Rate your sexual activity after stent placement (if any)

Excellent	Good	Satisfactory	Not Satisfactory	Disabled	N/A
1	2	3	4	5	☐

*10. Rate your physical activity (walking, running, biking, driving etc.) after stent placement

Excellent	Good	Satisfactory	Not Satisfactory	Disabled	N/A
1	2	3	4	5	☐

*11. Rate your Quality of life after stent placement (subjective perception)

Excellent	Good	Tolerable	Bad	Unsatisfactory
1	2	3	4	5

2   Background

Urinary stents are used to alleviate obstruction along the urinary tract and prevent its complications, either as a temporary or a definitive treatment. There are stents for the upper urinary tract (ureteric stents) and for the lower urinary tract (urethral stents and catheters).

There are mandatory and relative indications for urinary stent placement. Mandatory relief of obstruction is indicated in obstructed pyelonephritis, bilateral ureteral obstruction with anuria, obstruction of a solitary functioning kidney, ureteric injuries, and post-operatively in some cases for the upper urinary tract, and for acute urinary retention for the lower urinary tract. Relative indications include the relief of pain associated with ureteral obstruction, relief of renal colic during pregnancy, significant ureteral edema after ureteroscopy, or anticipated ureteral obstruction from stone fragments during shockwave lithotripsy [1, 2].

Urinary stents have numerous side-effects affecting the patient both, physically and psychologically. Ideal or near ideal stent designs and models should aim to minimize these side effects and be as much tolerable, safe, and efficacious as possible [3, 4].

3   Clinical Evaluation in Urinary Stents Improvement

After evaluating the available evidence, we concluded that in order to assess whether a device is fit for purpose(s) and suitable for the patient population(s) it is intended for, there are two crucial steps needed for a clinical investigation:

to verify whether the stent in accordance with clinical guidelines for stent implantation and the manufacturer's instructions is fit for purpose, and

to determine any side effects following clinical guidelines for stent implantation and the manufacturer's instructions of use, and assess the risk—benefit balance for the stent under its intended use.

4   Design of Clinical Investigation(s)

The design of any clinical investigation must be based on the claims made by the manufacturer and, as part of the demonstration of compliance, with the essential requirements of the medical device directive (MDD) [5, 6]. Undoubtedly, controlled randomized studies are best suited to confirm or deny claims made by the manufacturer. Randomized-comparative studies are required to demonstrate the risk-benefit profile of the stents. Studies must include enough patients to allow assessment of the primary performance and safety end-points specified in the clinical investigation plan, with a 95% confidence interval [7]. Several criteria need to be met to conduct reliable studies with clear and valuable end-points:

Criteria for population selection in clinical investigations.
Criteria for duration of the clinical investigation.
Criteria for analysis of Quality of Life (QoL).
Criteria for post market clinical follow-up.

5 Population Selection in Clinical Investigations

It is important for the study population selection that there are well-defined eligibility criteria, considering the safety and performance claims and any other future marketing claims. Criteria such as site, length and type of the obstruction, ureteral or urethral diameter, and risk factors including but not limited to infection, previous instrumentation, and other defined conditions must be applied. All patients should be on well-defined medically recommended prophylaxis and/or therapy unless otherwise justified.

The number of patients to be enrolled should not only be based on a sound scientific rationale, but also on statistical calculations to support the hypotheses.

6 Duration of the Clinical Investigation

Timelines for an acceptable evaluation of the performance and safety will depend upon the characteristics of a urinary stent as well as the urinary pathologies and/or medical conditions for which it is intended. Timelines must always be justified. Appropriate endpoints must also take into consideration the time-frame around possible complications. Moreover, a long-term follow-up should be performed, and a post market clinical follow-up should be considered unless there are good reasons not to.

7 Analysis of Quality of Life (QoL)

It is of utmost importance to achieve an acceptable QoL in patients that undergo urinary stent placement. Side-effects need to be quantified to evaluate their impact on QoL. Efforts have been made by Joshi et al. to develop a validated tool in the form of a questionnaire called USSQ that assesses patient comfort after stent placement [8]. It is endorsed in different languages and has been used in many comparative studies. Some authors concluded that USSQ is more relevant in long-term trials [9]. Along this whole process, a thorough literature review is necessary. The scientific literature in this area is highly focused and specific. Before setting up any such study protocol, it would be expected that a critical evaluation of available evidence is performed by a suitably qualified person [10].

Stents need to be re-designed to improve patient tolerance and minimize side-effects. Obtaining adequate feedback from the end-users, namely stented patients, is therefore very important. For that reason, we support the creation of specific questionnaires for the evaluation of QoL in patients with urinary stents.

However, existing questionnaires are ambiguous and cumbersome. We suggest such questionnaires should be composed of a maximum of 10 questions addressing discomfort, abdominal pain, pain during voiding (in upper urinary stents), mood disturbances, sleep disturbances, sexual life, social life, physical activities and subjective perception of QoL.

All these questions should be evaluated at certain well-defined time points depending on the type of stent.

8   Development of Urinary Stent Related Health (UriSteRH) Questionnaire

In order to achieve information about the tools and questionnaires used so far, we made a literature search in Google Scholar database. The search phrase used was "Quality of life questionnaire", period of publishing was set "all to 2020" and it disposed 4,250,000 articles. After introducing advanced search i.e., exact phrase "urinary stent symptoms", only 71 articles were disposed. Of them only 14 articles were related to the questionnaires that were analyzing urinary stents related symptoms and the data from the patients were obtained through SF-36, USSQ and IPSS questionnaire (Fig. 1).

Questionnaire for quality of life SF-36 (original or modified) can be used as an assessment form for quality of life of the patients in both types of urinary stents regarding the part of urinary tract they are introduced in. The results obtained by these questionnaires deliver information about the patients' satisfaction after stent or catheter introduction [11, 12]. However, this information cannot provide specific knowledge of urinary stents and catheters efficacy, safety and tolerance. A psychometrically valid measure to evaluate symptoms and impact on quality of life of ureteral stents was developed in the form of the ureteral stent symptom questionnaire (USSQ) [8].

The original English language Ureteral Stent Symptom Questionnaire (USSQ) has been validated in various languages worldwide. Still this questionnaire is related only to upper urinary tract stents and has its own advantages and disadvantages. Some authors concluded that USSQ is more relevant in long-term trials [9]. Both SF-36 and USSQ are paper-based questionnaires that have their own advantages and disadvantages. As the first one quantifies the patient's life on general basis, the

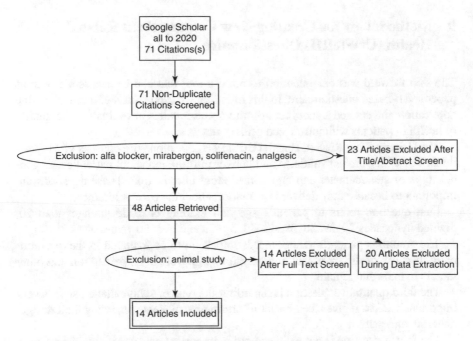

Fig. 1 PRISMA diagram of performed search of Google scholar database

second one is more specific and orients on patients with urinary stents. According to some experts in surveys and questionnaires development, it is best for a questionnaire to be as short as possible A long questionnaire leads to a long interview and this is open to the dangers of boredom on the part of the respondent (and poorly considered, hurried answers), interruptions by third parties and greater costs in terms of interviewing time and resources [13, 14].

The more reliable example of short and effective questionnaire is "The Satisfaction with Life Scale" (SWLS), developed to access an individual's cognitive judgment of their satisfaction with their life in general. The scale is a very simple, short questionnaire made up of only five statements [15].

It was our starting point to create a more specific variant of the questionnaire regarding patients with inserted urinary stents and catheters. In congruence with the World Health Organisation's definition of health, health-related quality of life refers to the overall conditions of the quality of life of ill or healthy individuals in accordance with the following eight domains: (1) limitations in physical activities because of health problems, (2) limitations in social activities because of physical or emotional problems, (3) limitations in role activities because of physical health problems, (4) bodily pain, (5) general mental health, (6) limitations in role activities because of emotional problems, (7) vitality, and (8) general health perceptions of an individual or a group measured in terms of feelings of satisfaction or dissatisfaction [16, 17].

9   Methodology for Creating New Urinary Stent Related Health (UriSteRH) Questionnaire

The step forward was our intention to build a tool that can be accessible both as paper and e-based questionnaire. In this intention we used "Survey Monkey" online application and created a short but specific questionnaire for evaluation the quality of health in patients with introduced urinary devices.

The Urinary Stent Related Health (UriSteRH) questionnaire consists of 11 questions, 4 of which are not validated and deliver information about patient's age, gender, type of stent/catheter and duration of stent introduction. These questions are important to because they deliver information about the patient him/herself.

First question refers to patient's age and grading is made younger than 20, divided in decades 20–29, 30–39, 40–49, 50–59 and over 60 years.

The second is patient's gender that is important to be included in the questionnaire, because of different anatomy, physiology, psychology, perception and other factors in male and female.

The third qualitative question is regarding the type of stent/catheter, so it is very important because it gives feed-back on certain type of stents regarding their design, material, and pattern.

The fourth question is not validated but is important because it obtain feed-back on the duration of stent/catheter introduction. Namely, the symptoms are not the same immediately after insertion and they tend to change in some manner after some time. We propose measurement of patients' stent related health after 24 h, 1 week, 1 month and 3 months.

Other seven questions in UriSteRH questionnaire are validated according Likert scale that in this case is a five-point scale which is used to allow the patient to make a numerical value which would be used to measure the attitude under investigation.

First two of these questions reveal to both suprapubic/flank and pain during voiding. Answers are graded such as 1 is no pain and 5 is extreme, intolerable pain.

The next question is related to patient's social life i.e. affection of urinary stent symptoms on social events (cinema, theatre, family matter events etc.) in patient's life. It is graded 1 for excellent social life a 5 for unsatisfactory social life.

Question number 8 quantifies patients' mood and sleep disturbances related to urinary stent symptoms. It is a very important question since patients with expressed symptoms become depressive, anxious and have sleep disturbances due to pain, frequency, and urgency.

Sexual activity has the important role in quality of life in stented patients and is evaluated in the questionnaire under number 9. The ratings include 1 for excellent activity to 5 for disabled. In the se we gave a N/A option for the patients that are not interested in answering.

As a question number 10 we introduced physical activity of stented patients regarding their everyday movement activities and hobbies, and we graded 1 for excellent activities and 5 for disabled. We also gave a N/A option for those patients that are not physically active (paraplegia, paresis etc.)

The last question (11) refer patient's subjective perception of the quality of life after stent placemen and it is graded 1 for excellent and 5 for extremely bad.

Total score classifies patients in three groups: score 5–13 = Good tolerance, satisfied patient, scores 14–24 = disturbing but tolerable, partially satisfied patient and score 25–35 = Bad tolerance, unsatisfied patient.

Regarding the total score and each question points, a correlation between the type of the stent, duration of its insertion and health repercussion can be obtained. These information are of great importance using as a patient feedback to inserted urinary stent or catheter.

10   Validation of UriSteRH Questionnaire

The questionnaire was evaluated by 15 urologists from North Macedonia in the network of Macedonian Urological Association of which 11 were male (73.3%) and 4 were female (26.7%), by nationality they were: 9 Macedonians (60%), 5 Albanians (33.3%) and one Turk (6.7%).

The questionnaire was translated from Macedonian and Bosnian to English language for the purposes of this report and language validation was done. Approval from the Ethical committee of Macedonian Urological Association was obtained in according to declaration from Helsinki in 1975, revised in Seoul 2008.

The questionnaire was evaluated by four domains

1. Relevance—does the questionnaire refer to the topic for which it is intended.
2. Availability—is the questionnaire easily available to the patients it is intended for.
3. Clarity—are the questions clearly defined without prejudicing the answer.
4. Design—does the questionnaire meet the needs of the examination after the initial examination, without quantification of the same.

For scoring a scale from 1 to 5 was used, 1 being the most negative and 5 the most positive characteristics score. The questionnaire received a perfect score of 5.0 by all 15 urologists regarding clarity, relevance, and design, where as a score of 4.67 ± 0.49 regarding availability, receiving a score of 4 by 5 urologists and score of 5 by 10. There were no significant differences in the scoring by gender and nationality of the evaluators. A correlation matrix and linear regression analysis could not be calculated due to 3 of 4 scoring characteristics being constants.

The validation of questionnaire was evaluated by 27 urologists from Bosnia and Herzegovina in the network of Urological Association of Federation of Bosnia and Herzegovina of which 25 were male and two were female.

Approval from the Ethical committee of Urologic Association of Federation of Bosnia and Herzegovina was obtained in according to declaration from Helsinki in 1975, revised in Seoul 2008.

Results of validation of questionnaire in Bosnia and Herzegovina was as the questionnaire received a perfect score of 5.0 by all 27 urologists regarding clarity and relevance, where as a score 4.73 ± 0.27 regarding availability and for design as 4.74 ± 0.26.

The statistical analysis was performed using IBM SPSS Statistics 20.0, Armonk, NY, U.S.

11 Post-Market Follow Up

A post market clinical follow-up is important for urinary implants to evaluate their long-term safety. Such a program must be planned and can take the form of a clinical investigation and/or registry where data obtained from the patients' feed-back are collected.

12 Discussion and Elaboration

The UriSteRH questionnaire is an easily accessible questionnaire related to patients with introduced urinary stents that can be distributed both as paper and e-based questionnaire. It is made according the World Health Organization's definition of health-related quality of life that refers to the overall conditions of the quality of life of ill or healthy individuals in accordance with the domains regarding bodily pain, limitations in physical activities because of health problems, limitations in social activities, general mental health, vitality (expressed throughout sexual life) and general health perceptions of an individual or a group measured in terms of feelings of satisfaction or dissatisfaction. These questions comply with the methodological guideline for closed-ended questions [17–19].

A short overview of each of the seven health-related quality of life dimensions assessed by the questionnaire is in accordance with WHO definitions.

1. Bodily pain (flank and/or abdominal): The scores on this dimension indicate to what extent the respondents' experience of bodily pain hinders their performance of daily activities, including work-related duties in the public domain and tasks within the home environment.
2. Related pain to voiding: The scores on this dimension indicate to what extent the respondents' experience the micturition pain that affects their satisfaction and disturb their daily activities and overnight rest.
3. Physical functioning and physical roles limitation: The scores on the physical functioning domain scale indicate the extent to which the respondents' perceptions of their quality of life are influenced by their physical condition. In the first place, physical functioning refers to the extent to which the respondents

can perform vigorous activities such as running, lifting heavy objects, participating in strenuous sports, climbing several flights of stairs and walking more
than a kilometer. In the second place, it entails the performance of moderate
activities such as bending, kneeling, or stooping, bathing, and dressing themselves. This dimension also refers to the extent to which respondents' performance of their roles in daily activities is impeded by their physical state of
health. For example, their ability to perform vigorous activities such lifting
heavy objects or to perform moderate activities such as moving a table or pushing a vacuum cleaner.

4. Social functioning refers to social activities and interaction with significant others such as family members, friends, neighbors, and other social relations.
5. The mental health dimension and psychology alterations of the respondent is measured in terms of the extent to which he/she is inter alia feeling full of pep, is
   happy, is feeling calm and peaceful, is very nervous, or is feeling worn out and tired.
6. The vitality dimension relates to the respondent's experience of feeling energetic
   and sexually active.
7. The perception of an individuals' general health is measured in terms of concepts such as excellent, very good, good, fair or poor, getting ill easier than other
   people, and just as healthy as anyone he/she knows.

Prior to the assessment of an individual's health-related quality of life, he/she
must be informed about and assured of several things. This information and assur-
ance can be verbally given by the fieldworker and includes the following:

- It must be clearly stated that, by completing the questionnaire, the respondent
  will be participating in research.
- The purpose of the research must be explained.
- An outline of the procedures of the research must be given.
- The respondent must be assured that the completion of the questionnaire is
  voluntary.
- It must be stated that the privacy of the respondents is preserved through ano-
  nymity and that no-one would be able to relate a given response to a given
  respondent.
- The respondent must be assured that the use of the data will be strictly
  confidential.
- It must be stated that the results will be reported accurately and that all shortcom-
  ings in the research, such as errors and limitations, will be disclosed [20].

13 Conclusion

As final part of the methodology on clinical evaluation of urinary stents, we suggest
definition of stent-related and procedure-related success endpoints. Such stent-
related endpoints should include but are not limited to successful delivery of the
stent bypassing the obstruction site, appropriate cuff expansion (in lower urinary
tract stents), appropriate stent deployment, successful removal of any delivery

system (if applicable) after correct stent placement and safe removal of the device in case of deployment failure.

Procedure related endpoints may include the above with additional criteria related to the clinical outcome of the procedure with the use of both, stents that are used only for diagnostic (short-term) and therapeutic purposes (longer indwelling time). We recommend choosing and defining well all necessary endpoints which may vary depending on the type of stent and the procedure it was used in.

In order to obtain feedback from patients with urinary stents, we need specific and good tools in the form of questionnaires who can quantify both, patients' safety and satisfaction with urinary stents/catheters. Any such data gathered from clinical practice should be used to establish clinical safety and fed back into the device labelling performance by manufacturers. The value of measuring patients' experiences of their health-related quality after introduction of urinary stent/catheter by making use of the UriSteRH questionnaire, is comprehensive.

The final goal of the clinical methodology is to identify specific problems, stent-health-related quality of life indicator. Based on these findings, interventions in stent design can then be done in order to improve individuals' quality of life. In that manner, the accessibility of the UriSteRH questionnaire allows more patients to be followed up and fourthly very quick presentation of results in electronic based distribution is enabled.

References

1. Sali GM, Joshi HB. Ureteric stents: overview of current clinical applications and economic implications. Int J Urol. 2020;27(1):7–15.
2. Oliver R, Wells H, Traxer O, Knoll T, Aboumarzouk O, Biyani CS, Somani BK, YAU Group. Ureteric stents on extraction strings: a systematic review of literature. Urolithiasis. 2018;46(2):129–36.
3. Al-Aown A, Kyriazis I, Kallidonis P, Kraniotis P, Rigopoulos C, Karnabatidis D, Petsas T, Liatsikos E. Ureteral stents: new ideas, new designs. Ther Adv Urol. 2010;2(2):85–92.
4. Tolley D. Ureteric stents, far from ideal. Lancet. 2000;356(9233):872–3.
5. Markiewicz K, van Til JA, IJzerman, M.J. Medical devices early assessment methods: systematic literature review. Int J Technol Assess Health Care. 2014;30(2):137–46.
6. Byrne RA, Serruys PW, Baumbach A, Escaned J, Fajadet J, James S, et al. Report of a European Society of Cardiology-European Association of Percutaneous Cardiovascular Interventions task force on the evaluation of coronary stents in Europe: executive summary. Eur Heart J. 2015;36:2608–20.
7. Nguyen T, Dave V, Jia S, Fang C, Wang L, Zhang C, Nguyen J, Fearnot N, Saito S. Practical clinical evaluation of stents. J Interv Cardiol. 1998;11:101–10.
8. Joshi HB, Newns N, Stainthorpe A, MacDonagh RP, Keeley FX Jr, Timoney AG. Ureteral stent symptom questionnaire: development and validation of a multidimensional quality of life measure. J Urol. 2003;169(3):1060–4.
9. Lingeman JE, Preminger GM, Goldfischer ER, Krambeck AE. Assessing the impact of ureteral stent design on patient comfort. J Urol. 2009;181:2581–7.
10. Park J, Kim E, Shin K. Developing an evaluation framework for selecting optimal medical devices. J Open Innov Technol Mark Complexity. 2019;5:64.
11. Jenkinson C, Coulter A, Wright L. Short form 36 (SF36) health survey questionnaire: normative data for adults of working age. BMJ. 1993;306:1437–40.

12. Ware J, Sherbourne C. The MOS 36-item short-form health survey (SF-36). I. Conceptual framework and item selection. Med Care. 1992;30:473–83.
13. Babbie E. The basics of social research. Belmont: Wadsworth; 2002.
14. Berg BL. Qualitative research methods for the social sciences. Boston: Allyn & Bacon; 1998.
15. Diener E, Emmons R, Larsen R, Griffin S. The satisfaction with life scale. J Pers Assess. 1985;49(1):71–5.
16. Preamble to the Constitution of the World Health Organization as adopted by the International Health Conference, New York, 19–22 June, 1946; signed on 22 July 1946 by the representatives of 61 States (Official Records of the World Health Organization, no 2, p. 100) and entered into force on 7 April 1948.
17. The WHOQOL Group. The World Health Organization Quality of Life Assessment (WHOQOL). Development and psychometric properties. Soc Sci Med. 1998;46:1569–85.
18. Frisch MB. Quality of life therapy and assessment in health care. Clin Psychol Sci Pract. 1998;5:19–40.
19. Baker F, Intagliata J. Quality of life in the evaluation of community support systems. Eval Program Plann. 1982;5:6–79.
20. Andersen ML, Taylor HF. Sociology: the essentials. Belmont: Wadsworth; 2002.

A Dynamically Degradable Surface: Can We *'Fool'* Bacteria to Delay Biofouling in Urinary Stents?

Syed A. M. Tofail

1 Introduction

Human body has evolved multiple strategies such as the development of a complex immune system and procurement of commensal microorganisms to deal with detrimental invasion by microbes. Despite this, biofilms pose an extremely difficult mechanism for humans to cope with infections caused by both pathogenic and opportunistically pathogenic microorganisms.

Ureteral stents are deployed using minimally invasive procedures in patients to prevent or treat the blockage of the flow of urine during or after treating kidney stones, tumours or other urinary incontinence. Paradoxically, the surface of a stent also offers a breeding ground for the adhesion and colonisation by uropathogens that create biofilms.

Biofilms on these stents can lead to patient-discomfort, urinary tract infection and bacteriuria, antimicrobial resistance, stent fouling (encrustation) and obstruction. Ultimately, these stents may require extracorporeal shock wave lithotripsy, ureteroscopy or even more invasive techniques for removal. While an 'ideal' ureteral stent should be free from any such complications. There is no 'ideal' ureteral stents, however.

A 'perfect' ureteral stent should be well tolerated by the patient while ensuring optimal urine flow, resistance to infection, corrosion and encrustation. Prevention and treatment of biofilms are thus crucial for long-term patency of ureteral stents and similar indwelling devices. 'Real stents' seldom have these and may need extracorporeal shock wave lithotripsy, ureteroscopy or even more invasive techniques for removal. These post-stenting procedures cause patient trauma and add to the cost of healthcare.

S. A. M. Tofail (✉)
Department of Physics and Bernal Institute, University of Limerick, Limerick, Ireland
e-mail: Tofail.Syed@ul.ie

© The Author(s) 2022
F. Soria et al. (eds.), *Urinary Stents*,
https://doi.org/10.1007/978-3-031-04484-7_16

One of the major problems associated with indwelling devices is that they present novel, non-host surfaces on which microbes can colonise and form biofilms. Biofilms, especially those formed in a nutrient-limiting environments, are complex, highly structured communities designed to maximise survival, reproduction and spread of the microorganism/s. The type of biofilm that will form largely depends on the properties of surface and the microorganism/s present, the ability of the surrounding milieu to support and inhibit the growth of microorganisms and the relationship the microorganisms have with each other. It is being now recognised that biofilm formation constitutes an 'intelligent' behaviour that involves cell-cell communication such as quorum sensing rather than a matter of a complex architecture. However, the complex three-dimensional architecture that biofilms often protects microorganisms from curative treatments e.g. through antimicrobial drugs.

Currently, biofilm prevention and treatment in ureteral stents are carried out using a 'static' coating of the stent with heparin or a pH control-buffer. They increase patency but still becomes colonised by bacteria leading to biofilms. In this chapter we outline a patent-pending first-principle design strategy for a stent-coating stents that has the potential of increasing the patency by manifold and, at will. This strategy involves delaying biofouling with a 'dynamically degradable surface' and will be described in this chapter.

2 The Surface, Biofilms and Response to Antibiotics

Microorganisms are long known as capable of attaching to and grow on surfaces exposed to them [1, 2]. Surface-associated microorganisms have exhibited a distinct phenotype with respect to gene transcription and growth rate when compared to their free-floating planktonic counterpart [3]. These adherent-microorganisms can elicit specific mechanisms for initial attachment to a surface, development of a community structure and ecosystem, and detachment [4].

A microbial biofilm can be broadly defined as microorganisms adherent to a surface and enveloped within a polymeric matrix, typically comprising exopolysaccharide and proteins that develops into a complex community. The composition is often heterogeneous with water channels occurring between matrix-enclosed microorganisms in stalk- or mushroom-like structures. The structure is also a dynamic one and may include single or multiple microbial species.

Biofilms have been identified in virtually every system in the human body especially involving mucosal surface. Indwelling devices for example artificial joints, urinary catheters and stents, heart valves, biliary stents are also highly susceptible to biofilm formation. In 2004, the Centres for Disease Control and Prevention (CDC) reported that approximately 65% of all infections in developed countries are caused by biofilms [5].

The growth of a biofilm almost always leads to a large increase in resistance to antimicrobial agents compared with cultures grown in suspension (planktonic) in conventional liquid media, with up to 1000-fold decreases in susceptibility. This poses a huge clinical problem as our current tools for fighting against infections are heavily dependent on the use of antimicrobial agents. The complex three-dimensional architecture of a biofilm, especially an extracellular polymer matrix with occasional biomineralisation makes it difficult to for antimicrobials to access the infection-causing microbes and destroy them.

Biofilms start with a conditioning film that leads to subsequent accumulation of organic and inorganic molecules [6–11]. The conditioning films alter the nature of the device surface and facilitate bacterial adhesion. After adhesion, the biofilm is formed by materials offered by the specific environment as well as extracellular polymeric substances produced by the microorganism. Bacteria can adhere to this initial biofilm and initiate the infection process.

Three mechanisms have been proposed to explain the general resistance of bio-films to antimicrobial agents [12, 13]:

the barrier properties of the slime matrix;

the creation of starved, stationary-phase dormant zones in biofilms; and

the existence of subpopulations of resistant phenotypes, which have been referred to as 'persisters'.

It is important to note that the eradication of infection by antibiotic treatment requires elimination of all the bacteria, typically assisted by the host defences. Specifically, biofilm-resistance can be determined by the susceptibility of the most resistant cells. The inhabitants of biofilms may be up to a thousand times more resistant to antimicrobial therapy than free-floating bacteria of the same species [14]. There is significant heterogeneity within biofilms, however, and it is not the case that all cells within a biofilm are always highly resistant to antimicrobial drugs. For example, planktonic cells that are derived from these biofilms are, in most cases, fully susceptible to antibiotics. Also, biofilms do not actually grow in the presence of elevated concentrations of systemically administered antibiotics.

Cells in the biofilm are slow-growing, and many are likely to be in the stationary phase of growth due to a nutrient-starving enveloped ecosystem. A small sub-population of cells (persisters) remain alive irrespective of the concentration of the antibiotic and the number of these persisters is greater in the non-growing stationary phase [15]. Lewis believes that the problem of antimicrobial resistance of biofilm is related to the presence of persisters [15].

Cells, whether they are rapidly dividing, slow- or non-growing cells in a bio-film, are generally susceptible to bactericidal agents such as fluoroquinolone anti-biotics or metal oxyanions [16, 17]. Antibiotic treatment will kill most biofilm and planktonic cells, leaving persisters alive. The immune system can kill remaining planktonic persisters and bacteriostatic antibiotic-treated non-growing cells. Biofilm exopolymer matrix, however, protects persisters and non-growing cells against immune cells against both antibiotic treatment and the immune system [18–20]. Persisters can repopulate the biofilm and shed off new planktonic cells when the concentration of antibiotic drops off. This will cause a relapse of biofilm infection.

3   Biofouling of Ureteral Stents

Microbial ureteral stent colonisation and subsequent development of biofilm is a multistep process starting with the formation of a conditioning film made of host proteins, electrolytes, and other substances [21]. The surface of any foreign material or object introduced to the urinary system can become coated with a biofilm composed of glycoproteins, matrix and exopolymers. This can take place within a few hours [22]. Nearly half to two-thirds of stents removed from patients displayed bacterial colonies [23] with over one-fifth of these patients had required treatment for bacteriuria infection [24, 25]. Most of these stents (75–100%) that were indwelling for a period of longer than 3 months had shown the highest rate of colonization, which could not be treated with systemic administration of oral antibiotics. All 93 stents from patients became colonized with bacteria despite antibiotic prophylaxis. Oral administration of common antibiotics such as fluoroquinolones, ciprofloxacin and ofloxacin, has not been proven to reduce colonization or infection despite being present at the stent surface at a dose level that has been sufficient to inhibit bacterial growth [26, 27]. Encrustation and bacterial colonization of stents and urinary catheters are problematic and may lead to further morbidity such as infection, sepsis or renal failure [28, 29]. Undetected biofilms may serve as a reservoir for microorganisms. During stent manipulation or instrumentation, biofilm pathogens could be shed into the urine and lead to bacteriuria or funguria or even to life-threatening urosepsis [30].

In a recent systematic review, Zumstein et al. thoroughly investigated the incidence, clinical impact and prevention of biofilm formation on ureteral stents [7]. According to the review, the conditioning film may form due to contact of the stent material with body fluids such as urine and blood, and uroepithelial tissue. Glycosylated uroepithelial cell–surface proteins such as cytokeratin, blood proteins such as haemoglobin and fibrinogen, and inflammatory proteins appear to be involved in conditioning film formation in the first 72 h after insertion. The conditioning film proteins are believed to facilitate the adsorption of various molecules such as collagen, fibrinogen and albumin from the surrounding fluids and tissues, which then alter the surface of the ureteral stent and may allow microorganisms attachment for which urinary pH, ionic strength, and electrostatic and hydrophobic interactions play an important role. Other adhesion strategies such as adhesion to secreted bacterial extracellular polymeric substances may also contribute to conditioning-film formation.

Five different proteins, namely, alpha-1 antitrypsin, immunoglobulin kappa (Ig kappa), immunoglobulin heavy chain G1 (IgH G1), histones H2b, and H3a are present in high numbers in encrustations and biofilms. *Pseudomonas aeruginosa* and *Proteus mirabilis* secrete urease, which increases the urine pH resulting in the precipitation of struvite and hydroxyapatite crystals, adhesion factors, transporters, transcription factors and enzymes. Complex biofilm structures are formed in the last stage of stent biofilm development. Colonies of bacteria are dispersed within spaces filled with fluid and open water channels that allow the transport of oxygen and nutrients to assure further cellular growth. Ureteral stent biofilms comprise of 10–25% cells and 75–90% of exopolysaccharide matrix characterised by a rough, and often mineralised, surface. Calcium oxalate and struvite dominate the mineralised biofilm. *Enterococcus faecalis* and *E. coli* are common pathogens colonising on ureteral stents [31]. Bacteria expressing urease, such as *Proteus* spp., *Providencia* or *Pseudomonas*, are also involved and can induce rapid growth of biofilms. Other bacteria that have been associated with stent biofilm formation are *Staphylococcus* and *Edwardsiella* spp.

As regard to the indwelling timeline, the review found that bacterial colonisation of stent was detectable 2 weeks after implantation, and that stent colonisation precedes urine colonisation. One study described an encrustation rate of 27% in < 6 weeks, 57% between 6 and 12 weeks, and 76% in > 12 weeks [32]. This compares with another study that reported a colonisation rate of 24% in < 4 weeks, 33% between 4 and 6 weeks, and 71% in over 6 weeks of indwelling time [33]. As it has been previously discussed, Riedl et al. reported 100% ureteral stent colonisation in permanently stented patients (mean stent indwelling time 39.5 days or 5–6 weeks) and 69% in the temporarily stented (mean 11 days or less than 1.5 weeks). The above also compare with a retrospective study of severely impacted ureteral stents requiring advanced removal procedures that found 43% and 76% of the stents had become encrusted within 4 months and 6 months respectively [34]. Patient risk factors such as diabetes mellitus, chronic renal failure and diabetic nephropathy can lead to a shorter stent indwelling times due to a significantly higher risk of colonisation and bacteriuria [35].

4　Resisting Biofouling of Ureteral Stents: Current and Emerging Approaches

New biomaterials, coatings and drug-eluting stents have been designed to reduce biofilm formation and subsequent infection and encrustation. Chew et al. have elaborated these approaches in terms of stent design, materials and coatings. The general strategy of protecting such stents from biofouling involved electronegative coating using heparin or a pH-buffer coating. Adhesion and colonisation by a multiplex of uropathogens (*P. mirabilis*, *E. coli*, *S. Aureus* among others) hosted within an extracellular polymeric matrix nourish and protect the pathogens at the later stages of biofilm formation.

Zumstein et al. summarises current state of the coating approaches. Heparin, hydrogel-based and diamond like coatings are commercially available as Radiance™, Hydroplus™, and VisioSafe DIAMOND™ coatings [7]. Oxalate degrading enzyme coatings and nanoscale body coatings are yet to be commercialised. So far, preventing and treating biofilms on ureteral stents have been challenging due to the conditioning film compromising the effectiveness of passive coatings (heparin, pH buffer-coat) and the involvement of multiple bacterial species. Although heparin-coated stents significantly reduced ureteral stent encrustation and offered a 12 months indwelling, no positive effect against bacterial adhesion was seen [36, 37]. In the past, hydrogel-based coatings raised expectations that they would effectively inhibit hydroxyapatite encrustation and bacterial biofilm colonisation, and reduce general stent-related morbidity [38]. However, bacterial adhesions were found to be similar in stents with and without hydrogel-based coatings [39].

A multi-stage approach of sterilisation following Bigger was proposed by Lewis to eradicate persisters in biofilms [40]. It was proposed to kill bacterial cells with a high initial dose of an antibiotic. The concentration of the antibiotic would then decrease to enable persisters to resuscitate and start to grow. If a second dose of antibiotic was then administered shortly after persisters had started to grow, a complete sterilization might have been achieved. While it was suggested for systemic pharmaceutical/biopharma treatment of biofilms, a similar approach can be adopted in coating designs using antiseptics/antimicrobials [41, 42]. Once attached to the surface, an antimicrobial molecule is immobilized and is unable to reach and kill the pathogen. Long, flexible polymeric chain linkers are needed to covalently anchor these antimicrobials to the surface of a material.

5 A Dynamically Degradable Surface

The coatings mentioned in the previous section are essentially 'static' means they degrade at a very slow rate. This allows sufficient time for the formation of the conditioning film and microbial attachment. In fact, micro-organisms are 'intelligent' to find mechanisms to colonise any abiotic surface that allows sufficient time to do so. This is because a 'static' surface offers to incoming molecules and microbes a relatively low-entropy boundary that eventually leads to a lowering of free energy for molecules and microbes to attach. If this 'static' condition of the coating surface could be replaced with a coating that is degrading at a constant or a variable speed, a relatively higher entropy condition can be created that would 'delay' the attachment of molecules and cells to the surface. This is analogous to a 'pulling the rug from under somebody's feet'. It would delay the formation of the conditioning films, and in turn delay the bacterial adhesion by constantly 'fooling' away bacteria from landing on a 'low-entropy' surface.

Biodegradation means that coatings do not have a static surface on which microbes can colonise to lead towards biofilm formation. The coating can be designed to suit the specific ecosystem in which it would have to prevent biofouling and its degradation rate tuned to suit the time it takes to form the conditioning film or the first few layers of microorganism colonisation.

Obviously, such a coating has to be degradable i.e. it would decay, corrode, erode or peel in response to its environment. The coating can also be multilayers or functionally graded to tune the degradation. Furthermore, the coating can itself be antimicrobial or can be loaded with antimicrobial, antiadhesive or cell-polarising agents.

A simple coating of electrically polar fluoropolymer (pyro and piezoelectric) can reduce encrustation significantly through mediating electrostatic interactions [7–9]. Biodegradable molecular crystals show very strong antimicrobial effects which can be engineered for sterilisation for clinical applications [43]. Polycationic or polyanionic surface offered by such polar molecular crystals can either cause cellular lysis or repulsion, respectively. Electrically polar biomolecules such as amino acids (e.g. glycine, cysteine), their derivatives (e.g. triglycine sulfate TGS), metabolites (e.g. peptide nanotubes) or enzymes (e.g. lysozyme) have also demonstrated very high electrically polar properties [10–14] which makes them responsive to changes in local environment such as pressure and temperature. Electrically polarised fluoropolymer, polyvinylidene difluoride (PVDF) stent has demonstrated 40% increase inhibition of calcification (oxalate and hydroxyapatite) after 30 days patency in ASME standard artificial urine in comparison to commercial polyurethane, unpoled PVDF, heparin coated polyurethane and hydrogel coated polyurethane. The use of an electrically polar, molecular crystals in the coating can produce a 'dynamic' surface that can combine biocompatibility with electro negativity and functional grading to reduce biofouling of ureteral stents. Biodegradable and functionally gradable polymers can also be used to create the 'dynamic' surface. Metallic materials such as magnesium and zinc-based coatings are also possible.

6 Conclusions

Biofouling complicates and compromises indwelling of ureteral stents. It causes patient discomfort, infection and trauma and its removal is expensive. Commercially available stents uses anti-fouling coatings with variable successes. These coatings are static and inadequate in resisting bacterial colonization that eventually leads to encrustation. In this chapter we introduced the concept of a dynamic surface which may be successful in 'fooling' bacteria due to constant degradation of the surface during indwelling. The concept is new and currently being experimented at the authors' group. It offers to use biodegradable, electrically polar molecular crystals as the anti-fouling coating, which can be functionally graded to tune the biodegradation and anti-encrustation effect.

References

1. Heukelekian H, Heller A. Relation between food concentration and surface for bacterial growth. J Bacteriol. 1940;40:547–58.
2. Zobell CE. The effect of solid surfaces on bacterial activity. J Bacteriol. 1943;46:39–56.
3. Donlan RM. Biofilms: microbial life on surfaces. Emerg Infect Dis. 2002;8(9):881–90.
4. Robin S, et al. Interactions of biofilm-forming bacteria with abiotic surfaces. In: Tofail SAM, editor. Biological interactions with surface charge in biomaterials. London: RSC Publishing; 2011.

5. Hall-Stoodley L, Costerton JW, Stoodley P. Bacterial biofilms: from the natural environment to infectious diseases. Nat Rev Microbiol. 2004;2:95–108.
6. Zelichenko G, Steinberg D, Lorber G, Friedman M, Zaks B, Lavy E, Hidas G, Landau EH, Gofrit ON, Pode D, Duvdevani M. Prevention of initial biofilm formation on ureteral stents using a sustained releasing varnish containing chlorhexidine: in vitro study. J Endourol. 2013;27:333–7.
7. Zumstein V, Betschart P, Albrich WC, Buhmann MT, Ren Q, Schmid HP, Abt D. Biofilm formation on ureteral stents—incidence, clinical impact, and prevention. Swiss Med Wkly. 2017;147:w14408.
8. Reid G, Denstedt JD, Kang YS, Lam D, Nause C. Microbial adhesion and biofilm formation on ureteral stents in vitro and in vivo. J Urol. 1992;148(5):1592–4.
9. Buhmann MT, Abt D, Altenried S, Rupper P, Betschart P, Zumstein V, Maniura-Weber K, Ren Q. Extraction of biofilms from ureteral stents for quantification and cultivation-dependent and -independent analyses. Front Microbiol. 2018;9:1470.
10. Zhang JM,·Liu J,·Wang K,·Zhang X, Zhao T,·Luo HMObservations of bacterial biofilm on ureteral stent and studies on the distribution of pathogenic bacteria and drug resistance Urol Int 2018, 101(3): 320-326
11. Gandhi AA, Korostynska O, Robin S, Laffir F, Soulimane T, Lavelle S, Tofail SAM. Contact poling of polyurethane, charge stability and interactions with *P. mirabilis*. In: Tofail SAM, Bauer J, editors. Electrically active materials for medical devices. Singapore: World Scientific; 2016.
12. Spoering AL, Lewis K. Biofilms and planktonic cells of *Pseudomonas aeruginosa* have similar resistance to killing by antimicrobials. J Bacteriol. 2001;183(23):6746–51.
13. Suci PA, Tyler BJ. A method for discrimination of subpopulations of *Candida albicans* biofilm cells that exhibit relative levels of phenotypic resistance to chlorhexidine. J Microbiol Methods. 2003;53(3):313–25.
14. Parsek MR, Singh PK. Bacterial biofilms: an emerging link to disease pathogenesis. Annu Rev Microbiol. 2003;57:677–701.
15. Lewis K. Persister cells, dormancy and infectious disease. Nat Rev Microbiol. 2007;5:48–56.
16. Harrison JJ, et al. Persister cells mediate tolerance to metal oxyanions in *Escherichia coli*. Microbiology. 2005;151:3181–95.
17. Harrison JJ, Turner RJ, Ceri H. Persister cells, the biofilm matrix and tolerance to metal cations in biofilm and planktonic *Pseudomonas aeruginosa*. Environ Microbiol. 2005;7:981–94.
18. Leid JG, Shirtliff ME, Costerton JW, Stoodley AP. Human leukocytes adhere to, penetrate, and respond to *Staphylococcus aureus* biofilms. Infect Immun. 2002;70:6339–45.
19. Jesaitis AJ, et al. Compromised host defense on *Pseudomonas aeruginosa* biofilms: characterization of neutrophil and biofilm interactions. J Immunol. 2003;171:4329–39.
20. Vuong C, et al. Polysaccharide intercellular adhesin (PIA) protects *Staphylococcus epidermidis* against major components of the human innate immune system. Cell Microbiol. 2004;6:269–75.
21. Bonkat G, Rieken M, Siegel FP, Frei R, Steiger J, Groschl I, Gasser TC, Dell-Kuster S, Rosenthal R, Gurke L, Wyler S, Bachmann A, Widmer AF. Microbial ureteral stent colonization in renal transplant recipients: frequency and influence on the short time functional outcome. Transpl Infect Dis. 2012;14:57–63.
22. Tieszer C, Reid G, Denstedt J. Conditioning film deposition on ureteral stents after implantation. J Urol. 1998;160:876–81.
23. Chew BH, Duvdevani M, Denstedt J. New developments in ureteral stent design, materials and coatings. Expert Rev Med Devices. 2006;3(3):395–403.
24. Riedl CR, Plas E, Hubner WA, Zimmerl H, Ulrich W, Pfluger H. Bacterial colonization of ureteral stents. Eur Urol. 1999;36(1):53–9.
25. Paick SH, Park HK, Oh SJ, Kim HH. Characteristics of bacterial colonization and urinary tract infection after indwelling of double-J ureteral stent. Urology. 2003;62(2):214–7.
26. Reid G, Habash M, Vachon D, Denstedt J, Riddell J, Beheshti M. Oral, fluoroquinolone therapy results in drug adsorption on ureteral stents and prevention of biofilm formation. Int J Antimicrob Agents. 2001;17(4):317–9.

27. Wollin TA, Tieszer C, Riddell JV, Denstedt JD, Reid G. Bacterial biofilm formation, encrustation, and antibiotic adsorption to ureteral stents indwelling in humans. J Endourol. 1998;12(2):101–11.
28. Damiano R, Oliva A, Esposito C, De Sio M, Autorino R, D'Armiento M. Early and late complications of double pigtail ureteral stent. Urol Int. 2002;69(2):136–40.
29. Singh I, Gupta NP, Hemal AK, Aron M, Seth A, Dogra PN. Severely encrusted polyurethane ureteral stents: management and analysis of potential risk factors. Urology. 2001;58(4):526–31.
30. Gautam G, Singh AK, Kumar R, Hemal AK, Kothari A. Beware! Fungal urosepsis may follow endoscopic intervention for prolonged indwelling ureteral stent. J Endourol. 2006;20(7):522–4.
31. Brotherhood H, Lange D, Chew BH. Advances in ureteral stents. Transl Androl Urol. 2014;3(3):314–9.
32. Kawahara T, Ito H, Terao H, Yoshida M, Matsuzaki J. Ureteral stent encrustation, incrustation, and coloring: morbidity related to indwelling times. J Endourol. 2012;26(2):178–82.
33. Rahman MA, Alam MM, Shamsuzzaman SM, Haque ME. Evaluation of bacterial colonization and bacteriuria secondary to internal ureteral stent. Mymensingh Med J. 2010;19(3):366–71.
34. Bultitude MF, Tiptaft RC, Glass JM, Dasgupta P. Management of encrusted ureteral stents impacted in upper tract. Urology. 2003;62(4):622–6.
35. Kehinde EO, Rotimi VO, Al-Awadi KA, Abdul-Halim H, Boland F, Al-Hunayan A, et al. Factors predisposing to urinary tract infection after J ureteral stent insertion. J Urol. 2002;167(3):1334–7.
36. Lange D, Chew BH. Update on ureteral stent technology. Ther Adv Urol. 2009;1(3):143–8.
37. Cauda F, Cauda V, Fiori C, Onida B, Garrone E. Heparin coating on ureteral double J stents prevents encrustations: an in vivo case study. J Endourol. 2008;22(3):465–72.
38. Lange D, Chew BH. Biomaterials and tissue engineering in urology. Amsterdam: Elsevier; 2009. p. 85–103.
39. John T, Rajpurkar A, Smith G, Fairfax M, Triest J. Antibiotic pretreatment of hydrogel ureteral stent. J Endourol. 2007;21(10):1211–6.
40. Bigger JW. Treatment of staphylococcal infections with penicillin. Lancet. 1944;244:497–500.
41. Tiller JC, Liao CJ, Lewis K, Klibanov AM. Designing surfaces that kill bacteria on contact. Proc Natl Acad Sci USA. 2001;98:5981–5.
42. Lewis K, Klibanov AM. Surpassing nature: rational design of sterile-surface materials. Trends Biotechnol. 2005;23:343–8.
43. McCloskey AP, Gilmore BF, Laverty G. Evolution of antimicrobial peptides to self-assembled peptides for biomaterial applications. Pathogens. 2014;3:791–821.

Biomaterials for Ureteral Stents: Advances and Future Perspectives

Margarida Pacheco, Joana M. Silva, Ivo M. Aroso, Estêvão Lima,
Alexandre A. Barros, and Rui L. Reis

1 Introduction

Ureteral stents play a fundamental role in the relief of several symptoms associated with common urinary diseases in the modern society, such as strictures, obstruction or promotion of ureteral healing [1, 2]. Even though ureteral stents have been used for more than 40 years and their performance had a huge development over time, they are still related with complications that include stent encrustation and urinary tract infections [1, 2]. Therefore, efforts from the research community still continue to better meet the clinical needs. Ureteral stent's materials have a great influence on their efficacy, mostly in terms of mechanical and physicochemical properties [3]. Thus, understanding the stent material's properties is fundamental to address problems of encrustation, bacterial adhesion, patient discomfort and the troubles during insertion, by working on the softness, flexibility and surface properties of the device [3].

Ureteral stents were described for the first time by Herdman back in 1949 [4]. Among the various biologically and chemically inert polymers that were popular at that time, polyethylene was used owing to its considerable tensile strength, flexibility, biocompatibility and hydrophobic properties. However, during the first animal

M. Pacheco · J. M. Silva · I. M. Aroso · A. A. Barros (✉) · R. L. Reis
3B's Research Group—Research Institute on Biomaterials, Biodegradables and Biomimetics, European Institute of Excellence on Tissue Engineering and Regenerative Medicine, University of Minho, Guimarães, Portugal

ICVS/3B's-PT, Government Associate Laboratory, Braga/Guimarães, Portugal
e-mail: joana.marques@i3bs.uminho.pt; ivo.aroso@i3bs.uminho.pt; ip@i3bs.uminho.pt; rgreis@i3bs.uminho.pt

E. Lima
School of Health Sciences, Life and Health Sciences Research Institute (ICVS), University of Minho, Braga, Portugal
e-mail: estevaolima@med.uminho.pt

© The Author(s) 2022
F. Soria et al. (eds.), *Urinary Stents*,
https://doi.org/10.1007/978-3-031-04484-7_17

studies tube blockages and hydronephrosis were detected as the main drawbacks [4]. Another suitable polymer that was at the time used for the manufacture of ureteral stents was silicone, which can withstand high temperatures, facilitating the sterilization process that, in turn, prevent infections [5, 6]. Silicone based stents were less likely to promote encrustations and infections while still being effective in different urological conditions. Nonetheless, due to the low radial strength, silicone-based stents were inefficient in bearing with high external compression [5, 6]. Thereby, the research efforts have turned the tide to merge the flexibility and elasticity of silicone with the rigidity of polyethylene, which resulted on the development of polyurethane as raw material for ureteral stents. Indeed, polyurethane mechanical properties were promissory, but this polymer also demonstrated higher predisposition for encrustation than silicone-based materials [7]. Metals and biodegradable materials have been also used for ureteral stents manufacturing due to their remarkable properties. Metallic ureteral stents are very efficient in situations of high compression forces and when long term treatments are required [1]. A recurrent disadvantage with metallic stents is tissue hyperplasia and increased propensity to develop encrustation due to longer indwelling time periods [3]. On the other side, biodegradable ureteral stents (BUS) provide the uniqueness of self-degradation but obtaining a controlled and homogeneous is still the main obstacle for development of BUS (Fig. 1). On the next sections of this chapter, the three main classes of

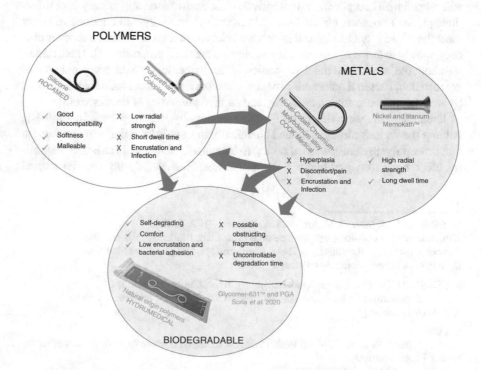

Fig. 1 Different materials used for ureteral stents development, including some examples of each class, the main advantages and disadvantages and how the different materials' properties complement each other

materials used for ureteral stents manufacture will be individually addressed and most recent findings will be discussed in order to shed the light on the advances and future perspectives in this field.

2 Materials for Ureteral Stents

2.1 Polymeric Materials

Polymers are attractive base materials for biomedical applications due to their inert nature, and constitute the first materials explored for ureteral stent development [8]. Currently, polymeric ureteral stents are the most common in the market, known by being inexpensive and well-tolerated by patients [3]. Certainly, the extensive research on polymers lead to a widespread understanding of their properties, the companies developed proprietary blends and high-quality polymeric ureteral stents are now commercially available [9]. The aim of the current studies on polymeric ureteral stents are focused on improving the biocompatibility, the indwelling time without significant encrustations and infections, and the ease of insertion and retrieval, maintaining the appropriate mechanical properties and radiopaque nature [3, 8]. Polyethylene was the first material employed on the design of ureteral stents, that is not used anymore due to the substantial drawbacks associated to it, namely the easy fragmentation caused by the brittleness of the material and the high rates of encrustation and infection [3, 10]. Currently, silicone and polyurethane are the most used polymers for ureteral stents manufacture [3, 8] (Fig. 1). Silicone has been extensively used, since the earlier beginning of ureteral stents production. Zimskind and colleagues, in 1967, studied for the first time the suitability of silicone for ureteral stents, describing the application of a piece of silicone tube with open ends and side holes to promote long term ureteral drainage of compromised ureters [6]. Nowadays, silicone is considered as a gold standard due to its unique properties, such as the less propensity of encrustation and bacteria contamination, non-toxicity and the improved comfort due to its softness and high lubricity [3, 11, 12]. Besides the aforementioned features, silicone is also easy to shape and process, facilitating the production phase. However, the high flexibility and elasticity is also a disadvantage during the placement on tight and tortuous ureters or when high compression (e.g. tumours) is present [3]. Additionally, difficulties in manoeuvring it with the guidewire were also reported [10]. The use of polyurethane in the urologic field is popular since the earlier beginning due to the suitable mechanical properties, however, as a stiff material, causes discomfort and pain to the patients, being also reported epithelial erosion and ulceration when compared to other materials [2]. The problems encountered in ureteral stents also instigated companies to develop optimized polyurethane-based proprietary formulations, like Sof-Flex®, Tecoflex®, Hydrothane® and ChronoFlex® [13]. Nowadays, polyurethane's chemical character-istics can be tuned, such as the surface wettability and surface energy, which allows the control of other properties like encrustation and bacterial adhesion propensity

[14]. Other polymers were also developed, such as the polyester copolymer, Silitek®, a proprietary polymer that becomes soft and flexible at body temperature, with a reported excellent biocompatibility, Perculfex®, polyethylene-vinyl acetate and styrene/ethylenebutylene/styrene block copolymers, F-Flex®, and poly(methyl methacrylate)/poly(hydroxyethyl methacrylate) (PMMA/pHEMA) with improved mechanical properties than silicone [15]. Albeit all the reported polymer's formulations, the available ureteral stents are not devoid of clinical complications, thereby, investigations aiming to modify the base polymers are still on going. A recent work presented by Rebl et al. addressed the influence of physical properties of different polymers' samples on their propensity to develop encrustation [14]. The data revealed that the encrustation degree is correlated with the surface charge and hydrophobicity of the polymer samples, a lower encrustation propensity was observed for polymers with strong negative surface charge and good hydrophilicity [14]. This behaviour is justified by the fact that the most common components of the infectious urinary stones are negatively charged, and, consequently, can be repelled by strongly negative charged polymers' samples [14]. Rosman et al. also explored the bacterial resistance and anti-biofilm properties of a polyacrylonitrile based ureteral stent (pAguaMedicina™, Pediatric Ureteral Stent, Q Urological) where a considerable reduction on bacterial colonization and biofilm formation in Broth (Trypticase Soy Agar broth), Broth with human urine, and Broth with swine blood was observed when compared with a commonly used commercial ureteral stent (Boston Scientific, USA) [16]. An interesting approach is a combinatorial approach of different materials, taking advantage of the properties of the individual counterparts. For example, Silhouette® ureteral stent consist on a nitinol wire covered with a synthetic polymer, thus this stent present an improved resistance due to the presence of metal on its structure and a good biocompatibility provided by the

Table 1 Polymeric ureteral stents available on the market

Commercial name	Company	Material
LithoStent	OLYMPUS	Tecoflex®
Classic closed tip ureteral stent	OLYMPUS	Silicone
UroGuide	OLYMPUS	Silicone
Lubri-Flex	OLYMPUS	Tecoflex®
Classic Double Pigtail	OLYMPUS	Tecoflex®
Sof-Curl™	OLYMPUS	Tecoflex®
Endosil® Silicone double loop ureteral stent	ROCAMED	Silicone
Amecath double loop stent	Amecath Medical Technologies	Tecoflex® (short term use) or Carbothane (long term use)
Silhouette® ureteral stent	Applied Medical	Synthetic polymers, proprietary materials and coil reinforced nitinol
Yellow Star Tumour Stents Green Star Stents White Star Stents	GBUK Healthcare	Aliphatic polyurethane
Ureteral stent medadvDJ	MEDAS INC	Polyurethane

Table 1 (continued)

Commercial name	Company	Material
Double pigtail ureteral stent	MEDNOVA	Polyurethane
MEDpro Ureteral Stents	MEDpro	Tecoflex® for short term use and Carbothane for tumour compression cases
Biosoft® duo ureter stent	Coloplast	Rigid proprietary material
Silicone double loop ureteral stent	Coloplast	Silicone
Polyurethane (PU-R and PU-S) double loop ureteral stents	Coloplast	Soft or rigid, proprietary polyurethane
Tumor stent	Coloplast	Proprietary formulation with a reinforced internal layer for excellent resistance to compression
Ureteral stent Polaris™ Ultra	Boston Scientific	Percuflex with dual durometer
Pyelostent	Coloplast	Silicone
Sof-Flex® Double Pigtail Stent	COOK Medical®	Proprietary radiopaque soft polyurethane
Percuflex®	Boston Scientific	Proprietary copolymer—modified polyurethane
Single J Urinary Diversion Stents	OLYMPUS	Silitek®

polymeric revetment [3, 17]. Table 1 presents examples of the polymeric commercial ureteral stents available on the market.

2.2 Metallic Materials

Metallic based ureteral stents were developed to treat ureteral obstruction caused by a malignant external compression, usually a tumour, and for patients needing chronical indwelling ureteral stents [18, 19]. In this context, polymeric ureteral stents are ineffective due to the inadequate drainage and requirement of replacement in a short time period, causing discomfort and extra hospital costs [19, 20] (Fig. 1). A metallic ureteral stent has an improved radial strength that provides long-lasting ureteral patency—12 months to 2 years—tackling the problem of low compression strength and shorter indwelling time—usually 3 months—of polymeric stents [21, 22]. The success rate of a treatment with a metallic stent is between 37 and 100% [19, 22, 23]. Current metallic ureteral stents could be double-J shaped as the traditional polymeric ones (Resonance®), self-expandable (Wallstent™, Allium), balloon expandable (Uventa™), thermo-expandable (Memokath 051) and/or covered with a polymer (Uventa™) [1, 24]. Resonance® has a double-J shape with an occluded lumen and, even though this exclusive design makes the stent insertion and retrieval more difficult, it assures ureteral patency and urine flow under high external compression [25]. Blaschko et al. have reported a significant higher flow rate for Resonance® when compared with a 6F standard stent under high extrinsic compression, 5.15 mL/min and 0.64 mL/min respectively [26]. In another exciting study, Christman et al.

compared the radial compression resistance of different ureteral stents—Silhouette®, Sof-Curl™, Resonance®, Polaris™ Ultra, and Percuflex®. The data indicated that Resonance® had a significant higher resistance to compression, followed by Silhouette®, which could be justified by the nitinol wire coil present on Silhouette® [17]. Resonance® is currently seen as a reference for malignant ureteral obstructions owing to the numerous advantages already reported, such as good biocompatibility, suitability for magnetic resonance imaging examination, inhibition of endogenous tissue growth and high flexibility due to the tightly coiled wire of the spiral shaped design [3, 27, 28]. Additionally, Resonance® is soft and, more importantly, has an indwelling time of more than 12 months, during which it retains its suitable features [27]. Chen et al. conducted a study where they compared the performance of Resonance® with an ordinary polymeric stent on patients with malignant ureteral obstruction [22]. The authors confirmed that after 1 year of stent placement, the stents patency decreased 60% in the polymeric stent group and only 9.3% metallic stent group, indicating that metallic stents with good drainage effect for a long period of time are superior to the traditional polymeric stents for patients who require long term stenting [22]. Up to now, different metallic ureteral stents were developed and accessible on ureteral stents market. Memokath 051 is a thermo-expandable nickel titanium alloy with a very tight coil design [20]. Memokath 051 deploys in warm saline and shrinks in cool saline, which is an attractive benefit for placing and retrieving them from the body [3]. Complications such as stent migration and encrustation were reported, together with tissue ingrowth and stent occlusion [15, 29]. Uventa is another commercially available metallic ureteral stent composed of a double layer of nickel and titanium alloys with polytetrafluoroethylene (PTFE) layer between them, designed to prevent migration and tissue adhesion [30]. The success rates of Uventa for malignant ureteral obstructions are between 64.8–81.7% and the associated complications include tumour progression beyond the stent, tissue ingrowth and pain [31]. Another metallic stent model is Wallstent, a self-expanding stent composed of cobalt-based microfilaments woven in crisscross pattern [32]. Unfortunately, Wallstent is also associated with pain, stent migration and tissue ingrowth [30]. Allium Ureteral Stent is made of nitinol and covered with a copolymer, with the purpose to prevent encrustation and tissue growth [33]. The major advantage of Allium Ureteral Stent is the easy removal owing to its particular design [33]. Passage™ is a coil-based metallic ureteral stent with improved flexibility and comfort and higher resistance to radial compression when compared with Resonance® and Silhouette® [1, 34]. Nitinol is a biocompatible material, composed of titanium oxide and nickel with a better

Table 2 Metallic ureteral stents available on the market

Commercial name	Company	Material
Resonance®	Cook Medical	Nickel–cobalt–chromium–molybdenum alloy
Allium Ureteral Stents	Allium™ Medical	Nitinol wire covered with a polytetrafluoroethylene (PTFE)
Passage™	Prosurg	Nitinol
WALLSTENT™	Boston Scientific	Cobalt-based microfilament
UVENTA™ Ureteral Stent	TaeWoong Medical	Double layer of nickel and titanium alloys with a layer of PTFE in between
Memokath 051	Memokath™	Nickel and titanium alloys

corrosion resistance than stainless steel—a material that was previously seen as a reference for stents—possessing also memory shape, i.e. it can be manipulated as needed for stent insertion and afterwards recovers its original shape [21]. Most of the currently available metallic ureteral stents are made of nitinol. Table 2 presents metallic ureteral stents currently available on the market and their composition.

2.3 Biodegradable Materials

Biodegradable ureteral stents are an appealing alternative since its use eliminates the need of a second surgery for the stent removal, avoid additional ureter damage, pain and discomfort, and diminishes the treatment costs [1, 3, 21], Table 3. These exceptional features and decreased propensity for bacterial adherence and encrustation motivated the investigations on biodegradable materials for ureteral stents development [1, 21] (Fig. 1). A crucial concern when producing a BUS is that the degradation profile of ureteral stents should occur in a controllable and adequate form, i.e. efficient mechanical properties must be assured during the treatment time and the degradation has to occur in an homogeneous way, avoiding additional ureteral obstruction [9, 21, 35]. In fact, these are very challenging features to obtain and constitute a critical point during the development process [3, 35]. BUS have been fabricated from synthetic polymers, naturally origin polymers, biodegradable metals or a combination of biodegradable polymers and metals [3, 35]. The concept of biodegradable material applied for ureteral stents date back to 1997, in which Schlick and Planz evaluated the degree of dissolution in acidic and alkaline artificial urine of two polymers (G100X-15LB and G100X-20LB) [36]. With these raw materials, they aimed at producing an ureteral stent with controlled degradation by alkalinizing the urine through medication. However, in clinical practice this concept is risky as a basic urine pH can lead to extra complications, such as precipitation of urine salts and also the development of a suitable environment for the growth of uropathogens growth [1, 21]. Olweny et al. in 2002 introduced the use of poly-L-lactide-*co*-glycolide (PLGA) as BUS material in a porcine model [37]. Other studies followed this direction and BUS were developed using PLGA, Poly-L,D-lactide (PLA), poly-L-lactic acid (PLLA), polycaprolactone (PCL) and poly-DL-lactic acid (PDLLA), nonetheless problems of inadequate degradation and toxicity were frequently found, with the exception of some promising results obtained in dogs with poly-L,D-lactide (SR-PLA96) where reduced inflammation and good biocompatibility was obtained [1, 21, 38–40]. Some concerns affecting the stent degradation are the size and shape, the molecular weight of the polymer, the presence of other ingredients and the respective proportions, among others, and improvements of

Table 3 Biodegradable ureteral stents available in the market

Commercial name	Company	Material
BraidStent	n/a	Glycomer-631™ and polyglycolic acid (PGA)
Uriprene™	Poly-Med Inc.	L-Glycolic acid
HydrUStent™	HYDRUMEDICAL	Natural origin polymers

BUS's characteristics are made by optimizing these features [1, 35]. Yang et al. proposed the use of PLGA for ureteral stents with a particular stent design that is different from the ones usually employed for BUS-braided and spiralled. The data suggested an homogeneous and controllable degradation and better radial compression strength when compared with a commercial stent [41]. This design is based on a multilayer immersion method using PGLA, zein-a natural protein- and barium sulfate [41]. Later on, Zhang et al. reported the use of a novel biodegradable polymer, methoxypoly(ethylene glycol)-*block*-poly(L-lactide-ran-ε-caprolactone) (mPEG-PLACL), that present less propensity for encrustation and superior biocompatibility [42]. Soria et al. scrutinised the performance of an innovative anti-reflux BUS, BraidStent, in 24 female pigs where only part of the ureter was intubated [43]. The stent degraded in 3–6 weeks without obstructive fragments and favourable anti-reflux properties [43]. Uriprene™ is a radiopaque glycolic acid-based stent that start the degradation process after 3 weeks, while after 7 and 10 weeks 60% and 100% of the stent was degraded, respectively, in porcine models [44]. This stent was designed to degrade in a specific direction, from the bladder to the kidney end, thereby preventing also the obstruction-formation fragments [1]. Uriprene™ provides similar drainage capacity as ordinary stents with less ureteral dilatation and microbial contamination [44]. The reported problem associated with this stent is the difficulty of insertion [21]. An improved version was later developed with a shorter degradation time (i.e., 4 weeks) [45]. Lingman et al. conducted clinical trial studies using a BUS produced from a proprietary formulation based on the natural origin polymer alginate [21, 46, 47]. The stent was biocompatible and presented appropriate patency up to 48 h, after that time the stent starts to degrade. The main problem of these stents is the permanence of fragments inside the patients for long periods, which required surgical intervention for removal. Recently, Barros et al. successfully reported the use of gelatin and alginate to produce an hydrogel BUS using the supercritical carbon dioxide technology in the production process, which proved to be beneficial for the mechanical properties [48]. In the first studies encouraging results in terms of biocompatibility and low propensity for bacterial contamination and encrustation were reported [48]. This model then showed good performance *in vivo*, in pig models, with better biocompatibility than a commercial ureteral stent and an homogeneous degradation profile [49, 50]. These works resulted in a patented BUS and the development of HydrUStent™, a biodegradable hydrogel stent for temporary treatments. HydrUStent™ was already validated in porcine model and is being currently preparing to start clinical trials [51].

Biodegradable metals can be used for prolonged time treatments, given the slower degradation rate when compared with biodegradable polymers. The potential of biodegradable metals for ureteral stents was studied for the first time by Lock et al. that investigated the antibacterial activity of magnesium (Mg)–4%Yttrium(Y), the Mg alloy AZ31 and commercially pure Mg. A decrease in *Escherichia coli* viable colonies was observed for all the tested Mg alloys when compared with commercial polyurethane stents [52]. Zang et al. studied the alloy ZK60 and pure Mg in terms of corrosion, in artificial urine, and histocompatibility in rat's bladder where they verified that ZK60 had a faster degradation both *in vitro* and in the animal's bladder and both metals reveal to be biocompatible [53]. Recently, Tie et al. reported for the first time the use of a Mg based alloy, ZJ31, in a large animal model for ureteral stent application [54]. The data indicated an homogeneous corrosion rate, good biocompatibility and antibacterial activity, when compared with stainless steel. The studies conducted up to now using biodegradable metals for ureteral stents application are still very scarce but promising. Thereby, it is envisioned the clinical translation of a biodegradable metallic ureteral stent in a near future.

Another appealing approach to improve the mechanical properties and degradation time of BUS is the combination of biodegradable polymers with biodegradable metals. Jin et al. evaluated the performance of a BUS based on filaments of Mg alloys covered with biodegradable polyurethane and a coating composed of a biodegradable polymer and barium sulphate [55]. The stents started to degrade after 1 week implantation on pig's ureter and degraded completely after 4 weeks. The degradation process is not explained but the authors highlight the better drainage ability of the developed stents [55].

3 Conclusions and Future Perspectives

Considerable progress has been done on ureteral stent's properties with the aim to meet the clinical problems encountered. Even though this progress does not end up with an ureteral stent without associated complications, it allows to understand the behaviour of different materials and designs in the urologic environment. Indeed, the vast amount of work done and respective outputs have been proven that the different materials can complement each other's disadvantages, for example, the metals can bear with the high compression that polymeric stents cannot. The goal is to combine the advantages of each material without their associated complications. Indeed, promising works have been validating the success of this approach, such as the combination of polymers and metals (Silhouette®) or biodegradable polymers and biodegradable metals. Biodegradable materials seem to be a superior alternative due to their undoubtedly outstanding advantages, the only concern that still needs to be optimized thorough is the degradation rate. However, it should be highlighted the outstanding progresses that have been made in the design of ureteral stents by tailoring their composition. Therefore, the use of biodegradable materials and combination of different raw materials and design adjustments appears to be the future of ureteral stents design.

References

1. Lange D, Bidnur S, Hoag N, Chew BH. Ureteral stent-associated complications—where we are and where we are going. Nat Rev Urol. 2015;12(1):17–25.
2. Ramachandra M, Mosayyebi A, Carugo D, Somani BK. Strategies to improve patient outcomes and QOL: current complications of the design and placements of ureteric stents. Res Rep Urol. 2020;12:303–14.

3. Zhang K, Cui H, Jiang H, Hao Y, Long R, Ma Q, et al. The current status and applications of ureteral stents. Int J Clin Exp Med. 2020;13(4):2122–33.
4. Herdman JP. Polythene tubing in the experimental surgery of the ureter. Br J Surg. 1949;37(145):105–6.
5. Williams KG, Blacker AJ, Kumar P. Ureteric stents: the past, present and future. J Clin Urol. 2018;11(4):280–4.
6. Zimskind PD, Fetter TR, Wilkerson JL. Clinical use of long-term indwelling silicone rubber ureteral splints inserted cystoscopically. J Urol. 1967;97(5):840–4.
7. Tunney M. Comparative assessment of ureteral stent biomaterial encrustation. Biomaterials. 1996;17(15):1541–6.
8. Khandwekar AP, Doble M. Physicochemical characterisation and biological evaluation of polyvinylpyrrolidone–iodine engineered polyurethane (Tecoflex®). J Mater Sci Mater Med. 2011;22(5):1231–46.
9. Forbes C, Scotland KB, Lange D, Chew BH. Innovations in ureteral stent technology. Urol Clin N Am. 2019;46(2):245–55.
10. Stoller ML, Meng MV, editors. Urinary stone disease the practical guide to medical and surgical management. New York: Springer Science & Business Media; 2007.
11. Gadzhiev N, Gorelov D, Malkhasyan V, Akopyan G, Harchelava R, Mazurenko D, et al. Comparison of silicone versus polyurethane ureteral stents: a prospective controlled study. BMC Urol. 2020;20(1):1–5.
12. Krasovskaya SM, Uzhinova LD, Andrianova MY, Prischenko AA, Livantsov MV, Lomonosov MV. Biochemical and physico-chemical aspects of biomaterials calcification. Biomaterials. 1991;12(9):817–20.
13. Chew BH, Denstedt JD. Technology Insight: novel ureteral stent materials and designs. Nat Clin Pract Urol. 2004;1(1):44–8.
14. Rebl H, Renner J, Kram W, Springer A, Fritsch N, Hansmann H, et al. Prevention of encrustation on ureteral stents: which surface parameters provide guidance for the development of novel stent materials? Polymers. 2020;12(3):558.
15. Liatsikos EN, Karnabatidis D, Katsanos K, Kallidonis P, Katsakiori P, Kagadis GC, et al. Ureteral metal stents: 10-year experience with malignant ureteral obstruction treatment. J Urol. 2009;182(6):2613–8.
16. Rosman BM, Barbosa JABA, Passerotti CP, Cendron M, Nguyen HT. Evaluation of a novel gel-based ureteral stent with biofilm-resistant characteristics. Int Urol Nephrol. 2014;46(6):1053–8.
17. Christman MS, L'Esperance JO, Choe CH, Stroup SP, Auge BK. Analysis of ureteral stent compression force and its role in malignant obstruction. J Urol. 2009;181(1):392–6.
18. Ganatra AM, Loughlin KR. The management of malignant ureteral obstruction treated with ureteral stents. J Urol. 2005;174(6):2125–8.
19. Asakawa J, Iguchi T, Tamada S, Ninomiya N, Kato M, Yamasaki T, et al. Outcomes of indwelling metallic stents for malignant extrinsic ureteral obstruction. Int J Urol. 2018;25(3):258–62.
20. Elsamra SE, Leavitt DA, Motato HA, Friedlander JI, Siev M, Keheila M, et al. Stenting for malignant ureteral obstruction: tandem, metal or metal-mesh stents. Int J Urol. 2015;22(7):629–36.
21. Barros AA, Oliveira C, Lima E, Duarte ARC, Healy K, Reis RL. Ureteral stents technology: biodegradable and drug-eluting perspective. In: Ducheyne P, editor. Comprehensive biomaterials II. 7th ed. Amsterdam: Elsevier; 2017. p. 793–812.
22. Chen Y, Liu C, Zhang Z, Xu P, Chen D, Fan X, et al. Malignant ureteral obstruction: experience and comparative analysis of metallic versus ordinary polymer ureteral stents. World J Surg Oncol. 2019;17(74):1–10.
23. Modi AP, Ritch CR, Arend D, Walsh RM, Ordonez M, Landman J, et al. Multicenter experience with metallic ureteral stents for malignant and chronic benign ureteral obstruction. J Endourol. 2010;24(7):1189–93.
24. Buchholz N, Hakenberg O, Bach C, Masood J, editors. Handbook of urinary stents: basic science and clinical applications. 1st ed. JP Medical Ltd: New York; 2016.
25. Turk T, Rao M, Polcari A. Updates on the use of ureteral stents: focus on the Resonance® stent. Med Devices Evid Res. 2011;4:11–5.

26. Blaschko SD, Deane LA, Krebs A, Abdelshehid CS, Khan F, Borin J, et al. In-vivo evaluation of flow characteristics of novel metal ureteral stent. J Endourol. 2007;21(7):780–3.
27. Miyazaki J, Onozawa M, Takahashi S, Maekawa Y, Yasuda M, Wada K, et al. The resonance® metallic ureteral stent in the treatment of malignant ureteral obstruction: a prospective observational study. BMC Urol. 2019;137:1–19.
28. Pedro RN, Hendlin K, Kriedberg C, Monga M. Wire-based ureteral stents: impact on tensile strength and compression. Urology. 2007;70(6):1057–9.
29. Agrawal S, Brown CT, Bellamy EA, Kulkarni R. The thermo-expandable metallic ureteric stent: an 11-year follow-up. BJU Int. 2009;103(3):372–6.
30. Kallidonis P, Kotsiris D, Sanguedolce F, Ntasiotis P, Liatsikos E, Papatsoris A. The effectiveness of ureteric metal stents in malignant ureteric obstructions: a systematic review. Arab J Urol. 2017;15(4):280–8.
31. Chung KJ, Park BH, Park B, Lee JH, Kim WJ, Baek M, et al. Efficacy and safety of a novel, double-layered, coated, self-expandable metallic mesh stent (Uventa™) in malignant ureteral obstructions. J Endourol. 2013;27(7):930–5.
32. Pollak JS, Rosenblatt MM, Egglin TK, Dickey KW, Glickman M. Treatment of ureteral obstructions with the wallstent endoprosthesis: preliminary results. J Vasc Interv Radiol. 1995;6(3):417–25.
33. Bahouth Z, Moskovitz B, Halachmi S, Nativ O. Allium stents: a novel solution for the management of upper and lower urinary tract strictures. Rambam Maimonides Med J. 2017;8(4):e0043.
34. Hendlin K, Korman E, Monga M. New metallic ureteral stents: improved tensile strength and resistance to extrinsic compression. J Endourol. 2012;26(3):271–4.
35. Wang L, Yang G, Xie H, Chen F. Prospects for the research and application of biodegradable ureteral stents: from bench to bedside. J Biomater Sci Polym Ed. 2018;29(14):1657–66.
36. Schlick RW, Planz K. Potentially useful materials for biodegradable ureteric stents. BJU Int. 1997;80(6):908–10.
37. Olweny EO, Landman J, Andreoni C, Collyer W, Kerbl K, Onciu M, et al. Evaluation of the use of a biodegradable ureteral stent after retrograde endopyelotomy in a porcine model. J Urol. 2002;167(5):2198–202.
38. Lumiaho J, Heino A, Tunnien V, Ala-Opas M, Talja M, Välimaa T, et al. New bioabsorbable polylactide ureteral stent in the treatment of ureteral lesions: an experimental study. J Endourol. 1999;13(2):107–12.
39. Li G, Wang Z-X, Fu W-J, Hong B-F, Wang X-X, Cao L, et al. Introduction to biodegradable polylactic acid ureteral stent application for treatment of ureteral war injury. BJU Int. 2011;108(6):901–6.
40. Lumiaho J, Heino A, Pietiläinen T, Ala-Opas M, Talja M, Välimaa T, et al. The morphological, in situ effects of a self-reinforced bioabsorbable polylactide (SR-PLA 96) ureteric stent; an experimental study. J Urol. 2000;164(4):1360–3.
41. Yang G, Xie H, Huang Y, Lv Y, Zhang M, Shang Y, et al. Immersed multilayer biodegradable ureteral stent with reformed biodegradation: an in vitro experiment. J Biomater Appl. 2017;31(8):1235–44.
42. Zhang Y, He J, Chen H, Xiong C. A new hydrophilic biodegradable ureteral stent restrain encrustation both in vitro and in vivo. J Biomater Appl. 2021;35(6):720–31.
43. Soria F, de la Cruz JE, Budia A, Serrano A, Galan-Llopis JA, Sanchez-Margallo FM. Experimental assessment of new generation of ureteral stents: biodegradable and antireflux properties. J Endourol. 2020;34(3):359–65.
44. Hadaschik BA, Paterson RF, Fazli L, Clinkscales KW, Shalaby SW, Chew BH. Investigation of a novel degradable ureteral stent in a porcine model. J Urol. 2008;180(3):1161–6.
45. Chew BH, Paterson RF, Clinkscales KW, Levine BS, Shalaby SW, Lange D. In vivo evaluation of the third generation biodegradable stent: a novel approach to avoiding the forgotten stent syndrome. J Urol. 2013;189(2):719–25.

46. Lingeman JE, Preminger GM, Berger Y, Denstedt JD, Goldstone L, Segura JW, et al. Use of a temporary ureteral drainage stent after uncomplicated ureteroscopy: results from a phase II clinical trial. J Urol. 2003;169(5):1682–8.
47. Lingeman JE, Schulsinger DA, Kuo RL. Phase I trial of a temporary ureteral drainage stent. J Endourol. 2003;17(3):169–71.
48. Barros AA, Rita A, Duarte C, Pires RA, Sampaio-Marques B, Ludovico P, et al. Bioresorbable ureteral stents from natural origin polymers. J Biomed Mater Res Part B Appl Biomater. 2015;103(3):608–17.
49. Barros AA, Oliveira C, Lima E, Duarte ARC, Reis RL. Gelatin-based biodegradable ureteral stents with enhanced mechanical properties. Appl Mater Today. 2016;5:9–18.
50. Barros AA, Oliveira C, Ribeiro AJ, Autorino R, Reis RL, Duarte ARC, et al. In vivo assessment of a novel biodegradable ureteral stent. World J Urol. 2018;36(2):277–83.
51. Reis R, Duarte AR, Barros A, Lima E, Oliveira C, Pinto J. An ureteral stent, methods and uses thereof. WO2016181371A1, 2016.
52. Lock JY, Wyatt E, Upadhyayula S, Whall A, Nuñez V, Vullev VI, et al. Degradation and antibacterial properties of magnesium alloys in artificial urine for potential resorbable ureteral stent applications. J Biomed Mater Res Part A. 2014;102(3):781–92.
53. Zhang S, Bi Y, Li J, Wang Z, Yan J, Song J, et al. Biodegradation behavior of magnesium and ZK60 alloy in artificial urine and rat models. Bioact Mater. 2017;2(2):53–62.
54. Tie D, Liu H, Guan R, Holt-Torres P, Liu Y, Wang Y, et al. In vivo assessment of biodegradable magnesium alloy ureteral stents in a pig model. Acta Biomater. 2020;116:415–25.
55. Jin L, Yao L, Yuan F, Dai G, Xue B. Evaluation of a novel biodegradable ureteral stent produced from polyurethane and magnesium alloys. J Biomed Mater Res Part B Appl Biomater. 2020;109(9):665–72.

Coatings for Urinary Stents: Current State and Future Directions

Beatriz Domingues, Joana M. Silva, Ivo M. Aroso, Estêvão Lima,
Alexandre A. Barros, and Rui L. Reis

1 Introduction

Urinary stent coatings are a strategy to tackle certain complications associated with the use of the materials previously mentioned on in previous chapters. The latest innovations in surface coatings focused on the prevention of those problems, thus reducing further costs with treatments. As previously mentioned on this book, device-associated infections and encrustation are considered the major challenges, and, in an attempt to prevent such morbidity, several strategies were developed. Hence, coatings have been designed to improve quality of life for patients, reducing the friction, inhibiting uropathogens survival or attachment on stents, and avoiding the deposition of urinary crystals that triggers encrustation [1–3]. In the light of current knowledge regarding biofilm formation mechanisms, coating solutions can be divided, according to its purpose, in anti-adhesive coatings and bactericidal coatings.

B. Domingues · J. M. Silva · I. M. Aroso · A. A. Barros (✉) · R. L. Reis
3B's Research Group, I3Bs – Research Institute on Biomaterials, Biodegradables and Biomimetics, European Institute of Excellence on Tissue Engineering and Regenerative Medicine, University of Minho, Guimarães, Portugal

ICVS/3B's–PT Government Associate Laboratory, Braga/Guimarães, Portugal
e-mail: beatriz.domingues@i3bs.uminho.pt; joana.marques@i3bs.uminho.pt;
ivo.aroso@i3bs.uminho.pt; abarros@hydrumedical.pt; rgreis@i3bs.uminho.pt

E. Lima
School of Health Sciences, Life and Health Sciences Research Institute (ICVS), University of Minho, Braga, Portugal
e-mail: estevaolima@med.uminho.pt

© The Author(s) 2022
F. Soria et al. (eds.), *Urinary Stents*,
https://doi.org/10.1007/978-3-031-04484-7_18

209

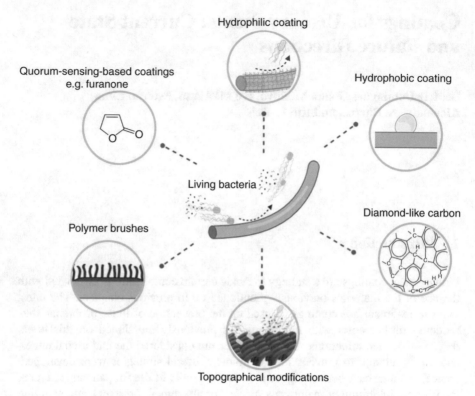

Fig. 1 Anti-adhesive coatings confer resistance to microorganism and protein adhesion. Distinct surface modifications can impair these processes, without directly causing bacterial death

2 Anti-adhesive Coatings

The anti-adhesive, or antifouling, strategies avoid the adhesion of microorganisms by preventing the attachment or allowing an easy detachment (Fig. 1). The key drive force to create these designs was the high resistance of biofilms to conventional antibiotic therapies. Therefore, the surface modification approaches usually provide the anti-adhesive properties with great antibacterial effects and low toxicity associated [4].

2.1 Hydrophilic and Hydrophobic Coatings

To prevent microorganism adhesion and encrustation on medical devices, both hydrophilic and hydrophobic solutions can be used [4, 5]. Hydrogels consist in hydrophilic crosslinked polymers, with ability to swell and retain large amounts of water [6]. When used as coatings for ureteral stents, hydrogels are exposed to urine, which allows its absorption by the polymeric structure. The hydration layer facilitates stent placement by reducing friction, potentially increasing patient comfort [2, 6]. This type of hydrogel on stent surface acts as a barrier, reducing adhesion of microorganisms and providing antifouling properties to the stent [6]. In an *in vitro* study, poly(*N*,*N*-dimethylacrylamide) (PDMAA) hydrogel network on ureteral stents reduced significantly the adherence of the most common uropathogens [7]. In a recent study with 104 patients, hydrogel-coated ureteral stents proved to be a superior option, comparing with uncoated commercial polyurethane ureteral stents. For treatments between 1 and 3 months, patients with hydrogel-coated stents reported lower side-effects rate and complications [8].

Similar to hydrogels, hydrophilic poly(vinyl pyrrolidone) (PVP) and polyethylene glycol (PEG) are capable of absorbing water, which provides a beneficial lubricious effect when used as coatings [9]. Besides that, after an *in vitro* study over a 14-week period with artificial urine, PVP-coated silicone and polyurethane stents presented significantly less encrustation than the uncoated ones [9]. PEG is also considered a antifouling agent for biomedical applications [10], however its thermal, oxidative, or hydrolytic degradation and the difficulty to generate a dense coating impair its utilisation. To overcome this, PEG can be conjugated with 3,4-dihydroxyphenylalanine (DOPA), an important amino acid in marine adhesive proteins [11]. *In vitro*, DOPA conjugated PEG coating proved to significantly resisted the attachment of uropathogens, comparing to control, while *in vivo*, using rabbit model, it was reported a reduction of 75% in the number of stent adherent organisms [12]. Although the potential of PVP and PEG for urological use has already been proven in studies [9, 11–13], validation in more complex models is still lacking.

Furthermore, antifouling hydrogel based on natural polysaccharide has a high clinical relevance in the urinary context. Polysaccharides are present on the surface of many microbial cells, mediating most of the cell–surface and cell–cell interactions that are highly responsible for biofilm formation [14]. However, it is also undoubtedly that several polysaccharides widely distributed in nature are actually able to inhibit or destabilize biofilm formation. Among polysaccharides, heparin, a highly-sulphated glycosaminoglycan, is widely known for its ability to inhibit bacterial attachment and its effects have been observed mostly on cardiovascular field but also on ureteral stents [15]. Heparin-coated stents were able to successfully remain encrustation-free during 6 weeks of indwelling time, while uncoated stents present biofilm formation only after 2 weeks [16]. In line with this study, in a long-term study involving patients, heparin-coated stents presented no signals of encrustation up to 10 months after insertion [17]. Besides heparin, hyaluronic acid is another polysaccharide tested as coating for urinary devices. Using a validated *in vitro* encrustation model, covalently bound hyaluronic acid catheters were associated with less encrustation than the control, silicone [18]. Despite these promising results, up to date, clinical relevance has never been assessed. Chitosan, a biodegradable polysaccharide, also displays antimicrobial properties and, due to its biocompatibility, it is possible to use it for biomedical applications [19]. Chitosan-based coating resisted biofilm formation by bacteria and yeast, over a 54-h experiment, with reductions in biofilm viable cell numbers ranging from 95 to ≈ 99.99%, comparing to control [20]. In another static study, the development of a chitosan/ poly(vinyl alcohol) (PVA) hydrogel successfully reduced protein absorption and provide antimicrobial properties to segmented polyurethane urethral catheters [21].

Due to its superhydrophilicity, zwitterionic coatings also emerged as highly effective antifouling strategy. Nowadays, there are three major classes of zwitterionic materials based on poly(phosphorylcholine), poly(sulfobetaine), and poly(carboxybetaine) [14, 22]. Zwitterionic coatings form a hydration layer surrounding the ionic surface, preventing non-specific protein adsorption and conferring a high resistance to microorganisms adhesion [23–27]. In an *in vitro* assay, a bioinspired surface functionalization with phosphorylcholine proved to enhanced lubrication and bacterial resistance to the surface of titanium alloy biomedical implants [28]. Recently, 2 zwitterionic polymers, poly(sulfobetaine methacrylate) (pSBMA) and poly(carboxybetaine methacrylate) (pCBMA), were used as coating for silicone surfaces. The coated material showed the antifouling properties provided by the zwitterionic polymers, proving that this is a promising approach for ureteral stent coatings [29]. Applying this rationale, Fan et al. [30] revealed that these type of coatings showed strong antimicrobial activity, as confirmed by the low number of viable adhered bacteria on silicone-based urinary devices. Another SBMA antifouling zwitterionic coating was tested in a urinary catheter for 1 week, using a dynamic system simulating the real usage conditions of the device. Besides increased hydrophilicity and reduced protein adsorption, results showed a biofilm formation reduction by 80% compared to the biofilm produced on the urethra of uncoated catheters, and by about 90% in the case of the biofilm produced on the catheter balloon. Moreover, this coating did not affect the viability of the human fibroblasts, showing increased potential for clinical use [23]. In addition, it is also possible to create layer-by-layer zwitterionic surface modification, as evidenced by Li et al. [31], using a polydopamine (PDA) layer, then a monolayer of 3-aminopropyl triethoxysilane (APTES) and finally the zwitterionic polysulfobetaine (PSB) layer. When tested *in vitro*, this construct dramatically reduced the protein and bacterial adhesion [31]. The research on hydrophilic coatings for ureteral medical devices is growing exponentially and it has already been translated nowadays in commercially available options, such as AQ® from Cook Urological, SL-6 from Applied Medical, HydroPlus™ from Boston Scientific, and heparin-based coating Endo-Sof™ Radiance™, from Cook Urological.

Hydrophobic coatings have also been applied on ureteral stents, among each polytetrafluoroethylene (PTFE) or teflon. Teflon has a wide range of applications, however, for this Chapter is only important to highlight its capacity to reduce biofilm development. This effect results from its resistance to Van der Waals forces, and, possibly, also due to the lower coefficient of friction [32]. Teflon-coated metal stents were associated with decreased reaction of epithelial cells to metal, resulting in increased biocompatibility. Additionally, an *in vivo* study performed in canine ureters with metallic self-expanding stents PTFE-covered proved that the benefits of this coating go beyond antimicrobial effects, as these formulations effectively prevented the luminal occlusion caused by urothelial hyperplasia [33]. The described results were obtained 5, 10, 15, and 30 weeks after insertion, suggesting that

PTFE-covered stents have clinical relevance for short and intermediate treatments [33]. More currently, superhydrophobic surfaces have become an emerging topic due to its water-repellent and self-cleaning properties [34]. Superhydrophobic soot coatings can be created by deposition via combustion flame synthesis, followed by functionalization using plasma polymerization and/or fluorination. In an *in vitro* assay, the anti-bioadhesion activity of these coatings was proven, since the proliferation of *Pseudomonas* species was significantly inhibited [35]. Although recent, this rationale is promising and it is a valid approach to investigate in the urological context.

Antifouling properties can also be provided by amphiphilic polymers, which combine both hydrophilic and hydrophobic parts. An amphiphilic polymer synthesized with dodecyl methacrylate (DMA), poly(ethylene glycol) methacrylate (PEGMA), and an acrylic acid (AA) successfully coated the surfaces of commercial catheter material and reduced bacterial adhesion, under static and dynamic conditions [36]. In a *in vivo* experiment, mice were observed over a 4-day period, and it was conclude that this amphiphilic coating effectively resisted *S. aureus* adhesion [36]. Nonetheless, further research is needed to fully assess the clinical relevance of this approach.

2.2 Diamond-Like Carbon Coatings

In 2004, Norbert Laube's research group [37] described for the first time the use of diamond-like carbon coatings (DLCs) on urological devices. This form of amorphous carbon material combines antimicrobial activity with its inert nature, biocompatibility, lubricity and durability features. The *in vivo* and *in vitro* studies demonstrated DLCs was capable of relieve patient symptoms, infections and encrustations [38, 39]. This coating was further tested in patients, during almost 7 years. With a stent removal frequency of less than 6 weeks, no crystalline biofilm formation was observed and due to the low friction, patients reported a less painful experience [5]. Nowadays, DLCs are a commercial option in the ureteral stent market (Ureteral Stent Set—CarboSoft), due to their promissory effect on reducing biofilm formation, the risk of encrustation and urinary tract infections, even for long-term treatments.

2.3 Topographical Modifications

As verified previously, nature is a valid source of inspiration to create new and improved solutions for medicine. Antifouling systems based on active topographies exist in nature, e.g. wings of insects, such as cicadas and dragonflies, and even in the human body, where the lung epithelial cells repel microbes with beating cilia [40]. Inspired by nature, topographical modifications, at micrometer and nanometer scale, can be engineered in urinary devices to provide the desired effect. This technology was tested in the urinary context by Gu et al. [41], that created a urinary catheter with micron-sized pillars that can beat at a programmable frequency. This active topographic design not only prevented biofilm formation, but also removed established biofilms of the studied uropathogens, including *E. coli*, *P. aeruginosa*, and *S. aureus*. Under flow of artificial urine, the coated catheters remained clean at least during 30 days, while control catheters were blocked by *E. coli* biofilms within 5 days [41]. While topographical modifications strategies are still relatively in its infancy, they represent a valid method to achieve the desired antifouling effects.

2.4 Polymer Brushes

Polymer brushes form an antifouling surface, since these structures impair the adsorption of biomolecules, decreasing the attachment of microorganisms and consequent biofilm formation [42, 43]. Alves et al. [44, 45] demonstrated the potential of this strategy for urinary tract devices, evaluating distinct polymer brushes, namely poly[*N*-(2-hydroxypropyl) methacrylamide] and also poly[oligo(ethylene glycol) methyl ether methacrylate], under adequate hydrodynamic conditions. The results showed that the surface area covered by bacteria was decreased up to 60% when compared with the control. Gultekinoglu et al. [46] designed polyurethane ureteral stents with polyethylenimine (PEI) brushes. In static conditions, this construct effectively presented bactericidal activity against *E. coli* and *P. mirabilis*, without any cytotoxic effect on L929 and G/G cells, proving to be a good candidate for antifouling and antimicrobial strategies for ureteral stents. Validation on more complex models is a key factor for the further development of this approach.

2.5 Quorum-Sensing-Based Coatings

In the light of current knowledge about bacterial mechanisms, it is possible to create a quorum-sensing-based solution to prevent bacterial adhesion on ureteral stents. Quorum-sensing is a cell–cell communication process used by bacteria to monitor cell population density, allowing bacteria to synchronize the gene expression as a group [47]. The disruption of this process impairs bacteria capacity to form biofilm, which may be used an alternative approach to tackle antimicrobial resistance [48]. Although the study of quorum-sensing-based coatings is still at an early stage, some auspicious results were already available [49, 50]. A layer-by-layer coating was developed comprising acylase and α-amylase, which are able to degrade bacterial quorum-sensing molecules and extracellular matrix, respectively. This multilayered coating demonstrated 30% higher antibiofilm efficiency against common uropathogens, such as *E. coli* and *P. aeruginosa* [49]. Additionally, under both static and dynamic conditions, this innovative coating on silicone urinary devices significantly reduced the occurrence of biofilms with single-specie and mixed-species, suggesting that it can be a suitable option for ureteral stents [49]. In an *in vivo* study, using rabbit as model, results proved that the quorum-quenching and matrix degrading enzyme construct inhibited the biofilm formation up to 7 days. Considering the resistance mechanisms of bacterial biofilms, it can be hypothesized that inhibiting biofilm formation would later increase the bacteria susceptibility to antimicrobials, even at subminimal inhibitory concentrations [49]. More recently, furanone, a quorum-sensing inhibitor, was used as a coating for urinary catheters, resulting in a complete blockage for *Candida* sp. adhesion, under static conditions [50]. This practice is still incipient and more validation is required in order to pass from the bench to the bedside.

3 Bactericidal Coating

In contrast to anti-adhesive coatings, bactericidal coatings prevent the attachment of microorganisms, but also trigger their death. In the case of ureteral coatings, most approaches are designed to trigger bacterial death, however, other uropathogens are also affected [4].

3.1 Release of Antimicrobial Agents

The successful development of an effective coating with eluting proprieties required the identification of the most promising antimicrobial agents, that for the urinary tract context may include antibiotics and metals composites (Fig. 2).

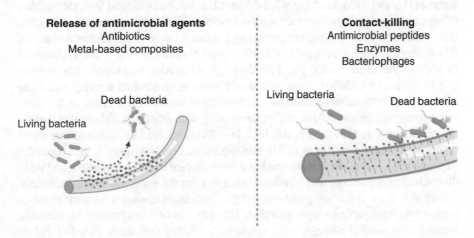

Fig. 2 Bactericidal coatings trigger bacterial death, either through the release of antimicrobials agents or by contact-killing approaches

3.1.1 Antibiotics

In case of ureteral stents-associated infections, the use of prophylactic antibiotics as a systemic therapy can trigger the development of further microbial resistance, without avoiding the attachment of the already resistant uropathogens [51]. The rationale behind the use of antibiotics in coatings consists in the opportunity of enhance the antimicrobial effects locally, without the adverse effects of a systemic therapy. Several antibiotics, such as ciprofloxacin, norfloxacin, ofloxacin, gentamicin, chlorhexidine, were incorporated on ureteral devices, and its efficacy was proven against the common uropathogens [52–54]. After a meta-analysis study, it was demonstrated that this strategy is effective for short-term implants, however the release profile of this type of compounds, with an initial burst release followed by concentrations that are not inhibitory, may not actually be translated into a favorable therapeutic effect [55]. In fact, for long-term implants, this strategy favors the development of microbial resistance, creating an infection even more difficult to treat [32].

3.1.2 Metal-Based Coatings

Metal, metal oxide, or composite nanoparticles are suitable alternatives as antimicrobial agents, being able to prevent biofilm-associated infections on medical implants [56]. The broad-spectrum antimicrobial mechanism of silver is well-known [57, 58] and it was one of the pioneer approaches in the urologic devices to prevent device-associated infections [59]. Its application is already approved by Food and Drug Administration (FDA) for the urinary context, namely for urinary catheters [26]. Over the years, numerous studies, including clinical trials, proved the effectiveness of the silver coatings against device-associated infections. In 2014, in a multicenter cohort study, Lederer et al. [60] reported that the silver alloy hydrogel catheter (Bardex I.C.), used for at least 3 months, inhibit in almost 50% the number of reported cases of symptomatic device-associated infections, comparing to standard catheters. Nonetheless, contradicting studies described the ineffectiveness of this strategy, reporting no significant differences between the use of the device with or without the silver coating [61, 62]. This type of coating was reported as ineffective in long-term catheterization, as it easily loses antimicrobial activity, and some clinical trials have demonstrated the occurrence of bacterial resistance in the intermittent catheterization. Additionality, comparing with other antimicrobial catheters, the cytotoxicity to host cells is still high [47–49]. This lead to conclude that silver could be a good candidate to tackle uroinfections, however there is still room for improvement. Novel silver materials have been studied over the last years, and up to date silver nanoparticles and silver nanoclusters are the most promising materials, within this area, for urinary stent coatings. Besides releasing antibacterial silver ions, silver nanoparticles with less than 100 nm can be incorporated by bacteria, leading to structural damages and, ultimately, causing cell death [63, 64]. Silver nanoclusters, due to its size < 2 nm, demonstrated an improved antimicrobial efficiency compared with the silver nanoparticles [26, 65–67]. An *ex vivo* study, using a set-up that mimics the biological conditions during stenting, silver nanoclusters were associated with less 45% of friction, comparing with the uncoated ones, which can indicate less pain to the patient [68].

Throughout the years, other metal-based approaches gained prominence due to their antibacterial properties, with emphasis on zinc oxide, with its intrinsic antimicrobial activity and biocompatibility [69]. Synergistically combination of zinc oxide films and the 2-hydroxyethyl methacrylate (HEMA) hydrogel by Laurenti et al. [69] created a barrier layer that *in vitro* prevented the unbeneficial burst release of zinc oxide. This advantageous effect results from the incorporation of a pH-triggered delivery system that controls the sustained release of this material. These findings indicated that the design is an encouraging candidate for urinary tract devices. Within metal-based coatings, a distinct concept using copper-bearing stainless steel was already evaluated in an *in vivo* rabbit model. Stents were analyzed 20, 40 and 80 days after implantation, and copper-bearing stainless steel coating was associated with less adherent microorganisms and deposited crystals, with significant differences comparing to uncoated control [70]. The conclusions drawn in this study represent a major advance for this strategy and further boost its use in urinary tract devices.

3.2 Contact-Killing

Within contact-killing coatings are included surfaces that exhibit antimicrobial activity without releasing antibiotics or other biocidal agents.

3.2.1 Antimicrobial Peptides (AMPs)

AMPs are antimicrobials effective against both Gram-negative and Gram-positive strains, viruses, and fungi, representing one of the most promising alternatives to conventional antimicrobial agents [71]. Usually, AMPs are short peptides with cationic charge and a great portion of hydrophobic residues, around 50%. This positive charge and amphiphilic nature allow AMPs to interact with several types of bacteria. The mechanisms of action are diversified, which confers AMPs a broad-spectrum of antimicrobial activity [71]. The disruption of cytoplasmic membrane [72], autolysin activation, inhibition of DNA, RNA, and protein synthesis [73] are some of the mechanisms already described in literature. A recent *in vitro* study of Wang et al. [74] revealed that AMPs can in fact reduce biofilm formation on medical tubes used in urology up to 7 days, which corroborates the use of this material in urological devices. *In vitro* assays demonstrated that chemo selective covalent immobilization of Dhvar5 AMP, a synthetic peptide derived from the histatins family, on thin chitosan coatings resulted in the decrease of bacterial colonization [75].

Wang et al. [74] demonstrated, in a 7-day *in vitro* test, that a customized and bought AMP, Bmap-28, incorporated into a biodegradable hydrophilic polyurethane was capable of inhibit bacterial biofilm formation of *P. mirabilis* and delay catheter obstruction caused by encrustation.

3.2.2 Enzyme-Containing Coatings

In the recent past, enzymes have been considered as a new generation of antimicrobial agents, targeting microbial growth and biofilm formation [76]. A cellobiose dehydrogenase functionalized urinary catheter was evaluated in artificial urine, over 16 days, resulting in the reduction of the viable *S. aureus* by 60%, and in the decrease of biofilm formation by 70%, comparing to control [77]. Other enzyme, the protease α-chymotrypsin (α-CT), was covalently immobilized on polyethylene surfaces. Using a Center for Disease Control (CDC) biofilm reactor it was proven that this strategy significantly impacted *E. coli* biofilm formation [78]. More studies will be further needed to fully validate this approach.

3.2.3 Bacteriophages

A recent and promising approach to prevent bacterial contamination on ureteral stents is the use of bacteriophages, i.e., viruses that infect bacteria, and then use bacterial cell as a factory to multiply themselves [79]. Bacteriophages are an attractive therapeutic agent, with highly specificity and very effective for the targeted pathogen. In case of lytic phages, the mechanism of action consist in the disturbance of the bacterial metabolism, inducing cellular lyses and consequent death [79]. Khawaldeh et al. [80] described a successful bacteriophage therapy for refractory *P. aeruginosa* urinary tract infection, in a 67-year-old woman that underwent extensive intra-abdominal resections and pelvic irradiation for adenocarcinoma, followed by bilateral ureteric stent placement to relieve obstruction. This patient has received multiple courses of gentamicin, ceftazidime, ciprofloxacin and meropenem over a 2-year period, with consecutive failures. During the study, no bacteriophage-resistant bacteria were reported, and the therapy resulted in symptomatic relief and microbiological cure, where repeated courses of antibiotics combined with stent removal had failed [80].

4   Conclusions and Future Perspectives

Coatings are an effective approach to improve urinary devices, reducing the most common complications experienced by patients during treatments and avoiding the even more challenging need to search for completely new materials associated with less morbidity. Currently for ureteral stents, hydrophilic and diamond-like carbon coatings are commercial options associated with an enhanced performance of devices, comparing with uncoated ones. These commercially available approaches are all anti-adhesive coatings, and, in the general overview, this type of strategy appears to be a superior alternative than bactericidal coatings. Designs that trigger uropathogen death are usually associated with higher toxicity, and, in some cases, it can even favor the development of microbial resistance, which can hamper the infection treatment. With the present knowledge about antimicrobial mechanisms and inspired by nature, more cutting-edge alternatives, able to confer antimicrobial properties to the inner and outer parts of stents, will surely appear. The correct validation of those strategies, according to international standards, is a very important step for the rise of innovative and effective solutions for urinary stents.

References

1. Ma X, Wu T, Robich MP. Drug-eluting stent coatings. Interv Cardiol. 2012;4(1):73–83.
2. Denstedt J, Atala A, editors. Biomaterials and tissue engineering in urology. 1st ed. Cambridge: Woodhead Publishing Limited; 2009.
3. Baum S, Pentecost MJ, editors. Abrams' angiography: interventional radiology. 2nd ed. Pennsylvania: Lippincott Williams & Wilkins; 2006.
4. Vladkova TG, Staneva AD, Gospodinova DN. Surface engineered biomaterials and ureteral stents inhibiting biofilm formation and encrustation. Surf Coat Technol. 2020;404:126424.
5. Liu L, Shi H, Yu H, Yan S, Luan S. The recent advances in surface antibacterial strategies for biomedical catheters. Biomater Sci. 2020;8(15):4074–87.
6. Mosayyebi A, Manes C, Carugo D, Somani BK. Advances in ureteral stent design and materials. Curr Urol Rep. 2018;19(5):35.
7. Szell T, Dressler FF, Goelz H, Bluemel B, Miernik A, Brandstetter T, et al. In vitro effects of a novel coating agent on bacterial biofilm development on ureteral stents. J Endourol. 2019;33(3):225–31.
8. Grigore N, Pirvut V, Mihai I, Hasegan A, Mitariu SIC. Side-effects of polyurethane ureteral stents with or without hydrogel coating in urologic pathology. Mater Plast. 2017;54(3):517–9.
9. Tunney MM, Gorman SP. Evaluation of a poly(vinyl pyrrolidone)-coated biomaterial for urological use. Biomaterials. 2002;23(23):4601–8.
10. Morra M. On the molecular basis of fouling resistance. Aust J Biol Sci. 2000;11(6):547–69.
11. Waite JH, Tanzer ML. The bioadhesive of *Mytilus byssus*: a protein containing L-dopa. Biochem Biophys Res Commun. 1980;96(4):1554–61.
12. Pechey A, Elwood CN, Wignall GR, Dalsin JL, Lee BP, Vanjecek M, et al. Anti-adhesive coating and clearance of device associated uropathogenic *Escherichia coli* cystitis. J Urol. 2009;182(4):1628–36.
13. Raut PW, Khandwekar AP, Sharma N. Polyurethane–polyvinylpyrrolidone iodine blends as potential urological biomaterials. J Mater Sci. 2018;53:11176–93.
14. Maan AMC, Hofman AH, Vos WM, Kamperman M. Recent developments and practical feasibility of polymer-based antifouling coatings. Adv Funct Mater. 2020;30(32):2000936.
15. Biran R, Pond D. Heparin coatings for improving blood compatibility of medical devices. Adv Drug Deliv Rev. 2017;112:12–23.
16. Stickler DJ, Evans A, Morris N, Hughes G. Strategies for the control of catheter encrustation. Int J Antimicrob Agents. 2002;19(6):499–506.

17. Cauda V, Cau F. Polyurethane in urological practice. In: Zafar F, Sharmin E, editors. Polyurethane. Rijeka: InTech; 2012. p. 123–46.
18. Choong SKS, Wood S, Whitfield HN. A model to quantify encrustation on ureteric stents, urethral catheters and polymers intended for urological use. BJU Int. 2002;86(4):414–21.
19. Junter GA, Thébault P, Lebrun L. Polysaccharide-based antibiofilm surfaces. Acta Biomater. 2016;30:13–25.
20. Carlson RP, Taffs R, Davison WM, Stewart PS. Anti-biofilm properties of chitosan-coated surfaces. J Biomater Sci Polym Ed. 2008;19(8):1035–46.
21. Yang S-H, Lee Y-SJ, Lin F-H, Yang J-M, Chen K. Chitosan/poly(vinyl alcohol) blending hydrogel coating improves the surface characteristics of segmented polyurethane urethral catheters. J Biomed Mater Res Part B Appl Biomater. 2007;83B(2):304–13.
22. Li B, Jain P, Ma J, Smith JK, Yuan Z, Hung HC, et al. Trimethylamine N-oxide—derived zwitterionic polymers: a new class of ultralow fouling bioinspired materials. Sci Adv. 2019;5(6):eaaw9562.
23. Diaz Blanco C, Ortner A, Dimitrov R, Navarro A, Mendoza E, Tzanov T. Building an anti-fouling zwitterionic coating on urinary catheters using an enzymatically triggered bottom-up approach. ACS Appl Mater Interfaces. 2014;6(14):11385–93.
24. Vaterrodt A, Thallinger B, Daumann K, Koch D, Guebitz GM, Ulbricht M. Antifouling and antibacterial multifunctional polyzwitterion/enzyme coating on silicone catheter material pre-pared by electrostatic layer-by-layer assembly. Langmuir. 2016;32(5):1347–59.
25. Tyler BJ, Hook A, Pelster A, Williams P, Alexander M, Arlinghaus HF. Development and characterization of a stable adhesive bond between a poly(dimethylsiloxane) cath-eter material and a bacterial biofilm resistant acrylate polymer coating. Biointerphases. 2017;12(2):02C412.
26. Zhu Z, Wang Z, Li S, Yuan X. Antimicrobial strategies for urinary catheters. J Biomed Mater Res A. 2019;107A:445–67.
27. Kovačevi D, Pratnekar R, Godič Torkar K, Salopek J, Draži G, Abram A, et al. Influence of polyelectrolyte multilayer properties on bacterial adhesion capacity. Polymers. 2016;8(10):345.
28. Liu S, Zhang Q, Han Y, Sun Y, Zhang Y, Zhang H. Bioinspired surface functionalization of tita-nium alloy for enhanced lubrication and bacterial resistance. Langmuir. 2019;35:13189–95.
29. Leigh BL, Cheng E, Xu L, Derk A, Hansen MR, Guymon CA. Antifouling photograftable zwitterionic coatings on PDMS substrates. Langmuir. 2019;35:1100–10.
30. Fan YJ, Pham MT, Huang CJ. Development of antimicrobial and antifouling universal coating via rapid deposition of polydopamine and zwitterionization. Langmuir. 2019;35:1642–51.
31. Li S, Huang P, Ye Z, Wang Y, Wang W, Kong D, et al. Layer-by-layer zwitterionic modification of diverse substrates with durable anti-corrosion and anti-fouling properties. J Mater Chem B. 2019;7:6024–34.
32. Lopez-Lopez G, Pascual A, Perea EJ. Effect of plastic catheter material on bacterial adherence and viability. J Med Microbiol. 1991;34(6):349–53.
33. Chung H-H, Seung AE, Ae HL, Bum S, Ae C, Suk H, et al. Comparison of a new polytetrafluoroethylene-covered metallic stent to a noncovered stent in canine ureters. Cardiovasc Intervent Radiol. 2008;31:619–28.
34. Zhu H, Guo Z, Liu W. Adhesion behaviors on superhydrophobic surfaces. Chem Commun. 2014;50(30):3900–13.
35. Esmeryan KD, Avramova IA, Castano CE, Ivanova IA, Mohammadi R, Radeva EI, et al. Early stage anti-bioadhesion behavior of superhydrophobic soot based coatings towards *Pseudomonas putida*. Mater Des. 2018;160:395–404.
36. Keum H, Yu B, Yu SJ. Prevention of bacterial colonization on catheters by a one-step coat-ing process involving an antibiofouling polymer in water. ACS Appl Mater Interfaces. 2017;9(23):19736–45.
37. Laube N. Diamonds are a urologist's best friend. EurekAlert! Science News AAAS; 2004. https://www.eurekalert.org/news-releases/897553.

38. Laube N, Kleinen L, Bradenahl J, Meissner A. Diamond-like carbon coatings on ureteral stents-a new strategy for decreasing the formation of crystalline bacterial biofilms? J Urol. 2007;177(5):1923–7.
39. Laube N, Bradenahl J, Meissner A, Rappard JV, Kleinen L, Müller SC. Plasma-deposited carbon coating on urological indwelling catheters: preventing formation of encrustations and consecutive complications. Urologe A. 2006;45(9):1163–9.
40. Tilley AE, Walters MS, Shaykhiev R, Crystal RG. Cilia dysfunction in lung disease. Annu Rev Physiol. 2015;77:379–406.
41. Gu H, Lee SW, Carnicelli J, Zhang T, Ren D. Magnetically driven active topography for long-term biofilm control. Nat Commun. 2020;11:2211.
42. Rodriguez-Emmenegger C, Brynda E, Riedel T, Houska M, Šubr V, Alles AB, et al. Polymer brushes showing non-fouling in blood plasma challenge the currently accepted design of protein resistant surfaces. Macromol Rapid Commun. 2011;32(13):952–7.
43. Nuzzo RG. Stable antifouling surfaces. Nat Mater. 2003;2:207–8.
44. Alves P, Gomes L, Vorobii M, Rodriguez-Emmenegger C, Mergulhão F. The potential advantages of using a poly(HPMA) brush in urinary catheters: effects on biofilm cells and architecture. Colloids Surf B Biointerfaces. 2020;191:110976.
45. Alves P, Gomes LC, Rodríguez-Emmenegger C, Mergulhão FJ. Efficacy of a poly(MeOEGMA) brush on the prevention of Escherichia coli biofilm formation and susceptibility. Antibiotics. 2020;9(5):216.
46. Gultekinoglu M, Sarisozen Y, Erdogdu C, Sagiroglu M, Aksoy EA, Oh YJ, et al. Designing of dynamic polyethyleneimine (PEI) brushes on polyurethane (PU) ureteral stents to prevent infections. Acta Biomater. 2015;21:44–54.
47. Ng W-L, Bassler BL. Bacterial quorum-sensing network architectures. Annu Rev Genet. 2009;43:197–222.
48. Salini R, Sindhulakshmi M, Poongothai T, Pandian SK. Inhibition of quorum sensing mediated biofilm development and virulence in uropathogens by Hyptis suaveolens. Antonie Van Leeuwenhoek. 2015;107(4):1095–106.
49. Ivanova K, Fernandes MM, Francesko A, Mendoza E, Guezguez J, Burnet M, et al. Quorum-quenching and matrix-degrading enzymes in multilayer coatings synergistically prevent bacterial biofilm formation on urinary catheters. ACS Appl Mater Interfaces. 2015;7(49):27066–77.
50. Devadas SM, Nayak UY, Narayan R, Hande MH, Ballal M. 2,5-Dimethyl-4-hydroxy-3(2H)-furanone as an anti-biofilm agent against non-Candida albicans Candida species. Mycopathologia. 2019;184:403–11.
51. Lo J, Lange D, Chew B. Ureteral stents and Foley catheters-associated urinary tract infections: the role of coatings and materials in infection prevention. Antibiotics. 2014;3(1):87–97.
52. Zelichenko G, Steinberg D, Lorber G, Friedman M, Zaks B, Lavy E, et al. Prevention of initial biofilm formation on ureteral stents using a sustained releasing varnish containing chlorhexidine: in vitro study. J Endourol. 2013;27(3):333–7.
53. Reid G, Sharma S, Advikolanu K, Tieszer C, Martin RA, Bruce AW. Effects of ciprofloxacin, norfloxacin, and ofloxacin on in vitro adhesion and survival of Pseudomonas aeruginosa AK1 on urinary catheters. Antimicrob Agents Chemother. 1994;38(7):1490–5.
54. Noimark S, Dunnill CW, Wilson M, Parkin IP. The role of surfaces in catheter-associated infections. Chem Soc Rev. 2009;38:3435–48.
55. Pietsch F, O'Neill AJ, Ivask A, Jenssen H, Inkinen J, Kahru A, et al. Selection of resistance by antimicrobial coatings in the healthcare setting. J Hosp Infect. 2020;106(1):115–25.
56. Naik K, Srivastava P, Deshmukh K, Monsoor MS, Kowshik M. Nanomaterial-based approaches for prevention of biofilm-associated infections on medical devices and implants. J Nanosci Nanotechnol. 2015;15(12):10108–19.

57. Dervisevic E, Dervisevic M, Nyangwebah JN, Şenel M. Development of novel amperometric urea biosensor based on Fc-PAMAM and MWCNT bio-nanocomposite film. Sens Actuators B. 2017;246:920–6.
58. Percival SL, Bowler PG, Russell D. Bacterial resistance to silver in wound care. J Hosp Infect. 2005;60(1):1–7.
59. Schaeffer AJ, Story KO, Johnson SM. Effect of silver oxide/trichloroisocyanuric acid antimicrobial urinary drainage system on catheter-associated bacteriuria. J Urol. 1988;139(1):69–73.
60. Lederer JW, Jarvis WR, Thomas L, Ritter J. Multicenter cohort study to assess the impact of a silver-alloy and hydrogel-coated urinary catheter on symptomatic catheter-associated urinary tract infections. J Wound Ostomy Cont Nurs. 2014;41(5):473–80.
61. Desai DG, Liao KS, Cevallos ME, Trautner BW. Silver or nitrofurazone impregnation of urinary catheters has a minimal effect on uropathogen adherence. J Urol. 2010;184(6):2565–71.
62. Stenzelius K, Laszlo L, Madeja M, Pessah-Rasmusson H, Grabe M. Catheter-associated urinary tract infections and other infections in patients hospitalized for acute stroke: a prospective cohort study of two different silicone catheters. Scand J Urol. 2016;50(6):483–8.
63. Sondi I, Salopek-Sondi B. Silver nanoparticles as antimicrobial agent: a case study on E. coli as a model for Gram-negative bacteria. J Colloid Interface Sci. 2004;275(1):177–82.
64. Kim JS, Kuk E, Yu KN, Kim JH, Park SJ, Lee HJ, et al. Antimicrobial effects of silver nanoparticles. Nanomedicine. 2007;3(1):95–101.
65. Zheng K, Setyawati MI, Lim TP, Leong DT, Xie J. Antimicrobial cluster bombs: silver nanoclusters packed with daptomycin. ACS Nano. 2016;10(8):7934–42.
66. Yuan X, Setyawati MI, Leong DT, Xie J. Ultrasmall Ag^+-rich nanoclusters as highly efficient nanoreservoirs for bacterial killing. Nano Res. 2014;7:301–7.
67. Yuan X, Setyawati MI, Tan AS, Ong CN, Leong DT, Xie J. Highly luminescent silver nanoclusters with tunable emissions: cyclic reduction-decomposition synthesis and antimicrobial properties. NPG Asia Mater. 2013;5:e39.
68. Carvalho I, Faraji M, Ramalho A, Carvalho AP, Carvalho S, Cavaleiro A. Ex-vivo studies on friction behaviour of ureteral stent coated with Ag clusters incorporated in a: C matrix. Diamond Relat Mater. 2018;86:1–7.
69. Laurenti M, Grochowicz M, Cauda V. Porous ZnO/2-hydroxyethyl methacrylate eluting coatings for ureteral stent applications. Coatings. 2018;8(11):376.
70. Zhao J, Cao Z, Lin H, Yang H, Li J, Li X, et al. In vivo research on Cu-bearing ureteral stent. J Mater Sci Mater Med. 2019;30:83.
71. Bahar A, Ren D. Antimicrobial peptides. Pharmaceuticals. 2013;6(12):1543–75.
72. Yu L, Guo L, Ding JL, Ho B, Feng S, Popplewell J, et al. Interaction of an artificial antimicrobial peptide with lipid membranes. Biochim Biophys Acta Biomembr. 2009;1788(2):333–44.
73. Nguyen LT, Haney EF, Vogel HJ. The expanding scope of antimicrobial peptide structures and their modes of action. Trends Biotechnol. 2011;29(9):464–72.
74. Wang J, Liu Q, Tian Y, Jian Z, Li H, Wang K. Biodegradable hydrophilic polyurethane PEGU25 loading antimicrobial peptide Bmap-28: a sustained-release membrane able to inhibit bacterial biofilm formation in vitro. Sci Rep. 2015;5:8634.
75. Costa FMTA, Maia SR, Gomes PAC, Martins MCL. Dhvar5 antimicrobial peptide (AMP) chemoselective covalent immobilization results on higher antiadherence effect than simple physical adsorption. Biomaterials. 2015;52:531–8.
76. Thallinger B, Prasetyo EN, Nyanhongo GS, Guebitz GM. Antimicrobial enzymes: an emerging strategy to fight microbes and microbial biofilms. Biotechnol J. 2013;8(1):97–109.
77. Thallinger B, Brandauer M, Burger P, Sygmund C, Ludwig R, Ivanova K, et al. Cellobiose dehydrogenase functionalized urinary catheter as novel antibiofilm system. J Biomed Mater Res Part B. 2016;104(7):1448–56.
78. Cattò C, Secundo F, James G, Villa F, Cappitelli F. α-Chymotrypsin immobilized on a low-density polyethylene surface successfully weakens Escherichia coli biofilm formation. Int J Mol Sci. 2018;19(12):4003.

79. Sulakvelidze A, Alavidze Z, Morris J. Bacteriophage therapy. Antimicrob Agents Chemother. 2001;45(3):649–59.
80. Khawaldeh A, Morales S, Dillon B, Alavidze Z, Ginn AN, Thomas L, et al. Bacteriophage therapy for refractory *Pseudomonas aeruginosa* urinary tract infection. J Med Microbiol. 2011;60(11):1697–700.

Bacterial Adhesion and Biofilm Formation: Hydrodynamics Effects

Luciana C. Gomes, Rita Teixeira-Santos, Maria J. Romeu, and Filipe J. Mergulhão

Abbreviations

3-D	Three-dimensional
AUM	Artificial urine medium
CFD	Computational fluid dynamics
CLSM	Confocal laser scanning microscopy
FC	Flow chamber
MRD	Modified Robbins device
PDMS	Polydimethylsiloxane
PPFC	Parallel-plate flow chamber
RD	Robbins device
UTD	Urinary tract device
UTI	Urinary tract infection

L. C. Gomes · R. Teixeira-Santos · M. J. Romeu
LEPABE-Laboratory for Process Engineering, Environment, Biotechnology and Energy,
Faculty of Engineering, University of Porto, Porto, Portugal
e-mail: luciana.gomes@fe.up.pt; ritadtsantos@fe.up.pt; mariaromeu@fe.up.pt

F. J. Mergulhão (✉)
LEPABE-Laboratory for Process Engineering, Environment, Biotechnology and Energy,
Faculty of Engineering, University of Porto, Porto, Portugal

ALiCE-Associate Laboratory in Chemical Engineering, Faculty of Engineering, University of
Porto, Porto, Portugal
e-mail: filipem@fe.up.pt

© The Author(s) 2022   225
F. Soria et al. (eds.), *Urinary Stents*,
https://doi.org/10.1007/978-3-031-04484-7_19

1 Introduction

The complications associated with indwelling ureteral stents, namely bacterial adhesion and biofilm formation, have been the main driving force for the development of new materials or coatings with antimicrobial and anti-adhesive properties. The first approach for testing and optimizing new biomedical surfaces usually consists of evaluating their *in vitro* efficacy under controlled experimental conditions that reflect the human physiological environment [1]. Consequently, several parameters, including the pathogenic species and their concentration, culture medium, temperature, and hydrodynamic conditions, must be considered when setting an *in vitro* experiment, hence increasing its predictive value and avoiding, during initial screening, expensive *in vivo* assays and animal sacrifice [1] without prior evidence of surface effectiveness. Among these parameters, hydrodynamic conditions have a prominent role in the experimental setup as assays performed in static conditions do not mimic the fluid flow that occurs at specific locations of the human body (e.g. urinary tract). Furthermore, it is well known that hydrodynamic conditions affect not only bacterial adhesion to biomedical surfaces [2], but also biofilm growth and architecture [3, 4]. In fact, flow determines the transport rate of planktonic cells to the surface and their subsequent interaction [5], as well as the transport of oxygen and nutrients to the biofilm [6]. Besides, flow influences both bacterial attachment and detachment rates [7].

The effectiveness of biomedical surfaces may also be highly affected by the hydrodynamic conditions [1]. Surfaces releasing antimicrobial substances when exposed to flow may exhibit shorter lifetimes than at static conditions [1]. Likewise, depending on the fluid flow surrounding the surface, contact-killing surfaces that are adhesive for bacterial cells may be covered by bacterial debris, which decreases their antimicrobial activity [1]. Lastly, non-adhesive coatings, such as polymer brush coatings, are generally sensitive to external stimuli, exhibiting higher antifouling performance at quasi-static conditions and more effective fouling release behavior under dynamic conditions [8].

Considering the importance of hydrodynamic conditions and their effects on bacterial adhesion and biofilm formation, a diversity of *in vitro* flow systems, including the Robbins device (RD) and modifications, the drip flow biofilm reactor, rotary biofilm reactors and flow chambers (FCs), have been developed and optimized to evaluate surfaces effectiveness under physiological conditions [9]. Certain flow systems enable real-time visualization of bacteria adhesion/biofilm development under controlled conditions (e.g. shear stress or shear rate, temperature), allow simultaneous testing of different materials, and can be used as high-throughput platforms [9], while others have some limitations in operating at highly controlled hydrodynamic conditions [1]. Hence, each platform presents advantages and disadvantages that must be considered before use.

In this chapter, the most commonly used platforms for the *in vitro* assessment of bacterial adhesion and biofilm formation under flow conditions—the modified Robbins device, flow chambers, and microfluidic devices—are introduced, and their main advantages and disadvantages discussed. These three testing platforms have been particularly used to evaluate the anti-adhesive and antibiofilm performance of novel surface materials for urinary tract devices (UTDs), including catheters and stents, due to their ability to control the hydrodynamics (shear stress and flow rate) and recreate *in vivo* flow conditions.

2 Robbins Device and Modifications

The Robbins device was initially developed by Jim Robbins and Bill McCoy to study biofilm formation in industrial water systems [10]. The RD consists of a pipe with several holes where coupons are mounted on the end of the screws and become in contact with the fluid. Thus, the RD generates submerged biofilms growing in aqueous systems that can be used for the investigation of multispecies communities [10].

Several modifications were later introduced to this design, including the use of a square-channel pipe where coupons are aligned with the inner surface without disturbing flow characteristics [11]. Other designs include a half-pipe geometry that more closely resembles the circular section of a tube [4]. With the modified Robbins devices (MRDs), the flow can be momentarily stopped to allow direct access to the coupons so that time-course experiments are also possible [3].

MRDs have been operated in conditions that mimic the flow in urinary catheters [12, 13] and stents [13, 14]. Tunner et al. [14] were among the first authors to use a continuous flow model based on an MRD to assess encrustation on silicone and polyurethane, the most widely used ureteral stent biomaterials. They revealed that the type and degree of encrustation produced were similar to those found *in vivo*, recommending this flow system for comparative evaluation of surface candidates for medical devices used in the urinary tract [14]. More recently, in our research group, a MRD (referred to as flow cell system) simulating the hydrodynamic conditions found in urinary catheters (shear rate of 15/s) [15] was used to characterize the microbial physiology of *Escherichia coli* and *Delftia tsuruhatensis* individually and in a consortium, in terms of growth kinetics and substrate uptake, when exposed to artificial urine medium (AUM) flow and silicone material [12]. Additionally, we used a custom-made semi-circular flow cell identical to that shown in Fig. 1 to assess the efficacy of different nanocomposite coatings in preventing urinary tract infections (UTIs) [13]. The hydrodynamics of this flow cell was fully characterized by computational fluid dynamics (CFD) [16], and it has been shown that the shear stress field is approximately the same in the curved and flat walls so that coupons can be placed on the flat wall for convenience and still be subjected to the same shear forces acting on the curved wall [17]. Moreover, this flow cell was constructed to have enough inlet length to allow for full flow development and a large surface area on which the hydrodynamic conditions remain constant for a wide range of flow velocities [16]. These dynamic systems are particularly useful for screening purposes as they enable the simultaneous testing of several surfaces [13, 14].

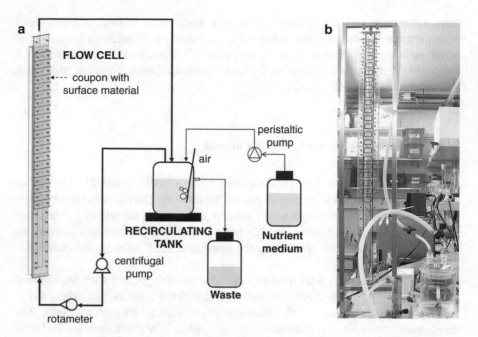

Fig. 1 (**a**) Schematic representation and (**b**) photograph of a MRD. The system is mainly composed by a recirculating tank, one vertical semi-circular flow cell (about a meter high) with removable coupons, and peristaltic and centrifugal pumps

Another advantage of MRDs is that coupons can be removed independently, for instance, at different experimental times [12].

3 Flow Chamber

Despite the many advantages of the MRDs, they are usually not suited for direct analysis of biofilm development [18], and they are not adequate to monitor cell adhesion to a surface. Nowadays, there are several models of flow chambers that can be mounted on a microscope stage and used with video capture systems, enabling real-time observation of microbial adhesion, particularly when used with transparent surfaces [18]. Different custom-made FCs have been used to evaluate the antiadhesive and antibiofilm properties of novel surfaces for UTDs, namely catheters and stents, in flow conditions that simulate those typically found in these medical devices [2, 15, 19, 20]. Table 1 summarizes several studies found in the literature where flow chamber assays were performed under fully characterized hydrodynamic conditions similar to those of urinary catheters and stents. Most of these studies aimed to monitor the initial adhesion of bacteria associated with UTIs (*E. coli, Enterococcus faecalis, Staphylococcus aureus* and *Pseudomonas aeruginosa*) to polymeric surfaces as polydimethylsiloxane (PDMS) [2, 9] and PDMS modified

Table 1 Flow chamber studies to evaluate the initial adhesion and biofilm formation under hydrodynamic conditions identical to those found in UTDs

Study aim	Surface material	Microorganisms	Culture conditions (medium, cell concentration, flow rate and/or Re, and time)	Shear stress and/or shear rate values	Major conclusions	Refs.
Initial adhesion	Smooth PDMS, smooth PDMS with peptide coating, micropatterned PDMS and micropatterned PDMS with peptide coating	E. coli	AUM 7.6 × 10⁷ cells/mL $Q = 2$ and 4 mL/s 30-min assay	0.010 and 0.024 Pa	The highest E. coli adhesion was obtained on the smooth PDMS, whereas the micropatterned PDMS coated with peptide totally inhibited adhesion. The peptide addition to the smooth PDMS reduced the adhesion by 43–58%, while the micropatterned PDMS reduced the adhesion by 99%.	[21]
	PDMS and CNT/PDMS composites	E. coli	Citrate buffer 7.6 × 10⁷ cells/mL $Q = 2$ mL/s 30-min assay	0.010 Pa 15/s	Introduction of the CNTs in the PDMS matrix yielded less bacterial adhesion than the PDMS alone. Less adhesion was obtained on the composites with pristine rather than functionalized CNTs. Incorporation of higher amounts of CNTs in polymer composites can affect bacterial adhesion by more than 40%. Composites enabling a 60% reduction in cell adhesion were obtained by CNT treatment by ball-milling.	[22, 23]
	Glass, poly(HPMA) and poly(MeOEGMA) brushes	E. coli	Citrate buffer 7.6 × 10⁷ cells/mL $Q = 2$ and 4 mL/s 30-min assay	0.010 and 0.024 Pa	The poly(MeOEGMA) and poly(HPMA) surfaces reduced the initial adhesion up to 90% when compared to glass.	[58]
	Glass, peptide-coated glass and PLLA	E. coli	Citrate buffer and enriched medium 7.6 × 10⁷ cells/mL $Q = 2$ and 4 mL/s 30-min assay	15 and 30/s	Adhesion reductions of 40–50% were attained at a shear rate of 15/s on the peptide-coated surfaces compared with bare glass. The performance of the peptide-based antifouling coating was superior to PLLA.	[26]
	Glass, PDMS and PLLA	E. coli	Citrate buffer 7.6 × 10⁷ cells/mL $Q = 2$ and 4 mL/s 30-min assay	0.01 and 0.022 ± 0.002 Pa (equivalent to 32/s)	Similar adhesion rates were obtained on glass and PDMS. The highest adhesion rates were obtained on glass and PDMS and the lowest on PLLA.	[2, 9]

(continued)

Table 1 (continued)

Study aim	Surface material	Microorganisms	Culture conditions (medium, cell concentration, flow rate and/or Re, and time)	Shear stress and/or shear rate values	Major conclusions	Refs.
	Silicone wafers, silicone rubber and PAAm brushes	S. aureus, Strep. salivarius, C. albicans	PBS or saliva, 3×10^8 bacteria/mL and 3×10^6 yeast/mL, 4-h assay	10/s	A high reduction (52–92%) in microbial adhesion to the surface-grafted PAAm brush was observed as compared with untreated silicon surfaces. PAAm brush coatings on silicone rubber inhibited microbial adhesion as well as PAAm brushes grafted from silicon wafers.	[59, 60]
	Glass and PEO-coated glass slide	S. epidermidis, S. aureus, Strep. salivarius, E. coli, Ps. aeruginosa, C. albicans, C. tropicalis	PBS, 3×10^8 bacteria/mL and 3×10^6 yeast/mL, $Q = 0.025$ mL/s, 4-h assay	10/s	The PEO brush yielded more than 98% reduction in bacterial adhesion, although for the more hydrophobic Ps. aeruginosa a smaller reduction was observed. For yeast species, adhesion suppression was less effective than for the bacteria, and here the more hydrophobic C. tropicalis showed less reduction than the more hydrophilic C. albicans.	[61]
	Silicone rubber	UTI isolates: E. coli, Ent. faecalis, S. epidermidis, Ps. aeruginosa, C. albicans	Human urine, 3×10^8 bacteria/mL and 3×10^6 yeast/mL, $Q = 0.034$ mL/s, 4-h assay	15/s	Cranberry and ascorbic acid supplementation can provide a degree of protection against adhesion and colonization of biomaterials by some uropathogens.	[20]
	Glass or silicone rubber coated with different concentrations of a biosurfactant	Ent. faecalis	PBS or pooled human urine, 3×10^8 cells/mL, $Q = 0.034$ mL/s, $Re = 1$, 4-h assay	15/s	Biosurfactant layers greatly inhibited the initial deposition rates (> 30%) and adhesion numbers (≈ 70–100%) in a dose-related way. This inhibition was stronger when buffer was used. For urine experiments, biosurfactant coatings on silicone caused higher adhesion reductions.	[15]
	Glass and FEP	Ent. faecalis	PBS or pooled human urine, 3×10^8 cells/mL, 4.5-h assay	15/s	Ent. faecalis was displaced by lactobacilli (31%) and streptococci (74%) from FEP in buffer and that displacement by lactobacilli was even more effective on glass in urine (54%). The passage of an air–liquid interface significantly impacted adhesion, especially when the surface had been challenged with lactobacilli (up to 100%) or streptococci (up to 94%).	[62]

Biofilm formation	PDMS, glass and the poly(HPMA) brush	E. coli	AUM 7.6 × 10^7 cells/mL Q = 2 mL/s 24 h biofilm formation (infection period) + 8 h fresh medium exposure (post-infection period)	15/s	Initial adhesion and surface coverage decreased on poly(HPMA) brush. This antifouling behavior was maintained during infection and post-infection period, when the reduction in total cell number reached 87%. VBNC cells were completely removed from the brush. Poly(HPMA) may reduce biofilm growth and antibiotic resistance in urinary catheters.	[19]
	PDMS, glass and poly(MeOEGMA) brush	E. coli	AUM 7.6 × 10^7 cells/mL Q = 2 mL/s 24 h biofilm formation + 8 h antibiotic treatment	15/s	The polymer brush reduced by 57% the surface area covered after 24 h, as well as the number of total adhered cells. The antibiotic treatment potentiated cell death and removal (88%). Poly(MeOEGMA) brush has the potential to prevent biofilm growth in UTDs, and in eradicating biofilms developed in these devices.	[24]
	Platinum electrodes	P. mirabilis	AUM 2 × 10^6 CFU/mL Q = 3333 mL/s 6 days	200/s	By applying alternating microcurrent densities, a self-regenerative surface is produced, which actively removed the conditioning film and significantly reduced bacterial adherence, growth, and survival.	[63]
	Silicone and silicone coated with ppVP	E. coli UTI isolates E. coli standard strain	Peptone-glucose nutrient medium 1 × 10^6 CFU/mL Q = 4 × 10^{-3} mL/s Re = 1.19 20–24 h	33/s	The temperature had a considerable influence upon the adhesion and biofilm-forming capacity of some of the isolates, and the influence of surface chemistry depended on temperature.	[25]

AUM artificial urine medium, *CNT* carbon nanotube, *FEP* fluorinated ethylene propylene, *PBS* phosphate-buffered saline, *PEO* poly(ethylene oxide), *PLLA* poly-L-lactic acid, *PAAm* polyacrylamide, *poly(HPMA)* poly[N-(2-hydroxypropyl) methacrylamide], *poly(MeOEGMA)* poly[oligo(ethyleneglycol) methyl ether methacrylate], *PDMS* polydimethylsiloxane, *ppVP* plasma polymerized vinylpyrrolidone, *Q* flow rate, *Re* Reynolds number, *UTDs* urinary tract devices, *VBNC* viable but nonculturable, *C. Candida*, *Ent. Enterococcus*, *E. Escherichia*, *P. Proteus*, *Ps. Pseudomonas*, *S. Staphylococcus*, *Strep. Streptococcus*

with antimicrobial substances (peptides and carbon nanotubes) [21–23] for 30 min to 4 h. In some instances, these systems were also used to investigate bacterial biofilm growth and survival for 24 h on novel surface coatings for UTDs [19, 24, 25].

A custom-made FC system (Fig. 2) was designed by our group to analyse cell adhesion [22, 26] and biofilm formation [19, 24]. This system includes a parallel-plate flow chamber (PPFC) coupled to a jacketed tank and connected to centrifugal pumps and a valve by a silicone tubing system. The valve allows the bacterial suspension to circulate through the system at a controlled flow rate, and the recirculating water bath is connected to the tank jacket to enable temperature control. To illustrate the type of data that can be obtained with this platform, biofilm formation experiments with *E. coli* were carried out for 24 h using PDMS as the test surface [27] and AUM recirculated through the FC system at 4 mL/s to mimic the urine flow behavior in ureteral stents (shear rate of 15/s). After 24 h, the system was stopped, and the biofilm formed on the PDMS surface was stained with a fluorescent dye and analysed by confocal laser scanning microscopy (CLSM) (Fig. 3 and Table 2).

CLSM is an optical imaging technique used to obtain high-resolution images of biofilms at various depths in their naturally hydrated form and to generate three-dimensional (3-D) reconstructions of the samples [28]. It is particularly well suited for monitoring 3-D structure formation in flow chamber-grown biofilms due to its non-invasive and non-destructive character [29, 30]. Early research investigating the use of CLSM in biofilm studies was more descriptive, using qualitative metrics to evaluate biofilm architecture [31]. The development of imaging software packages, specifically for biofilm samples, has enhanced the quantitative output from CLSM images of biofilms [32]. Among these, the COMSTAT ImageJ plugin [32] used in the present work (Table 2) or the PHLIP Matlab toolbox [33, 34] represent a set of reference tools that are efficient and reliable to characterize biofilms in terms of biomass, thickness distribution, surface coverage, roughness coefficient, or porosity.

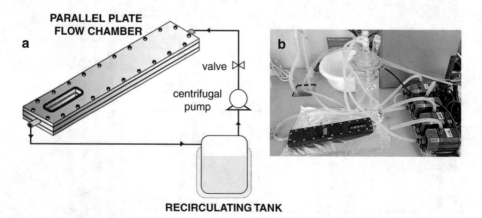

Fig. 2 (**a**) Schematic representation and (**b**) photograph of the FC system. The PPFC is coupled to a glass tank connected to four centrifugal pumps and a tubing system to conduct adhesion or biofilm formation assays

Fig. 3 3-D projection of biofilms formed on PDMS at a flow rate of 4 mL/s mimicking ureteral stents in the described PPFC system. Shown is an *E. coli* biofilm stained with SYTO 61 (633 nm laser line, LEICA HCX PL APO 10 ×/0.40 CS). This representative image was obtained using the "Easy 3D" tool of IMARIS 8.4.1 software (Bitplane, Switzerland) from a confocal *z* stack, and presents an aerial view of the biofilm structure with the shadow projection on the right

Table 2 Quantified data for *E. coli* biofilms grown on PDMS surfaces in the PPFC system. These parameters were obtained from confocal image series using the COMSTAT2 tool associated with the ImageJ software. The means (± standard deviations) for three independent experiments are presented

Biofilm parameters	
Biovolume ($\mu m^3/\mu m^2$)	29.99 (± 2.23)
Average thickness (μm)	72.99 (± 6.94)
Roughness coefficient	0.20 (± 0.02)

4 Microfluidic Devices

Microfluidic platforms have demonstrated high potential and versatility for the study of bacterial adhesion and biofilm formation under different growth conditions. These platforms allow the testing of different channel architectures and types of materials or surfaces at highly controlled flow conditions through a rapid and precise analysis [5]. For these reasons, microfluidic platforms have been used to explore the combined effect of several factors on the development of clinically relevant biofilms [35–37]. Table 3 lists several studies using microfluidic devices for the evaluation of bacterial adhesion and biofilm formation under flow conditions that represent relevant hydrodynamic regions of ureteral stents.

Although microfluidic devices can be constructed by different methodologies and from a diversity of materials, PDMS has been the material of choice for the construction of these devices, with most of the PDMS-based microfluidic devices

Table 3 Microfluidic platforms used for the study of bacterial adhesion and biofilm formation under hydrodynamic conditions identical to those found in ureteral stents

Microfluidic platform	Surface materials	Study aim	Microorganisms	Shear stress and/or shear rate values	Major conclusions	Refs.
PDMS-based microfluidic device	PDMS glass	Early-stage bacterial adhesion (25 min)	Ps. aeruginosa	0.05–10 Pa	The residence time increased with increasing shear stress linearly over a wide range of shear stresses (0.05–3.5 Pa).	[7]
	PA PDMS PEO PLLA PS	Development of a fabrication method to produce a microfluidic device to test cell adhesion (1800 s)	E. coli	0.01–1 Pa	Bacterial adhesion increased linearly over time. The evaluation performed with PDMS surfaces for shear stresses between 0.02 and 1 Pa showed that the lowered surface (inherent weakness of the fabrication method) did not influence adhesion.	[38]
	Glass	Short-term bacterial adhesion (1800 s)	E. coli	0.2–10 Pa	Bacterial adhesion increased in locations with a sudden increase in shear stress.	[39]
	Glass	Short-term bacterial adhesion (1 h)	B. subtillis Ps. aeruginosa	Up to 100/s	The flow produced a strong spatial heterogeneity in bacterial concentration, characterized by up to 70% cell depletion from low-shear regions due to "trapping" in high-shear regions. The maximal depletion occurred at intermediate shear rates. Surface coverage increased with increasing shear rate up to 20/s.	[40]
	PDMS	Short-term bacterial adhesion (1 h) in urinary stents	Ps. fluorescens	Up to 0.175 Pa	The unobstructed device showed no short-term bacterial attachment, including in regions of low WSS (< 0.04 Pa). For the obstructed devices, the cavity region, and the nearby proximal side-hole (WSS of 0.131–0.175 Pa) exhibited greater levels of bacterial attachment (18 ± 3%) compared to other regions of the model.	[5]
	PDMS	Bacterial attachment on curved surfaces (5 h)	E. coli Ps. aeruginosa	Up to 40/s	The bacterial attachment to a curved surface depends on the flow and in slower flow conditions can be up to two-fold higher.	[41]
	Glass	Initial biofilm formation (11 h)	E. coli	1.67, 8.33, 83.3 and 166.6/s	Bacteria were able to form communities at 8.33, 83.3, and 166.6/s. However, the multilayer growth was only visible at 166.6/s after 10 h.	[43]

Glass	Evaluation of bacterial colonization, competition, and dispersal (15 h)	*Ps. aeruginosa* *B. subtilis* *E. coli* *P. mirabilis* *S. aureus* *Sa. typhimurium*	0.02–2 Pa	The upstream movement was a direct response to surface shear stress and conferred to *Ps. aeruginosa* selective growth advantages.	[42]
Glass	Biofilm formation (24–48 h)	*Ps. aeruginosa*	0.002–0.014 Pa	Biofilm thickness was not affected by shear stress after 24 h, displaying on average 10 μm. At 48 h, the biofilm thickness increased significantly (36 ± 9 μm) at 0.0035 Pa and slightly at 0.0035 Pa (20 ± 4 μm). Contrary, no increase was observed for higher shear stress.	[44]
Uncoated and HBP-coated channels	Biofilm formation (16 h)	*S. aureus*	0.02–1 Pa	The flow was the major contributor to the shape of biofilm structures, whereas bacterial motility was less significant.	[45]
Channels coated with fibronectin solution from humans	Influence of constant or intermittent flow on QS-mediated communication during biofilm formation (16 h)	*S. aureus* *Vibrio cholerae*	0.003–0.3 Pa	QS was generally repressed by the flow. However, it could be locally activated in the downstream location of long channels and within the crevices of a groove-like surface.	[48]
Channels treated with octyl(tri-ethoxy)silane	Biofilm formation on intravascular catheters microenvironment (24 h)	*S. epidermidis*	0.065–1.14 Pa	Fluid shear alone induced the formation of polysaccharide intracellular adhesin-positive biofilms and influenced the biofilm structure.	[46]
Electrode surfaces	The effect of hydrodynamic stress on biofilm formation (71 h)	*P. fluorescens*	0.00535–0.0535 Pa	The complete removal of significant portions of biofilm outer layers occurred after the application of extreme shear stress and the structure of the remaining biofilm was susceptible to further changes.	[47]
PDMS	Biofilm growth and detachment (120 h)	*S. epidermidis*	0.01–0.15 Pa	*S. epidermidis* biofilm formation was affected by the local hydrodynamics conditions. Higher WSS conditions limited vertical biofilm growth, resulting in a monolayered structure, while cells growing in stagnant areas were able to divide and proliferate more freely, resulting in the formation of a large multilayered structure.	[35]

(continued)

Table 3 (continued)

Microfluidic platform	Surface materials	Study aim	Microorganisms	Shear stress and/or shear rate values	Major conclusions	Refs.
BioFlux microfluidic system	Glass	Biofilm formation (15 h)	A. baumannii	0.2 Pa	Bacteria attached to the glass surface at the start of the flow stayed attached and did not relocate.	[52]
	Glass	Gene expression during biofilm formation (18 h)	S. aureus	0.06 Pa	The cid and lrg expression was impaired during biofilm development under static conditions compared to flow conditions due to the hypoxic nature of static biofilms.	[49]
	Glass (dynamic) Polystyrene (static)	Biofilm formation (18 h)	Methicillin-resistant S. aureus	0.05 Pa	From tested isolates, 51% successfully formed biofilms under shear flow. However, differences in biofilm formation might also be due to the different adherent surfaces used in the static and dynamic systems.	[53]
	Glass	Gene expression during biofilm formation (18 h)	S. aureus	0.06 Pa	lytS and lytR deletion mutations did not have a visible effect on biofilm structure under microfluidic conditions, while LytR overactive strains induced differences in average biomass, average thickness, and roughness of biofilms formed under static conditions. The biofilm phenotypic differences may be related to the oxygen concentration in dynamic and static conditions.	[50]
	Glass and eukaryotic cells (HRT-18)	Biofilm formation (24 h)	E. coli	0.05–1 Pa	Biofilm formation on glass was observed for the most strains when they were grown in M9 medium at 30 °C but not in RPMI. Similar results were obtained for static conditions. HRT-18 cell monolayers enhanced E. coli binding and biofilm formation in RPMI medium.	[36]
	Glass	Effect of weaker biofilm-forming CNS isolates on the biofilm formation of other staphylococcal isolates (24 h)	Coagulase-negative staphylococci	0.05 Pa	CNS with weak-biofilm phenotype did not inhibit the growth of isolates with a strong-biofilm phenotype either under static or flow conditions.	[54]

CNS coagulase-negative staphylococci, HBP human blood plasm, PA polyamide, PDMS polydimethylsiloxane, PEO polyethylene oxide, PLLA poly-l-lactide acid, PS polystyrene, QS quorum sensing, WSS wall shear stresses, A. Acinetobacter, B. Bacillus, E. Escherichia, P. Proteus, Ps. Pseudomonas, S. Staphylococcus, Sa. Salmonella

being designed for a specific purpose. Several studies have investigated the initial bacterial adhesion on different materials using microfluidic platforms [5, 7, 38–41]. In general, the bacterial residence time and surface coverage increased linearly up to 3.5 Pa [7] and 20/s [40], respectively, and the adhesion rates were higher in locations with a sudden increase in shear forces [39]. For the particular case of ureteral stents, De Garcia et al. [5] demonstrated that unobstructed devices (wall shear stress ≤ 0.0875 Pa) showed no short-term bacterial adhesion, while in obstructed devices, the cavity region and nearby proximal side-hole (wall shear stress of 0.131–0.175 Pa) exhibited higher levels of bacterial attachment compared to other regions of the model. Although channel architecture and geometry affect bacterial adhesion [41], these findings indicate that flow influences both attachment and detachment rates [7].

PDMS-based microfluidic devices have also been applied to explore how bacterial colonization, competition, and dispersal occur at flow conditions. Indeed, flow can confer growth advantages to pathogens by allowing the bacteria upstream movement [42]. Similarly, the study of biofilm development is also possible using these microfluidic platforms [35, 43–48]. Several authors revealed that flow alone was able to induce the formation of polysaccharide intracellular adhesins [46] and was the major modulator of the biofilm structures [45]. Additionally, Lee et al. [35] demonstrated that the morphology of *Staphylococcus epidermidis* biofilm formation was influenced by local hydrodynamic conditions. While higher wall shear stress limited vertical biofilm growth, resulting in a monolayer structure, cells growing in stagnant areas were able to proliferate rapidly, resulting in the formation of a large multilayer structure [35]. Likewise, biofilm thickness was also affected by flow after 48 h, increasing significantly at 0.010 Pa (36 ± 9 µm) and slightly at 0.0035 Pa (20 ± 4 µm). Contrarily, no increase was detected for higher shear stresses [44]. Accordingly, Kim et al. [48] revealed that quorum sensing-mediated communication during biofilm formation was generally repressed by flow, impairing biofilm growth. The comprehensive analysis of gene expression during *S. aureus* biofilm formation was successfully conducted by Moormeier et al. [49, 50] using a different microfluidic device, the BioFlux system (Fluxion Systems, South San Francisco, CA), and compared with static conditions. The BioFlux system was presented as the most prominent commercial microfluidic platform that overcomes the limitations of static well plates and conventional laminar flow chambers. In this system, biofilm formation can be followed by light microscopy in microfluidic wells, allowing rapid screening of the effects of several compounds on the viability of biofilms under hydrodynamic conditions [51]. One of the early studies performed on this platform evaluated the effect of several antimicrobials on 8 h-developed *P. aeruginosa* biofilms under controlled hydrodynamic conditions at 37 °C. Results suggested that biofilm viability measured with the plate reader agreed with those determined using plate counts and with the results of fluorescence microscope image analysis. Since then, the BioFlux system has been considered a high-throughput methodology for the study of biofilm development under defined hydrodynamic conditions [36, 49, 50, 52–54].

Although only 1 of 21 analysed studies had the specific objective of evaluating bacterial adhesion in urinary stents, all provided a comprehensive analysis of adhesion and biofilm formation at flow conditions representative of relevant hydro-dynamic regions of ureteral stents [55] and should be considered when testing a new surface or coating for these medical settings.

5 Operating Conditions

As previously shown, MRDs, flow chambers and microfluidic devices have been used to study bacterial adhesion and biofilm formation under hydrodynamic conditions that simulate the UTDs. Because the flow rate by itself provides little information about shear without taking into account the geometry of the *in vitro* flow system, it is crucial to mimic the flow conditions in a catheter or stent by using either the wall shear stress or the shear rate [1]. The wall shear rate (σ, with unit/s) is a measure of change of the fluid velocity near the wall of the tube in the radial direction toward the center of the tube. In laminar conditions, the shear rate is related to the force which the fluid flow exerts on the wall, expressed as shear stress (τ, with unit Pa), through $\tau = \mu \times \sigma$, where μ is the dynamic viscosity of the fluid (10^{-3} Pa s for water). In the flow systems under study, the flow rate should be adjusted to approach an average shear rate of around 15/s as an estimate of the intraluminal urine flow, based on predictable daily urine production and internal catheter diameter [15]. Nevertheless, urinary output values are highly variable and may reach more than 10 times the mean value [56], yielding a proportional increase in wall shear rate. Some authors performed FC tests at a shear rate of 33/s, which is higher than mean values but still within the range of shear rates found in urinary catheters [25].

Regarding the flow chamber system described in this work (Fig. 2), the numerical simulations indicated that the shear rate of 15/s reported for urinary flow in catheters can be attained at a flow rate of 2 mL/s [2, 9]. On the other hand, the average shear stress in problematic zones of ureteral stents that are prone to encrustation (0.024 Pa) [55] can be obtained by operating the PPFC system at a flow rate of 4 mL/s [21]. In the case of MRDs used by our research group, the recirculation flow rates can range from 5 [12] to 53 mL/s [13] to mimic the shear forces on urinary catheters, depending on the geometry of the flow cell.

PDMS-based microfluidic devices are usually designed for a particular application, having their own architecture and geometry with specific operating conditions. In the case of the commercially available BioFlux system, numerical simulations revealed that the average shear stress value of 0.02 Pa reported for ureteral stents [55] can be reached at a flow rate of 66 μL/h [52].

6   Strengths and Limitations of Flow Platforms

Among the advantages of flow systems are the ability to compare, for instance, the effect that different substrates, media and hydrodynamic conditions exert on a biofilm at different developmental stages. These dynamic models may also provide an evaluation of the effect that transiently occurring molecules, such as antibiotics or adherence inhibitors, have on biofilms. However, the technical disadvantages of flow reactors include increased experimental complexity as well as possible formation/trapping of air bubbles in the setup tubing (particularly severe in microfluidic systems), as this can affect flow and biofilm architecture [57].

Choosing the experimental platform for flow experiments determines what kind of data can be extracted, and care must be taken to ensure that the selected reactor fulfills the objectives of the experiments. The three platforms covered in this chapter (modified Robbins device, flow chamber and microfluidics-based device) have benefits and limitations, which are summarized in Table 4.

Table 4   Advantages and disadvantages of dynamic biofilm cultivation devices

Platform	Advantages	Disadvantages
Modified Robbins device	Large biomass produced	Low to medium throughput
	Large number of sampling ports available for analysis	Limited *in situ* biofilm visualization
	Can run for very long periods without intervention	Biofilm destruction during sampling for quantitative analysis
Flow chamber	Allows direct and nondestructive observation of biofilm development	Low throughput
	Optimized for online *in situ* microscopy	Inability to study adhesion to nontransparent surfaces
Microfluidics-based device	Noninvasive technique	Requires special equipment for manufacturing and running systems
	Allows real-time visualization of biofilm development	Clogging can occur due to small dimensions
	Requires small volumes	Laborious operation
	Can be custom-made for specific purposes	
	Rapid and precise analysis	
	Compatible with single cells analysis	

7 Conclusions

To evaluate the anti-adhesive and antimicrobial performance of novel biomedical materials, a number of flow devices have been designed to recreate *in vivo* flow conditions. Shear stress and flow rate can be accurately controlled and varied in these *in vitro* flow systems, which requires prior knowledge of the flow dynamics inside the platform. After limiting their operational range, modified Robbins devices, flow chambers and microfluidic devices are suggested as experimental set-ups to mimic the flow behavior in urinary catheters and stents.

Acknowledgements This work was financially supported by: LA/P/0045/2020 (ALiCE), UIDB/00511/2020, and UIDP/00511/2020 (LEPABE), funded by national funds through the FCT/ MCTES (PIDDAC); Project PTDC/CTMCOM/4844/2020 funded by the Portuguese Foundation for Science and Technology (FCT); and by Project 2SMART (NORTE-01-0145-FEDER-000054), supported by Norte Portugal Regional Operational Programme (NORTE 2020), under the PORTUGAL 2020 Partnership Agreement, through the European Regional Development Fund (ERDF). L. C. Gomes and M. J. Romeu acknowledge FCT for the financial support of her work contract through the Scientific Employment Stimulus—Individual Call—[CEECIND/01700/2017] and for a PhD grant (SFRH/BD/140080/2018), respectively. R. Teixeira-Santos acknowledges the receipt of a junior researcher fellowship from the Project PTDC/BII-BIO/29589/2017—POCI-01-0145-FEDER-029589. Support from the EU COST Action ENIUS (CA16217) is also acknowledged.

References

1. Ramstedt M, Ribeiro IAC, Bujdakova H, Mergulhão FJ, Jordao L, Thomsen P, et al. Evaluating efficacy of antimicrobial and antifouling materials for urinary tract medical devices: challenges and recommendations. Macromol Biosci. 2019;19(5):e1800384.
2. Moreira JMR, Araújo JDP, Miranda JM, Simões M, Melo LF, Mergulhão FJ. The effects of surface properties on *Escherichia coli* adhesion are modulated by shear stress. Colloids Surf B Biointerfaces. 2014;123:1–7.
3. Teodósio JS, Simões M, Melo LF, Mergulhão FJ. Flow cell hydrodynamics and their effects on *E. coli* biofilm formation under different nutrient conditions and turbulent flow. Biofouling. 2011;27(1):1–11.
4. Pereira MO, Kuehn M, Wuertz S, Neu T, Melo LF. Effect of flow regime on the architecture of a *Pseudomonas fluorescens* biofilm. Biotechnol Bioeng. 2002;78(2):164–71.
5. De Grazia A, LuTheryn G, Meghdadi A, Mosayyebi A, Espinosa-Ortiz EJ, Gerlach R, et al. A microfluidic-based investigation of bacterial attachment in ureteral stents. Micromachines. 2020;11(4):408.
6. Pousti M, Zarabadi MP, Abbaszadeh Amirdehi M, Paquet-Mercier F, Greener J. Microfluidic bioanalytical flow cells for biofilm studies: a review. Analyst. 2019;144(1):68–86.
7. Lecuyer S, Rusconi R, Shen Y, Forsyth A, Vlamakis H, Kolter R, et al. Shear stress increases the residence time of adhesion of *Pseudomonas aeruginosa*. Biophys J. 2011;100(2):341–50.
8. Yang W, Zhou F. Polymer brushes for antibiofouling and lubrication. Biosurf Biotribol. 2017;3(3):97–114.
9. Moreira JMR, Ponmozhi J, Campos JBLM, Miranda JM, Mergulhão FJ. Micro- and macroflow systems to study *Escherichia coli* adhesion to biomedical materials. Chem Eng Sci. 2015;126:440–5.

10. McCoy WF, Bryers JD, Robbins J, Costerton JW. Observations of fouling biofilm formation. Can J Microbiol. 1981;27(9):910–7.
11. Stoodley P, Warwood BK. Use of flow cells an annular reactors to study biofilms. In: Lens P, O'Flaherty V, Moran AP, Stoodley P, Mahony T, editors. Biofilms in medicine, industry and environmental biotechnology: characteristics, analysis and control. 1st ed. Cornwall: IWA Publishing; 2003. p. 197–213.
12. Azevedo AS, Almeida C, Gomes LC, Ferreira C, Mergulhão FJ, Melo LF, et al. An *in vitro* model of catheter-associated urinary tract infections to investigate the role of uncommon bacteria on the *Escherichia coli* microbial consortium. Biochem Eng J. 2017;118:64–9.
13. Vladkova T, Angelov O, Stoyanova D, Gospodinova D, Gomes LC, Soares A, et al. Magnetron co-sputtered $TiO_2/SiO_2/Ag$ nanocomposite thin coatings inhibiting bacterial adhesion and biofilm formation. Surf Coat Technol. 2020;384:125322.
14. Tunney MM, Keane PF, Gorman SP. Assessment of urinary tract biomaterial encrustation using a modified Robbins device continuous flow model. J Biomed Mater Res. 1997;38(2):87–93.
15. Velraeds MMC, Van Der Mei HC, Reid G, Busscher HJ. Inhibition of initial adhesion of uropathogenic *Enterococcus faecalis* to solid substrata by an adsorbed biosurfactant layer from *Lactobacillus acidophilus*. Urology. 1997;49(5):790–4.
16. Teodósio JS, Simões M, Alves MA, Melo LF, Mergulhão FJ. Setup and validation of flow cell systems for biofouling simulation in industrial settings. Sci World J. 2012;2012:361496.
17. Teodósio JS, Silva FC, Moreira JMR, Simões M, Melo LF, Alves MA, et al. Flow cells as quasi-ideal systems for biofouling simulation of industrial piping systems. Biofouling. 2013;29(8):953–66.
18. Azeredo J, Azevedo NF, Briandet R, Cerca N, Coenye T, Costa AR, et al. Critical review on biofilm methods. Crit Rev Microbiol. 2017;43(3):313–51.
19. Alves P, Gomes LC, Vorobii M, Rodriguez-Emmenegger C, Mergulhão FJ. The potential advantages of using a poly(HPMA) brush in urinary catheters: effects on biofilm cells and architecture. Colloids Surf B Biointerfaces. 2020;191:110976.
20. Habash MB, Mei HCV, Busscher HJ, Reid G. The effect of water, ascorbic acid, and cranberry derived supplementation on human urine and uropathogen adhesion to silicone rubber. Can J Microbiol. 1999;45(8):691–4.
21. Dolid A, Gomes LC, Mergulhão FJ, Reches M. Combining chemistry and topography to fight biofilm formation: fabrication of micropatterned surfaces with a peptide-based coating. Colloids Surf B Biointerfaces. 2020;196:111365.
22. Vagos MR, Gomes M, Moreira JMR, Soares OSGP, Pereira MFR, Mergulhão FJ. Carbon nanotube/poly(dimethylsiloxane) composite materials to reduce bacterial adhesion. Antibiotics. 2020;9(8):434.
23. Vagos MR, Moreira JMR, Soares OSGP, Pereira MFR, Mergulhão FJ. Incorporation of carbon nanotubes in polydimethylsiloxane to control *Escherichia coli* adhesion. Polym Compos. 2019;40(S2):E1697–E704.
24. Alves P, Gomes LC, Rodríguez-Emmenegger C, Mergulhão FJ. Efficacy of a poly(MeOEGMA) brush on the prevention of *Escherichia coli* biofilm formation and susceptibility. Antibiotics. 2020;9(5):216.
25. Andersen TE, Kingshott P, Palarasah Y, Benter M, Alei M, Kolmos HJ. A flow chamber assay for quantitative evaluation of bacterial surface colonization used to investigate the influence of temperature and surface hydrophilicity on the biofilm forming capacity of uropathogenic *Escherichia coli*. J Microbiol Methods. 2010;81(2):135–40.
26. Alves P, Nir S, Reches M, Mergulhão FJ. The effects of fluid composition and shear conditions on bacterial adhesion to an antifouling peptide-coated surface. MRS Commun. 2018;8(3):938–46.
27. Gomes M, Gomes LC, Teixeira-Santos R, Mergulhão FJ. PDMS in urinary tract devices: applications, problems and potential solutions. In: Carlsen PN, editor. Polydimethylsiloxane: structure and applications. New York: Nova Science Publishers; 2020. p. 95–144.

28. Cattò C, Cappitelli F. Testing anti-biofilm polymeric surfaces: where to start? Int J Mol Sci. 2019;20(15):3794.
29. Tolker-Nielsen T, Sternberg C. Growing and analyzing biofilms in flow chambers. Curr Protoc Microbiol. 2011;21(1):1B.2.1–B.2.17.
30. Reichhardt C, Parsek MR. Confocal laser scanning microscopy for analysis of *Pseudomonas aeruginosa* biofilm architecture and matrix localization. Front Microbiol. 2019;10(677):677.
31. Thomas RN. *In situ* cell and glycoconjugate distribution in river snow studied by confocal laser scanning microscopy. Aquat Microb Ecol. 2000;21(1):85–95.
32. Heydorn A, Nielsen AT, Hentzer M, Sternberg C, Givskov M, Ersbøll BK, et al. Quantification of biofilm structures by the novel computer program COMSTAT. Microbiology. 2000;146(Pt10):2395–407.
33. Mueller LN, de Brouwer JFC, Almeida JS, Stal LJ, Xavier JB. Analysis of a marine phototrophic biofilm by confocal laser scanning microscopy using the new image quantification software PHLIP. BMC Ecol. 2006;6(1):1.
34. Gomes LC, Deschamps J, Briandet R, Mergulhão FJ. Impact of modified diamond-like carbon coatings on the spatial organization and disinfection of mixed-biofilms composed of *Escherichia coli* and *Pantoea agglomerans* industrial isolates. Int J Food Microbiol. 2018;277:74–82.
35. Lee JH, Kaplan JB, Lee WY. Microfluidic devices for studying growth and detachment of *Staphylococcus epidermidis* biofilms. Biomed Microdevices. 2008;10(4):489–98.
36. Tremblay YD, Vogeleer P, Jacques M, Harel J. High-throughput microfluidic method to study biofilm formation and host–pathogen interactions in pathogenic *Escherichia coli*. Appl Environ Microbiol. 2015;81(8):2827–40.
37. Shields RC, Burne RA. Growth of *Streptococcus mutans* in biofilms alters peptide signaling at the sub-population level. Front Microbiol. 2016;7:1075.
38. Ponmozhi J, Moreira JMR, Mergulhão FJ, Campos JBLM, Miranda JM. Fabrication and hydrodynamic characterization of a microfluidic device for cell adhesion tests in polymeric surfaces. Micromachines. 2019;10(5):303.
39. Neves SF, Ponmozhi J, Mergulhão FJ, Campos JBLM, Miranda JM. Cell adhesion in microchannel multiple constrictions—evidence of mass transport limitations. Colloids Surf B Biointerfaces. 2020;198:111490.
40. Rusconi R, Guasto JS, Stocker R. Bacterial transport suppressed by fluid shear. Nat Phys. 2014;10(3):212–7.
41. Secchi E, Vitale A, Miño GL, Kantsler V, Eberl L, Rusconi R, et al. The effect of flow on swimming bacteria controls the initial colonization of curved surfaces. Nat Commun. 2020;11(1):2851.
42. Siryaporn A, Kim MK, Shen Y, Stone HA, Gitai Z. Colonization, competition, and dispersal of pathogens in fluid flow networks. Curr Biol. 2015;25(9):1201–7.
43. Zhang XY, Sun K, Abulimiti A, Xu PP, Li ZY. Microfluidic system for observation of bacterial culture and effects on biofilm formation at microscale. Micromachines. 2019;10(9):606.
44. Janakiraman V, Englert D, Jayaraman A, Baskaran H. Modeling growth and quorum sensing in biofilms grown in microfluidic chambers. Ann Biomed Eng. 2009;37(6):1206–16.
45. Kim MK, Drescher K, Pak OS, Bassler BL, Stone HA. Filaments in curved streamlines: rapid formation of *Staphylococcus aureus* biofilm streamers. New J Phys. 2014;16(6):065024.
46. Weaver WM, Milisavljevic V, Miller JF, Di Carlo D. Fluid flow induces biofilm formation in *Staphylococcus epidermidis* polysaccharide intracellular adhesin-positive clinical isolates. Appl Environ Microbiol. 2012;78(16):5890–6.
47. Zarabadi MP, Paquet-Mercier F, Charette SJ, Greener J. Hydrodynamic effects on biofilms at the biointerface using a microfluidic electrochemical cell: case study of *Pseudomonas* sp. Langmuir. 2017;33(8):2041–9.
48. Kim MK, Ingremeau F, Zhao A, Bassler BL, Stone HA. Local and global consequences of flow on bacterial quorum sensing. Nat Microbiol. 2016;1:15005.
49. Moormeier DE, Endres JL, Mann EE, Sadykov MR, Horswill AR, Rice KC, et al. Use of microfluidic technology to analyze gene expression during *Staphylococcus aureus* biofilm formation reveals distinct physiological niches. Appl Environ Microbiol. 2013;79(11):3413–24.

50. Lehman MK, Bose JL, Sharma-Kuinkel BK, Moormeier DE, Endres JL, Sadykov MR, et al. Identification of the amino acids essential for LytSR-mediated signal transduction in *Staphylococcus aureus* and their roles in biofilm-specific gene expression. Mol Microbiol. 2015;95(4):723–37.
51. Benoit MR, Conant CG, Ionescu-Zanetti C, Schwartz M, Matin A. New device for high-throughput viability screening of flow biofilms. Appl Environ Microbiol. 2010;76(13):4136–42.
52. Feng SH, Stojadinovic A, Izadjoo M. Distinctive stages and strain variations of *A. baumannii* biofilm development under shear flow. J Wound Care. 2013;22(4):173–4.
53. Vanhommerig E, Moons P, Pirici D, Lammens C, Hernalsteens J-P, De Greve H, et al. Comparison of biofilm formation between major clonal lineages of methicillin resistant *Staphylococcus aureus*. PLoS One. 2014;9(8):e104561.
54. Goetz C, Tremblay YDN, Lamarche D, Blondeau A, Gaudreau AM, Labrie J, et al. Coagulase-negative staphylococci species affect biofilm formation of other coagulase-negative and coagulase-positive staphylococci. J Dairy Sci. 2017;100(8):6454–64.
55. Mosayyebi A, Yue QY, Somani BK, Zhang X, Manes C, Carugo D. Particle accumulation in ureteral stents is governed by fluid dynamics: in vitro study using a "stent-on-chip" model. J Endourol. 2018;32(7):639–46.
56. Fallis WM. Indwelling Foley catheters: is the current design a source of erroneous measurement of urine output? Crit Care Nurse. 2005;25(2):44–6.
57. Magana M, Sereti C, Ioannidis A, Mitchell CA, Ball AR, Magiorkinis E, et al. Options and limitations in clinical investigation of bacterial biofilms. Clin Microbiol Rev. 2018;31(3):e00084–16.
58. Lopez-Mila B, Alves P, Riedel T, Dittrich B, Mergulhão FJ, Rodriguez-Emmenegger C. Effect of shear stress on the reduction of bacterial adhesion to antifouling polymers. Bioinspir Biomim. 2018;13(6):065001.
59. Fundeanu I, van der Mei HC, Schouten AJ, Busscher HJ. Polyacrylamide brush coatings preventing microbial adhesion to silicone rubber. Colloids Surf B Biointerfaces. 2008;64(2):297–301.
60. Cringus-Fundeanu I, Luijten J, van der Mei HC, Busscher HJ, Schouten AJ. Synthesis and characterization of surface-grafted polyacrylamide brushes and their inhibition of microbial adhesion. Langmuir. 2007;23(9):5120–6.
61. Roosjen A, Kaper HJ, van der Mei HC, Norde W, Busscher HJ. Inhibition of adhesion of yeasts and bacteria by poly(ethylene oxide)-brushes on glass in a parallel plate flow chamber. Microbiology. 2003;149(11):3239–46.
62. Millsap K, Reid G, van der Mei HC, Busscher HJ. Displacement of *Enterococcus faecalis* from hydrophobic and hydrophilic substrata by *Lactobacillus* and *Streptococcus* spp. as studied in a parallel plate flow chamber. Appl Environ Microbiol. 1994;60(6):1867–74.
63. Gabi M, Hefermehl L, Lukic D, Zahn R, Vörös J, Eberli D. Electrical microcurrent to prevent conditioning film and bacterial adhesion to urological stents. Urol Res. 2011;39(2):81–8.

Biomaterial-Associated Infection: Pathogenesis and Prevention

Martijn Riool and Sebastian A. J. Zaat

1 The Clinical Problem

The use of medical devices, such as urinary stents, catheters, artificial heart valves, prosthetic joints and other implants, collectively often referred to as "biomaterials" has increased dramatically over the past century, and has become a major part of modern medicine and our daily life. With the aging society, the higher demand on these devices to restore function and quality of life, combined with the ever improving technology within the medical field, the problem of biomaterial-associated infection (BAI) is expected to increase.

Catheters, and orthopedic devices are among the most frequently used devices in human medicine [1, 2]. Catheters suspected for infection are replaced by a new catheter at a different location, since using the original location for re-implantation over a guide-wire is strongly discouraged because of the high reinfection risk [3]. Primary implantation of prosthetic joints like prosthetic hips, knees, elbows and ankles, is considered a so-called clean procedure [4], however, in 0.5–1% (hip or knee) to over 5% (elbow or ankle) of cases, infections occur [5, 6]. Revision surgery is associated with higher frequencies of infection, due to the compromised condition of the tissue, longer procedures and more extensive tissue damage during surgery.

The most common causative microorganisms in BAI are *Staphylococcus aureus*, a major pathogen in wound infections, and *Staphylococcus epidermidis*, the harmless skin commensal [6–8]. Depending on the type of device and location of application, other pathogens such as coagulase-negative staphylococci, enterococci, streptococci, *Propionibacterium acnes* and yeast can also cause BAI [9, 10].

M. Riool (✉) · S. A. J. Zaat
Department of Medical Microbiology and Infection Prevention, Amsterdam UMC,
Amsterdam institute for Infection and Immunity, University of Amsterdam,
Amsterdam, The Netherlands
e-mail: m.riool@amsterdamumc.nl; s.a.zaat@amsterdamumc.nl

© The Author(s) 2022
F. Soria et al. (eds.), *Urinary Stents*,
https://doi.org/10.1007/978-3-031-04484-7_20

As early as in 1957, Elek and Conen studied the minimum infective dose of staphylococci for man in relation to suture infection [11]. In healthy volunteers, they estimated the minimum pus-forming dose of *S. aureus*—called *Staphylococcus pyogenes* in those days—on intradermal injections in absence of sutures to be 2–8 million bacteria, numbers which are improbable in case of a natural infection. However, the presence of a foreign body, a suture in this case, resulted in a dramatic reduction in the minimal inoculum required for pus production: a dose of 300 bacteria led to abscess formation. Higher inoculum doses even resulted in lesions with 'the size of an orange', caused fever and took over a week to resolve, in spite of penicillin therapy. Although this experiment clearly demonstrated the enhancing effect of the presence of a foreign body, but the authors stated that the outcome of the experiment "led to great difficulty in finding further volunteers". Nowadays, such an experimental set-up would not be easily approved by medical ethical committees, but it did provide crucial information on the pathogenesis of BAI. Thus, it has been recognized for at least 60 years that the presence of a foreign body predisposes for infection, and this has repeatedly been confirmed in animal studies [12–15]. In rabbits, for example, only 50 colony forming units (CFU) of *S. aureus* were sufficient for infection in the presence of a cemented hip implant, whereas 10,000 CFU were required in absence of the foreign body [16].

1.1 Biofilms

Bacterial biofilm formation is considered the major element in the pathogenesis of BAI [1, 10, 17]. Biofilm formation is initiated when planktonic bacterial cells attach to the surfaces of implants (Fig. 1). BAI are often caused by biofilm-forming bacterial strains able to cover the surface of the biomaterial, resulting in complex structures consisting of bacteria, extracellular polymeric substances (bacterial products like polysaccharides, proteins and DNA) and host proteins and cells [17]. Bacteria in biofilms behave differently from planktonic bacteria, particularly in response to antibiotic treatment [18]. The complex bacterial community of a biofilm is highly tolerant to antibiotics [19]. This is partly due to the complicated structure of the extracellular polymeric matrix of the biofilm, making the bacteria less accessible to many antibiotic agents [20]. As most antibiotics target active cell processes, the slow growth or starved state of the bacteria in a biofilm may also make them more tolerant. A subpopulation of these bacteria, the so-called persisters, reaches a dormant and drug-tolerant state. Such persisters are suggested to be largely responsible for the recalcitrance and recurrence of biofilm-associated infections [21]. Moreover, biofilm-entrapped bacteria are unreachable for the human immune system.

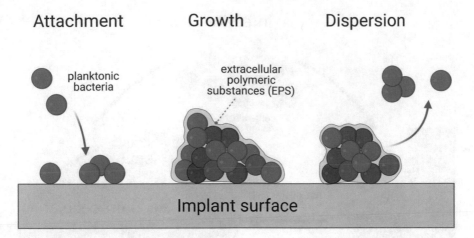

Fig. 1 Biofilm stages in biomaterials

1.2 Tissue Colonization

Next to biofilm formation, another important element in the pathogenesis of BAI is bacterial colonization of the tissue around implants (Fig. 2), due to dysregulation of the local immune response by the combined presence of bacteria and a foreign body [22–25]. Bacteria are inevitably introduced in the tissue wound during surgery, either originating from the patient's skin microflora or from the operation room [26]. Due to the implanted biomaterial, the efficacy of the host immune response is reduced. Already in the 1980s, Zimmerli *et al.* showed reduced neutrophil phago-cytic activity in guinea pig tissue cage models infected with *S. aureus* [27]. When different challenge doses of *S. epidermidis* were injected along subcutaneously implanted catheter segments at the back of mice, the bacteria were more often found in the peri-implant tissue than on the biomaterial itself, and persisted for longer periods in the tissue than on the implant [28]. Moreover, *S. epidermidis* survives inside macrophages in tissue surrounding implants in mice (Fig. 2) [25, 28].

In a mouse subcutaneous BAI model, the possible routes of infection at the inter-face between implants and the surrounding tissue were studied [29]. In this study, *S. epidermidis* bacteria applied on the surface of titanium implants, both adhering and as a biofilm, relocate from the material to the surrounding tissue (Fig. 2), which is accordance with earlier studies with other types of materials [25, 28]. This sug-gests that it is a more general phenomenon occurring around implants manufactured from biomaterials as diverse as polymer and titanium, and with different bacterial species. In a study by Broekhuizen *et al.*, mice were treated with dexamethasone and BrdU, a nucleotide analogue that is incorporated into DNA of dividing cells and can be detected immunohistologically. Analysis of tissue samples collected at 14

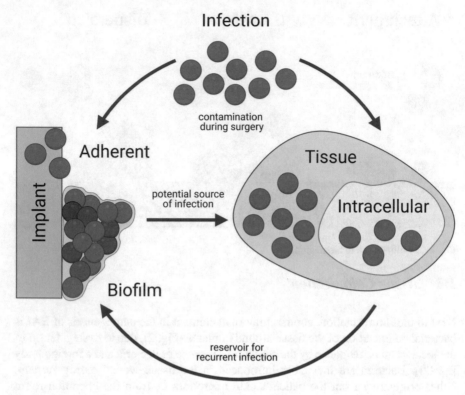

Fig. 2 Pathogenesis of the biomaterials associated infection

and 21 days after challenge with *S. epidermidis* showed regrowth of the bacteria with BrdU incorporated, which had apparently replicated between day 14 and 21, suggesting that tissue rather than the implant provides a hiding place for the bacteria [30]. Moreover, after incubation of peri-catheter tissue biopsies of deceased intensive care unit patients with BrdU, bacteria had incorporated BrdU *in situ*, proving that bacteria also reside and synthesize nucleic acids within tissue surrounding biomaterials in humans [30].

Bacteria colonizing the surface of a biomaterial not only are a focus of a localized biofilm infection, but can also be the source of tissue colonization (Fig. 2). Conversely, bacteria residing in the tissue can be a cause of infection after re-implantation, in experimental infection [31] as well as in patients [32].

Tissue-residing bacteria can be hard to eradicate by antibiotic treatment [33, 34]. For instance, when infected prosthetic joints are removed, patients usually require a prolonged regimen of systemic and local antibiotic treatment in order to reach and kill bacteria present in the tissue before re-implantation can be performed [6, 35]. In conclusion, next to the prevention of bacterial colonization of the implant and the subsequent biofilm formation, prevention of bacterial colonization of peri-implant tissue is of vital importance.

1.3 Intracellular Survival

In the subcutaneous mouse BAI model staphylococci predominantly co-localized with macrophages in the peri-implant tissue, even when the bacteria were present exclusively on the implant surface at the start of the experiment (Fig. 2) [29]. This interesting observation suggests that the bacteria were either removed from the implant by phagocytosis, or first detached and were subsequently phagocytosed. In this mouse model, both *S. epidermidis* [29] and *S. aureus* [36] were cultured in high numbers from the tissue and co-localized with macrophages in histology, particularly at 4 days after challenge, suggesting that these macrophages were not effectively killing the bacteria. Most likely, the local host immune response is impaired in presence of an implant, resulting in less or no clearance of bacteria. As mentioned before, neutrophils can have reduced phagocytic and bactericidal capacity in the vicinity of an implant [27, 37]. Moreover, the intracellular killing capacity of macrophages can be reduced due to altered cytokine tissue levels due to the presence of a biomaterial [25, 30, 37–39]. Staphylococci may even form small colony variants to adapt to this micro-environment, which are more resistant to antimicrobial compounds [40, 41]. Apparently, when bacteria are initially present near or on the surface of implants this results in ineffective eradication by phagocytes. This might lead to persistence of (intracellular) bacteria in the peri-implant tissue.

1.4 Antimicrobial Resistance

In addition to the difficulty of treating biofilm-encased or intracellularly residing bacteria with conventional antibiotic therapy, treating BAI is further hindered by the rising antibiotic resistance among pathogens. The World Health Organization recently endorsed a global action plan to tackle antibiotic resistance [42]. One of the key objectives of this plan is to develop novel antimicrobial drugs. The emergence of multidrug-resistant (MDR), extensively drug-resistant (XDR) and pandrug-resistant (PDR) pathogens, accelerated by the selective pressure exerted by extensive use and misuse of antimicrobials, further underscores the very pressing need for the discovery of novel treatment strategies to replace or complement the conventional antibiotics. Magiorakos *et al.* defined MDR bacteria as non-susceptible to at least one agent in three or more antimicrobial categories, XDR bacteria as non-susceptible to at least one agent in all but two or fewer antimicrobial categories, meaning bacterial isolates which remained susceptible to only one or two categories, and PDR bacteria as non-susceptible to all agents in all antimicrobial categories [43]. The occurrence of XDR and PDR strains illustrates the clinical challenges that we will be facing in the dark scenario of a possible "post-antibiotic era". Antimicrobial resistance causing limited or no treatment options in critically ill patients, stresses the importance of the development of new agents that can be used against drug-resistant bacteria. Clearly, it is vital that novel antimicrobial agents are also effective against drug-resistant Gram-negative bacteria belonging to the so-called ESKAPE panel (*Enterococcus faecium*, *S. aureus*, *Klebsiella pneumoniae*, *Acinetobacter baumannii*, *Pseudomonas aeruginosa*, and *Enterobacter* species [44]), which cause the majority of US hospital infections [45] and are associated with high morbidity and mortality [46].

2 Preventive Strategies

As explained above, in addition to biofilm formation on the implant, colonization of peri-implant tissue is an important factor in the pathogenesis of BAI. Therefore, this niche needs to be taken into consideration when designing preventive strategies against BAI. Current strategies mainly focus on the development of four types of antimicrobial surfaces: (1) antifouling/anti-adhesive surfaces, (2) tissue-integrating surfaces, (3) contact-killing surfaces, and (4) surfaces which incorporate and release antimicrobials (Fig. 3) [47]. These approaches all have their benefits and limitations, which need to be taken into account when designing an antimicrobial strategy for a particular device [48].

2.1   Anti-adhesive

Implant surfaces are ideal substrates for opportunistic bacteria to attach to, colonize, and form biofilms on. Surface properties of the implant, like surface charges, hydrophobicity/hydrophilicity and surface chemistry play a major role in initial bacterial adhesion and proliferation. Already in 1987, Gristina suggested that tissue cell integration and bacterial adhesion compete for a spot on the implant's surface, summarized as the so-called 'race for the surface' concept [49]. In case the bacteria win this race, infection instead of tissue integration would be the end result. In addition,

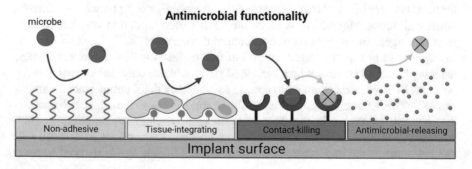

Fig. 3 Antimicrobial functionality in implant surface

Gristina also suggested that colonization of the tissue around implants was a possible mechanism of infection [49]. Bacterial adhesion and subsequent biofilm formation may be prevented by modifying the physicochemical surface properties of biomaterials, for instance by using hydrophilic polymer coatings, *e.g.* immobilized poly(ethylene glycol) (PEG), as applied on contact lenses, shunts, endotracheal tubes and urinary catheters [47, 50]. Functionalization of the surface with a dense layer of polymer chains commonly known as polymer brush coatings, is another approach [34, 51]. Large exclusion volumes of tethered polymer chains result in surfaces difficult to approach by proteins or bacteria, and these brush coating molecules may even possess antimicrobially active functional groups.

2.2 Antibiotics

In general, antibiotics are selected based on their capacity to prevent biofilm formation, but not on their ability to kill bacteria in the other niches relevant for BAI, like in peri-implant tissue and intracellularly in host cells [47]. Antibiotics often used in the treatment of BAI, such as vancomycin and gentamicin, have low or hardly any penetration into host cells, and are thereby not active against intracellular bacteria. On the other hand, rifampicin (against staphylococci) or fluoroquinolones (against Gram-negative bacilli) do target these intracellularly localized bacteria, but resistance develops rapidly against these antibiotics. The combination of vancomycin and rifampicin is often used to treat BAI, but—as vancomycin does not reach intracellular bacteria—this likely results in a high risk of resistance development towards rifampicin.

Coatings releasing antibiotic are widely used for medical devices, like in sutures and central venous and urinary tract catheters. These coatings have two major disadvantages: (1) a patient can be infected with a bacterium resistant to the released antibiotic, and (2) due to the local release a gradient of the antibiotic will be created near the implant, which increases the risk to select for resistant bacteria. In view of the increasing development of resistance, the use of antibiotics for medical device is discouraged by government regulatory agencies like the American Food and Drug Administration (FDA) [48, 52].

2.3 Antiseptics

As an alternative to antibiotics, commonly used antiseptics and disinfectants may be used, as they are less known to induce resistance and in general have a broader spectrum of activity than antibiotics. These biocides, such as alcohols, aldehydes and biguanides, are extensively used in hospitals and other health care settings, and also by the general public, as an essential part of infection control practices [53]. Probably the most widely used biocide in antiseptic products (*e.g.* hand wash and oral products) is chlorhexidine, owing to its broad spectrum activity, low toxicity and good tolerability of soft tissue. Moreover, resistance development is extremely rare and chlorhexidine has been shown to prevent infection in animal models [36] and in patients [54]. It is used topically, for surgical site preparation, and also intracorporeally [55], and as dental irrigant fluid [56]. Chlorhexidine is currently FDA approved for coatings on intravenous catheters, and these catheters have been shown to be effective in decreasing catheter-related infection in humans [57, 58].

2.4 Antimicrobial Peptides

As discussed earlier, due to the major problems arising from resistance to conventional antibiotics, there is a strong need for antimicrobials not associated with resistance development. Antimicrobial peptides (AMPs) are innate defence molecules of animals, plants and microorganisms. These amphipathic, cationic peptides commonly have antimicrobial activity against a wide variety of pathogens, including bacteria, fungi and viruses, and low risk of resistance development [59, 60]. In addition, many AMPs have immune-modulatory and wound healing activities [61]. The low risk of resistance development is due to the fact that AMPs interact with microbial membranes, mostly resulting in membrane depolarisation, permeabilization and/or disruption leading to rapid cell death, or passing of the membrane to reach intracellular targets [62]. Naturally occurring human AMPs are considered excellent templates for the development of novel synthetic antimicrobials. Indeed, native AMPs have been used as design templates for a large variety of synthetic AMPs, some of which have now entered phase 2 and 3 clinical trials [63, 64].

For biomaterials, the predominant AMP-related antimicrobial strategies are coating by tethering AMPs to the surface, or to apply the peptides in controlled release coatings. Immobilisation of AMPs on surfaces has been performed with a variety of peptides, and with many different chemistries [65–68]. Peptides should retain the structural characteristics important for their antimicrobial activity after immobilisation, to be effective on a surface. Length, flexibility, and kind of spacer connecting the peptide to the surface, the AMP surface density and the orientation of the immobilised peptides are other decisive factors for success [69]. Interestingly, even short surface-attached peptides, which are unlikely to have a free interaction with the bacterial membrane, have antimicrobial activity [70], probably due to destabilisation of the membrane by displacement of positively charged counter-ions, changing bacterial surface electrostatics and activating autolytic enzymes or disrupting the ionic balance [70].

Surface attachment of peptides may have certain disadvantages. Firstly, chemical procedures of tethering AMPs to surfaces may cause strong decrease in their antimicrobial activity, or even their inactivation [71, 72] depending on the combination of peptides and immobilization technology. Secondly, proteins, blood platelets and dead bacteria may block the antimicrobial groups on the surface. Lastly, since the antimicrobial activity is restricted to the surface of the implant, there is a lack of antimicrobial impact on bacteria in the tissue surrounding the implant.

Incorporation of AMPs in controlled release coatings has not yet been extensively developed, although AMPs such as OP-145 [73], IB-367 (Iseganan) [74] and Omiganan [75] have already reached clinical phase 2 or 3 testing for infections not associated with biomaterials [64]. Application of AMPs in antimicrobial surface coatings is however a subject of increasing interest [65–67, 76, 77].

In addition to direct antimicrobial activity, AMPs can prevent excessive activation of pro-inflammatory responses by binding bacterial endotoxins such as lipopolysaccharide (LPS) of Gram-negative bacteria, and peptidoglycan (PG) and lipoteichoic acid (LTA) of Gram-positive bacteria, which leads to their neutralization. This way, AMPs combine the desired characteristics of both direct antimicrobial agents and immune-modulators. The immunomodulatory activity may be used to increase efficacy of clearance of bacterial biofilm infection [78, 79], and might help to prevent derangement of immune responses which increase susceptibility to infection [22, 80, 81].

3 Conclusions and Future Perspective

Prevention of BAI is a challenging problem, in particular due to the increased risk of resistance development associated with current antibiotic-based strategies. Here we showed the evidence of biofilms as a source for peri-implant tissue colonization, clearly showing the importance of preventive measures to be able to act both against implant and tissue colonization. Subsequently, we described different strategies to prevent BAI and other difficult-to-treat biofilm infections. Therefore we conclude that future research should focus on the development of combination devices with both anti-fouling or contact-killing capacities—to protect the implant—and controlled release of an antimicrobial agent to protect the surrounding tissue.

References

1. Anderson JM, Patel JD. Biomaterial-dependent characteristics of the foreign body response and *S. epidermidis* biofilm interactions. In: Moriarty TF, SAJ Z, Busscher HJ, editors. Biomaterials associated infection. New York: Springer; 2013. p. 119–49.
2. Kwakman PHS, Zaat SAJ. Preventive measures against transcutaneous device infections. In: Moriarty TF, Zaat SAJ, Busscher HJ, editors. Biomaterials associated infection. New York: Springer; 2013. p. 229–48.
3. Safdar N, Kluger DM, Maki DG. A review of risk factors for catheter-related bloodstream infection caused by percutaneously inserted, noncuffed central venous catheters: implications for preventive strategies. Medicine (Baltimore). 2002;81(6):466–79.
4. Evans RP. Current concepts for clean air and total joint arthroplasty: laminar airflow and ultraviolet radiation: a systematic review. Clin Orthop Relat Res. 2011;469(4):945–53.
5. Krenek L, Farng E, Zingmond D, SooHoo NF. Complication and revision rates following total elbow arthroplasty. J Hand Surg Am. 2011;36(1):68–73.

6. Zimmerli W, Trampuz A, Ochsner PE. Prosthetic-joint infections. N Engl J Med. 2004;351(16):1645–54.
7. Anderson JM, Marchant RE. Biomaterials: factors favoring colonization and infection. In: Waldvogel FA, Bisno AL, editors. Infections associated with indwelling medical devices. 3rd ed. Washington, DC: American Society of Microbiology; 2000. p. 89–109.
8. O'Gara JP, Humphreys H. *Staphylococcus epidermidis* biofilms: importance and implications. J Med Microbiol. 2001;50(7):582–7.
9. Waldvogel FA, Bisno AL. Infections associated with indwelling medical devices. 3rd ed. Washington, DC: American Society of Microbiology; 2000.
10. Holmberg A, Lood R, Mörgelin M, Söderquist B, Holst E, Collin M, et al. Biofilm formation by *Propionibacterium acnes* is a characteristic of invasive isolates. Clin Microbiol Infect. 2009;15(8):787–95.
11. Elek SD, Conen PE. The virulence of *Staphylococcus pyogenes* for man; a study of the problems of wound infection. Br J Exp Pathol. 1957;38(6):573–86.
12. James RC, Macleod CJ. Induction of staphylococcal infections in mice with small inocula introduced on sutures. Br J Exp Pathol. 1961;42:266–77.
13. Noble WC. The production of subcutaneous staphylococcal skin lesions in mice. Br J Exp Pathol. 1965;46(3):254–62.
14. Taubler JH, Kapral FA. Staphylococcal population changes in experimentally infected mice: infection with suture-adsorbed and unadsorbed organisms grown in vitro and in vivo. J Infect Dis. 1966;116(3):257–62.
15. Zimmerli W, Waldvogel FA, Vaudaux P, Nydegger UE. Pathogenesis of foreign body infection: description and characteristics of an animal model. J Infect Dis. 1982;146(4):487–97.
16. Southwood RT, Rice JL, McDonald PJ, Hakendorf PH, Rozenbilds MA. Infection in experimental arthroplasties. Clin Orthop Relat Res. 1987;224:33–6.
17. Costerton JW, Stewart PS, Greenberg EP. Bacterial biofilms: a common cause of persistent infections. Science. 1999;284(5418):1318–22.
18. Chen M, Yu Q, Sun H. Novel strategies for the prevention and treatment of biofilm related infections. Int J Mol Sci. 2013;14(9):18488–501.
19. Otto M. *Staphylococcus epidermidis*—the "accidental" pathogen. Nat Rev Microbiol. 2009;7(8):555–67.
20. Flemming H-C, Wingender J. The biofilm matrix. Nat Rev Microbiol. 2010;8(9):623–33.
21. Gerdes K, Semsey S. Microbiology: pumping persisters. Nature. 2016;534(7605):41–2.
22. Zaat S, Broekhuizen C, Riool M. Host tissue as a niche for biomaterial-associated infection. Future Microbiol. 2010;5(8):1149–51.
23. Boelens JJ, Zaat SAJ, Murk JL, Weening JJ, van der Poll T, Dankert J. Enhanced susceptibility to subcutaneous abscess formation and persistent infection around catheters is associated with sustained interleukin-1beta levels. Infect Immun. 2000;68(3):1692–5.
24. Boelens JJ, Zaat SAJ, Meeldijk J, Dankert J. Subcutaneous abscess formation around catheters induced by viable and nonviable *Staphylococcus epidermidis* as well as by small amounts of bacterial cell wall components. J Biomed Mater Res. 2000;50(4):546–56.
25. Boelens JJ, Dankert J, Murk JL, Weening JJ, van der Poll T, Dingemans KP, et al. Biomaterial-associated persistence of *Staphylococcus epidermidis* in pericatheter macrophages. J Infect Dis. 2000;181(4):1337–49.
26. Fitzgerald RH. Microbiologic environment of the conventional operating room. Arch Surg. 1979;114(7):772–5.
27. Zimmerli W, Lew PD, Waldvogel FA. Pathogenesis of foreign body infection. Evidence for a local granulocyte defect. J Clin Investig. 1984;73(4):1191–200.
28. Broekhuizen CAN, de Boer L, Schipper K, Jones CD, Quadir S, Feldman RG, et al. Peri-implant tissue is an important Niche for *Staphylococcus epidermidis* in experimental biomaterial-associated infection in mice. Infect Immun. 2007;75(3):1129–36.

29. Riool M, de Boer L, Jaspers V, van der Loos CM, van Wamel WJB, Wu G, et al. *Staphylococcus epidermidis* originating from titanium implants infects surrounding tissue and immune cells. Acta Biomater. 2014;10(12):5202–12.
30. Broekhuizen CAN, Sta M, Vandenbroucke-Grauls CMJE, Zaat SAJ. Microscopic detection of viable *Staphylococcus epidermidis* in peri-implant tissue in experimental biomaterial-associated infection, identified by bromodeoxyuridine incorporation. Infect Immun. 2010;78(3):954–62.
31. Engelsman AF, Saldarriaga-Fernandez IC, Nejadnik MR, van Dam GM, Francis KP, Ploeg RJ, et al. The risk of biomaterial-associated infection after revision surgery due to an experimental primary implant infection. Biofouling. 2010;26(7):761–7.
32. Moriarty TF, Kuehl R, Coenye T, Metsemakers W-J, Morgenstern M, Schwarz EM, et al. Orthopaedic device-related infection: current and future interventions for improved prevention and treatment. EFORT Open Rev. 2016;1(4):89–99.
33. Broekhuizen CAN, de Boer L, Schipper K, Jones CD, Quadir S, Vandenbroucke-Grauls CMJE, et al. *Staphylococcus epidermidis* is cleared from biomaterial implants but persists in peri-implant tissue in mice despite rifampicin/vancomycin treatment. J Biomed Mater Res Part A. 2008;85A(2):498–505.
34. Nejadnik MR, Engelsman AF, Saldarriaga Fernandez IC, Busscher HJ, Norde W, van der Mei HC. Bacterial colonization of polymer brush-coated and pristine silicone rubber implanted in infected pockets in mice. J Antimicrob Chemother. 2008;62(6):1323–5.
35. Walenkamp GHIM. Gentamicin PMMA beads and other local antibiotic carriers in two-stage revision of total knee infection: a review. J Chemother. 2001;13(sup4):66–72.
36. Riool M, Dirks A, Jaspers V, de Boer L, Loontjens T, van der Loos C, et al. A chlorhexidine-releasing epoxy-based coating on titanium implants prevents *Staphylococcus aureus* experimental biomaterial-associated infection. Eur Cells Mater. 2017;33(4):143–57.
37. Zimmerli W, Sendi P. Pathogenesis of implant-associated infection: the role of the host. Semin Immunopathol. 2011;33(3):295–306.
38. Boelens JJ, van der Poll T, Dankert J, Zaat SAJ. Interferon-γ protects against biomaterial-associated *Staphylococcus epidermidis* infection in mice. J Infect Dis. 2000;181(3):1167–71.
39. Boelens JJ, van Der Poll T, Zaat SAJ, Murk JL, Weening JJ, Dankert J. Interleukin-1 receptor type I gene-deficient mice are less susceptible to *Staphylococcus epidermidis* biomaterial-associated infection than are wild-type mice. Infect Immun. 2000;68(12):6924–31.
40. Tuchscherr L, Heitmann V, Hussain M, Viemann D, Roth J, von Eiff C, et al. *Staphylococcus aureus* small-colony variants are adapted phenotypes for intracellular persistence. J Infect Dis. 2010;202(7):1031–40.
41. Zaat SAJ. Tissue colonization in biomaterial-associated infection. In: Moriarty TF, Zaat SAJ, Busscher HJ, editors. Biomaterials associated infection. New York: Springer; 2013. p. 175–207.
42. Chan M. Global action plan on antimicrobial resistance. Geneva: World Health Organization; 2015.
43. Magiorakos A-P, Srinivasan A, Carey RB, Carmeli Y, Falagas ME, Giske CG, et al. Multidrug-resistant, extensively drug-resistant and pandrug-resistant bacteria: an international expert proposal for interim standard definitions for acquired resistance. Clin Microbiol Infect. 2012;18(3):268–81.
44. Rice LB. Federal funding for the study of antimicrobial resistance in nosocomial pathogens: no ESKAPE. J Infect Dis. 2008;197(8):1079–81.
45. Boucher HW, Talbot GH, Bradley JS, Edwards JE, Gilbert D, Rice LB, et al. Bad bugs, no drugs: no ESKAPE! An update from the Infectious Diseases Society of America. Clin Infect Dis. 2009;48(1):1–12.
46. Paramythiotou E, Routsi C. Association between infections caused by multidrug-resistant Gram-negative bacteria and mortality in critically ill patients. World J Crit Care Med. 2016;5(2):111.

47. Busscher HJ, van der Mei HC, Subbiahdoss G, Jutte PC, van den Dungen JJ, Zaat SA, Schultz MJ, et al. Biomaterial-associated infection: locating the finish line in the race for the surface. Sci Transl Med. 2012;4(153):153rv10.
48. Brooks BD, Brooks AE, Grainger DW. Antimicrobial medical devices in preclinical development and clinical use. In: Moriarty TF, Zaat SAJ, Busscher HJ, editors. Biomaterials associated infection. New York: Springer; 2013. p. 307–54.
49. Gristina A. Biomaterial-centered infection: microbial adhesion versus tissue integration. Science (80-). 1987;237(4822):1588–95.
50. Banerjee I, Pangule RC, Kane RS. Antifouling coatings: recent developments in the design of surfaces that prevent fouling by proteins, bacteria, and marine organisms. Adv Mater. 2011;23(6):690–718.
51. Neoh KG, Shi ZL, Kang ET. Anti-adhesive and antibacterial polymer brushes. In: Moriarty TF, Zaat SAJ, Busscher HJ, editors. Biomaterials associated infection. New York: Springer; 2013. p. 405–32.
52. FDA. Draft guidance for industry and FDA Staff—premarket notification [510(k)] submissions for medical devices that include antimicrobial agents, vol. 510. Rockville: FDA; 2007.
53. McDonnell G, Russell AD. Antiseptics and disinfectants: activity, action, and resistance. Clin Microbiol Rev. 1999;12(1):147–79.
54. Rupp ME, Lisco SJ, Lipsett PA, Perl TM, Keating K, Civetta JM, et al. Effect of a second-generation venous catheter impregnated with chlorhexidine and silver sulfadiazine on central catheter-related infections: a randomized, controlled trial. Ann Intern Med. 2005;143(8):570–80.
55. Wilkins RG, Unverdorben M. Wound cleaning and wound healing. Adv Skin Wound Care. 2013;26(4):160–3.
56. Iqbal A. Antimicrobial irrigants in the endodontic therapy. Int J Health Sci (Qassim). 2012;6(2):1–7.
57. Campbell AA, Song L, Li XS, Nelson BJ, Bottoni C, Brooks DE, et al. Development, characterization, and anti-microbial efficacy of hydroxyapatite–chlorhexidine coatings produced by surface-induced mineralization. J Biomed Mater Res. 2000;53(4):400–7.
58. Darouiche RO, Raad II, Heard SO, Thornby JI, Wenker OC, Gabrielli A, et al. A comparison of two antimicrobial-impregnated central venous catheters. N Engl J Med. 1999;340(1):1–8.
59. Zasloff M. Antimicrobial peptides of multicellular organisms. Nature. 2002;415(6870):389–95.
60. Hancock REW, Sahl H-G. Antimicrobial and host-defense peptides as new anti-infective therapeutic strategies. Nat Biotechnol. 2006;24(12):1551–7.
61. Nakatsuji T, Gallo RL. Antimicrobial peptides: old molecules with new ideas. J Investig Dermatol. 2012;132(3 Pt 2):887–95.
62. Pasupuleti M, Schmidtchen A, Malmsten M. Antimicrobial peptides: key components of the innate immune system. Crit Rev Biotechnol. 2012;32(2):143–71.
63. Fox JL. Antimicrobial peptides stage a comeback. Nat Biotechnol. 2013;31(5):379–82.
64. Greber KE, Dawgul M. Antimicrobial peptides under clinical trials. Curr Top Med Chem. 2016;17(5):620–8.
65. Gao G, Lange D, Hilpert K, Kindrachuk J, Zou Y, Cheng JTJ, et al. The biocompatibility and biofilm resistance of implant coatings based on hydrophilic polymer brushes conjugated with antimicrobial peptides. Biomaterials. 2011;32(16):3899–909.
66. Yazici H, O'Neill MB, Kacar T, Wilson BR, Oren EE, Sarikaya M, et al. Engineered chimeric peptides as antimicrobial surface coating agents toward infection-free implants. ACS Appl Mater Interfaces. 2016;8(8):5070–81.
67. Rai A, Pinto S, Evangelista MB, Gil H, Kallip S, Ferreira MGSS, et al. High-density antimicrobial peptide coating with broad activity and low cytotoxicity against human cells. Acta Biomater. 2016;33:64–74.
68. Silva RR, Avelino KYPS, Ribeiro KL, Franco OL, Oliveira MDL, Andrade CAS. Chemical immobilization of antimicrobial peptides on biomaterial surfaces. Front Biosci (Schol Ed). 2016;1(8):129–42.
69. Costa F, Carvalho IF, Montelaro RC, Gomes P, Martins MCL. Covalent immobilization of antimicrobial peptides (AMPs) onto biomaterial surfaces. Acta Biomater. 2011;7(4):1431–40.

70. Hilpert K, Elliott M, Jenssen H, Kindrachuk J, Fjell CD, Körner J, et al. Screening and characterization of surface-tethered cationic peptides for antimicrobial activity. Chem Biol. 2009;16(1):58–69.
71. Bagheri M, Beyermann M, Dathe M. Immobilization reduces the activity of surface-bound cationic antimicrobial peptides with no influence upon the activity spectrum. Antimicrob Agents Chemother. 2009;53(3):1132–41.
72. Onaizi SA, Leong SSJ. Tethering antimicrobial peptides: current status and potential challenges. Biotechnol Adv. 2011;29(1):67–74.
73. Nell MJ, Tjabringa GS, Wafelman AR, Verrijk R, Hiemstra PS, Drijfhout JW, et al. Development of novel LL-37 derived antimicrobial peptides with LPS and LTA neutralizing and antimicrobial activities for therapeutic application. Peptides. 2006;27(4):649–60.
74. Mosca DA, Hurst MA, So W, Viajar BSC, Fujii CA, Falla TJ. IB-367, a protegrin peptide with in vitro and in vivo activities against the microflora associated with oral mucositis. Antimicrob Agents Chemother. 2000;44(7):1803–8.
75. Sader HS, Fedler KA, Rennie RP, Stevens S, Jones RN. Omiganan pentahydrochloride (MBI 226), a topical 12-amino-acid cationic peptide: spectrum of antimicrobial activity and measurements of bactericidal activity. Antimicrob Agents Chemother. 2004;48(8):3112–8.
76. Ma M, Kazemzadeh-Narbat M, Hui Y, Lu S, Ding C, Chen DDY, et al. Local delivery of antimicrobial peptides using self-organized TiO_2 nanotube arrays for peri-implant infections. J Biomed Mater Res Part A. 2012;100A(2):278–85.
77. Riool M, de Breij A, de Boer L, Kwakman PHSS, Cordfunke RA, Cohen O, et al. Controlled release of LL-37-derived synthetic antimicrobial and anti-biofilm peptides SAAP-145 and SAAP-276 prevents experimental biomaterial-associated *Staphylococcus aureus* infection. Adv Funct Mater. 2017;27(20):1606623.
78. Mansour SC, de la Fuente-Núñez C, Hancock REW. Peptide IDR-1018: modulating the immune system and targeting bacterial biofilms to treat antibiotic-resistant bacterial infections. J Pept Sci. 2015;21(5):323–9.
79. Mansour SC, Pena OM, Hancock REW. Host defense peptides: front-line immunomodulators. Trends Immunol. 2014;35(9):443–50.
80. Heim CE, Vidlak D, Scherr TD, Kozel JA, Holzapfel M, Muirhead DE, et al. Myeloid-derived suppressor cells contribute to *Staphylococcus aureus* orthopedic biofilm infection. J Immunol. 2014;192(8):3778–92.
81. Heim CE, Vidlak D, Scherr TD, Hartman CW, Garvin KL, Kielian T. IL-12 promotes myeloid-derived suppressor cell recruitment and bacterial persistence during *Staphylococcus aureus* orthopedic implant infection. J Immunol. 2015;194(8):3861–72.

Antibiotic-Free Solutions for the Development of Biofilm Prevention Coatings

Bruna Costa, Joana Barros, and Fabíola Costa

1 Introduction

Stents and urinary catheters are commonly used medical devices, whose need is forecasted to grow considering not only the world population increase but also its aging and sedentary lifestyle [1].

Independently of the great development on biomaterials and device design, infection represents still a major cause of failure of these devices, with undeniable humane and economical costs. Different antibiotic-based solutions have appeared in the market to try to address the matter. However, there is growing evidence on the impact of antibiotic-resistant microorganisms on urinary tract medical-devices infections, and respective outcomes [2]. Within this chapter, several antibiotic-free alternatives, dedicated to the urinary tract, will be discussed.

Most device associated-infections are originated by biofilm establishment. Bacterial colonization through irreversible attachment, allows the production of extracellular matrix, forming ultra-organised three-dimensional bacterial structures, with orchestrated phenotypes that provide microorganisms resistance mechanisms to survive both the immune system and conventional antibiotics [3]. From the knowledge of these bacterial constructs, researchers have been exploring different angles of action that enforce the balance towards the infection obliteration and host recovery (Fig. 1).

B. Costa
i3S – Instituto de Investigação e Inovação em Saúde, Universidade do Porto, Porto, Portugal

INEB – Instituto de Engenharia Biomédica, Universidade do Porto, Porto, Portugal

FEUP–Faculdade de Engenharia, Universidade do Porto, Porto, Portugal
e-mail: bruna.costa@i3s.up.pt

J. Barros · F. Costa (✉)
i3S – Instituto de Investigação e Inovação em Saúde, Universidade do Porto, Porto, Portugal

INEB – Instituto de Engenharia Biomédica, Universidade do Porto, Porto, Portugal
e-mail: joana.barros@ineb.up.pt

© The Author(s) 2022
F. Soria et al. (eds.), *Urinary Stents*,
https://doi.org/10.1007/978-3-031-04484-7_21

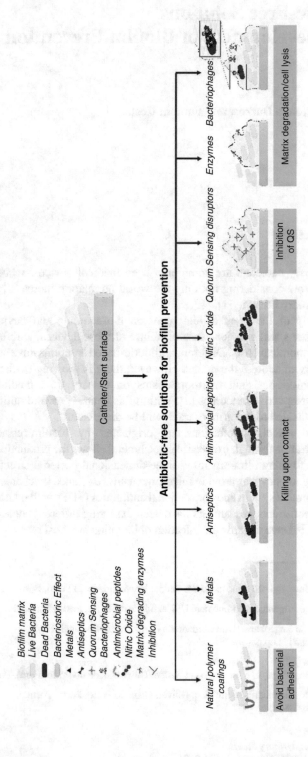

Fig. 1 Antibiotic-free strategies for combating biofilms on urinary stent or catheter surfaces

2 Natural Polymer Coatings

Apart from the different synthetic polymers with non-fouling properties described in previous chapters, naturally-occurring polysaccharides are presently being explored to design environmentally friendly and non-toxic materials. Several examples can be found in the literature, ranging from hyaluronic acid, heparin to ulvan or dextran [4–10], with potential for urinary applications. Gadenne et al., explored ulvans, with different molecular weight and sulfate ratio, for bacterial adhesion inhibition. Ulvans inhibited 36–88% of *Staphylococcus aureus* adhesion comparing to control [7]. Ruggieri et al., showed that latex catheters coated with a complex of heparin with tridodecylmethylammonium chloride were capable of reducing 53–84% *Escherichia coli* adherence comparing to controls: untreated latex, teflon coated latex (Bardex) and vinyl catheter [10]. Tenke et al., performed a 20 patients pilot assay and claimed that heparin-coated ureteral stents remained unaffected by encrustations and biofilm after 6 weeks [11]. Later, Lange et al., showed that heparin-coated Radiance © ureteral stents (Cook® Medical) failed in the prevention of *E. coli*, *Klebsiella pneumoniae*, *Enterococcus faecalis*, *S. aureus* and *Pseudomonas aeruginosa* adhesion and biofilm formation, while triclosan-eluting stents had an evident inhibitory effect on bacterial adherence for 7 days [8]. So further studies are needed to conclude about heparin coatings potential. A copolymer of polyurethane with dermatan sulfate (DS) was developed as new non-adhesive material, showing a significant *E. coli* adhesion decrease (29–57%) with increasing DS content [12].

Carboxymethyl chitosan was explored as an antimicrobial coating onto medical-grade silicone. Higher anti-biofilm efficiency was found against *E. coli* than *P. mirabilis* under flow-conditions. This effect can be explained by *P. mirabilis* high motility, which favors biofilms establishment downstream of an infected site [13]. Bracic et al., evaluated the anti-biofilm properties of colloidal polysaccharide complexes [chitosan, carboxymethyl chitosan, and hyaluronic acid in combination with a lysine-based surfactant (HA-MKM)] grafted on silicone sheets and tubes. All coatings showed antibacterial and antifungal properties, being HA-MKM the only solution capable of suppressing biofilm growth by ~ 50–75% during 18 h [14].

Recently, the anti-adhesive potential of cyanobacteria-based polymer coating (CyanoCoating) was reported against *Proteus mirabilis*, *E. coli*, *P. aeruginosa*, *K. pneumoniae*, Methicillin-resistant *Staphylococcus aureus* (MRSA) and *Candida albicans*. CyanoCoating hydrophilicity, negative charge and smooth surface may explain its broad anti-adhesive efficiency against all the uropathogens tested (68–95%), even in the presence of artificial urine (58–100%) [4]. Also, this anti-adhesive coating prevented big crystals deposition, reducing encrustation. CyanoCoating could also withstand ethylene oxide sterilization [5].

Biosurfactants represent an alternative strategy to promote anti-adhesiveness to the surfaces, which is thoroughly explained at Chap. 20.

3 Metal Alternatives

Metal alternatives such as silver (Ag), gold nanoparticles, copper oxide (CuO) or zinc (Zn), have been explored for urinary medical devices. The use of Ag or Ag alloys has been broadly exploited, having a wide expression in the market.

Gold nanoparticles antimicrobial effect is associated to bacterial membrane potential disruption, ATP levels reduction and tRNA inhibition [15]. Gold nanoparticles have been tested against important uropathogens, including *S. aureus*, *K. pneumonia*, *P. aeruginosa*, and *E. faecalis*, suppressing their bacterial growth at 24 h. However, the antimicrobial effectiveness diminished when used at longer-term, raising concerns about possible gold-resistance emergence [16].

Copper (Cu) promotes bacterial DNA degradation, enzymes inactivation and cell wall disruption [17–19]. Agarwala et al., tested CuO against *E. coli*, *P. mirabilis*, *E. faecalis*, *Pseudomonas* sp., MRSA and *S. epidermidis*, showing promising anti-biofilm activity even at sub-Minimum Inhibitory Concentrations (MIC) [20]. Rtimi et al., incorporated Cu alone or in combination with Ag onto polyurethane catheter surfaces using a new magnetron sputtering coating technique [21]. Cu–Ag hybrid coating catheters accelerated *E. coli* K12 inactivation (≤ 5 min) compared to Cu or Ag coating catheters (30 min) [21].

Zinc antimicrobial activity has been associated with hydrogen peroxide production [22]. Zn has been combined with CuO to mitigate bacterial colonization [17]. Shalom et al., showed that Zn-doped CuO nanoparticles coated catheters reduced *E. coli*, *S. aureus*, and *P. mirabilis* biofilm formation (> 90%) under flow conditions for 24 h [23]. Moreover, these coated catheters prevented biofilm formation over 7 days in a catheter-associated urinary tract infection (CAUTI) rabbit model [23].

Despite, the promising antimicrobial effects, well-designed toxicity and irritation studies are still needed.

4 Chlorhexidine

Chlorhexidine (CHX) is a well-known antiseptic agent used for skin, dentistry, and in medical devices [24]. CHX is broad-spectrum bacteriostatic at low and bactericidal at high concentrations [24]. Recently, CHX has also been tested as a coating on urinary catheters [25–27]. Shapur et al., explored a CHX-releasing ethylcellulose varnish as antimicrobial coating, showing a 94% reduction of *P. aeruginosa* biofilm formation on catheters coated with 1% CHX [26]. Later, Segev et al., proved the anti-biofilm effectiveness of 1% CHX ethylcellulose-varnish coated urinary catheters using a dog model [25]. Zelichenko et al., evaluated growth inhibition on ureteral stent segments coated with 1% and 2% CHX, showing that 2% CHX-varnish prevented $\geq 99.9\%$ biofilm formation of *E. faecalis*, *P. aeruginosa* and *E. coli* up to 2 weeks [28]. Gefter et al., compared anti-biofilm properties and dissolution kinetic of two sustained-release CHX-varnishes (ethylcellulose or Eudragit® RL) under the static or flow-conditions [27]. In both situations, ethylcellulose coatings had longer sustained release of CHX (for at least 2 weeks), which resulted in an inhibition of $\geq 90\%$ *P. aeruginosa* biofilm formation at 24 h [27]. Wood et al., developed a CHX hematophosphate nanoparticles (NP) ethylene-vinyl acetate-based coating [29]. The NP-coated surfaces inhibited MRSA and *P. aeruginosa* growth (measured at 24 h), and allowed for CHX sustained release over 56 days [29]. Phuengkham et al., spray-coated CHX-loaded polycaprolactone nanospheres onto silicone surface, reducing *S. aureus* (3 logs), *S. epidermidis* (2 logs) and *E. coli* (3 logs) biofilm formation over 7 days [30]. Then, Srisang et al., using the same coating reported 4 logs of reduction after 4 days, and 2 logs after 12 days of *E. coli*, *S. aureus*, and *C. albicans* tested in artificial urine [31]. Gaonkar et al., compared *in vitro* three different impregnated silicone catheters on urinary tract model: CHX–triclosan, CHX–Ag–sulfadiazine–triclosan, and nitrofurazone-coated catheters. CHX–triclosan catheter suppressed *P. mirabilis* growth for 20–30 days, compared to 4–10 days observed on the CHX–Ag–sulfadiazine–triclosan or nitrofurazone-coated catheters [32].

Despite, the extended protection period and promising antimicrobial effects, well-designed toxicity and safety studies are desirable to validate these coatings safety to patients.

5 Triclosan

Triclosan was the first compound to be approved for clinical use in ureteral stents, having potent broad-spectrum antimicrobial and anti-inflammatory activity. Cadieux et al., first tested triclosan impregnated ureteral stents on a *P. mirabilis* rabbit urinary tract infection model: 69% triclosan-stents showed no CFU counts and the remaining 31% had fewer CFU than controls. Also, triclosan group presented bladders with significantly less inflammation, although no significant difference in encrustation was observed among the groups [33]. However, in a long-term application (3 months) no clinical benefit was observed in terms of urine and stent cultures or overall subject symptoms in triclosan-eluting stents patients. Nevertheless, their use did result in decreased antibiotic usage and fewer symptomatic infections [34]. Later, a prospective randomized trial, reported that triclosan-eluting stent cannot reduce infection rates alone compared with antibiotic use [35]. This stent can, however, reduce several stent-related symptoms, and may have a role in combination with standard antibiotherapy.

6 Antimicrobial Peptides

Antimicrobial peptides (AMPs) may constitute an alternative to fight antibiotic resistance [36–39]. AMPs are part of the innate immune system of many organisms, having broad-spectrum, high anti-biofilm activity, and even immunomodulatory potential [40–43]. Due to an unspecific mode of action, targeting the bacterial membrane or affecting multiple targets within bacteria, AMPs are much less likely to induce resistance [44]. Monteiro et al., immobilized the AMP Chain201D on model self-assembled monolayers [45]. Chain201D has broad antimicrobial activity against relevant uropathogens (bacteria and yeast), being highly stable in a wide range of temperatures, pH and salt concentrations [45]. Increased amounts of grafted AMP led to higher numbers of adhered/dead bacteria, revealing a concentration-dependent behavior. Chain201D surfaces could bind and contact kill 89% of *E. coli* and 99% of *S. aureus* adherent bacteria, suggesting a good candidacy for urinary applications [45].

Minardi et al., compared the efficacy of the AMP Tachyplesin III-coated ureteral stent alone or combined with piperacillin–tazobactam (TZP) intraperitoneal injection in the prevention of *P. aeruginosa* biofilm in a rat model. Tachyplesin III combined with TZP showed efficacies higher (3 logs of reduction) than each single therapy [46].

Lim et al., conjugated an engineered arginine–tryptophan rich AMP (CWR11) onto polymethylsiloxane (PDMS) surfaces and catheters through different chemistries [47, 48]. The CWR11-PDMS slides displayed excellent bactericidal effect against *E. coli*, *S. aureus* and *P. aeruginosa*, preventing ~ 92% *P. aeruginosa* biofilm formation after 24 h. The CWR11-silicone Foley catheter antimicrobial properties were retained for at least 21 days, with negligible cytotoxicity [47].

Li et al., grafted two broad-spectrum and salt-tolerant arginine/lysine/tryptophan-rich AMP (RK1 and RK2), onto PDMS surfaces via an allyl glycidyl ether (AGE) polymer brush interlayer. AMP-PDMS killed over 80% of *E. coli*, *S. aureus*, and *C. albicans* in either media, PBS or urine, and impaired biofilm formation for up to 3 days [49].

Mishra et al., developed a Lasioglossin III AMP chemically modified with a cysteine residue (CysLasio-III) to selectively immobilize covalently onto commercial silicone catheter [50]. CysLasio-III-catheter showed significant anti-biofilm properties, reducing 40% and 60% of *E. coli* and *E. faecalis* biofilm, respectively [50].

Lo et al., used polymer brushes to graft different AMPs (E6, Tet20, Kai13, and Tet26) to surfaces. *In vitro* tests revealed E6 was the most effective against *P. aeruginosa*, decreasing ~ 94.1% of bacterial adhesion [51]. Later, Yu et al., similarly grafted E6 on polyurethane tubing, reporting a > 4 logs reduction in *P. aeruginosa* adhesion to the tube and 3 logs in the bladder in a CAUTI mouse model [52].

Pinese et al., developed a silylated analogue of the AMP Palm–Arg–Arg–NH$_2$ [1], to directly graft onto a plasma-activated PDMS catheter [53]. The authors suggested a dual anti-adhesive/bactericidal effect of the coating, since a decrease of ~ 75% *E. coli*, *P. aeruginosa* and *S. aureus* adhesion was observed and 92% of bacteria were killed on peptide-grafted catheters within 1 h. This AMP-catheter was superior to a commercial Ag-based silicone catheter (Covidien) against *S. aureus*, with earlier and persisting activity over 2 weeks [53].

Chua et al., compared an AMP CP11-6A-coated silicone catheter to an Ag-hydrogel-coated and an uncoated catheter using *E. coli* inoculated human urine. Within 3 days, both uncoated and Ag-coated catheters were heavily colonized, while CP11-6A-coated catheter showed negligible biofilm colonization and no detectable "bacteriuria" [54].

Although progress has been made, and many AMP-based coatings have impressive antimicrobial activity, further studies are needed to establish clinical significance.

7 Nitric Oxide

Nitric oxide (NO) has been used as an antimicrobial, showing great potential for biomedical applications [55], although poorly explored for urinary devices [56–58]. NO covalently binds DNA, proteins and lipids, thus inhibiting or killing pathogens [59]. NO-donating polymers may provide localized treatment with minor toxicity. Nevertheless, further studies are needed to understand the NO effects in the bladder, since it is known that NO plays an important role in other biological conditions (e.g. vasodilatation, neurotransmission) [56]. Regev-Shoshani et al., showed that gaseous NO-impregnated catheters have a sustained NO release over 14 days with stable storage. The NO release was faster in urine than in water, suggesting pH influence in the release, which might have implications at patient level [56]. Colletta et al., developed *S*-nitroso-*N*-acetyl-D-penicillamine impregnated Foley catheters with outstanding anti-biofilm effect, reducing *S. epidermidis* (3.7 logs) and *P. mirabilis* (6 logs) biofilm formation after 14 days [60]. Later, Ketchum et al., applied tertiary *S*-nitrosothiol and *S*-nitroso-*tert*-dodecyl mercaptan (SNTDM) as NO donors onto catheter tubings. NO-tubings reduced *S. aureus* colonization (4 logs) on SNTDM-impregnated catheters at 1 week, maintaining high anti-biofilm efficacy (3 logs of reduction) even after 3 weeks [61].

8 Quorum-Sensing Disrupters

Quorum-sensing (QS) corresponds to a cell–cell communication process, based on signaling molecules secreted by adhered bacteria to determine if a sufficient number of microorganisms is present that can initiate the expression of a particular biofilm-associated phenotype [62]. Quorum quenching, can severely hinder biofilm formation, diminishing bacteria antimicrobial resistance [63].

Ureteral stents coated with QS-inhibitor RNAIII-inhibiting peptide (RIP) reduced *S. aureus* adhesion (2 logs) to stents implanted in rat bladders. No bacteria were detected either on the stent or urine when the peptide treatment was combined with teicoplanin (which achieved only 3 logs reduction in single teicoplanin therapy) [64].

A combination of alpha-amylase and acylase was tested as a layer-by-layer coating on silicone urinary catheters [65, 66]. Alpha-amylase interferes with assembly of the extracellular matrix and acylase degrades small quorum signaling molecules. When tested *in vitro*, this coating reduced *P. aeruginosa* (> 40%), *S. aureus* (> 30%) and mixed-species biofilms (> 50%), although planktonic growth was not inhibited. *In vivo* (rabbit model) biofilm formation on the catheter's balloon section was decreased by 90%, although this was not seen in the lumen of the catheter. Furthermore, the quorum quenching action of single acylase, reduced significantly *P. aeruginosa* biofilm formation on a catheter under static and dynamic conditions [66].

Recently, furanone, a QS-inhibitor, was also tested as a coating for urinary catheters (latex, silicone and polyurethane), preventing *Candida* sp. biofilm formation in more than 80% [63].

9 Extracellular Matrix Degrading Enzymes

Exopolysaccharides are a crucial component of biofilm architecture, providing protection against drugs and host immunity [67]. Therefore, enzymes capable of degrading one of biofilm matrix components (proteins, extracellular DNA, polysaccharides), would impact on biofilm establishment [68].

Alpha-chymotrypsin (α-CT), a serine endopeptidase that cleaves peptide bonds [69, 70], was grafted on polyethylene surfaces, significantly reducing adherent cells, affecting the biofilm thickness, roughness and coverage. Additionally, the biovolume of the polysaccharide matrix decreased [70].

Also, recombinant human DNase (rhDNase), has efficiently inhibited *S. aureus* biofilm formation at 1–4 µg/L [71].

Cellobiose dehydrogenase (CDH), an oxidative enzyme that produces hydrogen peroxide, was grafted CDH onto PDMS catheters by ultrasonic waves, reducing *S. aureus* growth (60%), biomass deposition (30%), and biofilm production (70%) when compared to control catheters [72]. Thallinger *et al.*, tested CDH-grafted urinary catheter in artificial urine, over 16 days, observing a 60% reduction of the viable *S. aureus*, and a 70% biofilm formation decrease, comparing to control [73].

Glycoside hydrolases (Ghs) selectively target and hydrolyze the glycosidic bonds of exopolysaccharide components of the biofilm matrix [74, 75]. Asker et al., used Ghs that specifically targets Psl, a neutral exopolysaccharide, grafted to silica glass, PDMS, or polystyrene surfaces. PslGh-grafted surfaces reduced adhered *P. aeruginosa* in 3 logs up to 8 days, suggesting this strategy keeps bacteria in a planktonic state more susceptible to antimicrobials [76].

More studies might further validate this strategy, alone or in combination with other antimicrobials [75].

10 Bacteriophages

Bacteriophage (phage) therapy is proposed as a safe and effective strategy to address biofilms and multidrug-resistant pathogens, without impairing the resident microbiota [77, 78]. Lytic phages infect and kill specific bacteria, so their spectrum can be tuned creating a phage cocktail [77–80]. Phages are self-replicating at infection sites, producing new phage progeny that can migrate to a new focus of infection. Additionally, phages encode enzymes that degrade biofilm matrix [77, 78, 80]. Phages-impregnated catheters have been used against common uropathogens [78, 80–83].

Curtin et al., reported a significant reduction of coagulase-negative *S. epidermidis* biofilm formation (2.34 logs) over 24 h on hydrogel Foley catheter impregnated with phage 45,682. Later, Carson et al., showed that T4 or coli–proteus phages impregnated hydrogel-coated Foley catheters were able to reduce 90% of *P. mirabilis* or *E. coli* biofilm formation over 24 h, respectively [78].

Lehman et al., showed hydrogel catheters pretreated with anti-Pseudomonas and anti-Proteus phage cocktails have anti-biofilm activity against single- (1.5 logs *P. aeruginosa* and 2.5 logs *P. mirabilis*) and dual-species (4 logs and 2 logs, respectively) biofilms, over 48 h [77]. Previously, the same group reported that anti-Pseudomonas phage cocktail catheters is more effective than single phage-loaded catheters [82].

Milo et al., showed that the dual-layered polymeric coating, based on PVA hydrogel impregnated with phage, capped by a pH-sensitive polymer (EUDRAGIT S 100), was able to prevent *P. mirabilis*-associated encrustation of the catheter lumen through the pH-triggered release of phage [80].

Liao et al., compared the efficacy of 4 silicone catheter segments pretreated with sterile media, *E. coli* HU2117, anti-pseudomonal phage (ΦE2005-A) and *E. coli* HU2117 plus phage ΦE2005-A, on prevention *P. aeruginosa* biofilm formation for 72 h. A synergistic effect between pre-established biofilm of *E. coli* HU2117 and phage ΦE2005-A was observed, reducing efficiently (4 logs after 24 h and 3 logs after 72 h) *P. aeruginosa* adherence to catheters [83].

11 Conclusions

The urinary tract device-associated infections prevalence and the rise of multidrug-resistant microorganisms have prompt researchers towards the development of antibiotic-free solutions. A broad number of alternatives have been proposed, however, given the wide variability of results for different strategies, there remains a tremendous need to validate their clinical significance, particularly assuring patient safety. Additionally, most of these strategies might be advantageous while in combination with current therapies, so further studies are needed.

References

1. Anjum S, Singh S, Benedicte L, Roger P, Panigrahi M, Gupta B. Biomodification strategies for the development of antimicrobial urinary catheters: overview and advances. Glob Chall. 2018;2(1):1700068.
2. Koves B, Magyar A, Tenke P. Spectrum and antibiotic resistance of catheter-associated urinary tract infections. GMS. Infect Dis. 2017;5:Doc06.
3. del Pozo JL, Patel R. The challenge of treating biofilm-associated bacterial infections. Clin Pharmacol Ther. 2007;82(2):204–9.
4. Costa B, Mota R, Parreira P, Tamagnini P, Martins MCL, Costa F. Broad-spectrum anti-adhesive coating based on an extracellular polymer from a marine cyanobacterium. Mar Drugs. 2019;17(4):243–60.
5. Costa B, Mota R, Tamagnini P, Martins MCL, Costa F. Natural cyanobacterial polymer-based coating as a preventive strategy to avoid catheter-associated urinary tract infections. Mar Drugs. 2020;18(6):279–95.
6. Gadenne V, Lebrun L, Jouenne T, Thebault P. Antiadhesive activity of ulvan polysaccharides covalently immobilized onto titanium surface. Colloids Surf B Biointerfaces. 2013;112:229–36.
7. Gadenne V, Lebrun L, Jouenne T, Thebault P. Role of molecular properties of ulvans on their ability to elaborate antiadhesive surfaces. J Biomed Mater Res A. 2015;103(3):1021–8.
8. Lange D, Elwood CN, Choi K, Hendlin K, Monga M, Chew BH. Uropathogen interaction with the surface of urological stents using different surface properties. J Urol. 2009;182(3):1194–200.
9. Morra M, Cassineli C. Non-fouling properties of polysaccharide-coated surfaces. J Biomater Sci Polym Ed. 1999;10(10):1107–24.
10. Ruggieri MR, Hanno PM, Levin RM. Reduction of bacterial adherence to catheter surface with heparin. J Urol. 1987;138(2):423–6.
11. Tenke P, Riedl CR, Jones GL, Williams GJ, Stickler D, Nagy E. Bacterial biofilm formation on urologic devices and heparin coating as preventive strategy. Int J Antimicrob Agents. 2004;23(Suppl 1):S67–74.
12. Xu F, Flanagan CE, Ruiz A, Crone WC, Masters KS. Polyurethane/dermatan sulfate copolymers as hemocompatible, non-biofouling materials. Macromol Biosci. 2011;11(2):257–66.
13. Wang R, Neoh KG, Shi Z, Kang ET, Tambyah PA, Chiong E. Inhibition of *Escherichia coli* and *Proteus mirabilis* adhesion and biofilm formation on medical grade silicone surface. Biotechnol Bioeng. 2012;109(2):336–45.
14. Bracic M, Sauperl O, Strnad S, Kosalec I, Plohl O, Zemljic LF. Surface modification of silicone with colloidal polysaccharides formulations for the development of antimicrobial urethral catheters. Appl Surf Sci. 2019;463:889–99.
15. Cui Y, Zhao Y, Tian Y, Zhang W, Lü X, Jiang X. The molecular mechanism of action of bactericidal gold nanoparticles on *Escherichia coli*. Biomaterials. 2012;33(7):2327–33.
16. Annamalai DSK, Arunachalam PK, Arunachalam A, Raghavendra R, Kennedy S. One step green synthesis of phytochemicals mediated gold nanoparticles from *Aegle marmelos* for the prevention of urinary catheter infection. Int J Pharm Pharm Sci. 2014;6(1):700–6.
17. Dizaj SM, Lotfipour F, Barzegar-Jalali M, Zarrintan MH, Adibkia K. Antimicrobial activity of the metals and metal oxide nanoparticles. Mater Sci Eng C Mater Biol Appl. 2014;44:278–84.
18. Borkow G, Gabbay J. Putting copper into action: copper-impregnated products with potent biocidal activities. FASEB J. 2004;18(12):1728–30.
19. Borkow G, Gabbay J. Biocidal textiles can help fight nosocomial infections. Med Hypotheses. 2008;70(5):990–4.
20. Agarwala M, Choudhury B, Yadav RN. Comparative study of antibiofilm activity of copper oxide and iron oxide nanoparticles against multidrug resistant biofilm forming uropathogens. Indian J Microbiol. 2014;54(3):365–8.
21. Rtimi S, Sanjines R, Pulgarin C, Kiwi J. Quasi-instantaneous bacterial inactivation on Cu–Ag nanoparticulate 3D catheters in the dark and under light: mechanism and dynamics. ACS Appl Mater Interfaces. 2016;8(1):47–55.

22. Zhang L, Ding Y, Povey M, York D. ZnO nanofluids—a potential antibacterial agent. Prog Nat Sci. 2008;18(8):939–44.
23. Shalom Y, Perelshtein I, Perkas N, Gedanken A, Banin E. Catheters coated with Zn-doped CuO nanoparticles delay the onset of catheter-associated urinary tract infections. Nano Res. 2016;10:1–14.
24. Jones CG. Chlorhexidine: is it still the gold standard? Periodontol 2000. 1997;15(1):55–62.
25. Segev G, Bankirer T, Steinberg D, Duvdevani M, Shapur NK, Friedman M, et al. Evaluation of urinary catheters coated with sustained-release varnish of chlorhexidine in mitigating biofilm formation on urinary catheters in dogs. J Vet Intern Med. 2013;27(1):39–46.
26. Shapur NK, Duvdevani M, Friedman M, Zaks B, Gati I, Lavy E, et al. Sustained release varnish containing chlorhexidine for prevention of biofilm formation on urinary catheter surface: in vitro study. J Endourol. 2012;26(1):26–31.
27. Gefter Shenderovich J, Zaks B, Kirmayer D, Lavy E, Steinberg D, Friedman M. Chlorhexidine sustained-release varnishes for catheter coating—dissolution kinetics and antibiofilm properties. Eur J Pharm Sci. 2018;112:1–7.
28. Zelichenko G, Steinberg D, Lorber G, Friedman M, Zaks B, Lavy E, et al. Prevention of initial biofilm formation on ureteral stents using a sustained releasing varnish containing chlorhexidine: in vitro study. J Endourol. 2013;27(3):333–7.
29. Wood NJ, Maddocks SE, Grady HJ, Collins AM, Barbour ME. Functionalization of ethylene vinyl acetate with antimicrobial chlorhexidine hexametaphosphate nanoparticles. Int J Nanomedicine. 2014;9:4145–52.
30. Phuengkham H, Nasongkla N. Development of antibacterial coating on silicone surface via chlorhexidine-loaded nanospheres. J Mater Sci Mater Med. 2015;26(2):78.
31. Srisang S, Nasongkla N. Spray coating of Foley urinary catheter by chlorhexidine-loadedpoly(epsilon-caprolactone) nanospheres: effect of lyoprotectants, characteristics, and antibacterial activity evaluation. Pharm Dev Technol. 2019;24(4):402–9.
32. Gaonkar TA, Caraos L, Modak S. Efficacy of a silicone urinary catheter impregnated with chlorhexidine and triclosan against colonization with Proteus mirabilis and other uropathogens. Infect Control Hosp Epidemiol. 2007;28(5):596–8.
33. Cadieux PA, Chew BH, Knudsen BE, Dejong K, Rowe E, Reid G, et al. Triclosan loaded ureteral stents decrease Proteus mirabilis 296 infection in a rabbit urinary tract infection model. J Urol. 2006;175(6):2331–5.
34. Cadieux PA, Chew BH, Nott L, Seney S, Elwood CN, Wignall GR, et al. Use of triclosan-eluting ureteral stents in patients with long-term stents. J Endourol. 2009;23(7):1187–94.
35. Mendez-Probst CE, Goneau LW, MacDonald KW, Nott L, Seney S, Elwood CN, et al. The use of triclosan eluting stents effectively reduces ureteral stent symptoms: a prospective randomized trial. BJU Int. 2012;110(5):749–54.
36. Jenssen H, Hamill P, Hancock RE. Peptide antimicrobial agents. Clin Microbiol Rev. 2006;19(3):491–511.
37. Volejnikova A, Melichercik P, Nesuta O, Vankova E, Bednarova L, Rybacek J, et al. Antimicrobial peptides prevent bacterial biofilm formation on the surface of polymethylmethacrylate bone cement. J Med Microbiol. 2019;68(6):961–72.
38. Rodriguez Lopez AL, Lee MR, Ortiz BJ, Gastfriend BD, Whitehead R, Lynn DM, et al. Preventing S. aureus biofilm formation on titanium surfaces by the release of antimicrobial beta-peptides from polyelectrolyte multilayers. Acta Biomater. 2019;93:50–62.
39. D'Este F, Oro D, Boix-Lemonche G, Tossi A, Skerlavaj B. Evaluation of free or anchored antimicrobial peptides as candidates for the prevention of orthopaedic device-related infections. J Pept Sci. 2017;23(10):777–89.
40. van der Does AM, Bogaards SJ, Ravensbergen B, Beekhuizen H, van Dissel JT, Nibbering PH. Antimicrobial peptide hLF1-11 directs granulocyte-macrophage colony-stimulating factor-driven monocyte differentiation toward macrophages with enhanced recognition and clearance of pathogens. Antimicrob Agents Chemother. 2010;54(2):811–6.
41. Zasloff M. Antimicrobial peptides of multicellular organisms. Nature. 2002;415(6870):389–95.

42. Bahar AA, Ren D. Antimicrobial peptides. Pharmaceuticals (Basel). 2013;6(12):1543–75.
43. Magana M, Pushpanathan M, Santos AL, Leanse L, Fernandez M, Ioannidis A, et al. The value of antimicrobial peptides in the age of resistance. Lancet Infect Dis. 2020;20(9):e216–e30.
44. Raheem N, Straus SK. Mechanisms of action for antimicrobial peptides with antibacterial and antibiofilm functions. Front Microbiol. 2019;10:2866.
45. Monteiro C, Costa F, Pirttila AM, Tejesvi MV, Martins MCL. Prevention of urinary catheter-associated infections by coating antimicrobial peptides from crowberry endophytes. Sci Rep. 2019;9(1):10753.
46. Minardi D, Ghiselli R, Cirioni O, Giacometti A, Kamysz W, Orlando F, et al. The antimicrobial peptide tachyplesin III coated alone and in combination with intraperitoneal piperacillin–tazobactam prevents ureteral stent *Pseudomonas* infection in a rat subcutaneous pouch model. Peptides. 2007;28(12):2293–8.
47. Lim K, Chua RR, Bow H, Tambyah PA, Hadinoto K, Leong SS. Development of a catheter functionalized by a polydopamine peptide coating with antimicrobial and antibiofilm properties. Acta Biomater. 2015;15:127–38.
48. Lim K, Chua RR, Saravanan R, Basu A, Mishra B, Tambyah PA, et al. Immobilization studies of an engineered arginine–tryptophan-rich peptide on a silicone surface with antimicrobial and antibiofilm activity. ACS Appl Mater Interfaces. 2013;5(13):6412–22.
49. Li X, Li P, Saravanan R, Basu A, Mishra B, Lim SH, et al. Antimicrobial functionalization of silicone surfaces with engineered short peptides having broad spectrum antimicrobial and salt-resistant properties. Acta Biomater. 2014;10(1):258–66.
50. Mishra B, Basu A, Yuan Chua RR, Saravanan R, Tambyah PA, Ho B, Chang MW, Jan Leong SS. Site specific immobilization of a potent antimicrobial peptide onto silicone catheters: evaluation against urinary tract infection pathogens. J Mater Chem B. 2014;2:1706–16.
51. Lo JCY. Novel antimicrobial peptide coating to prevent catheter-associated urinary tract infections [Master's thesis]. 2015.
52. Yu K, Lo JC, Yan M, Yang X, Brooks DE, Hancock RE, et al. Anti-adhesive antimicrobial peptide coating prevents catheter associated infection in a mouse urinary infection model. Biomaterials. 2017;116:69–81.
53. Pinese C, Jebors S, Echalier C, Licznar-Fajardo P, Garric X, Humblot V, et al. Simple and specific grafting of antibacterial peptides on silicone catheters. Adv Healthc Mater. 2016;5(23):3067–73.
54. Chua RYR, Lim K, Leong SSJ, Tambyah PA, Ho B. An *in-vitro* urinary catheterization model that approximates clinical conditions for evaluation of innovations to prevent catheter-associated urinary tract infections. J Hosp Infect. 2017;97(1):66–73.
55. Yu H, Cui LX, Huang N, Yang ZL. Recent developments in nitric oxide-releasing biomaterials for biomedical applications. Med Gas Res. 2019;9(4):184–91.
56. Regev-Shoshani G, Ko M, Miller C, Av-Gay Y. Slow release of nitric oxide from charged catheters and its effect on biofilm formation by *Escherichia coli*. Antimicrob Agents Chemother. 2010;54(1):273–9.
57. Zhu ZL, Wang ZP, Li SH, Yuan X. Antimicrobial strategies for urinary catheters. J Biomed Mater Res A. 2019;107(2):445–67.
58. Carlsson S, Weitzberg E, Wiklund P, Lundberg JO. Intravesical nitric oxide delivery for prevention of catheter-associated urinary tract infections. Antimicrob Agents Chemother. 2005;49(6):2352–5.
59. Schairer DO, Chouake JS, Nosanchuk JD, Friedman AJ. The potential of nitric oxide releasing therapies as antimicrobial agents. Virulence. 2012;3(3):271–9.
60. Colletta A, Wu JF, Wo YQ, Kappler M, Chen H, Xi CW, et al. *S*-Nitroso-*N*-acetylpenicillamine (SNAP) impregnated silicone Foley catheters: a potential biomaterial/device to prevent catheter-associated urinary tract infections. ACS Biomater Sci Eng. 2015;1(6):416–24.
61. Ketchum AR, Kappler MP, Wu J, Xi C, Meyerhoff ME. The preparation and characterization of nitric oxide releasing silicone rubber materials impregnated with *S*-nitroso-*tert*-dodecyl mercaptan. J Mater Chem B. 2016;4(3):422–30.

62. Ng WL, Bassler BL. Bacterial quorum-sensing network architectures. Annu Rev Genet. 2009;43:197–222.
63. Devadas SM, Nayak UY, Narayan R, Hande MH, Ballal M. 2,5-Dimethyl-4-hydroxy-3(2*H*)-furanone as an anti-biofilm agent against non-*Candida albicans Candida* species. Mycopathologia. 2019;184(3):403–11.
64. Cirioni O, Ghiselli R, Minardi D, Orlando F, Mocchegiani F, Silvestri C, et al. RNAIII-inhibiting peptide affects biofilm formation in a rat model of staphylococcal ureteral stent infection. Antimicrob Agents Chemother. 2007;51(12):4518–20.
65. Ivanova K, Fernandes MM, Francesko A, Mendoza E, Guezguez J, Burnet M, et al. Quorum-quenching and matrix-degrading enzymes in multilayer coatings synergistically prevent bacterial biofilm formation on urinary catheters. ACS Appl Mater Interfaces. 2015;7(49):27066–77.
66. Ivanova K, Fernandes MM, Mendoza E, Tzanov T. Enzyme multilayer coatings inhibit *Pseudomonas aeruginosa* biofilm formation on urinary catheters. Appl Microbiol Biotechnol. 2015;99(10):4373–85.
67. Limoli DH, Jones CJ, Wozniak DJ. Bacterial extracellular polysaccharides in biofilm formation and function. Microbiol Spectr. 2015;3(3):3.
68. Thallinger B, Prasetyo EN, Nyanhongo GS, Guebitz GM. Antimicrobial enzymes: an emerging strategy to fight microbes and microbial biofilms. Biotechnol J. 2013;8(1):97–109.
69. Appel W. Chymotrypsin: molecular and catalytic properties. Clin Biochem. 1986;19(6):317–22.
70. Catto C, Secundo F, James G, Villa F, Cappitelli F. alpha-Chymotrypsin immobilized on a low-density polyethylene surface successfully weakens *Escherichia coli* biofilm formation. Int J Mol Sci. 2018;19(12):4003.
71. Kaplan JB, LoVetri K, Cardona ST, Madhyastha S, Sadovskaya I, Jabbouri S, et al. Recombinant human DNase I decreases biofilm and increases antimicrobial susceptibility in *Staphylococci*. J Antibiot. 2012;65(2):73–7.
72. Lipovsky A, Thallinger B, Perelshtein I, Ludwig R, Sygmund C, Nyanhongo GS, et al. Ultrasound coating of polydimethylsiloxanes with antimicrobial enzymes. J Mater Chem B. 2015;3(35):7014–9.
73. Thallinger B, Brandauer M, Burger P, Sygmund C, Ludwig R, Ivanova K, et al. Cellobiose dehydrogenase functionalized urinary catheter as novel antibiofilm system. J Biomed Mater Res Part B Appl Biomater. 2016;104(7):1448–56.
74. Baker P, Hill PJ, Snarr BD, Alnabelseya N, Pestrak MJ, Lee MJ, et al. Exopolysaccharide biosynthetic glycoside hydrolases can be utilized to disrupt and prevent *Pseudomonas aeruginosa* biofilms. Sci Adv. 2016;2(5):e1501632.
75. Snarr BD, Baker P, Bamford NC, Sato Y, Liu H, Lehoux M, et al. Microbial glycoside hydrolases as antibiofilm agents with cross-kingdom activity. Mycoses. 2017;114(27):7124–9.
76. Asker D, Awad TS, Baker P, Howell PL, Hatton BD. Non-eluting, surface-bound enzymes disrupt surface attachment of bacteria by continuous biofilm polysaccharide degradation. Biomaterials. 2018;167:168–76.
77. Lehman SM, Donlan RM. Bacteriophage-mediated control of a two-species biofilm formed by microorganisms causing catheter-associated urinary tract infections in an *in vitro* urinary catheter model. Antimicrob Agents Chemother. 2015;59(2):1127–37.
78. Carson L, Gorman SP, Gilmore BF. The use of lytic bacteriophages in the prevention and eradication of biofilms of *Proteus mirabilis* and *Escherichia coli*. FEMS Immunol Med Microbiol. 2010;59(3):447–55.
79. Sulakvelidze A, Alavidze Z, Morris JG Jr. Bacteriophage therapy. Antimicrob Agents Chemother. 2001;45(3):649–59.
80. Milo S, Hathaway H, Nzakizwanayo J, Alves DR, Esteban PP, Jones BV, et al. Prevention of encrustation and blockage of urinary catheters by *Proteus mirabilis* via pH-triggered release of bacteriophage. J Mater Chem B. 2017;5(27):5403–11.

81. Curtin JJ, Donlan RM. Using bacteriophages to reduce formation of catheter-associated bio-films by *Staphylococcus epidermidis*. Antimicrob Agents Chemother. 2006;50(4):1268–75.
82. Fu WL, Forster T, Mayer O, Curtin JJ, Lehman SM, Donlan RM. Bacteriophage cocktail for the prevention of biofilm formation by *Pseudomonas aeruginosa* on catheters in an *in vitro* model system. Antimicrob Agents Chemother. 2010;54(1):397–404.
83. Liao KS, Lehman SM, Tweardy DJ, Donlan RM, Trautner BW. Bacteriophages are synergistic with bacterial interference for the prevention of *Pseudomonas aeruginosa* biofilm formation on urinary catheters. J Appl Microbiol. 2012;113(6):1530–9.

Plasma Based Approaches for Deposition and Grafting of Antimicrobial Agents to Polymer Surfaces

Todorka Gancheva Vladkova and Dilyana Nikolaeva Gospodinova

1 Introduction

Improved protection of urinary stents against infections is a significant current challenge because of the increasing microbial resistance to the conventional antibiotics and negative issues for the patients. Formation of crystalline biofilms of pathogenic microbial cells is the leading cause of urinary stent associated infections.

On many parameters polymeric materials satisfy the basic requirements and are widely used for the fabrication of urinary stents, silicones and polyurethanes being preferable ones currently [1]; and biodegradables attracting interest lately. However, the nonsufficient microbial resistance, biofilm formation and encrustation are their common gap.

A lot of approaches, antimicrobial agents and techniques are under a study to mitigate the problem by creation of contact killing, releasing or low adhesive surfaces do not allowing attachment of microbial cells [2–4].

The plasma treatment has a number of advantages that make it preferable in many strategies for the development of antimicrobial biomaterials. The control over the plasma processing parameters allows control over the surface chemistry, charge, structure, morphology, hydrophilic/hydrophobic balance, etc. Due to a variety of biomaterials and bacteria, causing urinary tract infections, plasma assisted antibacterial strategies need in tailoring to each specific surface [5–8].

T. G. Vladkova (✉)
Department of Polymer Engineering, University of Chemical Technology and Metallurgy, Sofia, Bulgaria
e-mail: tgv@uctm.edu

D. N. Gospodinova
Department of Electrical Apparatus, Faculty of Electrical Engineering, Technical University of Sofia, Sofia, Bulgaria

© The Author(s) 2022
F. Soria et al. (eds.), *Urinary Stents*,
https://doi.org/10.1007/978-3-031-04484-7_22

273

2   Physical Plasma and Plasma Processes

Plasma is a multicomponent system obtained by a partial ionization of gas. The plasma consists of positively and negatively charged ions, negatively charged electrons, radicals, neutral and excited atoms, highly energetic molecules and molecular fragments [8–12]. According to the temperature of the ions, the plasma refers to *low temperature* (*cold*) or *high temperature plasma* [13].

Surface modification of polymeric biomaterials is performed in low temperature plasma created by ionization of inert (Ar, Ne, He) or reactive (O_2, N_2, NH_3, CO_2) gases or volatile monomers at low (RF) or atmospheric pressure by applying energy in the form of heat, direct or alternating electric current, radiation or laser light [8, 12].

Depending on the mode of plasma treatment, four types modification processes happen on the polymer surface: sputtering, etching, ion implantation and plasma polymer deposition [12].

Plasma sputtering is the plasma physical degradation, limited to the outermost layer of the polymeric biomaterial, as it simplified presented in Fig. 1.

Plasma sputtering is used for sterilization of sensitive to temperature or radiation biomaterials, removal of surface contaminations and deposition of sputtered thin coatings [12, 14].

Plasma etching (Fig. 2) is a process at which the loss of the exposed polymeric material is deeper and the adsorption of energetic species is followed by a product formation, prior to a product desorption.

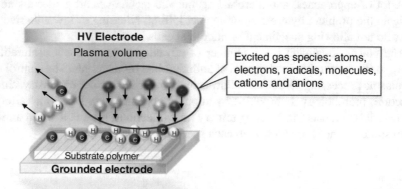

Fig. 1 Simplified presentation of plasma sputtering: the plasma degradation is limited to the outermost layer of the polymeric material

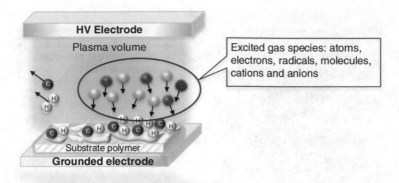

Fig. 2 Simplified presentation of plasma etching: the loss of the exposed polymeric biomaterial is deeper and the adsorption of energetic species is followed by a product formation, prior to a product desorption

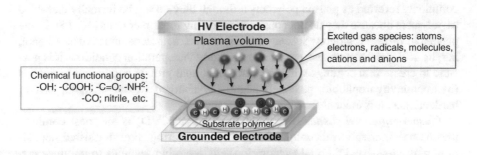

Fig. 3 Simplified presentation of plasma ion implantation: the presenting in the plasma excited species react directly with the polymer surface and induce grafting of new functional groups

Plasma etching is aimed at: removal of impurities, surface nanopatterning, cross-linking of surface polymer chains and generation of surface functional groups [11, 15].

Plasma ion implantation is a process at which the presenting in the plasma excited species react directly with the polymer surface and induce grafting of new chemical groups (amine, hydroxyl and others), Fig. 3 [11, 15].

Plasma polymer deposition (PPD) is a process in which a thin polymer-like film is formed over the surface of the substrate polymer (Fig. 4).

PPD happens inside the plasma reactor but outside the plasma zone where activated gas species polymerize onto the cold substrate. The generated films are

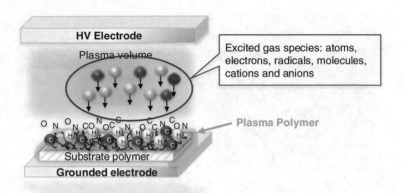

Fig. 4 Simplified presentation of plasma polymer deposition: a thin polymer-like film is formed over the surface of the original biomaterial

commonly referred as plasma polymers although they do not be formally classified as polymers because they do not consist of repeating monomer units [10, 15]. Using plasma of different gaseous substances: allylamine, octadiene, aldehydes, ethanol, acrylic acid, perfluorooctane, etc.) and optimizing the operation conditions it is possible to create thin coatings with different functional groups and varied properties (hydrophilic/hydrophobic, positively/negatively charged or non-charged, soft or hard, etc.), as it is evident from Fig. 5.

Plasma-enhanced chemical vapor deposition (PECVD) is the most common plasma polymerization technique. Magnetron sputtering, liquid-assisted deposition, plasma-assisted thermal evaporation, etc. are other technics to polymer surface modification [11, 15–17]. *Ion beam processing* includes: ion implantation; ion beam texturing and sputtering, etc. The ion-beam modification is durable and no surface "reconstruction" happens in contrary to the plasma treated surface. Plasma immersion ion implantation and ion treatment by plasma exposure are two relative new possibilities. The above methods could be utilized in antimicrobial approaches to the creation of functionalized, or low adhesive surfaces with controlled topography and surface energy [11, 18]. Some examples of plasma treatments are: ion-plasma modification of polyvinylchloride microfiltration membranes [19]; treatment of polyacrylonitrile membranes in DBD discharge in air (including magnet stimulated), [20–22]; electron beam cross-linking of silicone rubber [23], plasma pre-treatment of collagen and keratin base materials [24]; generation of self-organized patterns in cold atmospheric plasma-activated liquids [25] etc.

Fig. 5 Chemical composition (based on results from XPS) of RF vacuum plasma deposited films of different monomers: diaminocyclohexane (DACH), hydroxyethylmethacrylate (HEMA), hexamethyldisiloxane (HMDS), acrylic acid (AA), methane (CH₄) and polyethylene oxide (PEO) (from. T. Vladkova, Surface Engineering of Polymeric Biomaterials, Smithers Rapra, UK, 2013)

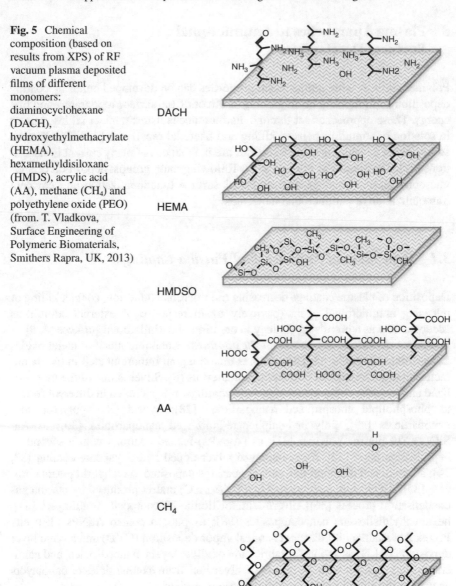

3   Plasma Approaches to Antimicrobial Surfaces Development

Polymer surfaces with antimicrobial properties can be developed either by coating deposition, antimicrobial agent grafting or affecting the surface topography and free energy. These approaches act through distinct mechanisms: contact killing, killing in solution or stimuli responsive killing and bacterial repellence [3, 4, 26]. Plasma strategies for developing of such surfaces are in the focus of many current investigations [27]. They could be referred to the following main groups: deposition of antimicrobial plasma coatings, plasma based surface functionalization and covalent immobilization of antimicrobial molecules.

3.1   Deposition of Antimicrobial Plasma Coatings

Deposition of plasma coatings decreasing the microbial adhesion, contact killing or releasing antimicrobial agent (passively or in response of external stimuli) is accepted now as a promising strategy to creation of antimicrobial surfaces [4, 8].

Plasma *deposition of nanocomposite coatings*, containing metal or metal oxides nanoparticles (Ag, Cu, Ti, TiO_2, etc.), is becoming an important step in the manufacturing of antimicrobial polymeric biomaterials [8]. Silver is one of the most utilized antibacterial components of plasma coatings. It is included in different forms: as phospholipid encapsulated nanoparticles [28]; hybrid silver-poly(*l*-lactide) nanoparticles [29]; polyvinyl-sulphonate-stabilized nanoparticles [30]; as Ag/ SiO(x)C(y) plasma polymer [31]; as (AgNPs)-loaded coatings with a second *n*-heptylamine layer [32]; plasma-sprayed silver-doped hydroxyapatite coating [33, 34]; silver-doped diamond-like carbon coatings deposited via a hybrid plasma process [35]; Ag clusters incorporated in a:C (Ag/a:C) matrix produced by plasma gas condensation process [36]; silver/montmorillonite biocomposite multilayers [37], hexamethyldisiloxane nanocomposites [38]; as plasma coated AgNPs [39]; etc. Piszek and Radtke [40] discuss chemical vapor deposition (CVD) and atomic layer deposition (ALD) as a tools for fabrication of silver layers, nanoparticles, and nanocomposites together with the release of silver ions from nanoparticles or nanolayers as well as the antimicrobial activity of these materials.

Vladkova et al. [41] developed new functional coatings for medical devices, employing magnetron co-sputtering to deposit triple $TiO_2/SiO_2/Ag$ nanocomposite thin films. Combining the antimicrobial activity of the TiO_2 and Ag with the dispersing effect of the SiO_2 these coatings demonstrate strong inhibitory effect toward *E. coli* and *P. aeruginosa* growth. Direct contact and eluted silver mediated killing were experimentally demonstrated as mechanism of antibacterial action of these coatings [41]. Kredl et al. [42] use DC plasma air jet to deposit Cu coating on PDMS and acrylonitrile butadiene styrene ABS triple co-polymer surfaces. Good antimicrobial activity against Gram-negative and Gram-positive test bacteria with clinical significance was found by Stoyanova et al. [43] for RF magnetron co-sputtered Ag and Cu doped TiO_2 coatings. Woskowicz et al. [44] just reported MS-PVD plasma treatment of polypropylene surface utilizing sputtering of Ag, Cu and their oxides in order to impart antimicrobial activity [44].

Deposition of *plasma coatings releasing antimicrobial agents either passively or in response to external stimuli* is another option to limit bacterial colonization. Releasing metal nanoparticles (silver, coper or tin), amino-hydrocarbon coatings, prepared by plasma immersion ion implantation are an example discussed as alternative of the antibiotics releasing ones [12].

Plasma coatings that *release antimicrobials in response to external stimuli* are produced by 'sandwiching' of antimicrobials between two plasma polymer layers, plasma polymer over coating or nano-templating for creation of antimicrobial reservoirs [45–47]. A novel approach to generate hydrogel coatings through atmospheric-pressure plasma polymerization includes: plasma pre-treatment of the substrate leaving reactive surface radicals; plasma-induced polymerization of the monomer units and cross-linking the polymer chains into a polymer network [48].

Plasma coatings inhibiting bacterial adhesion are based on the idea for creation of surfaces decreasing microbial adhesion down to levels do not allowing attachment or allowing easy detachment of microbial cells. Non-toxicity is the main advantage of this strategy together with some others. Ykada et al. [49] proved that the work of adhesion in aqueous media, $W_{1,2w}$ approaches to zero when the water contact angle (WCA) or surface tension, γ_c approaches to zero, i.e. low adhesive are strong hydrophilic or strong hydrophobic surfaces. Surface enrichment of relevant functional groups and topographical modifications are main ways to creation of such by plasma treatment [4, 11]. When plasma processes are combined with nano-texturing, remarkable wetting states such as superhydrophobicity and superhydrophilicity can be achieved [50–52]. Nwankire et al. [53] deposited superhydrophobic (WCA above 150°) siloxane coatings using atmospheric pressure plasma jet system and hexamethyldisiloxane (HMDSO), tetramethyl cyclotetrasiloxane (Tomcats) or a mixture of Tomcats and fluorosiloxane as liquid precursors [53].

Diamond like carbon (DLC) plasma coatings are also used for creation of low adhesive polymer surfaces. A fluid precursor, generally used for production of DLC is hydrocarbon (methane) or silicone. The hydrogen to carbon ratio has a dramatic influence on the characteristics of the DLC coatings. But overall they characterize by excellent biocompatibility and low friction coefficient [11, 54]. In 2007, Laube et al. [55] discuss DLC coatings as a new strategy for decreasing the formation of crystalline bacterial biofilms on ureteral stents. A preliminary study with ten patients having indwelled DLC coated stent demonstrates quite promising results: significantly decreased friction, encrustation and biofilm formation. It was concluded that further investigation in larger patient groups is necessary for their confirmation. Unfortunately, no reports were found about that [55]. The doping with antimicrobial metals (copper, silver, and other) or elements increasing the hydrophobicity are conventional tools to improve the DLC coatings resistance to bacterial biofilms formation. Ren [56] reports increased resistance to bacterial colonization of anti-adhesive Si-and F-Doped DLC coatings and micro-nanostructured surfaces than non-doped DLC coatings.

Another promising candidate for antimicrobial protection of biomaterial are *oxazoline-derived plasma polymer (PPOx) coatings*. Bacteria may attach in small numbers to the deposited under appropriate conditions PPOx coatings but would not proliferate to form biofilms, that is very interesting for development of low fouling coatings to indwelling medical devices [57, 58]. A simple and efficient strategy for preparation of poly(2-oxazoline)-based coatings on polytetrafluoroethylene (PTFE) substrate, using diffuse coplanar surface barrier discharge (DCSBD) as a cold plasma source was just reported [59].

3.2 Plasma-Based Surface Functionalization and Antimicrobial Agents' Immobilization

Plasma deposited antimicrobial coatings improve the antibacterial activity but the effect is not enough durable for some applications and toxicity concerns remain. Covalent grafting of antimicrobial agents is a subject of many investigations aimed at a long-lasting efficacy and a reduced toxicity [5]. Plasma treatment is an easy way to creation of functionalized surfaces with antimicrobial activity or such that can be utilized for covalent immobilization of antimicrobial agents including on nanoscale topographies [4, 60].

Conventionally, an antimicrobial agent immobilization is carried out in two steps: enriching the topmost polymer surface with reactive functional groups by cold plasma treatment (RF or atmospheric pressure plasma, lately preferable) followed by covalent binding using known chemical reactions [4, 60].

The oxygen-rich surfaces, containing hydroxyl, carboxyl and carbonyl groups promote the cellular attachment because of ionic interactions with molecules, mediating the cell adhesion [61]. The amine-rich polymer surfaces created by plasma treatment, using allylamine, ethylendiamine, propylamine, butlyamine or heptylamine as starting monomer are positively charged and facilitate the electrostatic adsorption of negatively charged proteins, that maybe confer their biocompatibility [62].

Plasma deposition of ring opening monomers (oxazolines, pyrrole, furfuryl, thiophene, aniline, etc.) generates surface chemistries that are not achievable via other ways. Careful tuning the plasma deposition condition is very important to tailor the amount of functionality suit for any specific application and to ensure that film reactivity can be maintained for relevant time [57, 63–67]. Plasma deposited polyoxazolines (POx) contain isocyanate-, nitrile groups and intact oxazoline rings. This provides unique opportunities to carry out binding reactions with biomolecules, nanoparticles and various ligands that contain carboxyl groups in their structures [57, 68]. Plasma-assisted processing and catechol chemistry as well as the use of natural antimicrobial agents to produce synthetic antibiotic-free antibacterial surfaces are a particularly hot topic discussed now [69].

Immobilization of biologically active molecules (antibiotics and other antimicrobial agents) to polymer surfaces is for a long time studied [4].

Examples of plasma assisted *attachment of antibiotics* are grafting of triclosan and bronopol on oxygen plasma pre-treated polyvinylchloride; grafting of gentamycin to polyvinylidene fluoride after plasma-induced graft polymerization of acrylic acid; etc. [27]. The efficacy of cold plasma for direct deposition of antibiotics is discussed lately as a novel approach for localized delivery and retention of the effect. Ampicillin and gentamicin, deposited onto two types of surfaces: polystyrene micro-titer plates and stainless steel coupons confirmed that the plasma process bonds the antibiotics to the surfaces and ensures localized retention of the antibiotic activity against planktonic and sessile *E. coli* and *P. aeruginosa* [70].

Plasma treated polymer surfaces, enriched with reactive functional groups are utilized in other bioactive molecules immobilization such as peptides, proteins, quaternary ammonium compounds, etc. via corresponding chemical reactions [11, 60]: Plasma pre-treated expanded poly(tetra fluoro ethylene) (PTFE) was peptide immobilised after acrylic acid (AA) grafting and diNH$_2$PEG coupling [71]; RF acrylic acid plasma treated silicone surface was immobilized with avidin protein [72].

Plasma treatments, opening a way to biofunctionalization of chemically inert polymers (such as PDMS is) are of especial interest. Trying to combine some advantages of both: ion-beam and plasma treatment, namely the durability of the modifying effect of the ion-beam with the simplicity of the plasma as compared to ion-beam equipment, we developed a special irradiation technique, plasma based Ar$^+$ beam, to activate the PDMS surface for further hybrid functionalization [18, 73, 74]. Assuming that the existence of an ion-flow in the plasma volume could strength the surface modifying effect including its durability, a parallel plate reactor equipped with a serial capacitance (Fig. 6) was employed to obtain an ion flow in the plasma volume. The vary of the discharge power ensures varied density of the ion flow [10].

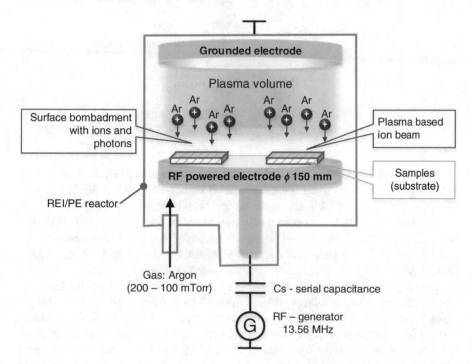

Fig. 6 Parallel plate single-wafer reactor in variant of plasma based Ar$^+$ beam mode of surface treatment

Fig. 7 Principle scheme of plasma based Ar⁺ beam initiated multistep surface modification of cross-linked polydimethylsiloxane (PDMS)

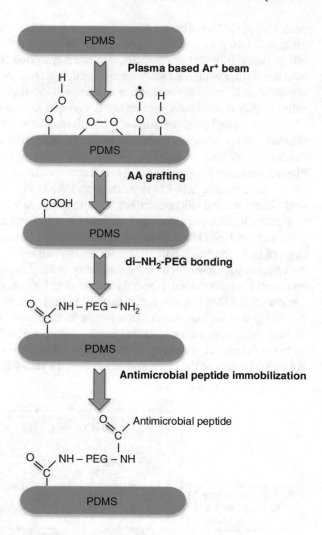

Plasma based Ar⁺ beam can initiate multistep surface modification procedure including antimicrobial agent (peptide/protein) immobilization via flexible spacer. The principle scheme of this experimental approach is presented in Fig. 7.

This multistep procedure opens a new way to obtain four types modified PDMS surfaces: (1) partially mineralised (moderate hydrophilic, with O-containing groups and free radicals); (2) chemically grafted with AA (moderate hydrophilic, with –COOH functional groups); (3) diNH₂PEG-coupled (strong hydrophilic, with –NH₂ functional groups; PEG acting as flexible spacer); and (4) biomolecules immobilized (collagen, antimicrobial peptide, or other). The chemical composition, surface topography and roughness as well as the surface hydrophilic/hydrophobic balance, surface free energy, its components and polarity were controlled on every stage of the modification procedure by means of XPS, AFM, SEM and equilibrium contact angle measurements.

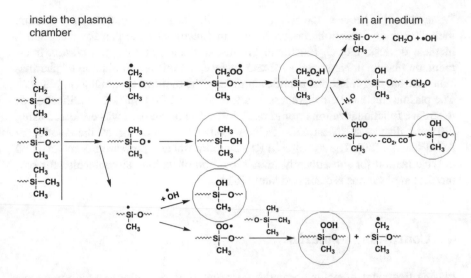

Fig. 8 A simplified sketch of the cascade process that results in a partial mineralization and O-containing functional groups formation on the PDMS surface due to a plasma Ar⁺ beam treatment

Figure 8 demonstrates the cascade process of partial mineralization and functionalization of cross-linked PDMS. It is evident where and how appear a number of active centres such as free radicals and oxygen-containing gropes that could be utilised in further chemical grafting of desired functionalities.

The partially mineralized surface layer was similar to that obtained after a conventional ion-beam. The PDMS surface hydrophilisation was due to surface polarity increase as a result of polar groups' accumulation, this effect depending on the discharge power. The above presented multi-step procedure has a potential to be used whenever need arises to control chemical activity, hydrophilic/hydrophobic balance and biocontact properties of chemically inert polymers for application as antimicrobial biomaterials for cells culture, processing of biosensors, indwelling medical devices, etc.

In 2019, Tran et al. [75] develop a single step plasma process for covalent binding of antimicrobial peptides on catheters to suppress bacterial adhesion. Plasma immersion ion implantation (PIII) was demonstrated as a single step treatment leading to covalent coupling of antimicrobial peptides to both internal and external surfaces of PVC catheter tubing, reducing 99% of bacterial adhesion. Ye et al. [76] created self-sterilizing surfaces using a single-step solvent less grafting method. A grafting process was conducted by vapor deposition of a crosslinked poly(dimethylaminomethyl styrene-*co*-ethylene glycol diacrylate) (P(DMAMS-*co*-EGDA)) prime layer, followed by *in situ* grafting of poly(dimethylaminomethyl styrene) (PDMAMS) from the reactive sites of the prime layer. This hybrid coating demonstrates more than 99% bacterial killing against both Gram-negative *E. coli* and Gram-positive *B. subtilis* [76]. Surface-grafted polymers, known as polymer brushes, become an important tool for surface modification and functionalization.

Wang et al. [77] review the recent progress in the surface-grafting of polymers, including their formation and utilization in functional materials for electronics, medical devices, etc. O_2-functional groups, introduced by oxygen-plasma treatment, on plasma polymerized HMDSO surface, are utilized in binding of pharmaceuticals and anti-microbial peptides inhibiting the biofilms accumulation [78, 79]. The plasma treatment effectiveness as a tool to direct PET surface modification or to surface functionalization prior to immobilization of chitosan was evaluated using different discharge types: DC-discharge (at the cathode or at the anode) or AC-discharge [80]. The use of cold RF- and atmospheric pressure plasma-assisted polymerization for subsequently immobilization of various biomolecules for biomedical applications is discussed lately [81].

4 Concluding Remarks

Plasma treatment of polymers under corresponding operation conditions allows deposition of contact killing, releasing (including controlled release) or low-adhesive antimicrobial coatings, as well as polymer surface functionalization and durable immobilization of antimicrobial molecules. Most of the plasma technologies are developed in laboratory conditions and the surface engineered biomaterials are tested *in vitro*.

The use of plasmas facilitates modifications which are difficult or unable to achieve by conventional physical or chemical methods, like for example the stable attachment of biologically active molecules onto chemically inert polymer surfaces.

For the step "from laboratory into clinical practice" it is essential to examine the *in vivo* antimicrobial action by using appropriate animal models and human groups.

References

1. Gadzhiev N, Gorelov D, Malkhasyan V, Akopyan G, Harchelava R, Mazurenko D, et al. Comparison of silicone versus polyurethane ureteral stents: a prospective controlled study. BMC Urol. 2020;20(1):10.
2. Mosayyebi A, Vijayakumar A, Yue QY, Bres-Niewada E, Manes C, Carugo D, et al. Engineering solutions to ureteral stents: material, coating and design. Cent Eur J Urol. 2017;70(3):270–4.
3. Zhang Z, Wagner VE. Antimicrobial coatings and modifications on medical device. Cham: Springer; 2017.
4. Vladkova TG, Staneva AD, Gospodinova DN. Surface engineered biomaterials and ureteral stents inhibiting biofilm formation and encrustation. Surf Coat Technol. 2020;404:126424.
5. Vasilev K, Griesser SS, Griesser HJ. Antibacterial surfaces and coatings produced by plasma techniques. Plasma Process Polym. 2011;8(11):1010–23.
6. Cvrček L, Horáková M. Plasma modified polymeric materials for implant applications. In Non-thermal plasma technology for polymeric materials. Amsterdam: Elsevier; 2019.

7. Múgica-Vidal R, Sainz-García E, Álvarez-Ordóñez A, Prieto M, González-Raurich M, López M, et al. Production of antibacterial coatings through atmospheric pressure plasma: a promising alternative for combatting biofilms in the food industry. Food Bioprocess Technol. 2019;12(8):1251–63.

8. Nikiforov A, Deng X, Xiong Q, Cvelbar U, Degeyter N, Morent R, et al. Non-thermal plasma technology for the development of antimicrobial surfaces: a review. J Phys D Appl Phys. 2016;49(20):204002.

9. Wikipedia. Plasma [Internet]. Plasma. https://bg.wikipedia.org/wiki/Плазма.

10. Hippler R, Pfau S, Schmidt M, Schoenbach KH. Low temperature plasma physics: fundamental aspects and applications. 2nd ed. New York: Wiley-VCH; 2008. p. 945. https://www.amazon.com/Low-Temperature-Plasmas-Fundamentals-Technologies-dp-3527406735/dp/3527406735/ref=dp_ob_image_bk.

11. Vladkova TG. Surface engineering of polymeric biomaterials. Shawbury: Smithers Rapra Technology; 2013. p. 590. https://www.amazon.co.uk/Surface-Engineering-Polymeric-Biomaterials-Vladkova/dp/1847356591.

12. Walschusp U, Schlosser K, Schroder M, Finke K, Nebe B, Meichsner B, et al. Application of low-temperature plasma processes for biomaterials. In Biomaterials applications for nanomedicine. London: IntechOpen; 2011.

13. Knowledge Computing. Plasma classification (types of plasma). https://www.plasma-universe.com/plasma-classification-types-of-plasma/.

14. Glow CB. Discharge processes: sputtering and plasma etching. 1st ed. New York: Wiley-Interscience; 1980. p. 432. https://www.wiley.com/en-bg/Glow+Discharge+Processes:+Sputtering+and+Plasma+Etching-p-9780471078289.

15. Yasuda H. Plasma polymerization. New York: Academic Press; 2012. p. 442. https://www.amazon.com/Plasma-Polymerization-H-Yasuda/dp/0123960916.

16. Hegemann D, Nisol B, Watson S, Wertheimer MR. Energy conversion efficiency in plasma polymerization—a comparison of low- and atmospheric-pressure processes. Plasma Process Polym. 2016;13(8):834–42. https://doi.org/10.1002/ppap.201500224.

17. Friedrich J. Mechanisms of plasma polymerization—reviewed from a chemical point of view. Plasma Process Polym. 2011;8(9):783–802. https://doi.org/10.1002/ppap.201100038.

18. Vladkova TG, Keranov IL, Dineff PD, Youroukov SY, Avramova IA, Krasteva N, et al. Plasma based Ar$^+$ beam assisted poly(dimethylsiloxane) surface modification. Nucl Instrum Methods Phys Res Sect B Beam Interact Mater Atoms. 2005;236(1):552–62.

19. Vladkova TG, Dineff P, Stojcheva R, Tomerova B. Ion-plasma modification of polyvinylchloride microfiltration membranes. J Appl Polym Sci. 2003;90(9):2433–40. https://doi.org/10.1002/app.12912.

20. Petrov S, Atanasova P, Dineff P, Vladkova T. Surface modification of polymeric ultrafiltration membranes I. Effect of atmospheric pressure barrier discharge in air onto some characteristics of polyacrylonitrile ultrafiltration membranes. High Energy Chem. 2012;46(4):283–91. https://doi.org/10.1134/S0018143912040145.

21. Atanasova P, Petrov S, Dineff P, Vladkova T. Surface modification of polymeric ultrafiltration membranes II. Effect of magnet stimulated atmospheric pressure barrier discharge in air onto some characteristics of polyacrylonitrile ultrafiltration membranes. High Energy Chem. 2012;46(5):1–8.

22. Vladkova T, Atanasova P, Petrov S, Dineff P. Surface modification of polymeric ultrafiltration membranes: III. Effect of plasma-chemical surface modification onto some characteristics of polyacrylonitrile ultrafiltration membranes. High Energy Chem. 2013;47(6):346–52. https://doi.org/10.1134/S0018143913060118.

23. Stelescu M, Manaila E, Vladkova T, Georgescu M. The influence of polyfunctional monomers on the mechanical properties of the silicone rubber cross-linked by irradiation with electron beam. Ecol Saf. 2012;6(1):323–9. https://www.scientific-publications.net/download/ecology-and-safety-2012-1.pdf.

24. Gaidau C, Petica A, Micutz M, Danciu M, Vladkova T. Progresses in treatment of collagen and keratin-based materials with silver nanoparticles. Open Chem. 2013;11(6):901–11. https://www.degruyter.com/view/journals/chem/11/6/article-p901.xml.
25. Chen Z, Xu RG, Chen P, Wang Q. Potential agricultural and biomedical applications of cold atmospheric plasma-activated liquids with self-organized patterns formed at the interface. IEEE Trans Plasma Sci. 2020;48(10):3455–71.
26. Singha P, Locklin J, Handa H. A review of the recent advances in antimicrobial coatings for urinary catheters. Acta Biomater. 2017;50:20–40.
27. Sardella E, Palumbo F, Camporeale G, Favia P. Non-equilibrium plasma processing for the preparation of antibacterial surfaces. Materials. 2016;9:515.
28. Taheri S, Cavallaro A, Christo SN, Majewski P, Barton M, Hayball JD, et al. Antibacterial plasma polymer films conjugated with phospholipid encapsulated silver nanoparticles. ACS Biomater Sci Eng. 2015;12:1278–86. https://doi.org/10.1021/acsbiomaterials.5b00338.
29. Taheri S, Baier G, Majewski P, Barton M, Förch R, Landfester K, et al. Synthesis and surface immobilization of antibacterial hybrid silver-poly(*l*-lactide) nanoparticles. Nanotechnology. 2014;25(30):305102. https://doi.org/10.1088/0957-4484/25/30/305102.
30. Vasilev K, Sah VR, Goreham RV, Ndi C, Short RD, Griesser HJ. Antibacterial surfaces by adsorptive binding of polyvinyl-sulphonate-stabilized silver nanoparticles. Nanotechnology. 2010;21(21):215102. https://doi.org/10.1088/0957-4484/21/21/215102.
31. Khalilpour P, Lampe K, Wagener M, Stigler B, Heiss C, Ullrich MS, et al. Ag/SiOxCy plasma polymer coating for antimicrobial protection of fracture fixation devices. J Biomed Mater Res Part B Appl Biomater. 2010;94(1):196–202. https://doi.org/10.1002/jbm.b.31641.
32. Ploux L, Mateescu M, Anselme K, Vasilev K. Antibacterial properties of silver-loaded plasma polymer coatings. J Nanomater. 2012;2012:674145. https://doi.org/10.1155/2012/674145.
33. Carmona VO, Martínez Pérez C, de Lima R, Fraceto LF, Romero García J, Ledezma Pérez A, et al. Effect of silver nanoparticles in a hydroxyapatite coating applied by atmospheric plasma spray. Int J Electrochem Sci. 2014;9:7471–94. http://www.electrochemsci.org/papers/vol9/91207471.pdf.
34. Roy M, Fielding GA, Beyenal H, Bandyopadhyay A, Bose S. Mechanical, in vitro antimicrobial, and biological properties of plasma-sprayed silver-doped hydroxyapatite coating. ACS Appl Mater Interfaces. 2012;4(3):1341–9. https://doi.org/10.1021/am201610q.
35. Cloutier M, Tolouei R, Lesage O, Lévesque L, Turgeon S, Tatoulian M, et al. On the long term antibacterial features of silver-doped diamondlike carbon coatings deposited via a hybrid plasma process. Biointerphases. 2014;9(2):29013. https://doi.org/10.1116/1.4871435.
36. Carvalho I, Faraji M, Ramalho A, Carvalho AP, Carvalho S, Cavaleiro A. Ex-vivo studies on friction behaviour of ureteral stent coated with Ag clusters incorporated in a: C matrix. Diam Relat Mater. 2018;86:1–7.
37. Iconaru SL, Groza A, Stan GE, Predoi D, Gaiaschi S, Trusca R, et al. Preparations of silver/montmorillonite biocomposite multilayers and their antifungal activity. Coatings. 2019;9:817.
38. Ionita MD, Ionita ER, Satulu V, De Vrieze M, Zille A, Modic M, et al. Antibacterial nanocomposites based on Ag NPs and HMDSO deposited by atmospheric pressure plasma. In: 23rd International symposium on plasma chemistry [Internet]. Montréal, Canada; 2014. http://repositorium.sdum.uminho.pt/handle/1822/57250.
39. Brobbey KJ, Haapanen J, Mäkelä JM, Gunell M, Eerola E, Rosqvist E, et al. Effect of plasma coating on antibacterial activity of silver nanoparticles. Thin Solid Films. 2019;672:75–82.
40. Piszczek P, Radtke A. Silver nanoparticles fabricated using chemical vapor deposition and atomic layer deposition techniques: properties, applications and perspectives: review. In: Seehra MS, Bristow AD, editors. Noble and precious metals-properties, nanoscale effects and applications. London: IntechOpen; 2018.
41. Vladkova T, Angelov O, Stoyanova D, Gospodinova D, Gomes L, Soares A, et al. Magnetron co-sputtered TiO$_2$/SiO$_2$/Ag nanocomposite thin coatings inhibiting bacterial adhesion and biofilm formation. Surf Coat Technol. 2020;384:125322.

42. Kredl J, Quade A, Mueller S, Peglow S, Polak M, Kolb JF, et al. Antimicrobial copper-coatings on temperature labile surfaces deposited with a DC plasma jet operated with air. 2014.
43. Stoyanova DS, Ivanova IA, Angelov OI, Vladkova TG. Antibacterial activity of thin films TiO$_2$ doped with Ag and Cu on gracilicutes and firmicutes bacteria. Biodiscovery. 2017;20:e15076. https://doi.org/10.3897/biodiscovery.20.e15076.
44. Woskowicz E, Łożynska M, Kowalik-Klimczak A, Kacprzyńska-Gołacka J, Osuch-Słomka E, Piasek A, et al. Plasma deposition of antimicrobial coatings based on silver and copper on polypropylene. Polimery. 2020;65(1):33–43. http://repo.bg.pw.edu.pl/index.php/en/r#/info/article/WUT7d3f00caa77d4cb1a07f2503c91147fe/Plasma+deposition+of+antimicrobial+coatings+based+on+silver+and+copper+on+polypropylene%23.X7pIVlUzaUk.
45. Simovic S, Losic D, Vasilev K. Controlled release from drug delivery systems based on porous platforms. Pharm Technol. 2011;35:68–71.
46. Vasilev K, Poulter N, Martinek P, Griesser HJ. Controlled release of levofloxacin sandwiched between two plasma polymerized layers on a solid carrier. ACS Appl Mater Interfaces. 2011;3(12):4831–6. https://doi.org/10.1021/am201320a.
47. Simovic S, Losic D, Vasilev K. Controlled drug release from porous materials by plasma polymer deposition. Chem Commun. 2010;46(8):1317–9. https://doi.org/10.1039/B919840G.
48. Levien M, Fricke K. Fabrication of hydrogel coatings by atmospheric-pressure plasma polymerization: function by structure and chemistry. Mater Today. 2020;41:316–7.
49. Ikada Y, Suzuki M, Tamada Y. Polymer surfaces possessing minimal interaction with blood components. In: Shalaby SW, Hoffman AS, Ratner BD, Horbett TA, editors. BT-Polymers as biomaterials. Boston: Springer; 1984. p. 135–47. https://doi.org/10.1007/978-1-4613-2433-1_10.
50. Choukourov A, Kylián O, Petr M, Vaidulych M, Nikitin D, Hanuš J, et al. RMS roughness-independent tuning of surface wettability by tailoring silver nanoparticles with a fluorocarbon plasma polymer. Nanoscale. 2017;9(7):2616–25. https://doi.org/10.1039/C6NR08428A.
51. Kuzminova A, Shelemin A, Kylián O, Petr M, Kratochvíl J, Solař P, et al. From super-hydrophilic to super-hydrophobic surfaces using plasma polymerization combined with gas aggregation source of nanoparticles. Vacuum. 2014;110:58–61.
52. Ramiasa-MacGregor M, Mierczynska A, Sedev R, Vasilev K. Tuning and predicting the wetting of nanoengineered material surface. Nanoscale. 2016;8(8):4635–42. https://doi.org/10.1039/C5NR08329J.
53. Nwankire CE, Favaro G, Duong Q-H, Dowling DP. Enhancing the mechanical properties of superhydrophobic atmospheric pressure plasma deposited siloxane coatings. Plasma Process Polym. 2011;8(4):305–15. https://doi.org/10.1002/ppap.201000069.
54. Vladkova TG. Surface engineered polymeric biomaterials with improved biocontact properties. Int J Polym Sci. 2010;2010:296094.
55. Laube N, Kleinen L, Bradenahl J, Meissner A. Diamond-like carbon coatings on ureteral stents—a new strategy for decreasing the formation of crystalline bacterial biofilms? J Urol. 2007;177(5):1923–7. https://doi.org/10.1016/j.juro.2007.01.016.
56. Ren D. Anti-adhesive Si-and F-doped DLC coatings and micro-nanostructured surfaces for medical implants. Dundee: University of Dundee; 2015. https://discovery.dundee.ac.uk/en/studentTheses/anti-adhesive-si-and-f-doped-dlc-coatings-and-micro-nanostructure.
57. Ramiasa MN, Cavallaro AA, Mierczynska A, Christo SN, Gleadle JM, Hayball JD, et al. Plasma polymerised polyoxazoline thin films for biomedical applications. Chem Commun. 2015;51(20):4279–82. https://doi.org/10.1039/C5CC00260E.
58. Visalakshan RM, Cavallaro A, Smith LE, MacGregor-Ramiasa M, Hayball J, Vasilev K. Downstream influences of oxazoline plasma polymerisation conditions on chemical and biological interactions. In CHEMECA 2016: Chemical engineering-regeneration, recovery and reinvention. Adelaide: CHEMECA; 2016. p. 840–8. https://search.informit.com.au/documentSummary;dn=410967258296456;res=IELENG;type=pdf.
59. Šrámková P, Zahoranová A, Kelar J, Kelar Tučeková Z, Stupavská M, Krumpolec R, et al. Cold atmospheric pressure plasma: simple and efficient strategy for preparation of poly(2-

oxazoline)-based coatings designed for biomedical applications. Sci Rep. 2020;10(1):9478. https://doi.org/10.1038/s41598-020-66423-w.

60. Hermanson GT. Chapter 4-Zero-length crosslinkers. 3rd ed. Boston: Academic Press; 2013. p. 259–73.

61. Ruiz J-C, Girard-Lauriault P-L, Wertheimer MR. Fabrication, characterization, and comparison of oxygen-rich organic films deposited by plasma- and vacuum-ultraviolet (VUV) photo-polymerization. Plasma Process Polym. 2015;12(3):225–36. https://doi.org/10.1002/ppap.201400146.

62. Lerouge S, Barrette J, Ruiz J-C, Sbai M, Savoji H, Saoudi B, et al. Nitrogen-rich plasma polymer coatings for biomedical applications: stability, mechanical properties and adhesion under dry and wet conditions. Plasma Process Polym. 2015;12(9):882–95. https://doi.org/10.1002/ppap.201400210.

63. Saboohi S, Al-Bataineh SA, Safizadeh Shirazi H, Michelmore A, Whittle JD. Continuous-wave RF plasma polymerization of furfuryl methacrylate: correlation between plasma and surface chemistry. Plasma Process Polym. 2017;14(3):1600054. https://doi.org/10.1002/ppap.201600054.

64. Kumar SD, Yoshida Y. Dielectric properties of plasma polymerized pyrrole thin film capacitors. Surf Coat Technol. 2003;169:600–3.

65. Silverstein MS, Visoly-Fisher I. Plasma polymerized thiophene: molecular structure and electrical properties. Polymer (Guildf). 2002;43(1):11–20.

66. Morales J, Olayo MG, Cruz GJ, Castillo-Ortega MM, Olayo R. Electronic conductivity of pyrrole and aniline thin films polymerized by plasma. J Polym Sci Part B Polym Phys. 2000;38(24):3247–55. https://doi.org/10.1002/1099-0488(20001215)38:24%3C3247::AID-POLB60%3E3.0.CO.

67. Jacob MV, Easton CD, Anderson LJ, Bazaka K. RF plasma polymerised thin films from natural resources. Int J Mod Phys Conf Ser. 2014;32:1460319. https://doi.org/10.1142/S2010194514603196.

68. Macgregor-Ramiasa MN, Cavallaro AA, Vasilev K. Properties and reactivity of polyoxazoline plasma polymer films. J Mater Chem B. 2015;3(30):6327–37. https://doi.org/10.1039/C5TB00901D.

69. Bazaka K, Jacob MV, Chrzanowski W, Ostrikov K. Anti-bacterial surfaces: natural agents, mechanisms of action, and plasma surface modification. RSC Adv. 2015;5(60):48739–59.

70. Los A, Ziuzina D, Boehm D, Han L, O'Sullivan D, O'Neill L, et al. Efficacy of cold plasma for direct deposition of antibiotics as a novel approach for localized delivery and retention of effect. Front Cell Infect Microbiol. 2019;9:428. https://doi.org/10.3389/fcimb.2019.00428.

71. Baquey C, Palumbo F, Porte-Durrieu MC, Legeay G, Tressaud A, d'Agostino R. Plasma treatment of expanded PTFE offers a way to a biofunctionalization of its surface. Nucl Instrum Methods Phys Res Sect B Beam Interact Mater Atoms. 1999;151(1):255–62. http://www.sciencedirect.com/science/article/pii/S0168583X99001068.

72. Costa LT, Vilani C, Peripolli S, Stavale F, Legnani C, Achete CA. Direct immobilization of avidin protein on AFM tip functionalized by acrylic acid vapor at RF plasma. J Mol Recognit. 2012;25(5):256–61. https://doi.org/10.1002/jmr.2189.

73. Keranov I, Vladkova TG, Minchev M, Kostadinova A, Altankov G, Dineff P. Topography characterization and initial cellular interaction of plasma-based Ar+ beam-treated PDMS surfaces. J Appl Polym Sci. 2009;111(5):2637–46. https://doi.org/10.1002/app.29185.

74. Keranov I, Vladkova T, Minchev M, Kostadinova A, Altankov G. Preparation, characterization, and cellular interactions of collagen-immobilized PDMS surfaces. J Appl Polym Sci. 2008;110(1):321–30. https://doi.org/10.1002/app.28630.

75. Tran C, Yasir M, Dutta D, Eswaramoorthy N, Suchowerska N, Willcox M, et al. Single step plasma process for covalent binding of antimicrobial peptides on catheters to suppress bacterial adhesion. ACS Appl Biol Mater. 2019;2(12):5739–48. https://doi.org/10.1021/acsabm.9b00776.

76. Ye Y, Song Q, Mao Y. Solventless hybrid grafting of antimicrobial polymers for self-sterilizing surfaces. J Mater Chem. 2011;21(35):13188–94. https://doi.org/10.1039/C1JM12050F.

77. Wang S, Wang Z, Li J, Li L, Hu W. Surface-grafting polymers: from chemistry to organic electronics. Mater Chem Front. 2020;4(3):692–714. https://doi.org/10.1039/C9QM00450E.

78. Yoshinari M, Matsuzaka K, Inoue T. Surface modification by cold-plasma technique for dental implants—bio-functionalization with binding pharmaceuticals. Jpn Dent Sci Rev. 2011;47(2):89–101. http://www.sciencedirect.com/science/article/pii/S1882761611000287.

79. Mon H, Chang Y-R, Ritter AL, Falkinham JO, Ducker WA. Effects of colloidal crystals, antibiotics, and surface-bound antimicrobials on *Pseudomonas aeruginosa* surface density. ACS Biomater Sci Eng. 2018;4(1):257–65. https://doi.org/10.1021/acsbiomaterials.7b00799.

80. Demina TS, Piskarev MS, Romanova OA, Gatin AK, Senatulin BR, Skryleva EA, et al. Plasma treatment of poly(ethylene terephthalate) films and chitosan deposition: DC- vs. AC-discharge. Materials (Basel, Switzerland). 2020;13(3):508.

81. Ramkumar MC, Trimukhe AM, Deshmukh RR, Tripathi A, Melo JS, Navaneetha PK. Immobilization of biomolecules on plasma-functionalized surfaces for biomedical applications. In: Tripathi A, Melo JS, editors. BT-immobilization strategies: biomedical, bioengineering and environmental applications. Singapore: Springer; 2021. p. 305–33. https://doi.org/10.1007/978-981-15-7998-1_8.

Antimicrobial Biosurfactants Towards the Inhibition of Biofilm Formation

Inês Anjos, Ana F. Bettencourt, and Isabel A. C. Ribeiro

1 Introduction

Nowadays, infections associated with urinary tract medical devices, have become a common health issue. The fact that their surfaces are prone to microbial colonization and biofilm formation is certainly a problem. As a result, these medical devices usage can be a source of extreme concern, especially for critically ill patients [1].

Urinary tract related infections (UTIs) are among the most frequent HAIs comprising 27% in Europe and 36–40% in the USA [2, 3]. Unfortunately, intensive care units (ICU) also have become a stage of HAIs events where several reported infections among ICU patients can be attributed to catheter-related urinary tract infections (CRUTIs) [4, 5]. UTIs in ICUs have been reported as 1.1 per 1000 patient-days in Europe and most of these are, CRUTIs i.e.97.4% [3]. Nevertheless, device-associated UTI are not exclusively catheter-related. Consequently, among patients undergoing ureteral stents, 38% develop UTI while 45–100% of them have bacteriuria [3].

The incidence of UTIs calls for a well understanding of their pathogenesis, alongside with rapid interventions before and after bacterial colonization and biofilm formation to prevent such infections and to diminish its negative impacts.

Biofilm is a mono or multilayer of interconnected microorganisms surrounded with extracellular matrix (ECM) interfacing a liquid medium. Scientists have described biofilm formation as a process of multi-steps including adhesion, aggregation, maturation, and detachment. Drawbacks associated with biofilm development are substantial and compose a challenge for UTIs management and prevention. In addition to their ability to detach as planktonic to colonize on other surfaces inside the body systems, the diversity of biofilm microorganisms also contributes to

I. Anjos · A. F. Bettencourt · I. A. C. Ribeiro (✉)
Research Institute for Medicines (iMed.ULisboa), Faculty of Pharmacy,
Universidade de Lisboa, Lisbon, Portugal
e-mail: ii.anjos@campus.fct.unl.pt; asimao@ff.ul.pt; iribeiro@ff.ulisboa.pt

© The Author(s) 2022
F. Soria et al. (eds.), *Urinary Stents*,
https://doi.org/10.1007/978-3-031-04484-7_23

the failure of antimicrobial treatment [6]. Additional potential protection of bacteria is provided by the biofilm composition which acts as a guard against antibiotics and immunity system.

Due to the resistance of mature biofilms and the risks associated to biofilm manipulation or eradication, prevention of biofilm generation is advantageous. Therefore, the majority of the strategies that have been proposed aim at preventing the early stages of biofilm formation on the catheter surface [7]. A possible strategy may be the use of surface active molecules with antimicrobial activity such as biosurfactants.

Biosurfactants are surface-active molecules that have granted priority in research and industrial studies. They are identified as amphiphilic biomolecules produced by a wide range of microorganisms as secondary metabolites, owning the ability of surface tension reduction like the industrial surfactants but with the advantage of being eco-friendly molecules that can be produced from renewable resources. Moreover features associated with biosurfactants include low toxicity, biodegradability, cost-effectiveness, and biocompatibility [8]. Due to their unique properties, biosurfactants can be used in several applications regarding pharmaceutical, food, agriculture, petroleum and cosmetic industries [9, 10].

According to their structure, biosurfactants have been classified into glycolipids (e.g. rhamnolipids and sophorolipids), lipoproteins or lipopeptides (e.g. surfactin), conjugated phospholipids and fatty acids (e.g. polymyxin) and polymeric biosurfactant (e.g. liposan) [8].

Glycolipids are the most used biosurfactants due to their surface-active properties, e.g. dispersion, emulsion, foaming, solubilization, wetting and penetration [8, 11]. In glycolipids monosaccharide residues are linked to an hydrophobic group [12] and this class comprises sophorolipids, rhamnolipids, trehalose lipids, cellobiose lipids and mannosylerythritol lipids, which are the most studied [8, 13].

Besides their surface-active properties, some biosurfactants also detain interesting biological activities and the most studied have been sophorolipids and rhamnolipids.

Among the glycolipid class, sophorolipids have been assigned for antimicrobial properties and are also considered as potential anticancer candidates considering their ability for apoptosis induction among different types of cells such as liver and leukemia cancer cells [14, 15]. Additional sophorolipids revealed sperm immobilization and death through micelles formation combined with anti-HIV via inhibition of virus duplication [16]. Also, rhamnolipids have been pointed to present antifungal, antimicrobial, antiviral and anti-adhesive properties which makes them suitable for a variety of industrial, environmental, agricultural or medical applications [17].

2   Sophorolipids and Rhamnolipids Antimicrobial Activity

To understand why sophorolipids and rhamnolipids have been proposed for biofilm inhibition or disruption it is important to study their antimicrobial properties.

2.1 Sophorolipids

Sophorolipids can be produced by several microorganisms with a considerable yield [13] and present the favorable characteristics of being antibacterial, antiviral, antimycoplasma, antifungal and antialgal agents. Furthermore, sophorolipids can occur either in an acidic (non-esterified) or lactonic (esterified) form as illustrated in Fig. 1. Usually, lactonic sophorolipids present higher antimicrobial activity while acidic SLs display higher solubility and foaming characteristics [13, 18].

Sophorolipids' antimicrobial activity effect is assigned to their ability to change the hydrophobic properties of bacterial surfaces and to burst the cellular membrane resulting in the release of intracellular content and death. Sophorolipids may act also as antifungal since they are able to inhibit their movement and induce their lysis [14, 15].

An example of sophorolipids' antimicrobial activity can be verified in Lydon et al. studies [19] when investigating the antimicrobial potential of sophorolipids produced by *Starmerella bombicola*. The acidic sophorolipids proved to have antimicrobial activities against the nosocomial infective agents *Enterococcus faecalis* and *Pseudomonas aeruginosa*, with significant reduction in colony forming units (CFU) at concentrations of 5 mg/mL. In addition, *in vivo* experiments using a mouse skin wounding assay revealed that acidic sophorolipids could be used as a component of antimicrobial creams to reduce the risk of wound infection during healing [19]. Moreover, the antimicrobial activity of sophorolipids was also shown by Dangle-Pulate et al. [20]. The biosurfactants obtained from *Candida bombicola*, with glucose and lauryl alcohol media supplementation, were able to prevent bacterial colonization of *Escherichia coli* (30 μg/mL and 2 h) and *P. aeruginosa* (1 μg/mL and 4 h) as well as *Staphylococcus aureus* (6 μg/mL and 4 h). The suggested mode of action of antibacterial sophorolipids was pointed out as cellular membrane disruption causing the loss of all cytoplasmic components leading to cellular death [20].

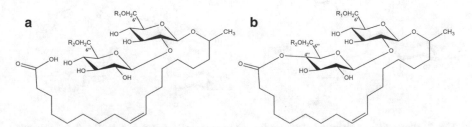

Fig. 1 Illustration of the chemical structure of acidic (**a**) and lactonic (**b**) sophorolipids. R₁=R₂=H; R₁=H and R₂=COCH₃; R₁=COCH₃ and R₂=H; R₁=R₂=COCH₃

2.2 Rhamnolipids

In the past three decades, rhamnolipids have also acquired some recognition for presenting some valuable characteristics, such as antifungal, antimicrobial, antiviral and antimycoplasma activity [21, 22]. Besides presenting antimicrobial activity, rhamnolipids also present antiadhesive properties that can be used as an antimicrobial strategy by coating the surface of medical devices and perform changes on surface's hydrophobicity [18].

Rhamnolipids have structures (Fig. 2) and properties similar to that of detergents and have been reported to intercalate into the membrane phospholipid bilayer, facilitating the permeability of the membrane and flow of metabolites [23].

Their antimicrobial mechanism can explain the results of the antimicrobial activity of the rhamnolipid extract, obtained by Ndlovu et al. [23], observing pronounced activity against a broad spectrum of opportunistic and pathogenic microorganisms, including antibiotic resistant *S. aureus* and *E. coli* strains and the pathogenic yeast *Candida albicans*, when using the agar disc susceptibility method [23]. Moreover, the antimicrobial properties of these compounds were also evaluated by Lotfabad et al. [24] who studied rhamnolipids produced by two indigenous *P. aeruginosa* strains. In this study, preliminary disc diffusion assay showed that all examined Gram-positive bacteria (i.e. *S. aureus* ATCC 29213, *Staphylococcus epidermidis* ATCC 12228 and *Bacillus cereus* ATCC 6051) were inhibited by biosurfactants produced by both MR01 and MASH1 strains [24]. Another study, conducted by de Freitas Ferreira et al. [25] investigated the antimicrobial activity of rhamnolipids under different pH values and assessed an antimicrobial activity against the Gram-positive pathogens, *Listeria monocytogenes*, *B. cereus* and *S. aureus*. *B. cereus* was the most sensitive bacteria showing a MIC value of 19.5 µg/mL, and a bactericidal activity at 39.1 µg/mL of rhamnolipids [25].

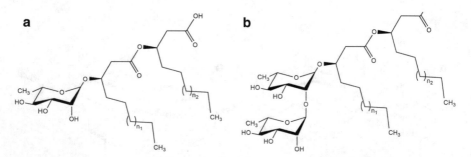

Fig. 2 Illustration of chemical structure for mono-rhamnolipids (**a**) and di-RLs (**b**). Fatty acid moieties may present a length that usually ranges from 8 to 14 carbon atoms ($1 < n_1$ and $n_2 < 7$)

3 Fighting Biofilm Formation with Biosurfactants

Biosurfactants are molecules that have amphipathic structures, which allow the interaction with cellular membranes, such as the bilayer membrane [24, 26]. The interaction of the biosurfactants with the cellular membrane causes changes and perturbations that will lead eventually to the disruption of the cellular membrane and ultimately the release of the cytoplasmic content of the cell and consequently important metabolites [24, 27]. These properties can be used to prevent biofilm formation on medical devices surfaces with the intention of reducing their related infections.

Due to presenting antimicrobial activity, sophorolipids have been explored on biofilm inhibition studies (Table 1). These studies have been developed mostly *in vitro* (e.g. using common microtiter plates) by evaluating the ability of sophorolipids' biofilm disruption or biofilm formation inhibition. Examples include the study of Mukherji and Prabhune [28] that observed the ability of sophorolipid mixtures, produced by *C. bombicola* when the media was supplemented with different plant essential oils, to inhibit *Vibrio cholerae* biofilm formation on glass slides [28]. Moreover, Sen et al. [29] investigated the efficacy of a sophorolipid mixture (SL-YS3) produced by *Rhodotorula babjevae* YS3 towards *Trichophyton mentagrophytes* biofilm. In this study a biofilm eradication around 80% was observed on microtiter plate assays when a concentration of 2 mg/mL was used. Moreover, when observing biofilms disruption on pre-sterilized glass coverslips by scanning electron microscopy (SEM) or confocal laser scanning microscopy (CLSM) a considerable reduction was also observed. The therapeutic efficacy of this sophorolipid mixture on experimentally induced dermatophytosis in mice infected with *T. mentagrophytes* was also evaluated. SL-YS3 showed therapeutic effects and also its ability to regulate collagen deposition together with proper matrix and spatial arrangement, thereby contributing to the healing of the infected skin tissue as compared to the untreated control [29].

The use of these natural biosurfactants to prevent biofilm formation on the surface of medical grade silicone, a common material used in catheters and stents fabrication has also been studied in order to evaluate its potential to reduce related infections. This was first investigated by Pontes et al. [30] who observed that sophorolipids when adsorbed to silicone could reduce *S. aureus* and *E. coli* biofilm formation. Comparing to plain silicone a reduction of 3 log units on *S. aureus* surface colonization was observed when using a solution with a concentration of 1.5 mg/mL to promote sophorolipids adsorption. Moreover, a 50% decrease on *E. coli* biofilm formation was also observed (Fig. 3, [30]).

More recently, Ceresa et al. [31] studied the effect of acidic congeners, C18 lactonic sophorolipids and mixture of acidic and lactonic sophorolipids on the disruption of *S. aureus* ATCC 6538, *P. aeruginosa* ATCC 10145 and *C. albicans* IHEM 2894 pre-formed biofilms on medical grade silicone. All three tested mixtures (when at a concentration > 0.1% w/v) were able to disrupt biofilms up to 70%, 75%

Table 1 Examples of research studies presenting the potential application of the biosurfactants (BS) sophorolipids (SLs) and rhamnolipids (RLs) in preventing biofilm formation

BS	BS Producer	Biofilm producer	Method	Results	Refs.
SLs	R. babjevae YS3	T. mentagrophytes	Biofilm eradication. Crystal violet stain, SEM or CLSM *In vivo* assay: experimentally induced dermatophytosis in mice	Biofilm eradication. Around 80% with of 2 mg/mL *In vivo* assay: SLs contributed to the healing of the infected skin tissue comparing to untreated control	[29]
SLs	S. bombicola	S. aureus ATCC 25923 and E. coli ATCC 25922	Biofilm inhibition. Crystal violet staining and CFU counts. Silicone coated with SLs, static assay. Concentration range 0.10–3 mg/mL	3 log units reduction S. *aureus* colonization 1.5 mg/mL to promote adsorption. A 50% decrease on E. coli biofilm formation with all concentrations	[30]
SLs	C. bombicola	C. albicans IHEM 2894, S. aureus ATCC 6538 and P. aeruginosa ATCC 10145	Anti-adhesion and antibiofilm activity. SLs-coated discs were evaluated using the crystal violet assay	75% and 68–70% inhibition on the cell attachment for S. *aureus* and C. *albicans*. No anti-adhesive effect on cells of P. aeruginosa	[31]
SLs	C. bombicola	P. aeruginosa PAO1 (WT) and ΔwspF deletion mutant (PAO1)	Biofilm eradication. Addition of SLs to formed biofilms, 5 h incubation. Response through OD_{600} and CLSM	SLs tested against a EPS overexpression mutant biofilms disrupts ~ 70% of the biofilm at a concentration of 0.1% and nearly 90% at 1%	[32]
RLs	P. aeruginosa LBI	L. monocytogenes ATCC 19112 and S. aureus ATCC 25923	Adhesion test. Crystal Violet staining. Different intervals, static. Concentration 0.25%, 0.5% and 1.0% (w/v)	Concentration 1.0% reduced 57.8% adhesion of L. *monocytogenes* and by 67.8% adhesion of S. *aureus*	[39]
		L. monocytogenes ATCC 19112 S. aureus ATCC 25923 and S. enteritidis PNCQ030	Disruption of biofilms. 24 h, static. Concentration 0.25% and 1.0% (w/v) aqueous solutions	At 0.25% RLs removed 58.5% the biofilm of S. *aureus*, 26.5% of L. *monocytogenes*, 23.0% of S. *enteritidis* and 24.0% of the mixed culture	[39]
RLs	P. aeruginosa	H. pylori, E. coli, P. aeruginosa, S. aureus and S. mutans	Biofilm inhibition	Biofilm inhibition for five bacterial strains in a dose-dependent manner	[43]

Table 1 (continued)

BS	BS Producer	Biofilm producer	Method	Results	Refs.
RLs	P. aeruginosa	S. epidermidis, S. salivarius, S. aureus, C. tropicalis, C. albicans, and R. dentocariosa	Biofilm inhibition and anti-adhesion. Crystal violet staining and phase-contrast microscopy	Reductions of 50% on bacteria was achieved for S. epidermidis, S. salivarius, S. aureus and C. tropicalis. C. albicans, R. dentocariosa showed a decrease after 4 h of 20–28%	[44]
RLs	P. aeruginosa	S. epidermidis	Biofilm inhibition. Flow-cell model in combination with CLSM and AFM	90% of biofilm inhibition	[45]
RLs	P. aeruginosa 89	S. aureus ATCC® 6538 and S. epidermidis ATCC® 35984	Biofilm disruption and inhibition. Crystal Violet staining and MTT assay. RLs at a concentration 0.06–2 mg/mL for disruption and 2 mg/mL for inhibition assays. End points at 24, 48 and 72 h of incubation	Biofilm disruption ranged from 68 to 89% for S. aureus and from 44 to 96% for S. epidermidis. Pre-treatment of silicone with R89BS resulted in a biofilm inhibition of 76% for S. aureus and of 63% for S. epidermidis	[46]
RLs	P. aeruginosa	S. aureus ATCC 25923	Biofilm inhibition. After incubation at 37 °C for 24 h, biofilm assessment was performed by colony forming units (CFU) count	A biofilm inhibition of 99% was achieved with rhamnolipid–chitosan nanoparticles	[47]

and 80% regarding *S. aureus*, *P. aeruginosa* and *C. albicans*, respectively. Moreover, acidic sophorolipid (0.8% w/v) pre-coated silicone discs reduced *S. aureus* biofilm by 75% while *C. albicans* reached 68–70% [31].

It is also of great importance to study the development and ways to prevent biofilm formation onto microfluidic systems. Nguyen et al. [32] demonstrated that sophorolipids had a stronger effect than chemical surfactants such as sodium dodecyl sulphate, Tween20 and Tween80 when disrupting established *P. aeruginosa* PAO1 biofilms grown in microfluidic channels. The authors noticed that although presenting antibiofilm properties, sophorolipids did not seem to have antibacterial effects on PAO1. When testing these compounds on a mutant strain that overexpresses extracellular polymeric substances they observed that sophorolipids detached and disintegrated biofilms from glass surfaces [32].

Rhamnolipids have been recognized for their antiadhesive and biofilm dispersion effects. It is suggested that the antibiofilm activity of rhamnolipids occurs through

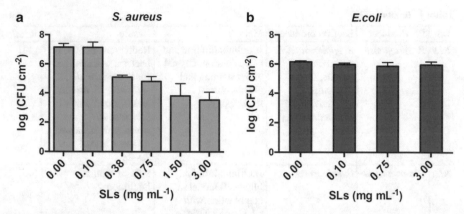

Fig. 3 Anti-sessile activity of silicone specimens adsorbed with sophorolipids towards *S. aureus* (**a**) and *E. coli* (**b**). Sessile cells CFU counts were performed when different concentrations of SLs were tested (0.1–3 mg/mL). (*Reproduced with permission* [30] *Copyright 2016, Elsevier*)

interference with quorum sensing of biofilm cells, which leads to detachment of microorganisms. This interference has been attributed to the inhibition of intracellular lipidic signals, however, it is also reported that rhamnolipids solubilize ECM proteins via micelles formation [8, 33]. Furthermore, other investigations have pointed out that rhamnolipids can manipulate biofilm-associated channels, altering the oxygen and nutrient supply for sessile microorganisms. Moreover, it has been observed that they may enhance interconnections changes as well, so they affect not only quorum sensing of bacteria but also, they do not allow them to develop genetic mutations or resistance [34]. A previous study of Davey et al. [35] mentioned that rhamnolipids can inhibit both intracellular contact and cell–surface contact allowing the detachment and preventing attachment of microorganisms [35]. Other studies pointed out that the mechanism of action of rhamnolipids is through modification of bacterial surface components. These studies proved that rhamnolipids could sharply increase the hydrophobicity of the cell surface by removing out the lipopolysaccharides parts from the outer membrane. Also, they showed that a low concentration of rhamnolipids is required to induce the disruption of cells [36, 37]. Similarly, the antifungal activity of rhamnolipids was explained by the disruption of the cytoplasmic membrane [38]. Additional investigations regarding the antibacterial effect of rhamnolipid showed that monorhamnolipids exhibit bacteriostatic effect while dirhamnolipids were able to kill the bacteria and show bactericidal effect [34].

Due to their antimicrobial and antiadhesive properties rhamnolipids have been the target of many studies focused on diminishing biofilm formation in different surfaces such as polystyrene, silicone and medical devices surfaces.

Different studies aiming the investigation of rhamnolipids antibiofilm, antiadhesive and biofilm dispersion effects have been performed and some examples can be found in Table 1. Gomes and Nitschke [39] used different concentrations of rhamnolipids from *P. aeruginosa* to evaluate their capacity in reducing the adhesion and biofilm formation on polystyrene surfaces. When using a rhamnolipids solution at 1% an adhesion reduction of 57.8 and 67.8% was observed for *L. monocytogenes* and *S. aureus*, respectively. Moreover, rhamnolipids were also effective in preventing the adhesion of bacterial mixed cultures. When at a concentration of 0.25%, rhamnolipids removed 58.5% of *S. aureus* biofilm, 26.5% of *L. monocytogenes* biofilm, 23.0% of *Salmonella enteritidis* and 24.0% of the mixed culture biofilm [39].

Moreover, Aleksik et al. [40] compared the antibiofilm ability against *P. aeruginosa* PAO1 of di-rhamnolipids produced by *Lysinibacillus* sp. BV152.1 with the commercial di-rhamnolipids. The authors observed that di-rhamnolipids produced by *Lysinibacillus* sp. BV152.1 were more effective in reducing biofilm than the commercial ones and an inhibition of 50% was observed with 50 μg/mL and 75 μg/mL, respectively. The authors also observed that amide derivatization of both di-rhamnolipids improved the inhibition of biofilm formation and dispersion, and that the morpholine derivative was the most active causing more than 80% biofilm inhibition at concentrations of 100 μg/mL [40].

Besides their activity towards bacterial biofilms, rhamnolipids, also have revealed activity on *C. albicans* biofilms. Di-rhamnolipids produced by *P. aeruginosa* when at a concentration of 0.16 or 5 mg/mL were able to reduce pre-formed biofilms on polystyrene by 50% and 90%, respectively. In this study the influence of rhamnolipids in disrupting *C. albicans* biofilms was proven and the authors suggested their exploration as a potential alternative to the available conventional therapies [41].

Comparison of rhamnolipids with other antimicrobial compounds or surfactants has also been performed. For example, Quinn et al. [42] compared rhamnolipids with antibiotics antibiofilm activity. The effect of a rhamnolipid mixture, containing mono- and di-rhamnolipids (20 μg/mL) in pre-existing biofilms was observed as a reduction of 88.4 ± 5.8, 74.5 ± 6.6% and 85.6 ± 3.9% against *B. subtilis*, *Micrococcus luteus* and *S. aureus*, respectively. A lower antibiofilm effect was observed with the antibiotics ampicillin, chloramphenicol and kanamycin (5 μg/mL) [42].

Moreover, Shen et al. [43] evaluated sodium lauryl sulfate, rhamnolipids, and N-acetylcysteine ability to eradicate mature biofilms and inhibit new biofilm formation of *Helicobacter pylori*, *E. coli*, *P. aeruginosa*, *S. aureus*, and *Streptococcus mutants*. The authors observed that sodium lauryl sulfate and rhamnolipids successfully inhibited the formation of those five bacterial biofilms in a dose-dependent manner even at concentrations below the minimal inhibitory concentrations. This suggests that their antibiofilm activities are unrelated to their antibacterial activities and that had already been observed by Quinn et al. [42] when comparing rhamnolipids antibiofilm activity to antibiotics [43].

These results have led to the hypothesis of using these biosurfactants on medical devices to prevent their related infections. Therefore, some papers have also investigated the potential of rhamnolipids inhibition of different strain biofilms on silicone rubber or medical grade silicone. For example, Rodrigues et al. [44] studied the ability of rhamnolipids to interfere in the adhesion of bacteria and yeasts isolated from explanted voice prostheses onto silicone rubber. The authors concluded that the number of cells adhering onto silicone rubber treated with biosurfactant was reduced and that declines of 50% on the number of cells were attained for *S. epidermidis*, *Streptococcus salivarius*, *S. aureus* and *C. tropicalis*. Nevertheless, *C. albicans* and the bacterial strain *Rothia dentocariosa* showed a lower decrease in the number of attached cells after 4 h (20–28%) [44].

Studies on antibiofilm activity of rhamnolipids have also been realized on other medical devices such as catheters. Biofilm formation by *S. epidermidis* is a cause of infections related to peritoneal dialysis. Pihl et al. [45] used a peritoneal dialysis catheter flow-cell model in combination with confocal scanning laser microscopy and atomic force microscopy to study biofilm formation by *S. epidermidis* and observed a reduction in the covering of biofilm with exposure to the supernatant from two *P. aeruginosa* strains (i.e. rhamnolipids). The exposure to this supernatant originated a coverage of only 10% in biofilm when compared to untreated samples [45].

Additionally, when adsorbed to silicone elastomeric discs the rhamnolipids 89, produced by *P. aeruginosa* 89, were able to reduce *Staphylococcus* spp. biofilm formation, by 70 and 50% regarding biomass and 72 and 63% regarding cell metabolic activity (at 72 h) for *S. aureus* and *S. epidermidis*, respectively. SEM analysis also corroborated these results making R89 a promising antibiofilm coating for silicon catheters [46].

Recently, Bettencourt et al. [47] developed chitosan–rhamnolipid nanoparticles intended to fight *S. aureus* infections. The obtained particles showed an antimicrobial synergic effect between chitosan and rhamnolipids produced by *P. aeruginosa* when testing their antimicrobial activity towards *S. aureus*. Regarding antibiofilm activity of the produced particles a reduction of 99% on biofilm formation on medical grade silicone could be observed making these particles an interesting approach to prevent *S. aureus* related infections such as the medical devices-related (Fig. 4) [47].

4 Conclusion

Infections associated with urinary tract medical devices are a common health concern, in particularly, when associated to biofilm formation on their surfaces.

Among multiple strategies to fight those infections, biosurfactants as glycolipids can be a valuable tool for biofilm inhibition or disruption. In particularly, multiple *in vitro* studies concerning sophorolipids and rhamnolipids confirms the antimicrobial activity of those compounds.

Further, sophorolipids or rhamnolipids potential role to prevent biofilm associated infections, using different surfaces like medical grade silicone as example of

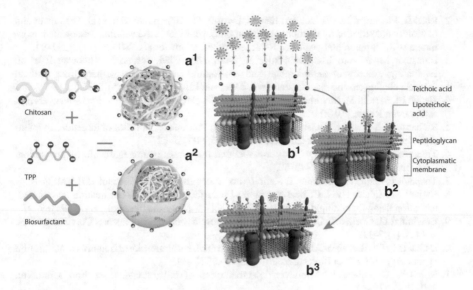

Fig. 4 Illustration of rhamnolipids–chitosan particles (RLs–CSp) antimicrobial mechanism of action towards *S. aureus*. Particles may deliver rhamnolipids as encapsulated onto RLs–CSp. (**A1**) or/and adsorbed to its surface (**A2**). First, electrostatic attraction of RLs–CSp (negatively charged) to *S. aureus* membranes (positively charged) takes place (**B1, B2**). Later, RLs are released from the particles, enter into membranes leading to cell damage and death (**B3**). (*Reproduced with permission* [47] *Copyright 2021, Elsevier*)

common material used in catheters and stents fabrication, shows the capacity of those biosurfactants in reducing the adhesion and biofilm formation.

Finally, new trends in the delivery of these biosurfactants, namely by their inclusion in nanoparticulate systems paves the way for newer clinical applications.

Overall, sophorolipids and rhamnolipids due to their multiple antimicrobial/anti-adhesive effects might be an interesting approach to fight urinary tract medical devices associated infections.

Acknowledgements The authors thank Fundação para a Ciência e Tecnologia (FCT) for the financial support under Project PTDC/BTM-SAL/29335/2017, UIDB/04138/2020 and UIDP/04138/2020 (iMed.ULisboa).

References

1. Muszanska AK, Nejadnik MR, Chen Y, Van Den Heuvel ER, Busscher HJ, Van Der Mei HC, et al. Bacterial adhesion forces with substratum surfaces and the susceptibility of biofilms to antibiotics. Antimicrob Agents Chemother. 2012;56(9):4961–4.

2. Raad II, Mohamed JA, Reitzel RA, Jiang Y, Dvorak TL, Ghannoum MA, et al. The prevention of biofilm colonization by multidrug-resistant pathogens that cause ventilator-associated pneumonia with antimicrobial-coated endotracheal tubes. Biomaterials. 2011;32(11):2689–94.
3. Ramstedt M, Ribeiro IAC, Bujdakova H, Mergulhão FJM, Jordao L, Thomsen P, et al. Evaluating efficacy of antimicrobial and antifouling materials for urinary tract medical devices: challenges and recommendations. Macromol Biosci. 2019;19(5):1–26.
4. Haque M, Sartelli M, Mckimm J, Bakar MA. Health care-associated infections—an overview. Infect Drug Resist. 2018;11:2321–33.
5. Richards M, Thursky K, Buising K. Epidemiology, prevalence, and sites of infections in intensive care units. Semin Respir Crit Care Med. 2003;24(1):3–22.
6. Trautner BW, Darouiche RO. Catheter-associated infections: pathogenesis affects prevention. Arch Intern Med. 2015;164:842–50.
7. Thebault P, Lequeux I, Jouenne T. Antibiofilm strategies. J Wound Technol. 2013;21:36–9.
8. Varjani SJ, Upasani VN. Critical review on biosurfactant analysis, purification and characterization using rhamnolipid as a model biosurfactant. Bioresour Technol. 2017;232:389–97.
9. Brackman G, Coenye T. Quorum sensing inhibitors as anti-biofilm agents. Curr Pharm Des. 2014;21(1):5–11.
10. Banat IM, De Rienzo MAD, Quinn GA. Microbial biofilms: biosurfactants as antibiofilm agents. Appl Microbiol Biotechnol. 2014;98(24):9915–29.
11. Ron EZ, Rosenberg E. Minireview natural roles of biosurfactants. Environ Microbiol. 2001;3(4):229–36.
12. Dìaz De Rienzo MA, Stevenson P, Marchant R, Banat IM. Antibacterial properties of biosurfactants against selected Gram-positive and-negative bacteria. FEMS Microbiol Lett. 2016;363(2):fnv224.
13. Malhotra R. Membrane glycolipids: functional heterogeneity: a review. Biochem Anal Biochem. 2012;1(2):1–5.
14. Van Bogaert INA, Saerens K, De Muynck C, Develter D, Soetaert W, Vandamme EJ. Microbial production and application of sophorolipids. Appl Microbiol Biotechnol. 2007;76(1):23–34.
15. Inès M, Dhouha G. Glycolipid biosurfactants: potential related biomedical and biotechnological applications. Carbohydr Res. 2015;416:59–69.
16. Kulakovskaya E, Kulakovskaya T. Biological activities of extracellular yeast glycolipids. In Extracellular glycolipids of yeasts. New York: Academic Press; 2014. p. 35–64.
17. Costa SGVAO, Nitschke M, Lépine F, Déziel E, Contiero J. Structure, properties and applications of rhamnolipids produced by *Pseudomonas aeruginosa* L2–1 from cassava wastewater. Process Biochem. 2010;45(9):1511–6.
18. Kim K, Dalsoo Y, Youngbum K, Baekseok L, Doonhoon S, Eun-Ki K. Characteristics of sophorolipid as an antimicrobial agent. J Microbiol Biotechnol. 2002;12(2):235–41.
19. Lydon HL, Baccile N, Callaghan B, Marchant R, Mitchell CA, Banat IM. Adjuvant antibiotic activity of acidic sophorolipids with potential for facilitating wound healing. Antimicrob Agents Chemother. 2017;61(5):e02547–16.
20. Dengle-Pulate V, Chandorkar P, Bhagwat S, Prabhune AA. Antimicrobial and SEM studies of sophorolipids synthesized using lauryl alcohol. J Surfactants Deterg. 2014;17(3):543–52.
21. Chong H, Li Q. Microbial production of rhamnolipids: opportunities, challenges and strategies. Microb Cell Fact. 2017;16(1):1–12.
22. Henkel M, Müller MM, Kügler JH, Lovaglio RB, Contiero J, Syldatk C, et al. Rhamnolipids as biosurfactants from renewable resources: concepts for next-generation rhamnolipid production. Process Biochem. 2012;47(8):1207–19.
23. Ndlovu T, Rautenbach M, Vosloo JA, Khan S, Khan W. Characterisation and antimicrobial activity of biosurfactant extracts produced by *Bacillus amyloliquefaciens* and *Pseudomonas aeruginosa* isolated from a wastewater treatment plant. AMB Express. 2017;7(1):1–19.
24. Lotfabad TB, Shahcheraghi F, Shooraj F. Assessment of antibacterial capability of rhamnolipids produced by two indigenous *Pseudomonas aeruginosa* strains. Jundishapur J Microbiol. 2013;6(1):29–35.

25. de Freitas Ferreira J, Vieira EA, Nitschke M. The antibacterial activity of rhamnolipid biosurfactant is pH dependent. Food Res Int. 2019;116:737–44.
26. Garg M, Priyanka CM. Isolation, characterization and antibacterial effect of biosurfactant from *Candida parapsilosis*. Biotechnol Rep. 2018;18:e00251.
27. Díaz De Rienzo MA, Banat IM, Dolman B, Winterburn J, Martin PJ. Sophorolipid biosurfactants: possible uses as antibacterial and antibiofilm agent. N Biotechnol. 2015;32(6):720–6.
28. Mukherji R, Prabhune A. Novel glycolipids synthesized using plant essential oils and their application in quorum sensing inhibition and as antibiofilm agents. Sci World J. 2014;2014:890709.
29. Sen S, Borah SN, Kandimalla R, Bora A, Deka S. Sophorolipid biosurfactant can control cutaneous dermatophytosis caused by *Trichophyton mentagrophytes*. Front Microbiol. 2020;11:1–15.
30. Pontes C, Alves M, Santos C, Ribeiro MH, Gonçalves L, Bettencourt AF, et al. Can sophorolipids prevent biofilm formation on silicone catheter tubes? Int J Pharm. 2016;513(1–2):697–708.
31. Ceresa C, Fracchia L, Williams M, Banat IM, Díaz De Rienzo MA. The effect of sophorolipids against microbial biofilms on medical-grade silicone. J Biotechnol. 2020;309:34–43.
32. Nguyen BVG, Nagakubo T, Toyofuku M, Nomura N, Utada AS. Synergy between sophorolipid biosurfactant and SDS increases the efficiency of *P. aeruginosa* biofilm disruption. Langmuir. 2020;36(23):6411–20.
33. Sodagari M, Wang H, Newby BMZ, Ju LK. Effect of rhamnolipids on initial attachment of bacteria on glass and octadecyltrichlorosilane-modified glass. Colloids Surf B Biointerfaces. 2013;103:121–8.
34. Diaz De Rienzo MA, Stevenson PS, Marchant R, Banat IM. Effect of biosurfactants on *Pseudomonas aeruginosa* and *Staphylococcus aureus* biofilms in a BioFlux channel. Appl Microbiol Biotechnol. 2016;100(13):5773–9.
35. Davey ME, Caiazza NC, O'Toole GA. Rhamnolipid surfactant production affects biofilm architecture in *Pseudomonas aeruginosa* PAO1. J Bacteriol. 2003;185(3):1027–36.
36. Al-Tahhan RA, Sandrin TR, Bodour AA, Maier RM. Rhamnolipid-induced removal of lipopolysaccharide from *Pseudomonas aeruginosa*: effect on cell surface properties and interaction with hydrophobic substrates. Appl Environ Microbiol. 2000;66(8):3262–8.
37. Sotirova A, Spasova D, Vasileva-Tonkova E, Galabova D. Effects of rhamnolipid-biosurfactant on cell surface of *Pseudomonas aeruginosa*. Microbiol Res. 2009;164(3):297–303.
38. Vatsa P, Sanchez L, Clement C, Baillieul F, Dorey S. Rhamnolipid biosurfactants as new players in animal and plant defense against microbes. Int J Mol Sci. 2010;11(12):5095–108.
39. do Valle Gomes MZ, Nitschke M. Evaluation of rhamnolipid and surfactin to reduce the adhesion and remove biofilms of individual and mixed cultures of food pathogenic bacteria. Food Control. 2012;25(2):441–7.
40. Aleksic I, Petkovic M, Jovanovic M, Milivojevic D, Vasiljevic B, Nikodinovic-Runic J, et al. Anti-biofilm properties of bacterial di-rhamnolipids and their semi-synthetic amide derivatives. Front Microbiol. 2017;8:1–16.
41. Singh N, Pemmaraju SC, Pruthi PA, Cameotra SS, Pruthi V. Candida biofilm disrupting ability of di-rhamnolipid (RL-2) produced from *Pseudomonas aeruginosa* DSVP20. Appl Biochem Biotechnol. 2013;169(8):2374–91.
42. Quinn GA, Maloy AP, Banat MM, Banat IM. A comparison of effects of broad-spectrum antibiotics and biosurfactants on established bacterial biofilms. Curr Microbiol. 2013;67(5):614–23.
43. Shen Y, Li P, Chen X, Zou Y, Li H, Yuan G, et al. Activity of sodium lauryl sulfate, rhamnolipids, and N-acetylcysteine against biofilms of five common pathogens. Microb Drug Resist. 2020;26(3):290–9.
44. Rodrigues LR, Banat IM, Van Der Mei HC, Teixeira JA, Oliveira R. Interference in adhesion of bacteria and yeasts isolated from explanted voice prostheses to silicone rubber by rhamnolipid biosurfactants. J Appl Microbiol. 2006;100(3):470–80.
45. Pihl M, Arvidsson A, Skepö M, Nilsson M, Givskov M, Tolker-Nielsen T, et al. Biofilm formation by *Staphylococcus epidermidis* on peritoneal dialysis catheters and the effects of extracellular products from *Pseudomonas aeruginosa*. Pathog Dis. 2013;67(3):192–8.

46. Ceresa C, Tessarolo F, Maniglio D, Tambone E, Carmagnola I, Fedeli E, et al. Medical-grade silicone coated with rhamnolipid R89 is effective against *Staphylococcus* spp. biofilms. Molecules. 2019;24(21):3843.
47. Bettencourt AF, Tomé C, Oliveira T, Martin V, Santos C, Gonçalves L, et al. Exploring the potential of chitosan-based particles as delivery-carriers for promising antimicrobial glyco-lipid biosurfactants. Carbohydr Polym. 2021;254:117433.

Novel Antimicrobial Strategies to Combat Biomaterial Infections

Zoran M. Marković and Biljana M. Todorović Marković

1 Introduction

Bacteria are present in nature everywhere and the combat with them has the major priority especially in various industrial settings (i.e. food industry) or medical devices [1]. It was established earlier that most of bacteria found in nature exist in the form of biofilms (attached to surface of different objects and not as free floating organisms). Therefore, biofilm formation can be defined as a multistage process. It starts with bacteria adhesion to surface and continues with the formation of extracellular matrix. This matrix is composed of one or more polymeric substances (proteins, polysaccharides, humic substances, extracellular DNA) [1, 2]. Bacteria adhesion to surfaces depends on different surface parameters: wettability, roughness, chemistry, and charge of materials as well as of the nature of bacterial surface, environmental factors and the associated flow conditions etc. [3, 4].

There are several possible strategies to reduce or prevent bacterial infections among different populations: patients and medical staff [5]. Traditional hospital sterilization strategies are based on usage of high level disinfectants: hydrogen peroxide, peracetic acid, glutaraldehyde and low level disinfectants: alcohols, hypochlorites, iodine and iodophor. Advanced sterilization technology focuses on chemical-free technology such as UV rays or gas plasma components. However, there are several disadvantages of both chemical and chemical-free approaches. Firstly, they are toxic to some extent so medical personnel and patients have to evacuate the premises. Secondly, the quality of sterilization is proportional to human labor invested by cleaning personnel [6]. One of the alternative strategies independent of human labor, is to produce antibacterial coatings to reduce or eliminate bacteria colonization on surfaces by leaching of biocides, antibacterial surfaces

Z. M. Marković (✉) · B. M. T. Marković
Vinča Institute of Nuclear Sciences—National Institute of the Republic of Serbia, University of Belgrade, Belgrade, Serbia
e-mail: biljatod@vin.bg.ac.rs

with deposited metals such as copper, silver or gold, formation of superhydrophobic surfaces and surfaces encapsulated by photoactive nanoparticles [7–12].

The major drawback of biocides and metal deposited surfaces is their leaching from the surface in the environment. In this way those surfaces lose their antibacterial properties after some time. Besides, these surfaces develop bacterial resistance which causes more than 33,000 deaths and costs 1.5 billion euros per year in Europe [13]. The increase of patients infected in hospitals (in the developing countries the infection rate is 75%) was noticed [14]. The cost and cytotoxicity of the agents mentioned above might be a problem as well. As the price of the best antimicrobial additives (silver, titanium, gold, chitosan) is too high, companies are looking for cheaper and safer additives with strong antimicrobial potential. Permanent cytotoxicity of certain antimicrobial agents in concentrations larger than needed for antimicrobial action may cause many problems. A further limited factor of these materials usage is that silver and copper nanoparticles are prone to oxidation. After a certain time they don't show antibacterial effects.

In recent years new types of antibacterial surfaces have been designed by encapsulation of different photoactive nanoparticles in polymer matrices (polyurethane or dimethylsiloxane) [5, 15, 16].

2   State of the Art

Photodynamic therapy (PDT) is a treatment which includes the usage of light sensitive drugs in the healing of various diseases (for example skin or eye cancers). Antibacterial PDT (APDT) is used to eliminate multidrug-resistance pathogenic bacteria [17]. Based on principles stated above it is possible to design antibacterial surfaces from photoactive nanoparticles (in the form of hybrids or thin films/coatings) or by encapsulation of photoactive nanoparticles into various polymer matrices. One of the properties of these nanoparticles is their ability to produce reactive oxygen species-ROS (singlet oxygen, superoxide, hydroxyl radicals, hydrogen peroxide) or heat [18, 19]. ROS eradicates multidrug resistant bacteria, quickly disappears and does not represent a danger to the environment. Heat causes denaturation of bacteria but requires additional means for its control.

Photoactive nanoparticles called photosensitizers (PSs) produce ROS by the following mechanism: PSs have been excited to a singlet excited state by ultraviolet or visible light. From this state electrons are moving to a triple state or return to a ground state. Singlet oxygen can be generated if they transfer their electrons or energy to molecular oxygen as shown in Fig. 1. Molecular oxygen causes oxidative damage of bacteria cells. Since molecular oxygen simultaneously attacks several sites in bacteria, the bacteria are unable to mutate and develop resistance [20–23].

Different nanoparticles can be used as PSs: pristine and doped carbon quantum dots (CQDs) and graphene quantum dots (GQDs), chitosan nanodots (ChiNDs), ultra short single wall carbon nanotubes (US SWCNTs), gold nanoparticles (AuNPs)—Fig. 2. It was earlier reported that polymers (polyurethane,

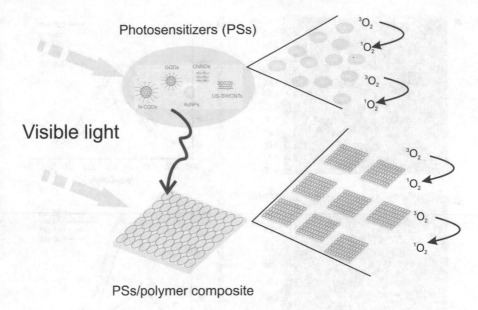

Fig. 1 Mechanism of singlet oxygen production by PSs

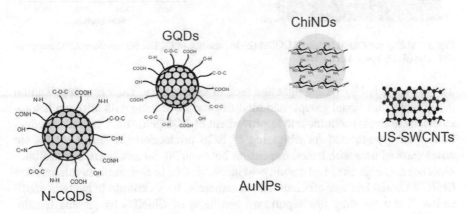

Fig. 2 Photoactive nanoparticles used potentially in APDT

polydimethylsiloxane) doped with different molecules and nanoparticles [porphyrin, methylene blue (MB), crystal violet (CV)/ZnO, Au–MB, CQDs/Ag] eradicate wide range of bacteria [*Staphylococcus aureus* (*S. aureus*), *Staphylococcus epidermidis* (*S. epidermis*), *Saccharomyces cerevisiae*, *Escherichia coli* (*E. coli*), *Bacillus subtilis* (*B. subtilis*)] effectively under visible light [12, 24–30].

CQDs and GQDs are zero dimensional carbon nanomaterials with lateral dimension smaller 10 nm. These materials have very interesting properties: high chemical stability, resistance to photo-bleaching, very good solubility in water or organic solvents, high photoluminescence and simple route for high yield synthesis—Fig. 3a, b. Most interesting biomedical property is their ability to generate ROS when

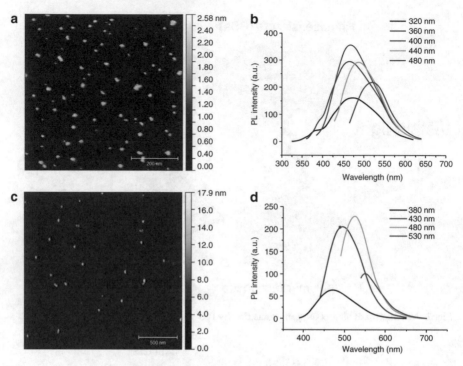

Fig. 3 (**a**) Top view AFM image of CQDs; (**b**) PL spectra of CQDs; (**c**) top view AFM image of ChiNDs; (**d**) PL spectra of ChiNDs

they are triggered by visible light and lack of cytotoxicity. Their functionalization (by different functional groups) and modification (by doping with different hetero-atoms for example) contribute to improvement of ROS generation as well as reduction of energy required for triggering of ROS production [31–36]. ChiNDs are novel class of dots with lateral dimension between 20–50 nm, tunable photoluminescence and high chemical stability—Fig. 3c, d. Due to high surface/volume ratio ChiNDs should be more efficient than commercial bulk chitosan in bacteria eradication. There are only few reports on synthesis of ChiNDs by gamma irradiation [37].

AuNPs have been widely studied in biomedicine due to their unique properties and multiple surface functionalities. Spherical AuNPs possess high surface-to-volume ratio, excellent biocompatibility, low toxicity, surface plasmon resonance and ability to quench fluorescence. Hybrids of AuNPs and CQDs produce ROS better than CQD alone [38].

US-SWCNTs are ultrashort 5–10 nm segments of single-walled carbon nanotubes (SWCNTs), with average width of 1 nm and semiconducting nature [39]. They are soluble in polar organic solvents, acids, and water. This high solubility in organic solvents coupled with their short length, should enable these US-SWNTs to be dispersed and incorporated as single tubes into other materials to form composites. Due to their similarity with CQDs and GQDs, US-SWCNTs should be potent ROS generators triggered by infrared light.

In our earlier investigation we established that pristine and doped CQDs and GQDs can be very toxic against different types of bacteria strains but only under blue light irradiation [34]. By depositing CQDs as very thin films (only 3 nm) on glass and SiO$_2$ substrates CQDs show good antibacterial activity against *S. aureus* and *E. coli* and moderate antibiofouling effect toward *Bacillus cereus* (*B. cereus*) and *Pseudomonas aeruginosa* (*P. aeruginosa*) under blue light [33]. By encapsulating CQDs in polyurethane and polydimethylsiloxane antibacterial activity of these nanocomposites enhances several orders of magnitude [5, 16]. Different authors reported earlier that CQDs/TiO$_2$, CQDs/Ag or CQDs/ZnO nanostructures as well as CQDs functionalized with (ethylenedioxy)bis(ethylamine)-EDA, N, S doped CQDs and CQDs @hematite composites show good antibacterial potentials against *S. aureus*, *E. coli*, *K. pneumoniae*, *B. subtilis* [30, 40–44]. CQDs/EDA nanostructures have higher fluorescence quantum yield compared to pristine CQDs and mixed with H$_2$O$_2$ show synergistic effect and thus can inhibit bacteria growth in smaller concentrations of each individual chemical [45].

3 Mechanism of Antibacterial Activity CQDs and Their Hybrids

Antibacterial activity of CQDs and their composites with different materials is based on the production of ROS. Generated singlet oxygen attacks bacterial wall membrane and contributes to lipid peroxidation. The bactericidal efficiency of CQDs/polymers depends on the lifetime of generated singlet oxygen [5, 16]. Luminescence method of singlet oxygen production indicates that luminescence of singlet oxygen come from the CQDs located in the interior of polymer matrix. Thus the contribution of the CQDs nearby polymer surface is negligible.

CQDs doping (for example with nitrogen) improves their antibacterial activity by the formation of amide and amino groups. Electrostatic interaction between protonated forms of amines and amides and the lipids of bacterial membrane induces bacterial dead [46].

In the case of CQDs/TiO$_2$ composites TiO$_2$ generates ROS-electrons of TiO$_2$ transfer from valence band to conduction band and thus form holes in the valence band whereas CQDs under visible light emit shorter wavelength and excite TiO$_2$ again [40]. Antibacterial effect of CQDs@hematite is achieved by electron–hole generation on the surface of this nanocomposite. The electrons in the conduction band react with molecular oxygen and thus produce hydroxyl radicals through an oxidative stress [44].

Agents applied in PDT should have low cytotoxicity. In our previous studies we established that CQDs had low dark cytotoxicity [47]. But it was also reported that cancer cells as well as normal cells might be less sensitive to phototoxicity of GQDs than bacteria strain due to different level of isocitrate dehydrogenase in the cells. Singlet oxygen affects the level of isocitrate dehydrogenase and the cells with lower level of isocitrate dehydrogenase are more sensitive to death by singlet oxygen [48].

Apart from ROS generation and surface functionalization of CQDs, surface wettability and roughness affect the bacterial death. But the effect of surface roughness is limited by the shape and size of bacteria. Namely, bacteria adhere to surfaces which features correspond to their own diameters [4].

4 Conclusion

In this chapter we discussed new light triggered strategies to combat bacterial infections and possible usage of photoactive polymers for these purposes. Photoactive antibacterial polymers are highly promising solution for novel medical devices. To enable their wise usage for the treatment of urinary infections some changes must be made. For example, the effectiveness of photoactive polymers inside human body can be increased by incorporation of micron sized electronic devices (light emitting diode, light detector, pH sensor, radio frequent device) into polymer matrices. The smart medical device should have multifunctional role: the detection of biofilm formation, the eradication of the formed biofilms by APDT and transferring information to medical staff in real time.

Acknowledgements Authors thank for support to the Ministry of Education, Science and Technological Development of the Republic of Serbia (451-03-2/2020-14/20-0302002) and for funding by a STSM grant from the COST Action CA16217 "ENIUS" and funded by the COST (European Cooperation in Science and Technology).

References

1. Azeredo J, Azevedo NF, Briandet R, Cerca N, Coenye T, Costa AR, et al. Critical review on biofilm methods. CRC Crit Rev Microbiol. 2017;43(3):313–51.
2. Flemming HC, Wingender J. The biofilm matrix. Nat Rev Microbiol. 2010;8:623–33.
3. Merritt K, An YH. Factors influencing bacterial adhesion. In: An YH, Friedman RJ, editors. Handbook of bacterial adhesion. Totowa: Humana Press; 2000. p. 53–72.
4. Katsikogianni M, Missirlis YF. Concise review of mechanisms of bacterial adhesion to biomaterials and of techniques used in estimating bacteria–material interactions. Eur Cells Mater. 2004;8:37–57.
5. Kovačova M, Marković ZM, Humpolíček P, MičuŠík M, Švajdlenková H, Kleinová A, et al. Carbon quantum dots modified polyurethane nanocomposites as effective photocatalytic and antibacterial agents. ACS Biomater Sci Eng. 2018;4(12):3983–93.
6. Abreu AC, Tavares RR, Borges A, Mergulhão F, Simõeset M. Current and emergent strategies for disinfection of hospital environments. J Antimicrob Chemother. 2013;68(12):2718–32.
7. Pietsch F, O'Neill AJ, Ivask A, Jenssen H, Inkinen J, Kahru A, et al. Selection of resistance by antimicrobial coatings in the healthcare setting. J Hosp Infect. 2020;106(1):115–25.

8. Tamayo L, Azócar M, Kogan M, Riveros A, Páez M. Copper–polymer nanocomposites: an excellent and cost-effective biocide for use on antibacterial surfaces. Mater Sci Eng C. 2016;69:1391–409.
9. Deshmukh SP, Patil SM, Mullani SB, Delekar SD. Silver nanoparticles as an effective disinfectant: a review. Mater Sci Eng C Mater. 2019;97:954–65.
10. Savelyev Y, Gonchar A, Movchan B, Gornostay A, Vozianov S, Rudenko A, et al. Antibacterial polyurethane materials with silver and copper nanoparticles. Mater Today Proc. 2017;4(1):87–94.
11. Zhang X, Wang L, Levänen E. Superhydrophobic surfaces for the reduction of bacterial adhesion. RSC Adv. 2013;3(30):12003–20.
12. Perni S, Piccirillo C, Pratten J, Prokopovich P, Chrzanowski W, Parkin IP, et al. The antimicrobial properties of light-activated polymers containing methylene blue and gold nanoparticles. Biomaterials. 2009;30(1):89–93.
13. Cassini A, Högberg LD, Plachouras D, Quattrocchi A, Hoxha A, Simonsen GS, et al. Attributable deaths and disability-adjusted life-years caused by infections with antibiotic-resistant bacteria in the EU and the European economic area in 2015: a population-level modeling analysis. Lancet Infect Dis. 2019;19(1):56–66.
14. Amos-Tautua BM, Songca SP, Oluwafemi OS. Application of porphyrins in antibacterial photodynamic therapy. Molecules. 2019;24(13):2456.
15. Marković Z, Kováčová M, Mičušík M, Danko M, Švajdlenková H, Kleinová A, et al. Structural, mechanical, and antibacterial features of curcumin/polyurethane nanocomposites. J Appl Polym Sci. 2019;136(13):47283.
16. Marković Z, Kováčová M, Humpolíček P, Budimir M, Vajďák J, Kubát P, et al. Antibacterial photodynamic activity of carbon quantum dots/polydimethylsiloxane nanocomposites against *Staphylococcus aureus*, *Escherichia coli* and *Klebsiella pneumoniae*. Photodiagn Photodyn Ther. 2019;26:342–9.
17. Liu Y, Qin R, Zaat SAJ, Breukink E, Heger M. Antibacterial photodynamic therapy: overview of a promising approach to fight antibiotic-resistant bacterial infections. J Clin Transl Res. 2015;1(3):140–67.
18. Marković Z, Trajković V. Biomedical potential of the reactive oxygen species generation and quenching by fullerenes (C_{60}). Biomaterials. 2008;29(26):3561–73.
19. Feng Y, Liu L, Zhang J, Aslan H, Dong M. Photoactive antimicrobial nanomaterials. J Mater Chem B. 2017;5(44):8631–52.
20. Marković Z, Todorović MB. Treating of aquatic pollution by carbon quantum dots. In: Gonçalves GAB, Marques P, editors. Nanostructured materials for treating aquatic pollution. Cham: Springer International Publishing; 2020. p. 129–32.
21. Jovanović S, Marković Z, Todorović MB. Carbon based nanomaterials as agents for photodynamic therapy. In: Fitzgerald F, editor. Photodynamic therapy (PDT): principles, mechanisms and applications. New York: Nova Science Publishers, Inc.; 2017. p. 35–108.
22. Dai T, Huang Y, Hamblin MR. Photodynamic therapy for localized infections—state of the art. Photodiagn Photodyn Ther. 2009;6(3–4):170–88.
23. Maisch T, Baier J, Franz B, Maier M, Landthaler M, Szeimies R, et al. The role of singlet oxygen and oxygen concentration in photodynamic inactivation of bacteria. Proc Natl Acad Sci. 2007;104(17):7223–8.
24. Felgenträger A, Maisch T, Spath A, Schroder JA, Baumler W. Singlet oxygen generation in porphyrin-doped polymeric surface coating enables antimicrobial effects on *Staphylococcus aureus*. Phys Chem Chem Phys. 2014;16(38):20598.
25. Walker T, Canales M, Noimark S, Page K, Parkin I, Faull J, et al. A light activated antimicrobial surface is active against bacterial, viral and fungal organisms. Sci Rep. 2017;7:15298.
26. Piccirillo C, Perni S, Gil-Thomas J, Prokopovich P, Wilson M, Pratten J, et al. Antimicrobial activity of methylene blue and toluidine blue O covalently bound to a modified silicone polymer surface. J Mater Chem. 2009;19(34):6167–71.

27. Sehmi K, Noimark S, Pike SD, Bear JC, Peveler WJ, Williams CK, et al. Enhancing the antibacterial activity of light-activated surfaces containing crystal violet and ZnO nanoparticles: investigation of nanoparticle size, capping ligand, and dopants. ACS Omega. 2016;1(3):334–43.

28. Naik AJT, Ismail S, Kay C, Wilson M, Parkin IP. Antimicrobial activity of polyurethane embedded with methylene blue, toluidene blue and gold nanoparticles against *Staphylococcus aureus* illuminated with white light. Mater Chem Phys. 2011;129(1–2):446–50.

29. Xing C, Xu Q, Tang H, Liu L, Wang S. Conjugated polymer/porphyrin complexes for efficient energy transfer and improving light-activated antibacterial activity. J Am Chem Soc. 2009;131:13117–24.

30. Duarah R, Singh YP, Gupta P, Mandal BM, Karak N. High performance biobased hyperbranched polyurethane/carbon dot-silver nanocomposite: a rapid self-expandable stent. Biofabrication. 2016;8(4):045013.

31. Ristić B, Milenkovic MM, Dakic IR, Todorovic-Markovic BM, Milosavljevic MS, Budimir M, et al. Photodynamic antibacterial effect of graphene quantum dots. Biomaterials. 2014;35(15):4428–35.

32. Jovanović S, Syrgiannis Z, Marković ZM, Bonasera A, Kepić DP, Budimir MD, et al. Modification of structural and luminescence properties of graphene quantum dots by gamma irradiation and their application in a photodynamic therapy. ACS Appl Mater Interfaces. 2015;7(46):25865–74.

33. Stanković NK, Bodik M, Šiffalovič P, Kotlar M, Mičušik M, Špitalsky Z, et al. Antibacterial and antibiofouling properties of light triggered fluorescent hydrophobic carbon quantum dots Langmuir–Blodgett thin films. ACS Sustain Chem Eng. 2018;6(3):4154–63.

34. Marković Z, Jovanović SP, MaŠković PZ, Danko M, Mičušik M, Pavlović VB, et al. Photo-induced antibacterial activity of four graphene based nanomaterials on a wide range of bacteria. RSC Adv. 2018;8(55):31337.

35. Marković Z, Jovanović SP, MaŠković PZ, Mojsin MM, Stevanović MJ, Danko M, et al. Graphene oxide size and structure pro-oxidant and antioxidant activity and photoinduced cytotoxicity relation on three cancer cell lines. J Photochem Photobiol B Biol. 2019;200:111647.

36. Stanković N, Todorović Marković B, Marković Z. Self-assembly of carbon-based nanoparticles films by the Langmuir–Blodgett method. J Serb Chem Soc. 2020;85(9):1095–127.

37. Pasanphan W, Rimdusit P, Choofong S, Piroonpan T, Nilsuwankosit S. Systematic fabrication of chitosan nanoparticle by gamma irradiation. Radiat Phys Chem. 2010;79(10):1095–102.

38. Sokolsky-Papkov M, Kabanov A. Synthesis of well-defined gold nanoparticles using pluronic: the role of radicals and surfactants in nanoparticles formation. Polymers. 2019;11(10):1553.

39. Li Y, Wu X, Kim M, Fortner J, Qu H, Wang YH. Fluorescent ultrashort nanotubes from defect-induced chemical cutting. Chem Mater. 2019;31(12):4536–44.

40. Hazarika D, Karak N. Photocatalytic degradation of organic contaminants under solar light using carbon dot/titanium dioxide nanohybrid, obtained through a facile approach. Appl Surf Sci. 2016;376:276–85.

41. Roy AK, Kim SM, Paoprasert P, Park SY. Preparation of biocompatible and antibacterial carbon quantum dots derived from resorcinol and formaldehyde spheres. RSC Adv. 2015;5(40):31677–82.

42. Kuang W, Zhong Q, Ye X, Yan Y, Yang Y, Zhang J, et al. Antibacterial nanorods made of carbon quantum dots-ZnO under visible light irradiation. J Nanosci Nanotechnol. 2019;19(7):3982–90.

43. Dong X, Al Awak M, Tomlinson N, Tang Y, Sun YP, Yang L. Antibacterial effects of carbon dots in combination with other antimicrobial reagents. PLoS One. 2017;12(9):e0185324.

44. Moradlou O, Rabiei Z, Delavari N. Antibacterial effects of carbon quantum dots@hematite nanostructures deposited on titanium against Gram-positive and Gram-negative bacteria. J Photochem Photobiol A Biol. 2019;379:144–9.

45. Al Awak MM, Wang P, Wang S, Tang Y, Sun YP, Yang L. Correlation of carbon dots' light-activated antimicrobial activities and fluorescence quantum yield. RSC Adv. 2018;7(48):30177–84.

46. Travlou NA, Giannakoudakis DA, Algarra M, Labella MA, Rodríguez-Castellón E, Bandosz TJ. S- and N-doped carbon quantum dots: surface chemistry dependent antibacterial activity. Carbon. 2018;135:104–11.
47. Marković Z, Ristić B, Arsikin K, Klisić D, Harhaji-Trajković L, Todorović-Marković B, et al. Graphene quantum dots as autophagy-inducing photodynamic agents. Biomaterials. 2012;33(29):7084–92.
48. Kim SY, Park JW. Cellular defense against singlet oxygen induced oxidative damage by cytosolic NADP⁺ dependent isocitrate dehydrogenase. Free Radic Res. 2003;37(3):309–16.

Light-Activated Polymer Nanocomposites Doped with a New Type of Carbon Quantum Dots for Antibacterial Applications

Mária Kováčová, Eva Špitalská, and Zdenko Špitálský

1 Introduction

Carbon quantum dots (CQDs) are relatively new carbon allotrope. The first mention dates from 2004 when Xu et al. described new fluorescent material after electrophoretic purification of carbon nanotubes [1]. It triggered an investigation of new CQD research of synthesis, properties CQDs, and applications. As can be seen from Fig. 1, the number of publications about CQDs is increasing exponentially during the last decade with 3419 papers in the last years according to Web of Science. Antibacterial properties of CQDs represent 3.2% of them; however, their citations are exponentially increasing exceeding the number over 2900 in last year. These data suggest a significant future of CQD as an antibacterial material.

CQDs are quasispherical carbon particles with a size less than 10 nm with crystalline sp^2 cores of graphite and quantum effects. A subclass of CQDs are graphene quantum dots (GQDs), and they have a structure of one or several graphene layers with diameter < 10 nm with higher crystallinity than CQDs. In both cases, however, CQDs are functionalized by functional groups on their surface, which can improve the optical properties, solubility, and chemical stability and generally increase the surface variability and complexity of CQDs.

CQDs have many hydrophilic functional groups at the edges or on the basal plane. Specific hydrophilic functional groups in the CQDs include epoxy and hydroxyl groups. Hydrophilic CQDs are very well soluble in water and other polar solvents due to their chemical composition; therefore, they differ from other

M. Kováčová · Z. Špitálský (✉)
Polymer Institute, Slovak Academy of Sciences, Bratislava, Slovakia
e-mail: m.kovacova@savba.sk; zdeno.spitalsky@savba.sk

E. Špitalská
Institute of Virology, Biomedical Research Center of the Slovak Academy of Sciences, Bratislava, Slovakia
e-mail: eva.spitalska@savba.sk

© The Author(s) 2022
F. Soria et al. (eds.), *Urinary Stents*,
https://doi.org/10.1007/978-3-031-04484-7_25

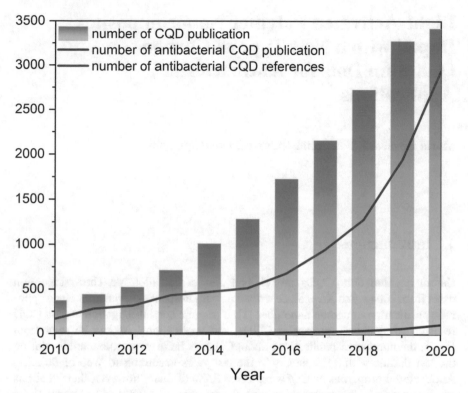

Fig. 1 Number of CQD publications (green bar), the number of antibacterial properties of CQDs publications (blue line) and their number of references (red line) according to Web of Science

carbon-based nanomaterials. Additional advantages of CQDs include their nontoxicity and biocompatibility. The second types of CQDs are hydrophobic CQDs containing carboxyl and carbonyl functional groups. In comparison to hydrophilic CQDs, hydrophobic CQDs are more effective in producing reactive oxygen species (ROS) responsible for the antibacterial activity of CQDs.

CQDs have extensive application usage from sensors through photoelectrochemical water splitting, chemiluminescence, LEDs, photovoltaic solar cells up to photocatalysis and readers can found several reviews about it [2–7]. CQDs also play an important role in medicine. CQDs are used in intracellular ion detection, toxin detection, pathogen, vitamin, enzyme, protein, nucleic acid, and biological pH value determination [8]. QDs also have great utility in bioimaging, biosensing (for example, QD modification with metal ions or biomolecules), fluorescence labelling of cellular proteins (biolabelling), genetic technologies, and cell motion tracking [9, 10]. Despite the broad range of biomedical applications, we would like to focus on antibacterial properties of pure CQDs and their polymer composites. The antibacterial effect of CQDs is based on noninvasive photodynamic therapy (PDT). PDT can cause a specific biological response on the cellular or subcellular level, such as apoptosis, programmed death, or necrosis, a nonprogrammed pathway [11]. During

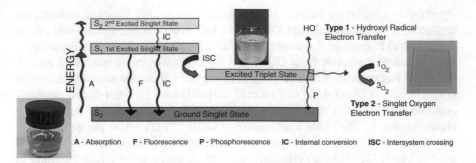

Fig. 2 Mechanism of photodynamic therapy, or so-called Jablonski diagram

this process, CQDs absorb light (photons). One electron absorbs this energy and moves into a higher excited single state. This state is in nanoseconds, and it can emit light and lose its energy or dissipate as heat. The excited photosensitizer (PS) in the singlet state may also undergo the process known as an intersystem crossing. The spin of the excited electron inverts to form the relatively long-lived (microseconds) excited triplet-state that has electron spins parallel. The long lifetime of the CQD triplet state is explained by the fact that the loss of energy by emission of light (phosphorescence) is a spin-forbidden process as the CQDs would move directly from a triplet to a singlet-state [12]. In the presence of molecular oxygen, part of the energy can be transformed into an oxygen molecule which changes to ROS. One of the most important types of ROS is singlet oxygen ($^1O_2$). Singlet oxygen and other ROS react with a wide range of biological targets and are known to be involved in cellular signalling and cell damage [13]. Therefore CQDs act as indirect antibacterial materials when after the illumination with light generates singlet oxygen. This whole process is presented in Fig. 2.

2 Antibacterial Effect of CQDs

2.1 Pure CQDs

Jhonsi et al. showed that antibacterial and antifungal activities of CQDs on *Escherichia coli* and *Candida albicans* increased linearly with an increase in CQDs' concentration. It reveals that CQDs can effectively inhibit the growth of the bacteria in a concentration-dependent manner. The results revealed that CQDs inhibit the growth of *E. coli* and *C. albicans* more effectively compared to other tested microbes, *Staphylococcus aureus, Klebsiella pneumoniae,* and *Pseudomonas aeruginosa* [14]. Nie et al. demonstrated that CQDs are effective photosensitizers for *in vitro* PDT, and revealed detection limit inactivation (99.9999 + %) of *E. coli* and *S. aureus* upon visible light illumination ($\lambda \geq 420$ nm, 65 ± 5 mW/cm^2; 60 min) [15]. The antibacterial effect of photoexcited GQDs using blue light (465–475 nm) significantly affected the viability of *E. coli* or *S. aureus* [16]. Sun et al. designed an antibacterial system combining GQDs with a low level of H_2O_2, which could inhibit the growth of *E. coli* and *S. aureus* (10^6 CFU/mL) bacteria and assessed the antibacterial efficacy of patches from GQDs *in vivo* using Kumming mice as a model. Results of that study indicated that GQDs have potential use for wound disinfection [17]. The results of the study of Kuo et al. showed that a nitrogen-doped graphene quantum dot (N-GQD), serving as a photosensitizer, was capable of generating a higher amount of ROS than a nitrogen-free GQD in PDT when photoexcited for only 3 min of 670 nm laser exposure, indicating highly improved antimicrobial effects. The N-GQD (5.1%) efficiently exerted an antibacterial effect, resulting in 100% elimination after a 3-min exposure [18]. Sulfur-doped CQDs (S-CQDs) and N-CQDs were evaluated for bactericidal activity against *E. coli* and *B. subtilis* subsp. *subtilis* (6×10^6 cells/mL). Antibacterial activity was slightly higher against *B. subtilis* than against *E. coli* for both S-CQDs and N-CQDs with greater effectiveness of N-CQDs compared to S-CQDs [19].

2.2 Doped CQDs

Nanorods of CQDs–ZnO had strong antibacterial activity under visible light irradiation, and a concentration of 0.1 mg/L was able to kill more than 96% of bacteria *E. coli* and *S. aureus* [20]. Feng et al. realized bacterial inactivation on a CQD/TiNT film. Use of CQD/TiNTs led to almost complete inactivation of *S. aureus* and *E. coli* (2×10^7 CFU/mL) within 10 min using 365 nm UV irradiation [21]. Nitrogen and zinc doped CDs displayed good bactericidal activity against *E. coli* (10^7 CFU/mL) and *S. aureus* (10^8 CFU/mL) under visible-light radiations [22].

Wang et al. compare photodynamic properties of GQDs, hollow mesoporous silica nanoparticles (hMSN) and GQDs@hMSN hybrid antimicrobial system triggered by commonly available LED lamps. GQDs@hMSN can produce singlet oxygen under light exposure to destroy bacteria's structure, thus achieving a highly efficient antimicrobial effect. However, GQDs@hMSN-erythromycin's antimicrobial efficacy was significantly better than that of GQDs@hMSN or erythromycin alone [23]. Kholikov et al. used GQDs and GQDs combined with methylene blue (MB) to eradicate *E. coli* (10^6 CFU/mL), and G+ *Micrococcus luteus* (10^6 CFU/mL) using irradiation with red LED light. Using MB-GDQ improved the deactivation rate more than twice compared with MB [24]. Similarly, Dong et al. evaluated the antimicrobial effects of the CQDs with surface passivation molecules 2,2'-(ethylenedioxy)bis(ethylamine) (EDA) in combination with MB or toluidine blue (TB) against *E. coli* cells with 1-h visible light illumination and showed their synergistic interaction. The combination treatment with 5 µg/mL CQDs combined with 1 µg/mL MB completely inhibited bacteria growth, resulting in 6.2-log viable cell number reduction. Similar results were observed using TB/CQDs combination [25]. Galdiero et al. evaluated the antimicrobial activity on *S. aureus, P. aeruginosa, E. coli* and *K. pneumoniae,* and the ecotoxicity of CQDs alone and coated with indolicidin and showed improved germicidal action and low ecotoxicity for modified CQDs compared to CQDs alone. Modified CQDs demonstrated a percentage of bacteria reduction related to an initial inoculum of 35.1 ± 3.0, 29.3 ± 2.7, and 39.3 ± 4.1, respectively, for *E. coli*, *P. aeruginosa*, and *K. pneumoniae*. Only for *S. aureus*, was observed a low killing ability of $12.3 \pm 1.0\%$ for modified CQDs, but this was always more significant than that for indolicidin alone and CQDs alone [26]. The antimicrobial activity of the as-synthesized spermidine-capped fluorescent CQDs (Spd–CQDs) (size ~ 4.6 nm) has been tested by Li et al. against non-multidrug-resistant *E. coli*, *S. aureus*, *B. subtilis*, and *P. aeruginosa* bacteria and also multidrug-resistant bacteria, *methicillin-resistant S. aureus* (MRSA). The minimal inhibitory concentration value of Spd–CQDs is much lower (> 25,000-fold) than that of spermidine. Spd–CQDs had promising antibacterial effects causing significant damage to the bacterial membrane with high biocompatibility, especially to multidrug-resistant bacteria [27]. Multi-walled carbon nanotubes filters incorporated with CQDs are highly effective to remove bacteria (*E. coli*, *B. subtilis*) from water and to inhibit the activities of the captured bacteria on filter surfaces [28]. The bactericidal function of EDA–CQDs to *B. subtilis* and *E. coli* (~ 10^6 CFU/mL) was evaluated under different light conditions, the bacteria-killing effect of EDA–CQDs treatment was possible increased dramatically to approximately 4-logs (~ 99.99) [29]. EDA–CQDs exhibited much greater antibacterial activity to *B. subtilis* cells compared to 3-ethoxypropylamine modified CQDs, treatment with EDA–CQDs resulted in an about 5.8-log reduction in viable cell number upon treatments under light illumination [30]. The CQDs–TiO$_2$ properties and their antimicrobial activity against *E. coli* and G+ *S. aureus* were evaluated by Yan et al. [31]. The antibacterial efficiency reached 90.9% and 92.8% toward *E. coli* and *S. aureus*, respectively, with 1 mg/mL CQDs–TiO$_2$ under visible light. Zhang et al. (2018) [32] showed that the bracket modified with ZnO/CQDs coating exhibited excellent antibacterial performance than the unmodified bracket (*Streptococcus mutans* 96.13%, *S. aureus* 90.28% and *E. coli* 92.35%) under natural light. Composite of CQDs/Na$_2$W$_4$O$_{13}$/WO$_3$ exhibited excellent antimicrobial activity against G− *E. coli* (10^7 CFU/mL) [33]. After visible light irradiation for 100 min, ~ 68.3% of the *E. coli* cells treated with Na$_2$W$_4$O$_{13}$ survived, which have no more than 1-log reduction. For treatment with the synthesized WO$_3$/Na$_2$W$_4$O$_{13}$ and WO$_3$ materials, approximately 72.6% and 0.6%, respectively, of the *E. coli* cells were alive. The CQDs-decorated Na$_2$W$_4$O$_{13}$ composite showed the best photocatalytic bactericidal activity, with approximately 2×10^7 CFU/mL of the *E. coli* cells completely inactivated within 100 min, which have 7-log reduction.

3   Antibacterial Effect of CQD Polymer Composites

As mentioned above, CQDs can be used in a wide range of applications, and especially in biomedicine for their antimicrobial, in the narrower sense—antibacterial effects. However, due to real use (catheters, stents, coatings, dressings, patches, textiles, etc.), CQDs need a certain carrier [34, 35]. The most common carrier solution is a polymer matrix (various kinds), and CQDs are incorporated in different ways onto the material's surfaces. Unfortunately, there is still a minimum of polymer composites with CQDs that would exhibit antibacterial activity without side effects.

For more comfortable mixing with polymers, pure hydrophobic CQDs (hCQDs) were invented. Their great advantage is also that, in contact with water or other biological fluids, they do not elute from the polymer matrix and do not degrade [36, 37]. The antibacterial effect of these hCQDs was tested against *S. aureus, E. coli*, and *K. pneumoniae* in combination with various polymers, as polyurethane (PU), polydimethylsiloxane (PDMS). PU and PDMS are frequently used in medicine as medical devices and tools for their biocompatibility and desired properties. Materials work on the principle of classic PDT and produce singlet oxygen—in Fig. 3. As the light source was used common blue LEDs at 470 nm, the power of 50 W, and the intensity of 700 μW/cm^2 on the sample surface placed at a distance of 50 cm from the LEDs. In both cases, the desired effect has been achieved. The nanocomposite hCQDs/PU has 100% bactericidal effectivity after 1 h of irradiation. Second polymer hCQDs/PDMS eradicated 100% bacterial colonies (5-logs) after 15 min of irradiation, because of its excellent oxygen diffusion [38, 39]. The bacterial reduction could be improved using diffuse coplanar dielectric barrier discharge. The plasma generated in atmospheric air oxidizes the surface of hCQDs and therefore enhances the energy transfer between the hCQDs and molecular oxygen. It means that the irradiation time is decreased, and material is suitable for faster disinfection [40]. Moreover, there is a possibility to create novel antibacterial textiles by a lamination process, using commercially-available transparent PUs and modified them with hCQDs [34].

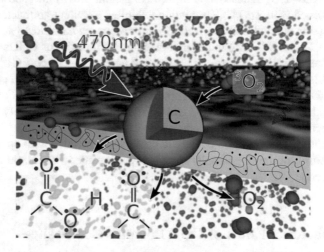

Fig. 3 Schematic view of light-triggered polymer nanocomposite with hCQDs

Also, there is another possibility to create antibacterial polymer by electrospinning nanofibers filled with hydrophilic CQDs. Nie et al. prepared such material with polyacrylonitrile (PAN) and CQDs (synthesized by a facile one-pot solvothermal method from citric acid and 1,5-diaminonaphthalene in ethanol), which works after visible light illumination. Antibacterial activity was performed against several types of G+ and G− bacteria (~ 6-log units inactivation). In all cases, they achieved a reduction in bacterial cultures, although only very weak in the case of G+ bacteria [41]. The same combination PAN/CQDs (but CQDs obtained from the hydrothermal method—citric acid and urea) could be useful as fluorescent scaffold reported in research Kanagasubbulakshmi et al. Scaffold has antimicrobial properties, and it was tested for reepithelialisation in albino Wistar rats [42]. CQDs could be used for modification of polymer membrane, for example, polysulfone polymer membranes embedded with CQDs (obtained from activated carbon) for antibacterial effect against *E. coli* and *S. aureus* (tested by disk diffusion method) with improved permeability, high hydrophilicity and porosity [43]. Moreover, polycaprolactone/CQDs electrospun nanofibers were used for improved wound healing with antibacterial properties [44].

Eco-friendly antimicrobial material was reported by Salimi et al. as nanocellulose sheets-CQDs. CQDs were prepared from white mulberry (*Morus alba L.*), and nanocellulose is a natural biopolymer. Antimicrobial effectiveness was performed against *L. monocytogenes* via disk-covering method [45].

Very recently, few antimicrobial polymer hybrids with CQDs are known. One example is Ag_2S–CQDs–PEI–GO composite material with strong antibacterial activity against *E. coli, S. aureus, P. aeruginosa,* and *E. faecalis*, which was evaluated by disk diffusion method [46].

4 Conclusion

CQDs are a very promising new antibacterial nanoparticles. Their antibacterial effect against different G+ and G− bacteria was confirmed. These nanoparticles work mainly as a photosensitiser and their antibacterial effect can be amplified by doping or surface modification. CQDs are very suitable for incorporation into different polymer matrices what makes them the antibacterial material with a very universal usage. Therefore, they can be used in almost any area.

Acknowledgements Authors thank for support to the COST Action CA16217 "ENIUS" funded by COST (European Cooperation in Science and Technology). The authors are also grateful for the financial support of Ministry of Education of the Slovak Republic and Slovak Academy of Sciences, Grant VEGA 2/0021/21 (Eva Spitalska) and VEGA 2/0051/20 (Zdenko Spitalsky) and APVV SK-SRB-21-0020 (Maria Kovacova).

References

1. Xu X, Ray R, Gu Y, Ploehn HJ, Gearheart L, Raker K, et al. Electrophoretic analysis and purification of fluorescent single-walled carbon nanotube fragments. J Am Chem Soc. 2004;126(40):12736–7.
2. Tian L, Li Z, Wang P, Zhai X, Wang X, Li T. Carbon quantum dots for advanced electrocatalysis. J Energy Chem. 2021;1(55):279–94.
3. Ghosh D, Sarkar K, Devi P, Kim KH, Kumar P. Current and future perspectives of carbon and graphene quantum dots: from synthesis to strategy for building optoelectronic and energy devices. Renew Sustain Energ Rev. 2021;1(135):110391.
4. Shaker M, Riahifar R, Li Y. A review on the superb contribution of carbon and graphene quantum dots to electrochemical capacitors' performance: synthesis and application. FlatChem. 2020;1(22):100171.
5. Rani UA, Ng LY, Ng CY, Mahmoudi E. A review of carbon quantum dots and their applications in wastewater treatment. Adv Colloid Interface Sci. 2020;1(278):102124.
6. Molaei MJ. Principles, mechanisms, and application of carbon quantum dots in sensors: a review. Anal Methods. 2020;12(10):1266–87.
7. He P, Shi Y, Meng T, Yuan T, Li Y, Li X, et al. Recent advances in white light-emitting diodes of carbon quantum dots. Nanoscale. 2020;12(8):4826–32.
8. Fitzgerald F. Photodynamic therapy (PDT): principles, mechanisms and applications. In: Photodynamic therapy (PDT): principles, mechanisms and applications. New York: Nova Biomedical; 2017. p. 1–209.
9. Wang J, Qiu J. A review of carbon dots in biological applications. J Mater Sci. 2016;51(10):4728–38.
10. Gomaa OM, Okasha A, Hosni HM, El-Hag AA. Biocompatible water soluble polyacrylic acid coated CdSe/Cu quantum dot conjugates for biomolecule detection. J Fluoresc. 2018;28(1):41–9.
11. Igney FH, Krammer PH. Death and anti-death: tumour resistance to apoptosis. Nat Rev Cancer. 2002;2(4):277–88.
12. Castano AP, Demidova TN, Hamblin MR. Mechanisms in photodynamic therapy: part one—photosensitizers, photochemistry and cellular localization. Photodiagn Photodyn Ther. 2004;1(4):279–93.
13. Briviba K, Klotz LO, Sies H. Toxic and signaling effects of photochemically or chemically generated singlet oxygen in biological systems. Biol Chem. 1997;378(11):1259–65.
14. Jhonsi MA, Ananth DA, Nambirajan G, Sivasudha T, Yamini R, Bera S, et al. Antimicrobial activity, cytotoxicity and DNA binding studies of carbon dots. Spectrochim Acta Part A Mol Biomol Spectrosc. 2018;5(196):295–302.
15. Nie X, Jiang C, Wu S, Chen W, Lv P, Wang Q, et al. Carbon quantum dots: a bright future as photosensitizers for in vitro antibacterial photodynamic inactivation. J Photochem Photobiol B Biol. 2020;206:111864.
16. Ristic BZ, Milenkovic MM, Dakic IR, Todorovic-Markovic BM, Milosavljevic MS, Budimir MD, et al. Photodynamic antibacterial effect of graphene quantum dots. Biomaterials. 2014;35(15):4428–35.
17. Sun H, Gao N, Dong K, Ren J, Qu X. Graphene quantum dots-band-aids used for wound disinfection. ACS Nano. 2014;8(6):6202–10.
18. Kuo WS, Chen HH, Chen SY, Chang CY, Chen PC, Hou YI, et al. Graphene quantum dots with nitrogen-doped content dependence for highly efficient dual-modality photodynamic antimicrobial therapy and bioimaging. Biomaterials. 2017;1(120):185–94.
19. Travlou NA, Giannakoudakis DA, Algarra M, Labella AM, Rodríguez-Castellón E, Bandosz TJ. S- and N-doped carbon quantum dots: surface chemistry dependent antibacterial activity. Carbon. 2018;1(135):104–11.
20. Kuang W, Zhong Q, Ye X, Yan Y, Yang Y, Zhang J, et al. Antibacterial nanorods made of carbon quantum dots-ZnO under visible light irradiation. J Nanosci Nanotechnol. 2019;19(7):3982–90.

21. Feng L, Sun H, Ren J, Qu X. Carbon-dot-decorated TiO_2 nanotube arrays used for photo/ voltage-induced organic pollutant degradation and the inactivation of bacteria. Nanotechnology. 2016;27(11):115301.
22. Tammina SK, Wan Y, Li Y, Yang Y. Synthesis of N, Zn-doped carbon dots for the detection of Fe^{3+} ions and bactericidal activity against *Escherichia coli* and *Staphylococcus aureus*. J Photochem Photobiol B Biol. 2020;1(202):111734.
23. Wang N, Xu H, Sun S, Guo P, Wang Y, Qian C, et al. Wound therapy via a photo-responsively antibacterial nano-graphene quantum dots conjugate. J Photochem Photobiol B Biol. 2020;1(210):111978.
24. Kholikov K, Ilhom S, Sajjad M, Smith ME, Monroe JD, San O, et al. Improved singlet oxygen generation and antimicrobial activity of sulphur-doped graphene quantum dots coupled with methylene blue for photodynamic therapy applications. Photodiagn Photodyn Ther. 2018;1(24):7–14.
25. Dong X, Bond AE, Pan N, Coleman M, Tang Y, Sun YP, et al. Synergistic photoactivated antimicrobial effects of carbon dots combined with dye photosensitizers. Int J Nanomed. 2018;27(13):8025–35.
26. Galdiero E, Siciliano A, Maselli V, Gesuele R, Guida M, Fulgione D, et al. An integrated study on antimicrobial activity and ecotoxicity of quantum dots and quantum dots coated with the antimicrobial peptide indolicidin. Int J Nanomed. 2016;26(11):4199–211.
27. Li YJ, Harroun SG, Su YC, Huang CF, Unnikrishnan B, Lin HJ, et al. Synthesis of self-assembled spermidine-carbon quantum dots effective against multidrug-resistant bacteria. Adv Healthc Mater. 2016;5(19):2545–54.
28. Dong X, Al Awak M, Wang P, Sun YP, Yang L. Carbon dot incorporated multi-walled carbon nanotube coated filters for bacterial removal and inactivation. RSC Adv. 2018;8(15):8292–301.
29. Al Awak MM, Wang P, Wang S, Tang Y, Sun YP, Yang L. Correlation of carbon dots' light-activated antimicrobial activities and fluorescence quantum yield. RSC Adv. 2017;7(48):30177–84.
30. Abu Rabe DI, Al Awak MM, Yang F, Okonjo PA, Dong X, Teisl LR, et al. The dominant role of surface functionalization in carbon dots' photo-activated antibacterial activity. Int J Nanomed. 2019;23(14):2655–65.
31. Yan Y, Kuang W, Shi L, Ye X, Yang Y, Xie X, et al. Carbon quantum dot-decorated TiO_2 for fast and sustainable antibacterial properties under visible-light. J Alloys Compd. 2019;10(777):234–43.
32. Zhang J, An X, Li X, Liao X, Nie Y, Fan Z. Enhanced antibacterial properties of the bracket under natural light via decoration with ZnO/carbon quantum dots composite coating. Chem Phys Lett. 2018;16(706):702–7.
33. Zhang J, Liu X, Wang X, Mu L, Yuan M, Liu B, et al. Carbon dots-decorated $Na_2W_4O_{13}$ composite with WO_3 for highly efficient photocatalytic antibacterial activity. J Hazard Mater. 2018;5(359):1–8.
34. Kováčová M, Kleinová A, Vajďák J, Humpolíček P, Kubát P, Bodík M, et al. Photodynamic-active smart biocompatible material for an antibacterial surface coating. J Photochem Photobiol B Biol. 2020;211:112012.
35. Kováčová M, Špitalská E, Markovic Z, Špitálský Z. Carbon quantum dots as antibacterial photosensitizers and their polymer nanocomposite applications. Part Part Syst Charact. 2019;37:1900348.
36. Bodik M, Siffalovic P, Nadazdy P, Benkovicova M, Markovic Z, Chlpik J, et al. On the formation of hydrophobic carbon quantum dots Langmuir films and their transfer onto solid substrates. Diam Relat Mater. 2018;83:170–6.
37. Stanković NK, Bodik M, Šiffalovič P, Kotlar M, Mičušik M, Špitalsky Z, et al. Antibacterial and antibiofouling properties of light triggered fluorescent hydrophobic carbon quantum dots Langmuir–Blodgett thin films. ACS Sustain Chem Eng. 2018;6(3):4154–63.
38. Kováčová M, Marković ZM, Humpolíček P, MičuŠík M, Švajdlenková H, Kleinová A, et al. Carbon quantum dots modified polyurethane nanocomposite as effective photocatalytic and antibacterial agents. ACS Biomater Sci Eng. 2018;4(12):3983–93.

39. Marković ZM, Kováčová M, Humpolíček P, Budimir MD, Vajďák J, Kubát P, et al. Antibacterial photodynamic activity of carbon quantum dots/polydimethylsiloxane nanocomposites against *Staphylococcus aureus*, *Escherichia coli* and *Klebsiella pneumoniae*. Photodiagn Photodyn Ther. 2019;26:342–9.

40. Kováčová M, Bodík M, Mičušík M, Humpolíček P, Šiffalovič P, Špitálsky Z. Increasing the effectivity of the antimicrobial surface of carbon quantum dots-based nanocomposite by atmospheric pressure plasma. Clin Plasma Med. 2020;20:100111.

41. Nie X, Wu S, Mensah A, Lu K, Wei Q. Carbon quantum dots embedded electrospun nanofibers for efficient antibacterial photodynamic inactivation. Mater Sci Eng C. 2020;108:110377.

42. Kanagasubbulakshmi S, Lakshmi K, Kadirvelu K. Carbon quantum dots-embedded electrospun antimicrobial and fluorescent scaffold for reepithelialization in albino Wistar rats. J Biomed Mater Res Part A. 2020;109(5):637–48.

43. Mahat NA, Shamsudin SA, Jullok N, Ma'Radzi AH. Carbon quantum dots embedded polysulfone membranes for antibacterial performance in the process of forward osmosis. Desalination. 2020;493:114618.

44. Ghosal K, Kováčová M, Humpolíček P, Vajďák J, Bodík M, Špitalský Z. Antibacterial photodynamic activity of hydrophobic carbon quantum dots and polycaprolactone based nanocomposite processed via both electrospinning and solvent casting method. Photodiagn Photodyn Ther. 2021;35:102455.

45. Salimi F, Moradi M, Tajik H, Molaei R. Optimization and characterization of eco-friendly antimicrobial nanocellulose sheet prepared using carbon dots of white mulberry (*Morus alba* L.). J Sci Food Agric. 2020;101(8):3439–47.

46. Wang K, Liang L, Xu J, Li H, Du M, Zhao X, et al. Synthesis and bacterial inhibition of novel Ag$_2$S–N–CQD composite material. Chem Pap. 2020;74(5):1517–24.

Nanoparticles. Potential for Use to Prevent Infections

Nenad Filipović, Nina Tomić, Maja Kuzmanović,
and Magdalena M. Stevanović

1 Introduction

According to the literature, one of the most common complications related to indwelling urinary stents is microbial adhesion to their surface which leads to biofilm formation, and often thereafter to infection and, in some patients, urosepsis [1–3]. Bacteria in a biofilm can be up to 1000-fold more resistant to antimicrobial drugs [4]. The traditional methodology of using therapeutic intervention for developing an antimicrobial urinary stent very often lacks clinically meaningful benefit [5]. For that reason, urinary stent modifications using alternative methods and materials with antimicrobial functionality such as nanoparticle-based systems are being intensively investigated. Coverings or coatings, functionalization, blending and drug impregnation based on nanoparticles are mainly applied for these purposes [6]. In such a system i.e. product, nanoparticles may be used as the primary ingredient, constituent, or sub-constituent. Nanoparticles have demonstrated a broad-spectrum of antimicrobial properties against both Gram-positive and Gram-negative bacteria [7–12]. The growing interest toward antimicrobial potential of nanoparticles within the scientific community can be easily evaluated by searching the appropriate keywords through some of the recognized literature databases. According to one of them, SCOPUS, in the last 30 years more than 14,000 peer-reviewed documents have been published containing keywords such as "antimicrobial" and "nanoparticles" (Fig. 1). Interestingly, in the more specified search which refers only to the utilization of nanoparticles in urinary infections, it could be observed a similar profile i.e. growing tendency, except with a significantly lower number of published documents, (less than 2%). Even more interesting is the fact that when this search is expanded on the keywords such as antimicrobial + nanoparticles + urinary

N. Filipović · N. Tomić · M. Kuzmanović · M. M. Stevanović (✉)
Institute of Technical Sciences of SASA, Belgrade, Serbia
e-mail: nenad.filipovic@itn.sanu.ac.rs; magdalena.stevanovic@itn.sanu.ac.rs

© The Author(s) 2022
F. Soria et al. (eds.), *Urinary Stents*,
https://doi.org/10.1007/978-3-031-04484-7_26

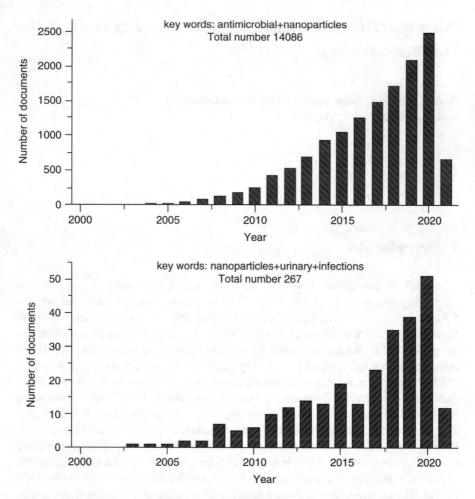

Fig. 1 Graphical presentation of documents that contain the mentioned keywords, published from 1987 up to now. Results are obtained from the SCOPUS database and the search is conducted on March 15th, 2021

(ureteral) + stents, only two documents are listed. Although this type of searching has some limitations, it is obvious that, so far, the potential of the nanoparticles is not sufficiently investigated in this field.

Until now, the antimicrobial mechanism of action of the nanoparticles is not fully explained but it is considered to be based either on induction of the oxidative stress [13], metal ion release [14], or non-oxidative mechanisms [15]. These mechanisms can occur also simultaneously (Fig. 2). In literature it has been anticipated that some nanoparticles neutralize the electric charge of the bacterial cell surface and consequently modify its penetrability, leading to bacterial death [16]. Also, nanoparticles may increase the production of reactive oxygen species resulting in constraints on the antioxidative defense system and thereafter mechanical

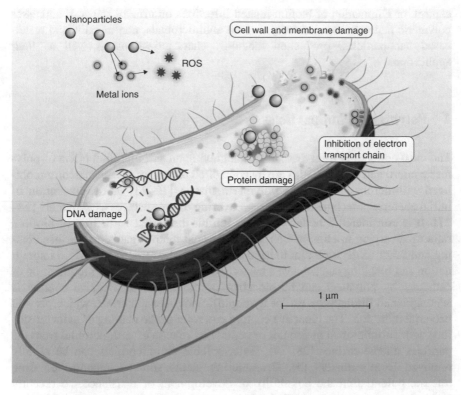

Fig. 2 Nanoparticles exhibit antimicrobial activity through multiple mechanisms: cell wall disruption and alteration in membrane permeability, generation of ROS, nucleus/DNA damage, protein denaturation, inhibition of electron transport chain; and consequently the humpering of bacterial metabolic processes

damage to the bacterial cell membrane. So, nanoparticles can disrupt and penetrate the bacterial cell membrane, induce the creation of reactive oxygen species, stimulate intracellular antibacterial activity, and interact with DNA and proteins [16] (Fig. 2).

All these led to their pronounced antibacterial properties. The effect of nanoparticles on biofilm formation depends on several parameters such as the type of the nanoparticles (metallic, nonmetallic, polymeric, etc.), their morphology (size and shape), electric charge, hydrophobicity, composition, polar interaction, etc. [17]. For example, Slomberg and coauthors examined the efficacy of silica nanoparticles containing nitric oxide against Gram-negative *Pseudomonas aeruginosa* and Gram-positive *Staphylococcus aureus* biofilms as a function of particle size and shape [18]. Smaller particles exhibited better nitric oxide delivery and enhanced bacteria killing compared to the larger ones. Also, the rod-like particles proved to be more effective than spherical particles in delivering nitric oxide and inducing greater antibacterial action throughout the biofilm. This chapter gives an extensive overview of the different types of nanoparticles and nanostructured materials for the prevention, control, or elimination of biofilm-related infections on urinary stents. It addresses polymeric nanoparticles, naturally derived antimicrobials, non-metallic and metal-based nanoparticles, production methods, characterizations as well as their applications.

2   Polymeric Nanoparticles

The most commonly used methods for achieving an antimicrobial effect of polymeric micro and nanoparticles are by controlled release of encapsulated/immobilized antimicrobial within the polymeric matrix [19–23] or by prevention of initial bacterial attachment by coating/covering of the surfaces by polymers [24–27]. It is considered a better option to inhibit the initial formation of biofilm, rather than trying to eliminate already colonized microorganisms. Surface coating and functionalization aim to have a bacteriostatic effect, while drug impregnation and blending can achieve a bactericidal effect [6]. Surface modification of catheters by polymers can be bioactive or biopassive. Biopassive coating is accomplished through the use of hydrophilic polymer materials, which prevent bacterial adhesion. The bioactive coating can refer to the coating of catheter surface with antimicrobial molecules or controlled release of antimicrobial from the particles on the surface [28, 29]. Water-soluble antimicrobials can be rapidly removed from catheters [5]. Drug-eluting stents showed uncontrolled drug release, potentiating the possibility of development of resistance, so recently researches focused on controlled release antibiotic, and antibiotic combination stent coatings.

Srisang et al. reported the synthesis of chlorhexidine loaded nanoparticles, in form of poly(-ethylene glycol)-block-poly(e-caprolactone) micelles, and poly(e-caprolactone) nanospheres, and coating of Foley catheter surface in multiple layers. In both cases, bacteria started to colonize the coated catheter only after 21 days, which indicates the prolonged release of chlorhexidine [30].

Non-adhesive hydrophilic implants are developed to prevent host irritation and bacterial adhesion [31]. Palmieri et al. designed a nanocomposite coating made of hydrophilic polymer polyethylene glycol and hydrophobic polyphenol curcumin deposited on the surface of graphene oxide nanoparticles. This coating decreased adherence and biofilm formation of *Candida albicans* on polyurethane catheters [32].

More research dealing with polymers such as poly(glycolic acid), poly(lactic-*co*-glycolic acid), polyamine, etc. are reported below since they are also involving non-metallic or metallic nanoparticles.

2.1 Naturally Derived Antimicrobials

Naturally derived antimicrobials such as essential oils, curcumin, enzymes, hyaluronic acid, and antimicrobial peptides in combination with synthetic antibiotics/nanoantibiotics [33, 34] are likely to exert sufficient inhibitory effect on uropathogens. These compounds are the basis of many modern pharmaceuticals, mainly antibiotics [35]. Due to low bioavailability, stability, and biocompatibility, they are often loaded into nanoparticles to improve their characteristics [36]. These nanosystems, comprised of phytochemicals or microbial metabolites, and especially in combination with nanoantibiotics [33], have the potential to be used as antimicrobial coating of urinary catheters [6].

Venkat Kumar et al. synthesized kanamycin–chitosan nanoparticles by ionic gelation, which were then covalently immobilized on polyurethane ureteral stents. These stents exhibited increased, synergistic antibacterial activity, which is suggested to be a result of the disruption of negatively charged bacterial membranes, due to the polycationic nature of these nanoparticles and therefore increased positive surface charge of stents [37].

Phenazine-1-carboxamide is an aromatic compound isolated from *P. aeruginosa*. It was used for functionalization of silica nanoparticles, which were then applied for coating of urethral stents, by Kanugala et al. They report promising antibacterial and antifungal activity on *S. aureus* and *C. albicans*, and also activity against mixed-species biofilms [38].

Kumar et al. reported functionalization of silver nanoparticles with Kocuran, an exopolysaccharide from *Kocuria rosea* [39]. These Kocuran-capped silver glyconanoparticles were used as a coating for silicone urethral catheters and showed significant antibacterial and antiadhesive properties against *E. coli* and *S. aureus*.

There have been attempts to inhibit biofilm growth by interfering with bacterial communication, quorum sensing. "Quorum quenching" molecules are compounds that interfere with quorum sensing by various mechanisms and can be utilized to create antibiofilm coatings. Nanocoatings made of α-amylase and acylase, capable of degrading bacterial exopolysaccharides and quorum sensing molecules, respectively, were deposited layer by layer on silicone urinary catheter surface. This coating exhibited inhibition of *P. aeruginosa* and *S. aureus* biofilms, consisting either of α-amylase or acylase, but especially in form of hybrid nanocoatings of both enzymes, which inhibited even mixed-species *P. aeruginosa* and *E. coli* biofilms [40]. NanoQuench was a European project for developing quorum quenching enzymes and nanoantibiotics for novel coatings, aiming to prevent biofilm formation on urinary catheters, with a focus on Gram-negative *P. aeruginosa* biofilms. One of the project's results is antibiofilm multilayer nanovancomycin and acylase coating, which was shown to be efficient in-vitro [41].

Nanobiosystem composed of magnetite nanoparticles coated with *Rosmarinus officinalis* essential oil was efficient in reducing adherence to catheter surface, and biofilm formation by *C. albicans* and *C. tropicalis* [42].

Phytochemicals-capped gold nanoparticles were synthesized using *Aegle marmelos* leaf extract, for the further purpose of prevention of urinary catheter infections. Obtained nanotriangles exhibited major antimicrobial activity against *S. aureus*, *P. aeruginosa*, *K. pneumoniae* and *E. faecalis* [43].

3   Non-metallic Nanoparticles

A wide class of oxides, nitrides, silicide and carbide, hydroxyapatite, diamond-like carbon, and others are used as antimicrobials [16, 44, 45]. Surface coatings with these nanomaterials have gained significant attention due to their antimicrobial activity. Graphene-based nanomaterials have different surface chemistry (graphite, graphene oxide GO, and reduced graphene oxide RGO) and different microbial activity mechanisms. GO has a more potent antimicrobial effect against *Escherichia coli* when compared to graphite and RGO [46]. Amorphous carbon was also used as a matrix material for the incorporation of metallic clusters [47].

Laube and co-workers used diamond-like carbon (DLC) material for coating ureteral stents. They published an in vitro and in vivo study in which they observed that there was a reduction in encrustation, biofilm formation, and patients' symptoms [48].

Nanostructured coatings of diamond-like carbon, molybdenum disulfide and tungsten disulfide nanoparticles were deposited on a polydimethylsiloxane substrate. These coatings were compared in terms of resistance to the formation of urinary deposits. It was found that tungsten disulfide was the most resistant to encrustations after 4 weeks of immersion in artificial urine [49].

To obtain functionalized catheter surface with improved resistance to microbial colonization and biofilm formation Fe_2O_3/C_{12} nanoparticles were coated on 2-((4-ethylphenoxy)   methyl)-*N*-(substituted-phenylcarbamothioyl)-benzamide used as adsorption shell. This material showed improved resistance to *Staphylococcus aureus* and *Pseudomonas aeruginosa*, and did not show cytotoxicity [50].

Boron nitride (BN) has physicochemical properties similar to graphene-based nanomaterial, but it holds an advantage in terms of biocompatibility with human cells. Boron nitride composite with polyethylene was studied for biomedical applications. It was demonstrated that bacterial activity of BN/PE composite correlates with BN concentration [51].

Nitric oxide (NO) has been a well-known antimicrobial agent. Commonly used NO donor in the medical research *S*-Nitroso-*N*-acetyl-DL-penicillamine (SNAP) was impregnated in commercial urinary catheters [52].

It was shown that catheters have very high antimicrobial efficacy and effectively reduce biofilm formation over a longer period. However, the issue of NO storage remains, as the polymers are limited reservoirs for NO.

3.1 Metal-Based Nanoparticles

Metal-based nanoparticles are very popular antimicrobials [53]. They do not bind to a specific receptor in the bacterial cell which makes them have non-specific bacterial toxicity mechanisms and consequently makes the development of resistance by bacteria to be difficult. As a result, a large majority of metal-based nanoparticle efficacy studies performed so far have shown promising results in both Gram-positive and Gram-negative bacteria [54, 55]. Several review papers can be found regarding this subject, among few of them have been published most recently [17, 56–58].

In the field of urinary catheters, silver-based coatings are in use for over 20 years but their true efficacy is still a matter of debate [59, 60]. The narrow boundary between beneficial and toxic effects, especially in the prolonged applications remains a major concern in Ag utilization. One of the promising approaches to overcome the toxicity issue of Ag, is to functionalize it with more biocompatible compounds. As already mentioned above, Kumar et al., proposed the usage of exopolysaccharide Kocuran, as a capping and reducing agent of silver nanoparticles [39]. Related to the subject of Ag NPs functionalization, Ashmore and colleagues manage to coat Ag NPs with polyvinylpyrrolidone (PVP) and compared the antibacterial efficacy with the non-coated AgNPs [61]. As a result, a significant improvement in antibacterial efficacy was achieved. It is worth noting that two types of Ag-PVP NPs were prepared, either containing 10% of Ag or 99% and both of them have shown better antimicrobial properties against *E. coli* than non-coated AgNPs. In addition, the authors reported that Ag-PVP NPs also promote downregulation of the expression of genes that are involved in the cellular growth *of E. coli*.

Based on *in vitro* investigations of Giri and colleagues [62] reducing the surface charge of AuNPs broadens the therapeutic window, so a higher concentration of these particles can be used without toxicity concerns.

I. Carvalho et al. reported in their study, that deposition of Ag and Ag–Au bimetallic clusters on thermoplastic polyurethane tape (as one of the materials used in the ureteral stent manufacture) have positive outcomes [47]. The coating was performed by physical methods (sputtering and plasma gas condensation) and the authors characterized it as a promising for long periods, since the release of silver in artificial urine did not reach the maximum amount of coating even after 30 days. Nevertheless, these released Ag were sufficient for the prevention of biofilm formation and achievement of antibacterial effect against *E. coli* while preserving good biocompatibility. Comparing the antibacterial effects, amount of released Ag, and morphology of deposited Ag and Ag–Au clusters, the authors concluded that the size of the deposited cluster determines the mechanism and release kinetic of Ag. In the case of smaller homogeneously distributed clusters, the release of Ag ions is favored, while in the case of larger deposits the release of Ag NPs is the dominant process. In both scenarios, the bactericidal effect against *E. coli* was very similar. The other coatings investigated in this study achieved a slow Ag release and no antibacterial effect, suggesting that the release kinetics of Ag is directly responsible for the antibacterial properties of coatings.

Rocca et al. performed an interesting strategy in the coating of silicone catheters. The authors described a simple method for producing Au nanoplates by reduction of Au salt with gentamycin at elevated temperature [63]. The coating was performed *in situ*, during the synthesis procedure, and lasted only 15 min. Regardless of the duration of coating, deposited Au nanoplates were efficient in preventing the growth of three bacterial strains (*S. aureus*, *P. aeruginosa* and *E. coli*) after 18 h of incubation. The observed anti-biofouling effect of Au nanoplates was explained through the topographic change at the nano-scale level, which disrupts attachments of the bacterial cells. Additionally, the authors also confirmed the effectiveness of coating by testing it in stimulated flow conditions, using the physiological solution and syringe pump [63].

In the work performed by Ron et al., encrustation of silicone catheters was remarkably prevented in *in vitro* conditions, by coating with rhenium-doped molybdenum disulfide (Re:IF-MoS$_2$) nanoparticles [64]. As the authors stated, these NPs displayed a unique tendency to self-assemble into mosaic-like arrangements, modifying the surface at the nanoscale to be encrustation-repellent. Encrustation investigation was conducted using a custom-built device and artificial urine. The effectiveness of Re:IF-MoS$_2$ nanoparticles coating lies in their specific physico-chemical properties such as negative charge, low surface free energy, and nanotexture, providing them a superior solid-lubrication behavior.

The second approach, besides stents coating, is the impregnation of nanoparticles in the drug-eluting stents. Recently, Gao et al. performed a thorough investigation of biodegradable stents with a renewable surface capable of contact killing of bacteria [65]. The renewable property was accomplished through surface degradation of poly(glycolic acid)/poly(lactic-*co*-glycolic acid) (PGA/PGLA) layer, while antibacterial properties were achieved by impregnation of hyperbranched poly(amide-amine)-capped Ag shell and Au core nanoparticles in PGA–PGLA. *In vitro* and *in vivo* testing have confirmed that this particular stent design provides good mechanical properties, high antibacterial activity, the low release of Ag ions, and good biocompatibility. According to the authors, the capping agent (poly(amide-amine) was most responsible for high bactericidal effects and low cytotoxicity of nanoparticles by providing a high-stabile structure. The stent degradation in artificial urine was gradual, constantly detaching adhered bacteria and proteins, and releasing enough amounts of nanoparticles. As a result, the authors reported good antibiofilm properties after 2 weeks-examination and lower levels of inflammatory and necrotic cells, 3 weeks after implantation.

A similar comprehensive approach in designing antibacterial and repellent coating was reported by Dayyoub et al. [66]. This group of scientists successfully developed a film of poly(lactic-*co*-glycolide) (PLGA) to release norfloxacin and Ag NPs, coated with tetraether lipid The strength of this multifunctional system lies in the fact that it consists of dual antimicrobial agents (norfloxacin is a broad-spectrum synthetic antibiotic almost exclusively indicated in the treatment of urinary tract infections) impregnated in the biodegradable matrix. The authors used this film to coat polyurethane and silicone sheets, which results in effective inhibition of bacteria adhesion, compared to uncoated sheets. Thanks to the fact that degradation of PLGA creates an acidic environment, it neutralizes alkali products of urea hydrolysis and thus reduces the encrustation, based on *in vitro* experiments in artificial urine that lasted two weeks.

Agarwala et al. investigated antibacterial/antibiofilm activity of iron oxide and copper oxide nanoparticles against multidrug-resistant biofilm forming uropathogens. They found that CuO nanoparticles are more effective as an antibacterial material than Fe_2O_3 nanoparticles [67].

Besides mentioned studies, a significant number of additional papers could be found regarding the antimicrobial activity of metal-based NPs and some of them are summarized in Table 1.

4 Conclusion

The effectiveness of nanoparticles against numerous bacterial strains including those that cause biofilm formations in urinary stents is well documented in many papers. However, the important issues that should be addressed in the nanoparticles utilization are the release from the inner surface of the stents and the stability of the coating. The harsh environment, to which the urinary stents are exposed, represents the obstacle that must be considered with great percussion when choosing the coating/impregnation technique and concentrations of nanoparticles. Literature data are constantly expanding with new findings regarding antibacterial activity, encrustation repellence, and biocompatibility, but lacking those regarding release profiles and how these profiles are influenced by the chemistry and flow conditions. Nevertheless, the reported studies have confirmed the nanoparticle-based strategy exhibit great potential and that it's a matter of time when it will find its way to commercially available product.

Acknowledgments Funds for the realization of this work were provided by the Ministry of Education, Science and Technological Development of the Republic of Serbia, Agreement on realization and financing of scientific research work of the Institute of Technical Sciences of SASA in 2021 (Record number: 451-03-9/2021-14/200175). We are also thankful to COST Action CA16217.

Table 1 Metal-based NPs used for prevention and treatment of UTI

Type of nanomaterials	Specific properties/findings	Microbial activity	Refs.
Green Ag NPs	*In situ* photo-assisted deposition of AgNPs on Foley catheter	*In vitro* (antibiofilm—*E. coli*)	[68]
Chrysophanol-Ag NPs	Coating on polystyrene and silicone surfaces; inhibition of quorum sensing	*In vitro* (the anti-adhesion and anti-biofouling—*P. aeruginosa* and *E. coli*; static + flow conditions) + *In vivo* (antibiofilm in mices)	[69]
Sp. platensis methanolic extract—Ag NPs	Coating on latex catheters; inhibition of rhamnolipid production	*In vitro* (antibiofilm—*P. aeruginosa*)	[70]
Ag–PolyRicinoleic acid–polystyrene NPs	Coating on polyurethane catheter modified with tetracycline hydrochloride	*In vitro* (antibacterial and antibiofilm—*E. coli* and *S. aureus*)	[71]
AgNPs	Layer-by-layer deposition on silicone cath. Using polydopamine and poly(sulfobetaine methacrylate-*co*-acrylamide)	*In vivo* (antibiofilm in mices and pigs, obs. period 14 and 21 days); comparison with uncoated and Dover™ Ag-coated catheters	[72, 73]
Polydopamine + AgNPs	Sustained release of Ag from polydopamine layer deposited on Foley catheter	*In vitro* (antibiofilm—*S. aureus* and *E. coli*)	[28]
AgNPs	Layer-by-layer deposition coating on silicone Foley catheter; superhydrophobicity	*In vitro* (antibacterial—*E. coli, P. mirabilis*; static + dynamic conditions)	[74]
HAp-Ag+ NPs	silico-latex two-way indwelling catheters	*In vivo* (occurrence of bacteriuria and biofilm in rabbits, obs. period 7 days)	[75]
Fe$_3$O$_4$@Au nanoeggs + Vancomycin	Phothermal effects	*In vitro* (antibacterial-clinical isolates of *S. saprophyticus, S. pyogenes, E. coli, A. baumannii*, VRE, MRSA, and PDRAB)	[76]
ZnO NPs	Reduction of biofilm biomass, formed on urinary catheters	*In vitro* (antimicrobial and antibiofilm—clinical isolates of *C. albicans*)	[77, 78]
Zn-doped CuO NPs	Sonochemical deposition on silicone catheters	*In vitro* (antibiofilm—*E. coli, S. aureus* and *P. mirabilis*) + *In vivo* (rabbits, obs. period 7 days)	[79]
Graphene and graphene–Ag nanoplatelets	Spray-coating on a Foley catheter	*In vitro* (antibiofilm-*S. epidermidis*)	[80]
TiO$_2$/SiO$_2$/Ag nanocomposite	Magnetron co-sputtering, triple layer deposition on glass substrate	*In vitro* (antibacterial and antibiofilm—*E. coli* and *P. aeruginosa*)	[81]
MgF$_2$ NPs	Coating on glass coupons; disruption in the membrane potential of bacteria	*In vitro* (antibacterial and antibiofilm—*E. coli* and *S. aureus*)	[82]

References

1. Kehinde EO, Rotimi VO, Al-Hunayan A, Abdul-Halim H, Boland F, Al-Awadi KA. Bacteriology of urinary tract infection associated with indwelling J ureteral stents. J Endourol. 2004;18(9):891–6. https://doi.org/10.1089/end.2004.18.891.
2. Azevedo AS, Almeida C, Melo LF, Azevedo NF. Impact of polymicrobial biofilms in catheter-associated urinary tract infections. Crit Rev Microbiol. 2017;43(4):423–39. https://doi.org/10.1080/1040841X.2016.1240656.
3. Kumon H, Hashimoto H, Nishimura M, Monden K, Ono N. Catheter-associated urinary tract infections: impact of catheter materials on their management. Int J Antimicrob Agents. 2001;17(4):311–6.
4. Soto SM. Importance of biofilms in urinary tract infections: new therapeutic approaches. Adv Biol. 2014;2:1–13.
5. Samuel U, Guggenbichler JP. Prevention of catheter-related infections: the potential of a new nano-silver impregnated catheter. Int J Antimicrob Agents. 2004;23(SUPPL. 1):75–8.
6. Anjum S, Singh S, Benedicte L, Roger P, Panigrahi M, Gupta B. Biomodification strategies for the development of antimicrobial urinary catheters: overview and advances. Glob Chall. 2018;2(1):1700068.
7. Filipović N, Ušjak D, Milenković MT, Zheng K, Liverani L, Boccaccini AR, et al. Comparative study of the antimicrobial activity of selenium nanoparticles with different surface chemistry and structure. Front Bioeng Biotechnol. 2021;8:1591.
8. Stevanović M, Filipović N, Djurdjević J, Lukić M, Milenković M, Boccaccini A. 45S5Bioglass®-based scaffolds coated with selenium nanoparticles or with poly(lactide-co-glycolide)/selenium particles: processing, evaluation and antibacterial activity. Colloids Surf B Biointerfaces. 2015;132:208–15.
9. Stanković A, Sezen M, Milenković M, Kaišarević S, Andrić N, Stevanović M. PLGA/nano-ZnO composite particles for use in biomedical applications: preparation, characterization, and antimicrobial activity. J Nanomater. 2016;2016:1–10.
10. Stevanović M, Bračko I, Milenković M, Filipović N, Nunić J, Filipič M, et al. Multifunctional PLGA particles containing poly(l-glutamic acid)-capped silver nanoparticles and ascorbic acid with simultaneous antioxidative and prolonged antimicrobial activity. Acta Biomater. 2014;10(1):151–62.
11. Stevanović M, Jordović B, Uskoković D. Morphological changes of poly(dl-lactide-co-glycolide) nano-particles containing ascorbic acid during in vitro degradation process. J Microsc. 2008;232(3):511–6.
12. Stevanović M, Lukić MJ, Stanković A, Filipović N, Kuzmanović M, Janićijević Ž. Biomedical inorganic nanoparticles: preparation, properties, and perspectives. In: Materials for biomedical engineering. Amsterdam: Elsevier; 2019. p. 1–46. https://linkinghub.elsevier.com/retrieve/pii/B9780081028148000019
13. Gurunathan S, Woong Han J, Abdal Daye A, Eppakayala V, Kim J. Oxidative stress-mediated antibacterial activity of graphene oxide and reduced graphene oxide in *Pseudomonas aeruginosa*. Int J Nanomed. 2012;7:5901. http://www.dovepress.com/oxidative-stress-mediated-antibacterial-activity-of-graphene-oxide-and-peer-reviewed-article-IJN
14. Nagy A, Harrison A, Sabbani S, Munson RS Jr, Dutta PK, WJW. Silver nanoparticles embedded in zeolite membranes: release of silver ions and mechanism of antibacterial action. Int J Nanomed. 2011;6:1833. http://www.dovepress.com/silver-nanoparticles-embedded-in-zeolite-membranes-release-of-silver-i-peer-reviewed-article-IJN
15. Leung YH, Ng AMC, Xu X, Shen Z, Gethings LA, Wong MT, et al. Mechanisms of antibacterial activity of MgO: non-ROS mediated toxicity of MgO nanoparticles towards *Escherichia coli*. Small. 2014;10(6):1171–83. https://doi.org/10.1002/smll.201302434.
16. Wang L, Hu C, Shao L. The antimicrobial activity of nanoparticles: present situation and prospects for the future. Int J Nanomed. 2017;12:1227–49. https://www.dovepress.com/the-antimicrobial-activity-of-nanoparticles-present-situation-and-pros-peer-reviewed-article-IJN

17. Han C, Romero N, Fischer S, Dookran J, Berger A, Doiron AL. Recent developments in the use of nanoparticles for treatment of biofilms. Nanotechnol Rev. 2017;6(5):383–404. https://doi.org/10.1515/ntrev-2016-0054/html.

18. Slomberg DL, Lu Y, Broadnax AD, Hunter RA, Carpenter AW, Schoenfisch MH. Role of size and shape on biofilm eradication for nitric oxide-releasing silica nanoparticles. ACS Appl Mater Interfaces. 2013;5(19):9322–9. https://doi.org/10.1021/am402618w.

19. Filipović N, Stevanović M, Nunić J, Cundrič S, Filipič M, Uskoković D. Synthesis of poly(ε-caprolactone) nanospheres in the presence of the protective agent poly(glutamic acid) and their cytotoxicity, genotoxicity and ability to induce oxidative stress in HepG2 cells. Colloids Surf B Biointerfaces. 2014;117:414–24.

20. Filipović N, Veselinović L, RaŽić S, Jeremić S, Filipič M, Žegura B, et al. Poly (ε-caprolactone) microspheres for prolonged release of selenium nanoparticles. Mater Sci Eng C. 2019;96:776–89.

21. Filipović N, Stevanović M, Radulović A, Pavlović V, Uskoković D. Facile synthesis of poly(ε-caprolactone) micro and nanospheres using different types of polyelectrolytes as stabilizers under ambient and elevated temperature. Compos Part B Eng. 2013;45(1):1471–9.

22. Stevanović M. Biomedical applications of nanostructured polymeric materials. In Nanostructured polymer composites for biomedical applications. Amsterdam: Elsevier; 2019. p. 1–19. https://linkinghub.elsevier.com/retrieve/pii/B9780128167717000016

23. Stevanović MMM, Uskoković DP. Poly(lactide-*co*-glycolide)-based micro and nanoparticles for the controlled drug delivery of vitamins. Curr Nanosci. 2009;5(1):1–14. http://www.eurekaselect.com/openurl/content.php?genre=article&issn=1573-4137&volume=5&issue=1&spage=1

24. Cano A, Ettcheto M, Espina M, López-Machado A, Cajal Y, Rabanal F, et al. State-of-the-art polymeric nanoparticles as promising therapeutic tools against human bacterial infections. J Nanobiotechnol. 2020;18(1):156. https://doi.org/10.1186/s12951-020-00714-2.

25. Venkatesan N, Shroff S, Jayachandran K, Doble M. Polymers as ureteral stents. J Endourol. 2010;24(2):191–8. https://doi.org/10.1089/end.2009.0516.

26. Škrlová K, Malachová K, Muñoz-Bonilla A, Měřinská D, Rybková Z, Fernández-García M, et al. Biocompatible polymer materials with antimicrobial properties for preparation of stents. Nanomaterials. 2019;9(11):1548. https://www.mdpi.com/2079-4991/9/11/1548

27. Stevanović M. Polymeric micro- and nanoparticles for controlled and targeted drug delivery. In Nanostructures for drug delivery. Amsterdam: Elsevier; 2017. p. 355–78. https://linkinghub.elsevier.com/retrieve/pii/B9780323461436000117

28. Yassin MA, Elkhooly TA, Elsherbiny SM, Reicha FM, Shokeir AA. Facile coating of urinary catheter with bio-inspired antibacterial coating. Heliyon. 2019;5(12):e02986. https://linkinghub.elsevier.com/retrieve/pii/S2405844019366459

29. Badran MM, Alomrani AH, Harisa GI, Ashour AE, Kumar A, Yassin AE. Novel docetaxel chitosan-coated PLGA/PCL nanoparticles with magnified cytotoxicity and bioavailability. Biomed Pharmacother. 2018;106:1461–8.

30. Srisang S, Wongsuwan N, Boongird A, Ungsurungsie M, Wanasawas P, Nasongkla N. Multilayer nanocoating of Foley urinary catheter by chlorhexidine-loaded nanoparticles for prolonged release and anti-infection of urinary tract. Int J Polym Mater Polym Biomater. 2020;69(17):1081–9.

31. Scotland KB, Lo J, Grgic T, Lange D. Ureteral stent-associated infection and sepsis: pathogenesis and prevention: a review. Biofouling. 2019;35(1):117–27.

32. Palmieri V, Bugli F, Cacaci M, Perini G, De Maio F, Delogu G, et al. Graphene oxide coatings prevent *Candida albicans* biofilm formation with a controlled release of curcumin-loaded nanocomposites. Nanomedicine. 2018;13(22):2867–79.

33. Manjula R, Chavadi M. Nanoantibiotics: the next-generation antimicrobials. Cham: Springer; 2020. p. 375–88. https://doi.org/10.1007/978-3-030-41464-1_16.

34. Bračič M, Fras-Zemljič L, Pérez L, Kogej K, Stana-Kleinschek K, Kargl R, et al. Protein-repellent and antimicrobial nanoparticle coatings from hyaluronic acid and a lysine-

derived biocompatible surfactant. J Mater Chem B. 2017;5(21):3888–97. http://xlink.rsc. org/?DOI=C7TB00311K

35. Dinic M, Pecikoza U, Djokic J, Stepanovic-Petrovic R, Milenkovic M, Stevanovic M, et al. Exopolysaccharide produced by probiotic strain *Lactobacillus paraplantarum* BGCG11 reduces inflammatory hyperalgesia in rats. Front Pharmacol. 2018;9:1.
36. Watkins R, Wu L, Zhang C, Davis RM, Xu B. Natural product-based nanomedicine: recent advances and issues. Int J Nanomed. 2015;10:6055–74.
37. Venkat Kumar G, Su CH, Velusamy P. Surface immobilization of kanamycin–chitosan nanoparticles on polyurethane ureteral stents to prevent bacterial adhesion. Biofouling. 2016;32(8):861–70.
38. Kanugala S, Jinka S, Puvvada N, Banerjee R, Kumar CG. Phenazine-1-carboxamide functionalized mesoporous silica nanoparticles as antimicrobial coatings on silicone urethral catheters. Sci Rep. 2019;9(1):1–16.
39. Kumar CG, Sujitha P. Green synthesis of Kocuran-functionalized silver glyconanoparticles for use as antibiofilm coatings on silicone urethral catheters. Nanotechnology. 2014;25(32):325101. https://doi.org/10.1088/0957-4484/25/32/325101.
40. Ivanova K, Fernandes MM, Francesko A, Mendoza E, Guezguez J, Burnet M, et al. Quorum-quenching and matrix-degrading enzymes in multilayer coatings synergistically prevent bacterial biofilm formation on urinary catheters. ACS Appl Mater Interfaces. 2015;7(49):27066–77.
41. NanoQuench Project. 2015. https://cordis.europa.eu/project/id/331416/reporting/it.
42. Chifiriuc C, Grumezescu V, Grumezescu A, Saviuc C, Lazǎr V, Andronescu E. Hybrid magnetite nanoparticles/*Rosmarinus officinalis* essential oil nanobiosystem with antibiofilm activity. Nanoscale Res Lett. 2012;7(1):209. https://doi.org/10.1186/1556-276X-7-209.
43. Arunachalam K, Annamalai SK, Arunachalam AM, Raghavendra R, Kennedy S. One step green synthesis of phytochemicals mediated gold nanoparticles from *Aegle marmales* for the prevention of urinary catheter infection. Int J Pharm Pharm Sci. 2014;6(1):700–6.
44. Karwowska E. Antibacterial potential of nanocomposite-based materials—a short review. Nanotechnol Rev. 2017;6(2):243–54. https://doi.org/10.1515/ntrev-2016-0046/html.
45. Ušjak D, Dinić M, Novović K, Ivković B, Filipović N, Stevanović M, et al. Methoxy-substituted hydroxychalcone reduces biofilm production, adhesion and surface motility of *Acinetobacter baumannii* by inhibiting ompA gene expression. Chem Biodivers. 2021;18(1):e2000786. https://doi.org/10.1002/cbdv.202000786.
46. Zou X, Zhang L, Wang Z, Luo Y. Mechanisms of the antimicrobial activities of graphene materials. J Am Chem Soc. 2016;138(7):2064–77. https://doi.org/10.1021/jacs.5b11411.
47. Carvalho I, Dias N, Henriques M, Calderon VS, Ferreira P, Cavaleiro A, et al. Antibacterial effects of bimetallic clusters incorporated in amorphous carbon for stent application. ACS Appl Mater Interfaces. 2020;12(22):24555–63. https://doi.org/10.1021/acsami.0c02821.
48. Laube N, Kleinen L, Bradenahl J, Meissner A. Diamond-like carbon coatings on ureteral stents-a new strategy for decreasing the formation of crystalline bacterial biofilms? J Urol. 2007;177(5):1923–7.
49. Cardona A, Iacovacci V, Mazzocchi T, Menciassi A, Ricotti L. Novel nanostructured coating on PDMS substrates featuring high resistance to urine. ACS Appl Biol Mater. 2019;2(1):255–65. https://doi.org/10.1021/acsabm.8b00586.
50. Anghel I, Limban C, Grumezescu AM, Anghel AG, Bleotu C, Chifiriuc MC. In vitro evaluation of anti-pathogenic surface coating nanofluid, obtained by combining Fe_3O_4/C12 nanostructures and 2-((4-ethylphenoxy) methyl)-*N*-(substituted-phenylcarbamothioyl)-benzamides. Nanoscale Res Lett. 2012;7(1):1–10.
51. Pandit S, Gaska K, Mokkapati VR, Forsberg S, Svensson M, Kádár R, et al. Antibacterial effect of boron nitride flakes with controlled orientation in polymer composites. RSC Adv. 2019;9(57):33454–9.
52. Colletta A, Wu J, Wo Y, Kappler M, Chen H, Xi C, et al. S-Nitroso-*N*-acetylpenicillamine (SNAP) impregnated silicone foley catheters: a potential biomaterial/device to prevent catheter-associated urinary tract infections. ACS Biomater Sci Eng. 2015;1(6):416–24. https://doi.org/10.1021/acsbiomaterials.5b00032.

53. Stevanovic M. Assembly of polymers/metal nanoparticles and their applications as medical devices. Adv Biomater Biodevices. 2014;18:343–66.
54. Sánchez-López E, Gomes D, Esteruelas G, Bonilla L, Lopez-Machado AL, Galindo R, et al. Metal-based nanoparticles as antimicrobial agents: an overview. Nanomaterials. 2020;10(2):292. https://www.mdpi.com/2079-4991/10/2/292
55. Stevanović M, Uskoković V, Filipović M, Škapin SD, Uskoković D. Composite PLGA/AgNpPGA/AscH nanospheres with combined osteoinductive, antioxidative, and antimicrobial activities. ACS Appl Mater Interfaces. 2013;5(18):9034–42.
56. Qindeel M, Barani M, Rahdar A, Arshad R, Cucchiarini M. Nanomaterials for the diagnosis and treatment of urinary tract infections. Nanomaterials. 2021;11(2):546.
57. Aderibigbe B. Metal-based nanoparticles for the treatment of infectious diseases. Molecules. 2017;22(8):1370.
58. Singh A, Gautam PK, Verma A, Singh V, Shivapriya PM, Shivalkar S, et al. Green synthesis of metallic nanoparticles as effective alternatives to treat antibiotics resistant bacterial infections: a review. Biotechnol Rep. 2020;25:e00427.
59. Beattie M, Taylor J. Silver alloy vs. uncoated urinary catheters: a systematic review of the literature. J Clin Nurs. 2011;20(15–16):2098–108. https://doi.org/10.1111/j.1365-2702.2010.03561.x.
60. Liu XS, Zola JC, McGinnis DE, Squadrito JF, Zeltser IS. Do silver alloy-coated catheters increase risk of urethral strictures after robotic-assisted laparoscopic radical prostatectomy? Urology. 2011;78(2):365–7.
61. Ashmore D, Chaudhari A, Barlow B, Barlow B, Harper T, Vig K, et al. Evaluation of *E. coli* inhibition by plain and polymer-coated silver nanoparticles. Rev Inst Med Trop Sao Paulo. 2018;60:e18. http://www.scielo.br/scielo.php?script=sci_arttext&pid=S0036-46652018005000209&lng=en&tlng=en
62. Giri K, Rivas Yepes L, Duncan B, Kolumam Parameswaran P, Yan B, Jiang Y, et al. Targeting bacterial biofilms via surface engineering of gold nanoparticles. RSC Adv. 2015;5(128):105551–9. http://xlink.rsc.org/?DOI=C5RA16305F
63. Rocca DM, Aiassa V, Zoppi A, Silvero Compagnucci J, Becerra MC. Nanostructured gold coating for prevention of biofilm development in medical devices. J Endourol. 2020;34(3):345–51. https://doi.org/10.1089/end.2019.0686.
64. Ron R, Zbaida D, Kafka IZ, Rosentsveig R, Leibovitch I, Tenne R. Attenuation of encrustation by self-assembled inorganic fullerene-like nanoparticles. Nanoscale. 2014;6(10):5251. http://xlink.rsc.org/?DOI=c3nr06231g
65. Gao L, Wang Y, Li Y, Xu M, Sun G, Zou T, et al. Biomimetic biodegradable Ag@Au nanoparticle-embedded ureteral stent with a constantly renewable contact-killing antimicrobial surface and antibiofilm and extraction-free properties. Acta Biomater. 2020;114:117–32. https://linkinghub.elsevier.com/retrieve/pii/S1742706120304116
66. Dayyoub E, Frant M, Pinnapireddy SR, Liefeith K, Bakowsky U. Antibacterial and anti-encrustation biodegradable polymer coating for urinary catheter. Int J Pharm. 2017;531(1):205–14. https://linkinghub.elsevier.com/retrieve/pii/S0378517317307792
67. Agarwala M, Choudhury B, Yadav RNS. Comparative study of antibiofilm activity of copper oxide and iron oxide nanoparticles against multidrug resistant biofilm forming uropathogens. Indian J Microbiol. 2014;54(3):365–8.
68. Chutrakulwong F, Thamaphat K, Tantipaibulvut S, Limsuwan P. In situ deposition of green silver nanoparticles on urinary catheters under photo-irradiation for antibacterial properties. Processes. 2020;8(12):1630.
69. Prateeksha P, Bajpai R, Rao CV, Upreti DK, Barik SK, Singh BN. Chrysophanol-Functionalized silver nanoparticles for anti-adhesive and anti-biofouling coatings to prevent urinary catheter-associated infections. ACS Appl Nano Mater. 2021;4(2):1512–28.
70. LewisOscar F, Nithya C, Vismaya S, Arunkumar M, Pugazhendhi A, Nguyen-Tri P, et al. In vitro analysis of green fabricated silver nanoparticles (AgNPs) against Pseudomonas aeruginosa PA14 biofilm formation, their application on urinary catheter. Prog Org Coatings. 2021;151:106058.

71. Koc H, Kilicay E, Karahaliloglu Z, Hazer B, Denkbas EB. Prevention of urinary infection through the incorporation of silver–ricinoleic acid–polystyrene nanoparticles on the catheter surface. J Biomater Appl. 2021;36(3):385–405.
72. Mandakhalikar KD, Wang R, Rahmat JN, Chiong E, Neoh KG, Tambyah PA. Restriction of in vivo infection by antifouling coating on urinary catheter with controllable and sustained silver release: a proof of concept study. BMC Infect Dis. 2018;18(1):370.
73. Wang R, Neoh KG, Kang E, Tambyah PA, Chiong E. Antifouling coating with controllable and sustained silver release for long-term inhibition of infection and encrustation in urinary catheters. J Biomed Mater Res Part B Appl Biomater. 2015;103(3):519–28.
74. Zhang S, Liang X, Gadd GM, Zhao Q. Superhydrophobic coatings for urinary catheters to delay bacterial biofilm formation and catheter-associated urinary tract infection. ACS Appl Bio Mater. 2020;3(1):282–91.
75. Evliyaoğlu Y, Kobaner M, Çelebi H, Yelsel K, Doğan A. The efficacy of a novel antibacterial hydroxyapatite nanoparticle-coated indwelling urinary catheter in preventing biofilm formation and catheter-associated urinary tract infection in rabbits. Urol Res. 2011;39(6):443–9.
76. Huang W-C, Tsai P-J, Chen Y-C. Multifunctional Fe3O4@Au Nanoeggs as photothermal agents for selective killing of nosocomial and antibiotic-resistant bacteria. Small. 2009;5(1):51–6.
77. Hosseini SS, Ghaemi E, Noroozi A, Niknejad F. Zinc oxide nanoparticles inhibition of initial adhesion and als1 and als3 gene expression in candida albicans strains from urinary tract infections. Mycopathologia. 2019;184(2):261–71.
78. Hosseini SS, Ghaemi E, Koohsar F. Influence of ZnO nanoparticles on Candida albicans isolates biofilm formed on the urinary catheter. Iran J Microbiol. 2018;10(6):424–32.
79. Shalom Y, Perelshtein I, Perkas N, Gedanken A, Banin E. Catheters coated with Zn-doped CuO nanoparticles delay the onset of catheter-associated urinary tract infections. Nano Res. 2017;10(2):520–33.
80. Dybowska-Sarapuk Ł, Kotela A, Krzemiński J, Wróblewska M, Marchel H, Romaniec M, et al. Graphene nanolayers as a new method for bacterial biofilm prevention: preliminary results. J AOAC Int. 2017;100(4):900–4.
81. Vladkova T, Angelov O, Stoyanova D, Gospodinova D, Gomes L, Soares A, et al. Magnetron co-sputtered TiO2/SiO2/Ag nanocomposite thin coatings inhibiting bacterial adhesion and biofilm formation. Surf Coatings Technol. 2020;384:125322.
82. Lellouche J, Kahana E, Elias S, Gedanken A, Banin E. Antibiofilm activity of nanosized magnesium fluoride. Biomaterials. 2009;30(30):5969–78.

Urinary Tract Infections and Encrustation in Urinary Stents

Roman Herout, Alina Reicherz, Ben H. Chew, and Dirk Lange

1 Introduction

Ureteral stents are hollow tubes that ensure urine flow from the kidney via the ureter into the bladder. First introduced by Zimskind in 1967, the modern "double pigtail" or "double J" ureteral stent, as we know it today, was developed by Finney et al. in 1978 [1, 2]. Since then, ureteral stents have been broadly used in the field of Urology for various indications such as blocking ureteral calculi, following endoscopic procedures, as well as reconstructive procedures such as uretero-ureterotomy or pyeloplasty. In addition, long-term stenting is frequently required in patients with malignancies to relieve obstruction of a compressed ureter. Besides warranting antegrade urine flow, these stents can also protect an anastomosis and serve as a scaffold in the healing process.

R. Herout
Department of Urologic Sciences, The Stone Centre at Vancouver General Hospital, University of British Columbia, Vancouver, BC, Canada

Department of Urology, University Hospital Carl Gustav Carus, Technische Universität Dresden, Dresden, Germany
e-mail: roman.herout@ukdd.de

A. Reicherz
Department of Urologic Sciences, The Stone Centre at Vancouver General Hospital, University of British Columbia, Vancouver, BC, Canada

Department of Urology, Ruhr-University of Bochum, Marien Hospital Herne, Herne, Germany
e-mail: alina.reicherz@rub.de

B. H. Chew · D. Lange (✉)
Department of Urologic Sciences, The Stone Centre at Vancouver General Hospital, University of British Columbia, Vancouver, BC, Canada
e-mail: ben.chew@ubc.ca; dirk.lange@ubc.ca

© The Author(s) 2022
F. Soria et al. (eds.), *Urinary Stents*,
https://doi.org/10.1007/978-3-031-04484-7_27

Regardless of their clinical benefits, these indispensable tools for everyday practice come with substantial hindrances as they can lead to stent-related symptoms, encrustation, hematuria, infection and hence to an overall reduction in the quality of life of patients [3].

2 The Complex Interaction Between Bacteria, Biofilm and Urinary Tract Infections

Bacterial colonization of foreign bodies has been a significant problem in Medicine in general and Urology in particular for decades. The formation of a biofilm typically consists of multiple, defined steps: First, a so-called conditioning film forms within minutes after insertion of the foreign body. Here, various constituents from urine, blood and surrounding tissues such as polysaccharides, ions and glycoproteins deposit to the surface of the stent. Hence, the surface properties of the foreign body are altered, which enables planktonic bacteria to adhere to the conditioning film [4–6].

Studies have shown that around 42–100% of all indwelling ureteral stents are colonized by bacteria [7–9]. Typically, the bacteria continue to form a more mature biofilm as large, structured communities of bacteria adhere onto surfaces and secret polysaccharides, nucleic acids, lipids and proteins that form an eminently protective cast around the bacteria. Bacteria manage to survive and proliferate in an otherwise hostile environment by enriching the matrix around them with DNA, proteins, and other organic material [10]. Also, the extracellular matrices shield bacteria from shear stress caused by urine flow, as well as from antibiotics [11, 12]. Other contributing factors to antibiotic resistance are the change in phenotype as bacteria transform from planktonic into stationary, biofilm-forming bugs and the tendency to slow down their metabolism hence evading antibiotic mechanisms of action [5].

Biofilm formation on ureteral stents is assumed to be initiated within minutes after insertion and has been proven to be established as early as 24 h after insertion [7]. In a study by Shabeena et al., longer indwelling times correlated with higher colonization rates and after 120 days, 90% of the stents were colonized [13]. Despite our knowledge of bacterial colonization and biofilm formation, the link to clinically significant urinary tract infections is poorly understood: even though most indwelling stents are colonized with bacteria, few patients with stents and positive urine cultures develop clinical symptoms. The complex interaction between the pathogen, the foreign body surface, and the host is the subject of numerous studies attempting to elucidate the problem. Altunal et al. prospectively evaluated 60 patients after ureteral stent placement and detected a clinically significant urinary tract infection in 11% of patients with a median follow-up of 111 days [14].

Recently, Salari et al. retrospectively investigated the link between urine culture, stent culture, and subsequent urinary tract infections. Of the 159 patients included in this study, 15% had positive urine and 45% had positive stent culture. Two-thirds of the patients with a positive stent culture had a negative urine culture. The calculated odds for patients with negative urine and positive stent culture were 5.7 and

13.6 for patients with both cultures positive to develop a urinary tract infection in the future, respectively [15].

3 Encrustation

Encrustation describes the process of mineral crystal deposition on the surfaces of a foreign body. Biofilm formation and encrustation are believed to be interdependent processes, with bacterial colonization being addressed as the primary culprit for both events.

Clinically, we often see markedly encrusted proximal and distal ends of ureteral stents, with the mid-section typically being unconcerned and the last part of the stent to encrust. Researchers hypothesized that a kind of "wiping" effect of ureteral peristalsis and that the curled proximal and distal ends are continually exposed to urine, and its contents might be responsible for this phenomenon [16]. In Fig. 1, an encrusted catheter harvested from a mouse bladder after 6-day dwelling time from our catheter-associated urinary tract infection mouse model is depicted.

As previously described, ureteral stents are almost instantaneously coated with a conditioning film of glycoproteins, polysaccharides and ions upon introduction in the urinary tract. From there, the fate of the indwelling stent depends on several factors, which can either leave the stent unchanged, initiate the formation of a biofilm or cause encrustation of the stent [3, 17, 18]. However, these different entities might

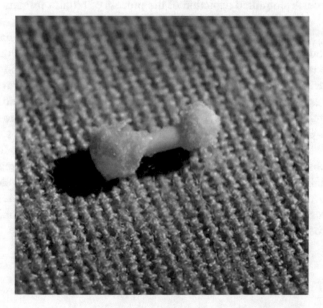

Fig. 1 Macroscopic appearance of catheter encrustation and stone formation after 6-day dwelling time. Biofilm and calculi were particularly noted on catheter lateral ends [42]

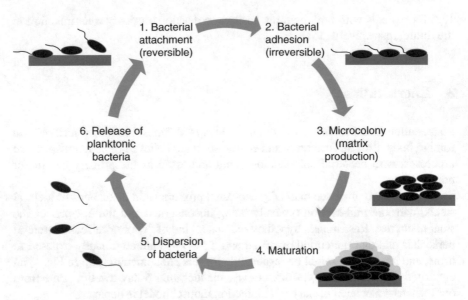

Fig. 2 The process of biofilm formation [41]

be encountered on the same stent and exist simultaneously. That being said, a biofilm with its exopolysaccharide matrix might serve as a scaffold for mineral crystals to be retained, hence serving as a nidus for encrustation. Conversely, crystals deposited on the conditioning film enlarge the surface enormously, thus facilitating bacterial adherence. A simplified depiction of the process of biofilm formation in shows in Fig. 2.

Large crystals can form rapidly with urease-positive bacteria, especially *Proteus mirabilis,* and cause significant problems in affected patients. These Gram-negative bacteria are notorious for their ability to form large infection stones in the urinary tract via elevation of the urine pH. An alkaline pH is essential, as struvite precipitates above a pH level of 7.2 [19]. With the enzyme urease, urea in urine is split into ammonia and CO_2. Because of high ammonia and CO_2 levels and the reaction of CO_2 with H_2O, which results in high bicarbonate levels, the pH level steadily rises and plateaus finally at 7.2–8.0. Ammonia continues to be hydrolyzed to form ammonia ions. Subsequently, "struvite-apatite dust" is formed around the urease-producing bacteria. Both in and around these bacteria, crystallization may develop and lead to crystal formation and finally encrustation. Urease positive bacteria tend to cause severe encrustation that often results in device failure with obstruction, leading to hydronephrosis and possibly urosepsis [20].

4   Risk Factors for Encrustation

Several risk factors, such as indwelling time, bacterial colonization, comorbidity of the patient, and the physical properties of the ureteral stent that lead to encrustation, have been established.

As with biofilm formation, studies have shown that with longer indwelling times, encrustation tends to increase. El-Fatiq et al. showed that 9% of stents had encrustations after an indwelling time of 6 weeks, 48% of patients after 6–12 weeks and 77% after 12 weeks [21]. Kawahara and colleagues evaluated 330 ureteral stents for encrustation and found 47% encrusted. A time-dependent encrustation rate was evident where 27% of stents with an indwelling time of fewer than 6 weeks showed encrustations. However, this rate increased to 57% after 6–12 weeks and 76% after more than 12 weeks. Their study could also demonstrate a correlation with ureteral stent size as higher rates of encrustation in ureteral catheter 6F or smaller were seen compared to 7F stents [22]. Kartal and coworkers came to the same conclusion in their study in 2018 that prolonged indwelling time in patients with stents and urolithiasis was associated with increased encrustation and stone burden [23].

Regarding patient-specific factors, diabetes mellitus, recurrent urinary tract infections, and chronic renal failure have shown to increase the risk of bacteriuria and possibly stent encrustation [24].

5 Strategies to Avoid Stent Encrustation

The complex nature of stent encrustation is reflected in the ubiquity of encrustations regardless of the stent materials used. There is a great incentive for companies to push advances in the field as the global ureteral stent market size was estimated at USD 422.9 million in 2019. However, due to the rise in urological and kidney-related diseases, the market is still growing and is expected to reach USD 723.6 million in 2027 [25].

Innovations that have been explored to diminish complications of ureteral stenting involve coating with antimicrobials, altering the material compounds or changing the stent architecture.

Today, most stents used in everyday practice are comprised of polymer blends. The majority of these stents are coated with bioactive compounds. However, the exact composition is unknown as these blends are typically proprietary.

5.1 Stent Coating

Several attempts have been made to develop stent coatings that prevent biofilm formation and encrustation. Initial attempts to coat ureteral stents with antibiotic agents have been abandoned due to high rates of antibiotic resistance and failed efficacy in clinical trials [26]. Another substance that has been investigated for its potential to prevent biofilm formation was heparin. For decades, this negatively charged glycosaminoglycan has been extensively used as an anticoagulant and was hypothesized to hamper bacterial adhesion and biofilm formation. However, the data for heparin are ambiguous as some authors found significantly decreased encrustation in heparin-coated stents as others failed to demonstrate a benefit [27, 28]. In a recently published work, Soria et al. tested a new heparin-coated biodegradable antireflux stent (BraidStent®-H) in a porcine model [29]. The newly developed stent could demonstrate an early decrease in bacterial load, but this effect did not prevail long-term.

5.2   Metal Stents

Metal-based stents have been introduced to tackle some of the significant draw-backs of polymer stents, such as encrustation, device failure resulting from external compression and the need for regular stent change. Various models with different mechanisms of action are currently on the market.

Resonance® (Cook Medical, USA) is a metal-based double-J stent composed of a proprietary nickel–cobalt chromium–molybdenum alloy [30]. Unlike conventional polymer stents, this metal stent is not a hollow tube with multiple holes but consists of tightly wound coils that help maintain continuous drainage by allowing urine to flow in and out of the coils. The Resonance® stent has proven to be safe and effective: Patel et al. reported successful treatment of hydronephrosis in 96% of patients in their series with median indwelling times of 19.5 months in non-malignant and 12 months in malignant ureteral obstruction [31]. The recommended indwelling time of the Resonance® stent is 12 months, hence reducing the frequency of stent changes markedly and making it more cost-effective when compared to conventional polymer stents that must be changed every 3–6 months [32]. However, in a series with a longer follow-up, a failure rate of 28% due to pain, recurrent infections, stent migration, hematuria and encrustation was reported [33].

A different method of action is adopted by the Allium® ureteral stent (Allium Medical Solutions, Israel), a self-expanding large caliber stent (24–30 Fr in diameter) of a nitinol alloy which is covered by a proprietary polymer to avoid tissue ingrowth and encrustation. According to the manufacturer, these stents are intended for short- and long-term use with a recommended maximum indwelling time of 3 years. The nitinol stents come mounted on a 10 Fr delivery system for antegrade or retrograde insertion. Moskovitz et al. first published their results on 49 Allium® stents in 40 patients in 2013 [34]. They reported successful stent placement of the stent in all patients, and after a mean indwelling time of 17 months and a mean follow-up of 21 months, stent migration occurred in 14.2%, one stent was occluded, and an uncomplicated removal with no evidence of obstruction hereafter was performed in eight patients.

Memokath™ (PNN Medical, Denmark) is a self-expanding stent comprised of a nickel-titanium alloy. The nickel content of Memokath™ is very low and encased in an inactive protective layer of biocompatible titanium oxide, making it suitable for people with a nickel allergy. The stent is thermally malleable so that upon insertion, the stent needs to be flushed with heated saline (60 °C) to expand. Agrawal et al. reported on their outcomes of 74 stents inserted in 55 patients [35]. They experienced 3 early complications (urinary extravasation, failed expansion and equipment failure) and 18 late complications, including stent migration in 13, stent encrustation in 2 and fungal infections in 3 patients. The authors concluded that the Memokath™ represents a valid alternative to conventional polymer stents with durable long-term relief from ureteric obstruction.

No prospective trials compare the various stents in patients with chronic ureteral obstruction. However, Khoo et al. recently reported on their single-center experience with the Resonance®, Allium® and Memokath-051™ stent [36]. Compared to the latter two, the Resonance® metallic ureteric stent showed superior functional stent survival. However, follow-up in this study was relatively short (median actual stent follow-up was less than 12 months for all stents), and the retrospective nature without randomization makes the study prone to selection bias.

In conclusion, metal stents represent viable alternatives for patients who require long-term stenting with comparatively low encrustation rates.

5.3 Biodegradable Stents

Biodegradable stents are ureteral stents that consist of materials that dissolve over time. This approach has several advantages as invasive removal is not required after the stents have completely dissolved over time. In addition, biodegradable materials tend to be softer, which may benefit stent tolerability and stent discomfort. Also, the ever-changing surface of the stent during dissolution might impede bacterial adhesion and encrustation. Various materials have been tested for this purpose, such as polyglycolic acid, polylactic acid, poly(lactic-co-glycolic acid) and alginate-based materials [3, 37, 38]. With some of the tested materials like polylactic acid, issues with incomplete degradation and biocompatibility prevented further development, while others showed promising preclinical utility but were not further investigated.

The Uriprene stent (Poly-Med, USA), comprised of a radiopaque, glycolic–lactic acid formula, is widely considered the most promising candidate for future clinical implementation. This degradable stent has the unique characteristic to degrade in the distal to proximal direction, which minimizes the risk of blocking fragments in the ureter and the time the renal coil could block the ureteropelvic junction. Experiments in porcine models have demonstrated good biocompatibility with less inflammation when compared to conventional non-degradable polymer stents. In a study by Chew et al., 90% of the stents were completely degraded after 4 weeks, and less hydronephrosis as compared to the biostable stents was observed [39].

The biodegradable stents could be beneficial in specific indications in the future, especially for patients after ureteroscopy and for short-term stenting. However, to date, there are no biodegradable stent solutions for long-term stenting on the horizon, which probably represent the patient cohort that suffers most from stent encrustation and its sequelae.

6 Conclusions

Due to the complex biology and interactions between foreign body surfaces, the host and microbes, a simple, one-fits-all solution is not very likely to be developed. Nonetheless, our knowledge of the underlying biology has dramatically expanded, and novel technologies are being tested. Probably the easiest solution is to appraise ureteral stenting critically and omit stenting whenever feasible. However, for patients in need of a ureteral stent the future might bring "ideal" stents that are biodegradable, coated to avoid biofilm formation and incrustation and ideally emit sufficient levels of specific drugs that prevent tissue ingrowth or even dissolve urinary calculi [40–42].

Key Points
- Ureteral stent encrustation is a significant problem in the field of Urology.
- Most ureteral stents to date are made of a polymer blend with a proprietary coating.
- Attempts have been made to reduce biofilm formation and encrustation via altering the stent surface, architecture and design.
- Biodegradable stents may help avoid the forgotten stent syndrome, especially in patients after endourologic procedures.
- For patients with malignant obstruction, metal stents have proven as a viable alternative to the conventional polymer stents with less encrustation.

References

1. Zimskind PD, Fetter TR, Wilkerson JL. Clinical use of long-term indwelling silicone rubber ureteral splints inserted cystoscopically. J Urol. 1967;97:840–4.
2. Finney RP. Experience with new double J ureteral catheter stent. J Urol. 1978;120: 678–81.
3. Lange D, Bidnur S, Hoag N, et al. Ureteral stent-associated complications—where we are and where we are going. Nat Rev Urol. 2015;12:17–25.
4. Costerton JW. Introduction to biofilm. Int J Antimicrob Agents. 1999;11:217–21.
5. Tenke P, Kovacs B, Jäckel M, et al. The role of biofilm infection in urology. World J Urol. 2006;24:13.
6. Elwood CN, Lo J, Chou E, et al. Understanding urinary conditioning film components on ureteral stents: profiling protein components and evaluating their role in bacterial colonization. Biofouling. 2013;29:1115–22.
7. Reid G, Denstedt JD, Kang YS, et al. Microbial adhesion and biofilm formation on ureteral stents in vitro and in vivo. J Urol. 1992;148:1592–4.
8. Riedl CR, Plas E, Hübner WA, et al. Bacterial colonization of ureteral stents. Eur Urol. 1999;36:53–9.
9. Kehinde EO, Rotimi VO, Al-Hunayan A, et al. Bacteriology of urinary tract infection associated with indwelling J ureteral stents. J Endourol. 2004;18:891–6.
10. Tenke P, Köves B, Nagy K, et al. Update on biofilm infections in the urinary tract. World J Urol. 2012;30:51–7.
11. Sutherland IWY. Biofilm exopolysaccharides: a strong and sticky framework. Microbiology. 2001;147:3–9.

12. Stewart PS, Costerton JW. Antibiotic resistance of bacteria in biofilms. Lancet. 2001;358:135–8.
13. Shabeena KS, Bhargava R, Manzoor MAP, et al. Characteristics of bacterial colonization after indwelling double-J ureteral stents for different time duration. Urol Ann. 2018;10:71–5.
14. Altunal N, Willke A, Hamzaoğlu O. Ureteral stent infections: a prospective study. Braz J Infect Dis. 2017;21:361–4.
15. Salari B, Khalid M, Ivan S, et al. Urine versus stent cultures and clinical UTIs. Int Urol Nephrol. 2021;53:2237–42.
16. Singh I, Gupta NP, Hemal AK, et al. Severely encrusted polyurethane ureteral stents: management and analysis of potential risk factors. Urology. 2001;58:526–31.
17. Gristina AG. Biomaterial-centered infection: microbial adhesion versus tissue integration. Science. 1987;237:1588–95.
18. Tomer N, Garden E, Small A, et al. Ureteral stent encrustation: epidemiology, pathophysiology, management and current technology. J Urol. 2021;205:68–77.
19. Schwartz BF, Stoller ML. Nonsurgical management of infection-related renal calculi. Urol Clin N Am. 1999;26:765–78.
20. Flannigan R, Choy WH, Chew B, et al. Renal struvite stones—pathogenesis, microbiology, and management strategies. Nat Rev Urol. 2014;11:333–41.
21. el-Faqih SR, Shamsuddin AB, Chakrabarti A, et al. Polyurethane internal ureteral stents in treatment of stone patients: morbidity related to indwelling times. J Urol. 1991;146:1487–91.
22. Kawahara T, Ito H, Terao H, et al. Ureteral stent encrustation, incrustation, and coloring: morbidity related to indwelling times. J Endourol. 2012;26:178–82.
23. Kartal IG, Baylan B, Gok A, et al. The association of encrustation and ureteral stent indwelling time in urolithiasis and KUB grading system. Urol J. 2018;15:323–8.
24. Akay AF, Aflay U, Gedik A, et al. Risk factors for lower urinary tract infection and bacterial stent colonization in patients with a double J ureteral stent. Int Urol Nephrol. 2007;39:95–8.
25. Anon: Ureteral Stents Market Size | Industry Report, 2020–2027. https://www.grandviewresearch.com/industry-analysis/ureteral-stents-market. Accessed 30 Nov 2021.
26. El-Nahas AR, Lachine M, Elsawy E, et al. A randomized controlled trial comparing antimicrobial (silver sulfadiazine)-coated ureteral stents with non-coated stents. Scand J Urol. 2018;52:76–80.
27. Riedl CR, Witkowski M, Plas E, et al. Heparin coating reduces encrustation of ureteral stents: a preliminary report. Int J Antimicrob Agents. 2002;19:507–10.
28. Lange D, Elwood CN, Choi K, et al. Uropathogen interaction with the surface of urological stents using different surface properties. J Urol. 2009;182:1194–200.
29. Soria F, de La Cruz JE, Fernandez T, et al. Heparin coating in biodegradable ureteral stents does not decrease bacterial colonization-assessment in ureteral stricture endourological treatment in animal model. Transl Androl Urol. 2021;10:1700–10.
30. Anon: Resonance® Metallic Ureteral Stent Set | Cook Medical. https://www.cookmedical.com/products/uro_rmsr_webds/, https://www.cookmedical.com/products/uro_rmsr_webds/. Accessed 01 Dec 2021.
31. Patel C, Loughran D, Jones R, et al. The resonance® metallic ureteric stent in the treatment of chronic ureteric obstruction: a safety and efficacy analysis from a contemporary clinical series. BMC Urol. 2017;17:16.
32. López-Huertas HL, Polcari AJ, Acosta-Miranda A, et al. Metallic ureteral stents: a cost-effective method of managing benign upper tract obstruction. J Endourol. 2010;24:483–5.
33. Kadlec AO, Ellimoottil CS, Greco KA, et al. Five-year experience with metallic stents for chronic ureteral obstruction. J Urol. 2013;190:937–41.
34. Moskovitz B, Halachmi S, Nativ O. A new self-expanding, large-caliber ureteral stent: results of a multicenter experience. J Endourol. 2012;26:1523–7.
35. Agrawal S, Brown CT, Bellamy EA, et al. The thermo-expandable metallic ureteric stent: an 11-year follow-up. BJU Int. 2009;103:372–6.
36. Khoo CC, Ho C, Palaniappan V, et al. Single-centre experience with three metallic ureteric stents (Allium® URS, Memokath™-051 and Resonance®) for chronic ureteric obstruction. J Endourol. 2021;35(12):1829–37.

37. Lingeman JE, Schulsinger DA, Kuo RL. Phase I trial of a temporary ureteral drainage stent. J Endourol. 2003;17:169–71.
38. Chew BH, Lange D, Paterson RF, et al. Next generation biodegradable ureteral stent in a Yucatan pig model. J Urol. 2010;183:765–71.
39. Chew BH, Paterson RF, Clinkscales KW, et al. In vivo evaluation of the third generation biodegradable stent: a novel approach to avoiding the forgotten stent syndrome. J Urol. 2013;189:719–25.
40. Venkatesan N, Shroff S, Jayachandran K, et al. Polymers as ureteral stents. J Endourol. 2010;24:191–8.
41. Khoddami S, Chew BH, Lange D. Problems and solutions of stent biofilm and encrustations: a review of literature. Turk J Urol. 2020;46:S11–8. https://doi.org/10.5152/tud.2020.20408.
42. Janssen C, Lo J, Jager W, et al. A high throughput, minimally invasive, ultrasound guided model for the study of catheter associated urinary tract infections and device encrustation in mice. J Urol. 2014;192:1856–63. https://doi.org/10.1016/j.juro.2014.05.0922.

Learning from Our Mistakes: Applying Vascular Stent Technologies to the Urinary Tract

Daniel Yachia

1 Introduction

In medicine a "stent" is a tube made of a polymer or a metal to be inserted into the lumen of an obstructed tubular organ to keep its lumen open. "Stenting" is the term of inserting such a device into the narrowed or occluded tubular organ due to either benign or malignant obstructive reasons.

The aim of preparing this chapter is to clarify certain points which are confusing many if not most of our urologist colleagues on the subject of "*stents* and *stenting* the urinary tract*". Another point of confusion in urology is the term of "chronic obstruction" describing an obstruction necessitating long-term stenting. Which stent to use? For how long? There are clear differences in the occlusion mechanisms of the ureters. These are either intrinsic pathologies causing a benign obstruction or a malignant obstruction. Benign obstructions are either traumatic fibrosis occurring after ureteral manipulations or iatrogenic trauma occurring during abdominal or pelvic surgeries. Such obstructions can be managed by inserting a large caliber JJ or even 2 JJs in tandem and left them in place until regeneration of the injury occurs. Malignant occlusions can be due a primary or infiltrating malignancies or because compression of the ureter by an extra-ureteral mass.

The fact is that the most used stent in the urinary tract is the *double-J stent* (JJ) or its variations such as the *pig-tail stents*. To reduce the confusion between the double-J and other urinary tract stents I will use the general term of *JJ stents* in this chapter.

D. Yachia (✉)
Department of Urology, Hillel Yaffe Medical Center, Hadera, Israel

Bruce Rappaport Faculty of Medicine, Technion, Haifa, Israel

Innoventions Ltd., Or Akiva, Israel
e-mail: dyachia@innoventions-med.com

© The Author(s) 2022
F. Soria et al. (eds.), *Urinary Stents*,
https://doi.org/10.1007/978-3-031-04484-7_28

Are there only JJs available to us? No. There are several other but much less used stents which are available for use in the urinary tract, such as large caliber metal coil stents or covered large caliber metal mesh stents. There are also self-expandable or balloon expandable metallic mesh stents originally developed for use in the vascular system.

The question is: Is it logical to insert a mesh stent when malignant tissues are compressing or infiltrating the ureteral lumen? Obviously, not. These are the reasons why there should be a separation between stenting ureters occluded by a *benign* or a *malignant* pathology for optimizing the outcome of the stenting.

In 1972, Goodwin described a stent being *"a mold made of a compound, for holding some form of a graft in place"* [1]. This was much before the wide use of the JJ which was invented by Finney in 1978 [2] and the other intraluminal stents developed since then and are in use in urology today.

One of the common mistakes we do as urologists is to think that any obstruction of the ureter can be managed by inserting a JJ. The truth is that in most cases the JJ provides an immediate but relatively short-term palliation for ureters obstructed by stones or by edema developing after endoscopic procedures. Their use becomes a discussion subject when we confront a chronic obstruction and our aim is to provide long term drainage to the kidneys. Even is such case the ethio-pathology causing the ureteral obstruction plays a role in our decision either using a JJ or another kind of stent. Today we pass a JJ beside a stone, or through the narrowed passage caused by a benign or malignant stricture either causing external compression or infiltrating the ureteral wall, for immediate relieve of the obstruction. The same is done in urethral obstructions. In such cases we pass a urethral catheter for draining the bladder. These are short-term *palliative* problem solving activities.

In cases of benign narrowing of the urethra like in BPH or external non-malignant ureteral compressions caused by retroperitoneal fibrosis, or in infiltrating or compressing malignant obstructions in the ureter, what is needed is insertion of a large caliber stent into the obstructed segment for long periods or even permanently for re-creating a large ureteral lumen. In benign, intrinsic ureteral stenosis the aim is to create not only long-term drainage but also re-shaping of the ureteric lumen, which can be accepted as *curative stenting*. The same occur also in urethral obstructions, either due to benign or malignant prostatic obstructions or in distal urethral strictures. All these are for allowing free flow of the urine.

The use of JJs in urology preceded the use of metallic mesh stents developed for the vascular system. However, the vascular stents became much more popular and common treatment option for opening occlusions of the coronary and cerebral arteries, the carotid, iliac and femoral arteries.

In the vascular system stents started to be used for ensuring the patency of compromised arteries to allow blood flow for bringing oxygen and other vital compounds to organs.

When we look to the history of vascular stents we see that it was Julio Palmaz, an interventional vascular radiologist, who invented the balloon-expandable stent in 1985 [3]. This was followed by the Wallstent which is a self-expanding vascular stent, invented by Hans Wallsten who was not a physician. The Wallstent was first used in the vascular system by Ulrich Sigwart in 1986 [4].

The successful use of vascular stents, gradually took the place of certain cardio-vascular surgical procedures, saving the lives of many patients in a minimally invasive way.

This great success induced an idea in urology that said: *"If it is good for the vascular system, it is also good for the urinary system"*. Based on this idea some urologists thought that such stents may have possible promising implications in urinary tract stenting. This was first described in 1991 by Lugmayr and Pauer who started a new approach for relieving ureteric obstruction [5]. Then several additional reports of successful placement of mesh stents in the urinary tract were published [6, 7].

However, these stents were used predominantly in patients with extrinsic malignant compression of the ureter who had limited life expectancy [8, 9]. Even at that time, Lugmayr and Pauer noted that at the site of the stent implantation they observed transient mucosal edema and tissue hyperplasia causing short term obstruction, and that these obstructions disappeared after the stent wires became fully incorporated into the urothelium. There were also early reports that showed, when used in the ureter the uncovered metal wires of these stents developed encrustations and created obstructions in the stent lumen [5, 10].

Others reported long-term urothelial hyperplasia resulting in obstruction, necessitating insertion of a double-J sent to reestablish lumen patency [11, 12] or removing the encrustations occluding the mesh stent [13]. A problem with bare metallic mesh stents used in the urinary tract is the bare wires remaining uncovered by urothelium, which frequently can happen at the ends of such stents, becoming a starting point for stone formation. A typical case was reported by Smrkolj and Šalinović, in which a patient was, inserted a nitinol mesh stent in the ureteropelvic junction in 2000 after failure of two pyeloplasty procedures. The patient returned 15 years later with a 35 mm stone encrusted on the mesh stent and a hardly functioning kidney [14].

Early experience also showed that balloon-expandable stents developed more urothelial hyperplasia, limiting their use in the ureter [15, 16]. There was even a report on the use of a high-frequency *rotablator* (a miniature drill capped with an abrasive, diamond-studded burr which is commonly used to pulverize hardened plaque within a coronary artery) for removing the occluding ingrown hyperplastic tissue in a ureteral mesh stent [17]. Despite the experience showing such complications, the enthusiasm around using metal mesh stents in arteries drove some urologists to use similar stents in the urinary tract. Such stents were implanted into the tubular structures of the urinary tract such as the ureter, the prostatic, bulbar and more distal parts of the urethra even in patients who had not a short life expectancy having benign narrowings [12, 18–20].

Then came the era of drug eluting vascular stents reducing hyperplastic reactions of the endothelium and resulting vascular re-stenosis. These encouraging results with the drug eluting vascular stents induced a new hope in urologists to use similar stents in the urinary tract [21, 22].

2   Vascular Tract vs. Urinary Tract

It is obvious that not all tubular organs in the body have the same anatomy/histology and physiology, and that the lumen narrowing seen in blood vessels are drastically different than the ones seen in the ureter, urethra, or in the bile duct or the esophagus. Each tubular organ in the body has a different anatomy and also different histological and functional properties. Although both the ureter and the urethra are tubular structures, they are NOT similar to an artery or to any other body tube.

Can we expect a stent designed for the vascular system be as effective in the ureter or the urethra as it is in an artery? It may be, but for only several hours, or until the ureteral or urethral tissues start to react to the geometry and to the material of a metallic mesh stent designed for the vascular system or until the malignant tissue infiltrates through the mesh of the stent.

The pathophysiology of lumen narrowing in arteries is completely different than the narrowing of the ureteral lumen. In arteries the narrowing is mainly caused by "*atheromatous plaques*" which are made up of cholesterol and calcified material build-up in the luminal wall or by neointimal hyperplasia caused by proliferation and migration of vascular smooth muscle cells that create a thickening of the arterial wall. Where ureteral occlusion or narrowing are entirely different pathologies. A ureter can be occluded by a stone and these occlusions is relieved by passing a JJ beside the stone until definitive treatment. Traumatic fibrosis of the ureter is mainly caused by diagnostic or therapeutic endo-ureteral manipulations. Rarer reasons are iatrogenic injuries during abdominal surgery, retroperitoneal fibrosis encasing the ureter or peri-ureteral tumors compression or infiltrating the ureters. Differing from the vascular system, the urinary tract is an actively functioning system where each part of it has different anatomies and functionalities.

In the urinary tract stents are used to ensure the patency of compromised urine flow. In the ureter they allow to drain urine from the kidneys to the bladder and all along the urethra to allow unobstructed bladder emptying.

Let's compare an artery with the ureter, which is the most stented part of the urinary tract, and also the urethral segments.

The urinary system has an entirely different anatomy and physiology than the vascular system. Starting from the ureteropelvic junction, down to the intravesical part, the ureter has different segments with varying diameters ever-changing with each passing peristaltic wave for moving forward the urine. Compared with the ureters, arteries with their very gradual decreasing lumen are almost inactive tubes allowing blood pumped by the heart to flow forward. Histologically the layers of the ureter are different than the arterial layers. The cross section of the ureter has a "star-shaped" lumen surrounded by 2–5 cell thick urothelium and 2 layers of smooth muscle for the proximal 2/3 of its length, and 3 layers of muscle for the final 1/3 of its length toward the bladder. These smooth muscles (muscularis propria) contracts in a peristaltic movement to advance the urine from the kidney to bladder. The *urothelium* covering the lumen of the urinary tract is the most impermeable epithelial barrier in the body. In contrast, the endothelium performs a vital task of providing nutrients to the underlying tissue as well as maintaining tissue oncotic pressure [23].

Although it never happens, in a living organism the lumen of an artery keeps its tubular shape with an open lumen even if no blood flows through it. Hydrodynamically urine acts different than the blood dynamics. Differing from the blood pressure that advances its flow, the pressure in the urine bolus is determined primarily by the pressure created by ureteral peristalsis needed to separate the walls of the collapsed ureter.

The lumen lining the urethra also varies depending on the anatomical section: The prostatic urethra is lined by urothelial cells with patches of stratified columnar epithelium. The membranous urethra which passes through the external sphincter and the penile urethra are lined by stratified columnar and pseudostratified columnar epithelium and the most distal penile urethra is lined with non-keratinized stratified squamous cells.

Can the flow dynamics of continuous arterial blood flow and the changes of intra-arterial pressure be compared with the dynamics of urine during urination which is initiated by bladder contraction and simultaneous relaxation of the urethral sphincters? Where the daily amount of urine transported through the ureters can change in each individual during a single day, depending on the liquid intake affecting the amount of urine excreted from the kidneys, also related to the body and environmental temperature etc. How the urethra through which urine passes once every 2–4 or 6 h can be compared to a blood vessel?

Blood flowing through the arteries has a viscosity and it contains a large collection of living cells that interact with one another. Changes in blood flow occur during systole and diastole. Blood flows quicker at peak-systole because it is physically thinner, and at end-diastole it flows slower because it becomes 2–4 times thicker because of the aggregation of the red cells [24, 25]. This occurs 50–70 times a minute, with blood advancing through the arteries even at diastole. In contrast, without a peristaltic wave moving a bolus of urine, the ureter is empty and in a collapsed state. Since its lumen calibre changes along all its length and during peristaltic movements, the chances of a bare metal stent being completely embedded into the ureteral wall by pushing itself into the wall are low. In most cases parts of the mesh stents remain bare in the ureteral lumen. Because its high lithogenicity, urinary crystals start to depose on the exposed stent wires and form a stone.

Another reason to my opposition for using a permanent stent in the urinary tract is that they become an implant. Even the best foreign body, with time start to cause problems. To believe that it will remain an "innocent implant" for long years is at least a wishful thinking. Even the most solid hip or knee joint implants have to be changed after 10–15 years. If we decide to implant a stent in a segment of the urinary tract, we have to take into account the possibility that in case of an obstructive complication we will have to excise the implanted segment of the ureter or the urethra and do a reconstructive surgery.

Vast experimental and then clinical work showed that the anti-proliferative drug eluting balloons and mesh stents could reduce most arterial re-stenoses. These results created the hope that drugs, like Zotarolimus or Paclitaxel coated stents can be used also in the urinary tract. A study done on porcine and rabbit ureter showed that compared with bare metal stents, these animals developed lower hyperplastic reactions in the ureter [26]. Additional studies were done by the same group to see distribution of Paclitaxel in porcine ureters and rabbit urethras [22, 27].

Both studies indicated that when Paclitaxel coated balloons were inflated in a healthy ureter or urethra, a distribution of the drug was observed in all its layers. The theory behind these experiments was to show the possible use of antiproliferative drugs eluted by high pressure balloons or by stents coated with such drugs in ureteral and urethral strictures, and expect the results obtained in stenosed arteries. Although these findings looked encouraging, they could not prove that the same distribution will occur in the tense fibrous tissues causing the ureteral and urethral strictures. Stent occlusion due to tumor in-growth as well as "overgrowth" was observed with bare metal mesh stents [28]. It is well known that in most recurrent urethral strictures, all urethral layers, and even the peri-urethral spongious tissues become fibrotic. The same deep fibrosis occurs in traumatic/iatrogenic ureteral strictures. These fibrotic scar tissues are entirely different than the connective tissue formation in the smooth muscle layer of an artery that can be managed by drug eluting balloons or stents.

3   Conclusions

In reality, most stents inserted into any place in the body are needed only for relatively short- or long-term. Then they need to be removed. This is true also for the stents used in the vascular tract. But since they are not easily accessible and since they are embedded in the vascular wall, they cannot be removed. In the vascular system, re-entry for stent removal is risky. So, nowadays vascular stents are permanently implanted. If they become occluded their patency are re-created by balloon dilatation with or without implantation of an additional stent (stent-in-stent).

I recommend to be realistic when looking to the facts and not be like typical parents believing that their baby *"is the most beautiful and smartest child"*.

Before using a permanent stent along the urinary tract we should think hard about what may happen to a ureter or urethra implanted with a permanent metallic mesh stent. This is especially important when something goes wrong like when the stent lumen becomes obliterated by hyperplastic or malignant tissues, the stent wires fracture, or tissue coverage over the stent wires is incomplete and the resulting stone formation on the wires, ureteral or urethral perforations etc.

My almost three decades long experience in using and developing two generations of stents thought me that all stents to be used in the urinary tract needs to be either removable or bioabsorbable/biodegradable. The current technology does not allow replacement of a part of the urinary tract with metal parts like doing a knee or hip joint replacement.

From the beginning of the early 1990s my approach was that, whatever their configuration, since the vascular stents are permanent implants, using them in the urinary tract is an erroneous concept. Even when the drug eluting mesh stents started to be used anywhere in the urinary tract my approach did not change.

Since my involvement with prostatic urethral stents started in the middle 1980s, first using the *Prostacath* in prostatic obstructions, and then the self-expandable metallic *ProstaCoil* or *UroCoil stents* in prostatic or urethral strictures. I defended my thesis that the urinary tract doesn't need a permanent stent, because the entire collecting system of the urinary tract is accessible, allowing their easy removal after a certain length of time. This become more possible with the introduction of the self-expanding covered Allium stents and the Uventa stent in the early 2010s.

Therapeutically when a large caliber stent is to be used in the urinary tract, the aim is not only allowing urine drainage through the narrowing but also re-shaping the narrowed segment by acting as a cast, when left in place until the ureter or urethra regenerates and its scarring process stabilizes. Those defending the use of permanent stents always mentioned their successful use in blood vessels, but less the complications they created even in them. It is wrong thinking that the various obstructive problems along the ureter can be solved by using a *single shape stent*, no matter from which material it is done or drug it is coated. Because, differing from the vascular system, in the urinary system *'one shape, does not fit all'*.

My approach is still that, since vascular stents are permanently implanted devices, before using them in the urinary tract, we need to have clear proofs that the urothelium will react the same way as the vascular endothelium reacts to the stent and that the stent will become completely covered. We should take great care in using even a drug coated metal stent before clear and approved studies on its efficacy to the urothelium are proved.

This is not so simple.

Biodegradable stents were tried in the past but they failed clinically. If such stents will be available and will show that they do not collapse and occlude the ureter or the urethra, then a new era in long-term ureteral or urethral stenting will start. So far stent technologists could not develop an effective dissolvable or absorbable vascular stent that will keep its physical properties until they disappear.

By adopting the vascular stent technologies, we were hoping that taking a single stent shape, changing its length and caliber they could be used all along the urinary tract. Then asking ourselves, *why the results were less than what we were expecting*. Here I would like to requote a sentence attributed to Albert Einstein: *"Insanity is doing the same thing over and over again and expecting different results."*

References

1. Goodwin WE. Splint, stent, stint. Urol Dig. 1972;11:13–4.
2. Finney RP. Experience with 'double J' ureteral catheter stent. J Urol. 1978;120:678–81.
3. Palmaz JC, Sibbitt RR, Reuter SR, Tio FO, Rice WJ. Expandable intraluminal graft: a preliminary study. Work in progress. Radiology. 1985;156:73–7.
4. Sigwart U, et al. Intravascular stents to prevent occlusion and restenosis after transluminal angioplasty. N Engl J Med. 1987;316:701–6.
5. Lugmayr H, Pauer W. Self-expanding metallic stents in malignant ureteral stenosis. Deutsche Medizinische Wochenschrift. 1991;116:573–6.
6. Flueckiger F, et al. Malignant ureteral obstruction: preliminary results of treatment with metallic self-expandable stents. Radiology. 1993;186:169–73.
7. Reinberg Y, Ferral H, Gonzalez R, et al. Intraureteral metallic self-expanding endoprosthesis (Wallstent) in the treatment of difficult ureteral strictures. J Urol. 1994;151(6):1619–22.

8. López-Martínez RA, et al. The use of metallic stents to bypass ureteral strictures secondary to metastatic prostate cancer: experience with 8 patients. J Urol. 1997;158:50–3.
9. Lang EK, et al. Placement of metallic stents in ureters obstructed by carcinoma of the cervix to maintain renal function in patients undergoing long-term chemo-therapy. Am J Roentgen. 1998;171:1595–9.
10. Pauer W, Lugmayr H. Metallic Wallstents: a new therapy for extrinsic ureteral obstruction. J Urol. 1992;148:281–4.
11. Burgos FJ, et al. Self-expanding metallic ureteral stents for treatment of ureteral stenosis after kidney transplantation. Transplant Proc. 2005;37:3828–9.
12. Daskalopoulos G, et al. Intraureteral metallic endoprosthesis in the treatment of ureteral strictures. Eur J Radiol. 2001;39:194–200.
13. Pauer W, Kerbl K. Self-expanding permanent endoluminal stents in the ureter: technical considerations. Tech Urol. 1995;1:67–71.
14. Smrkolj T, Šalinović D, et al. Endoscopic removal of a nitinol mesh stent from the ureteropelvic junction after 15 years. Case Rep Urol. 2015;2015:273614.
15. Barbalias GA, et al. Metal stents: a new treatment of malignant ureteral obstruction. J Urol. 1997;158:54–8.
16. Hekimoğlu B, et al. Urothelial hyperplasia complicating use of metal stents in malignant ureteral obstruction. Eur. Radiol. 1996;6:675–81.
17. Protzel C, et al. High frequency rotablation as a new therapeutic procedure for obstructed metallic ureter stents. J Urol. 2001;166:1399–400.
18. Barbalias GA, et al. Ureteropelvic junction obstruction: an innovative approach combining metallic stenting and virtual endoscopy. J Urol. 2002;168:2383–6.
19. Trinchieri A, Montanari E, Ceresoli A, et al. Permanent stenting in the treatment of ureteral strictures. Ann Urol. 1999;33:186–91.
20. Al-Aown A, et al. Ureteral stents: new ideas, new designs. Ther Adv Urol. 2010;2:85–92.
21. Liourdi D, et al. Evaluation of the distribution of paclitaxel by immunohisto-chemistry and nuclear magnetic resonance spectroscopy after the application of a drug-eluting balloon in the porcine ureter. J Endourol. 2015;29:580–9.
22. Barbalias D, et al. Evaluation of the distribution of paclitaxel after application of a paclitaxel-coated balloon in the rabbit urethra. J Endourol. 2018;32:381–6.
23. Sukriti S, et al. Mechanisms regulating endothelial permeability. Pulm Circ. 2014;4:535–51.
24. Letcher R, et al. Direct relationship between blood pressure and blood viscosity in normal and hypertensive subjects. Role of fibrinogen and concentration. Am J Med. 1981;70:1195–202.
25. Fowkes FGR, et al. The relationship between blood viscosity and blood pressure in a random sample of the population aged 55 to 74 years. Eur Heart J. 1993;14(5):597–601.
26. Kallidonidis P, et al. Evaluation of zotarolimus-eluting metal stent in animal ureters. J Endourol. 2011;25:1661–7.
27. Liourdi D, et al. Evaluation of the distribution of paclitaxel by immunohistochemistry and nuclear magnetic resonance spectroscopy after the application of a drug-eluting balloon in the porcine ureter. J Endourol. 2015;29:580–9.
28. Lang EK, et al. Long-term results of metallic stents for malignant ureteral obstruction in advanced cervical carcinoma. J Endourol. 2013;27:646–51.

Biodegradable Urinary Stents

Federico Soria, Julia E. de la Cruz, Marcos Cepeda, Álvaro Serrano,
and Francisco M. Sánchez-Margallo

1 Introduction

In the twenty-first century, it is difficult to understand that a medical device as
widely used as urinary stents require a second medical procedure for removal. When
both ureteral and urethral stents are in direct contact with a fluid like urine. These
characteristics should be used for their degradation by a simple controlled hydrolysis reaction.

Research in the development of biocompatible biodegradable urinary stents
(BUS) has been one of the most important research areas of innovation in the stent
technology. The main characteristics of a BUS are related to its ability to degrade
into non-obstructive fragments in a predefined time and to be removed through micturition, after providing an appropriate internal scaffold effect and urinary drainage
[1]. The main beneficial effect of this type of stent is the avoidance of a second
medical procedure for removal, which reduces stress for patients and makes them
less reluctant to undergo stenting in the future. It also overcomes the difficulties that
in some cases are associated with the removal of a conventional ureteral stent,
mainly in those with encrustations [2]. It should also be highlighted that, in the
subpopulation of children, where sedation is necessary for stent removal, the risks
and associated costs are reduced [1, 3]. Finally, another advantage provided by
BUSs is the decrease in indirect healthcare costs. First, by avoiding the classic cystoscopic removal procedure, and second, by lowering the costs associated with the

F. Soria (✉) · J. E. de la Cruz · F. M. Sánchez-Margallo
Foundation, Jesús Usón Minimally Invasive Surgery Center, Cáceres, Spain
e-mail: fsoria@ccmijesususon.com

M. Cepeda
Urology Department, Hospital Universitario Rio Hortega, Valladolid, Spain

Á. Serrano
Urology Department, Hospital Clínico San Carlos, Madrid, Spain

© The Author(s) 2022
F. Soria et al. (eds.), *Urinary Stents*,
https://doi.org/10.1007/978-3-031-04484-7_29

management of complications caused by urinary stents, particularly those related to the treatment of calcified or forgotten stents. The latter can be up to six times more expensive than uncomplicated cystoscopic removal of the ureteral stent [3, 4].

Specific circumstances occur in relation to urethral stents, as they are nowadays generally permanent, so their removal is not the main benefit sought with the development of these devices. The main indications are therefore to allow their temporary use and to reduce the side effects associated with urethral or prostate metallic stents, such as obstructive urothelial hyperplasia [5].

An important desired characteristic of the BUSs is to add to their predictable and controlled degradation capacity other beneficial characteristics, such as the possibility of local drug release or the possibility of becoming the first bio-coated urinary stent designs. In this way, they aim to combine the innovation of a biodegradable stent with the reduction of adverse effects, as well as properties that allow for the extension of stent-associated therapeutics. Biodegradable urethral stents with tissue therapy applications for adjuvant treatment of urethral strictures, as well as the delivery of chemotherapy to the upper urinary tract, are technological developments currently under discussion at [6].

2   Ideal Biodegradable Urinary Stent

The characteristics that a BUS must show are mainly a biodegradable character in relation to its indications. That is, it must show a stable and functional structure, which allows it to maintain its mechanical properties during the degradation time. It should also favour urinary drainage and its important function as a ureteral or urethral tutor as an internal scaffold [1, 7, 8]. It should be highlighted that a BUS is not degradable from the first moment of its placement, and therefore behaves in its first phases as a biostable stent, although once its degradation phase has begun, the biomaterials and their architecture should ensure its stability and functionality.

Obviously, the biomaterials of these stents must be stable and biocompatible in the urinary tract [1, 7]. Both the BUS biomaterials and its metabolites must not lack mutagenic, carcinogenic, antigenic, toxic effects, or present the possibility of being absorbed through the urothelium [1, 7, 8].

Its design and mechanical characteristics must ensure that the BUS remains in place without migration. But these characteristics must be compatible with easy insertion, both at ureteral and urethral lumen, as well as in urinary obstructions [7]. Furthermore, an important consideration for suitable patient follow-up is that an ideal BUS should show good tracing ability under X-ray and ultrasound (Fig. 1).

However, if there is one characteristic of an ideal BUS, it is that it should be completely biodegradable. In this regard, both the biomaterials and the design of the BUS must provide a predictable and controlled degradation in urinary tract. This controlled degradation phenomenon is the cornerstone of an ideal BUS, as its degradation rate must be predictable to fulfil its indication, but it must also be safe.

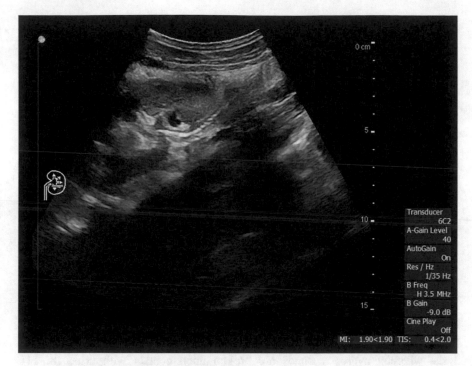

Fig. 1 Ultrasound ureteral BUS assessment. BraidStent®

Therefore, the degradation fragments must be easily washed out in the urine and never embedded or retained. Another ideal requirement is that once the degradation phase has started, the urine should be stained, never red, so that the degradation phase can be easily monitored by the patient [1, 7, 8].

Ideal BUSs should allow coating with antibacterial contamination inhibiting agents, as well as allow drug release for topical adjuvant therapy, or allow tissue engineering therapy. The ideal biodegradable stent should also maintain its characteristics unchanged after the required sterilisation process and have a reasonable manufacturing cost [8–10] (Table 1).

Unfortunately, none of the technological developments have provided the ideal BUS. Although many advances in design and improvements in mechanical characteristics and biocompatibility have been made in the last decade, one of the main drawbacks for the development of a clinically useful BUS is the lack of control and prediction of device degradation [1]. This is due to the fact that the urinary tract represents a changing environment, depending on each individual and the disease condition, and all these factors affect the degradation process of the BUS [8].

Table 1 Ideal biodegradable urinary stent

• Excellent biocompatibility
• Moderate mechanical properties
• Complete biodegradation without obstructive fragments
• Prevent migration
• Good flexibility for stent delivery
• Good tracing ability under X-ray and ultrasound
• Urine dye (never red)
• Control degradation rate
• No mutagenic, antigenic, carcinogenic or toxic degradation metabolites
• Be affordable
• The stent must retain all its characteristics after the sterilisation process
• Allow drug release

3   Biodegradables Biomaterials

As has been described in depth in previous chapters (Chapter "Biomaterials for ureteral stents: advances and future perspectives"), the main biomaterials used for the manufacture of BUS are summarised, as well as the degradation mechanisms. The main degradation mechanism of biomaterials used in the urinary tract is hydrolysis, whereby hydrogen bonds are broken upon contact with urine [8, 11]. Degradation by hydrolysis is influenced by a multitude of factors, including: changes in urinary pH, urine composition, variations in patients' fluid intake and the nature of those fluids, and the characteristics of the polymeric biodegradable biomaterial to absorb moisture into its interior, as this last characteristic is responsible for the degradation kinetics [8, 11]. The other main degradation mechanism of BUSs is the biological one that causes the breakdown of biodegradable polymers by enzymatic reactions. No BUS has an exclusive biodegradation mechanism, although there is always one of them that is responsible for the highest percentage of degradation.

So, in summary, biodegradable polymers in the urinary tract first undergo a destabilisation of their bonds causing fragmentation. In this first step, the biomaterial does not lose its biomechanical characteristics. However, further hydrolytic degradation of the chemical bonds causes a loss of molecular weight triggering polymer fragmentation.

The most common biomaterials are natural polymers, synthetics and metals.

3.1   Natural Biomaterials

The use of gelatine, alginate, gellan gum or their combinations has proven to be an attractive material due to its biocompatibility and low immunogenicity [12]. In particular, alginate, a linear polysaccharide from marine algae, due to its high capacity to form hydrogels, is frequently used in the manufacture of medical devices. The most recently described BUS from biomaterials of exclusively natural origin have been developed by the research group of Barros et al. in Portugal [10, 13–15].

3.2 Synthetic Biodegradable Biomaterials

Biodegradable polymers of synthetic origin are the most frequently used by BUS research groups. Their main advantages are their evident biocompatibility, as well as the absence of immunogenicity, carcinogenicity, teratogenicity and toxicity [16]. The most frequently used synthetic polymers are: polylactic acid (PLA), polyglycolic acid (PGA), PLGA, PCL and polydioxanone (PDX). PLA and PCL have excessively slow degradation times, while the degradation rates of PGA and PDX are relatively fast, with degradation times from weeks to months [1, 17]. PLA is a polymer that has been widely used for the manufacture of medical devices due to its low toxicity, as it generates lactic acid as a metabolite [18, 19]. In addition, it has good mechanical properties, but a degradation rate of 4–6 months is a limitation for clinical use [20–22]. PGA is a slow degrading linear aliphatic polyester that has shown very favourable results with regard to bacterial adhesion and encrustation [12, 22].

Regarding the copolymers, they are more easily degradable than the individual polymers [22]. PLGA is polymerised with glycolic acid and lactic acid in different proportions, thus combining the advantages of both compounds [1]. Due to its excellent properties, PLGA has been evaluated in combination with other polymers for the manufacture of BUS [22]. Recently, the combination of PLGA and PGA has been analysed in vitro, showing that by heat treatment of the polymer cross-linker an ideal crystallisation of PGA is achieved, providing longer degradation times [23]. As well as that the combinations in the ratio between PGA and PLGA allow to control the mechanical properties of the stent [24].

3.3 Metallic Biodegradable Biomaterials

Magnesium (Mg^{2+}) and its alloys have been widely investigated as a material for biodegradable medical devices. However, the fast degradation of Mg-based alloys in a physiological environment has hindered their widespread use [25]. Lock et al. confirmed the use of Mg^{2+} alloy for BUS development. Their results showed that Mg^{2+} has suitable mechanical and antimicrobial properties for manufacturing BUS ureteral stents. However, corrosion control of the Mg^{2+} alloy remains an challenge [26]. Although recently, it has been demonstrated the corrosion rate of magnesium can be tailored by alloying elements, surface treatments and heat treatments [25].

4   Biodegradable Ureteral Stent

The aims for the development of a ureteral BUS are very clear and have been described earlier in this chapter. However, currently the absence of ureteral BUSs in daily clinical practice is mainly due to the complicated degradation rate control, maintenance of mechanical properties and safe urinary excretion of stent fragments [27].

One of the barriers slowing down the progress of research was already described in 2000 and concerns the lack of agreement between in vitro and in vivo degradation rates demonstrated in a large number of experimental studies [21]. Mainly because research in animal models presents changing conditions of urine characteristics, interaction with the urothelium, bacterial contamination and because of the intrinsic hydrodynamic characteristics of the urinary tract that have been poorly investigated in vitro [8]. Fortunately, all biomaterials used in the development of ureteral BUSs have shown adequate biocompatibility, largely because synthetic polymers had already demonstrated their use in medical devices [8].

Nowadays, the research groups focused on this line of research are very well defined and, although they have not achieved a ureteral BUS for clinical use, they have made relevant advances in this area.

Early research (1999–2000) emerged from studies by the research group of Lumiaho et al., developing ureteral BUSs composed of SR-PLA and SR-PLGA polymers [27, 28]. The results showed good biocompatibility of the stents, but also a high tendency to migrate due to weaknesses in the mechanical properties of the stent. They also showed a long-term degradation time of more than 24 weeks with a high risk of hydronephrosis [21, 28]. Subsequently, another group developed a clinical trial with the placement of a ureteral BUS in patients undergoing percutaneous nephrolithotomy [29]. These stents showed proper urine drainage at 48 h and degraded at one month, with only distal migration [29]. However, a subsequent clinical trial did not yield satisfactory results, as 20% of the TUDS® ureteral stents (Boston Scientific Corporation, USA) migrated and 22% failed to maintain adequate urine drainage. Additionally, stent fragments were retained for more than 3 months, which required extracorporeal lithotripsy and ureteroscopy for resolution [30].

Progressing from the first innovations in this area of knowledge, one of the most important research groups should be highlighted. Chew and Lange et al., who have developed the Uriprene® BUS, having improved this stent after three generations of evolution [31–33]. The 2008 evaluation of the first generation of Uriprene® in a porcine model showed favourable biocompatibility and degradation without obstructive fragments [31]. Limitations of this first generation Uriprene® were a 16% migration rate, a degradation time of 10 weeks and a slight obstructive activity [31]. In addition, a drawback was that unlike standard stents, Uriprene® had to be inserted through a ureteral access sheath. In later studies, this research group developed two more generations that were evaluated in animal models, technological innovations focused on changing the ratio and composition of the biomaterials to achieve shorter degradation times and to provide sufficient strength for placement of the BUS coaxially to a guidewire [33]. Both the second and third generation Uriprene® had adequate axial and radial strength for successful insertion [32, 33].

Other groups have developed electrospinning ureteral BUSs made from PCL and PLGA [17]. Analysis of safety and degradation in vivo in a porcine model demonstrated that degradation begins at 4 weeks from the distal end of the stent and progresses proximally up to day 10 weeks, causing significantly less hydronephrosis, inflammation and urothelial irritation in a comparative study compared to a conventional ureteral stent [34]. Designs of this nature that allow control over the section of the stent that degrades is an important development in the design of BUSs, as it promotes the maintenance of the internal scaffold while allowing for controlled stent degradation.

One of the most promising groups in the development of ureteral BUSs is Barros et al., from 3B's Research Group and the company HydruMedical in Portugal. Their ureteral BUS is manufactured with polymers of natural origin, having completed extensive studies in vitro and in a porcine animal model [10, 13–15]. The stent showed homogeneous degradation without impairing urinary flow. Studies in a porcine model demonstrated better pathological results compared to a conventional ureteral stent, showing the ideal biocompatibility of these natural materials [14]. However, the problems that currently limit the therapeutic application of this device are its short time, its poor radiopacity and a progressive loss of stability during the degradation process. This same device has been modified by this group to give it the capacity to release ketoprofen, allowing the local application of substances to reduce the morbidity associated with ureteral stents in in vitro studies [35]. Another innovation of this research group is a drug-eluting ureteral BUS for the topical adjuvant treatment of low-grade upper urinary tract urothelial carcinoma, which has also been evaluated in tumoral cell culture studies [15].

The most widely described ureteral BUS in the scientific literature is the BraidStent® developed by our research group, Soria and de la Cruz. In contrast to other BUSs, our stent is intraureteral, which reduces the morbidity associated with ureteral stents, as it does not cause VUR (vesicoureteral reflux) or LUTS (lower urinary tract symptoms) [36, 37] (Fig. 2). This ureteral BUS is composed of a combination of polymers and copolymers of PGA and Glycomer 631 combined together and arranged in a braided design to provide a different degradation rate between both biomaterials, avoiding obstructive size fragments and the sudden loss of the mechanical properties of the stent [7, 37]. Its main indication is to promote upper urinary tract drainage and to serve as an internal scaffold for healing after ureteral surgery [8]. Early results from the evaluation of BraidStent® in a porcine model demonstrated a predictable and controlled degradation rate between the third and sixth week, with no evidence of obstructive events during the hydrolysis of the biomaterials [7, 38] (Figs. 3 and 4). These good results are due to the cross-linked stent architecture and the combination of two polymers with different degradation rates. A remarkable aspect of this BUS is that it does not affect distal ureteral peristalsis, preserving distal peristalsis in up to 83% of ureters. This is great progress for patients, as it would probably avoid ureteral spasm, which is one of the main causes

Fig. 2 Biodegradable
ureteral stent. BraidStent®

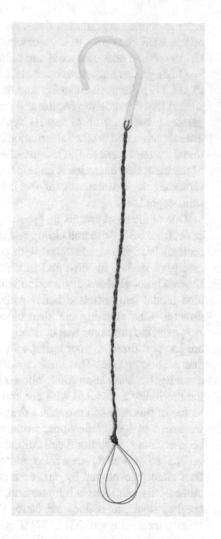

of pain in patients, as well as decrease the requirement for alpha-blockers or anti-muscarinic drugs [7]. These good results contrast with a high rate of migration and asymptomatic bacteriuria, never UTI, shown in early studies. To reduce these undesirable effects, the BraidStent® was coated with heparin, a well-know bacterial anti-adhesive agent. In the three experimental studies evaluating BraidStent®-H in 2021, in a comparative study versus a conventional ureteral stent, in the adjuvant treatment of ureteral perforation and after endourological treatment of ureteral strictures, the coated BUS maintains the positive characteristics previously shown [39–41]. However, although heparin coating reduces the early asymptomatic bacteriuria rate, it increases again in the long term. This demonstrates the inability of heparin to reduce bacterial contamination (Fig. 5).

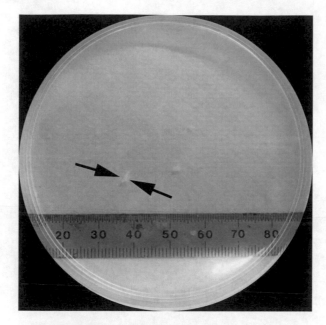

Fig. 3 In vitro assessment of degradation fragments. BraidStent®

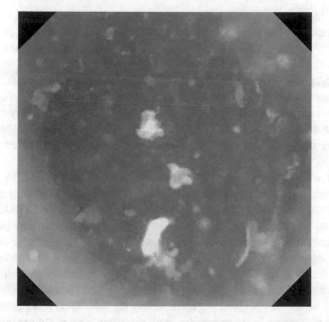

Fig. 4 Cystoscopic view. In vivo assessment of degradation fragments. BraidStent®

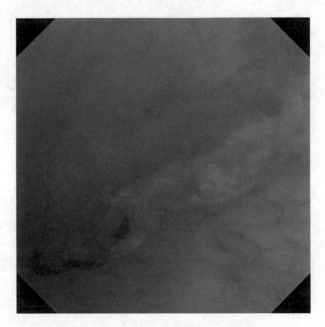

Fig. 5 Ureteroscopic view. Porcine animal model assessment of BraidStent®

In order to alleviate the weak mechanical properties of degradable biomaterials in recent years, in-depth research has been carried out on metallic BUS. In this respect, Mg^{2+} and its alloys (Mg–Sr–Ag), polyurethane and Magnesium alloys have been used in in vitro and in vivo studies. These metallic BUS demonstrate good biocompatibility, high strength and homogeneous corrosion rate. With degradation rates ranging from 4 to 14 weeks depending on the alloy [42, 43]. An important advantage of this type of BUS with Mg^{2+} alloys is that they show a significantly antibacterial activity in upper urinary tract. For these reasons, magnesium alloys have become excellent candidate material for manufacturing BUS [42–45].

Another area of current research is the emergence of ureteral BUS to provide a new approach for local drug delivery in upper urinary tract. Drugs may be released while the stent is degrading. In this regard, Barros et al. developed a BUS to deliver different anti-tumour agents: paclitaxel, doxorubicin, epirubicin and gemcitabine [15]. Cell culture studies confirmed that these drug-eluted degradable stents could efficiently suppress the growth of T24 urothelial cancer cells. Our group has also developed the biodegradable BraidStent®-MMC, which delivers Mitomycin C for the adjuvant treatment of low grade upper tract urothelial carcinoma (Fig. 6). These innovations, in addition to avoiding a secondary stent removal procedure, allow the release of anti-tumour drugs, preventing their systemic administration and their side effects [46]. Following the same line of innovation on BUS-DES (drug eluting stent), another design that has been evaluated in an animal model is a BUS with mTOR inhibitor-eluting to reduce the progression of fibrosis proteins in ureteral stricture by means of rapamicyn release [47].

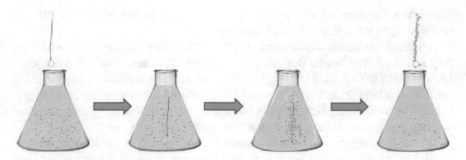

Fig. 6 BUS coating. BraidStent®-MMC

5   Biodegradable Urethral Stent

Despite their use to improve drainage of the lower urinary tract, metallic stents have shown significant side effects: migration, obstruction due to urothelial hyperplasia, encrustation and urinary tract infection. As a result, they cause a significant decrease in quality of life, thus reducing their therapeutic use [48].

In order to overcome the limitations of metallic stents, the development of BDG urethral stents was started. The main indications of these BUS devices are:

– Temporary treatment of urinary retention, pending prostate surgery.
– Treatment of urethral strictures, as an adjuvant to endoscopic urethrotomy or in cases of recurrence.
– After BPH treatment, to ensure urinary drainage [6].
– Scaffold for tissue engineering.

The first clinical efficacy studies of BUS prostatic coil stents were performed with PGA and initially achieved better voiding outcomes compared to a suprapubic catheter. However, the early loss of biomechanical properties inherent to this polymer caused voiding flow to decrease, concurrent with stent degradation [49]. To improve the results, another polymer with a slower degradation rate, PLA, was chosen. Showing good early results that were maintained over the long term, however, the degradation of this polymer was excessively long, 6 months [50]. Subsequently, other research groups demonstrated one of the main weaknesses of this type of urethral BUS, uncontrolled fragmentation of the stent caused infravesical obstruction.

After 10 years of clinical use of the urethral coil stent, a new braided tubular mesh design, similar to vascular stents, was developed to address the complications and weaknesses of early coil stent urethral BUS designs. These were mainly summarised as early migration; sudden collapse of the coil configuration in cases of recurrent stricture treatment, which induced urethral obstruction; fragments embedded in the mucosa after post-urethrotomy placement [51].

Early studies of this tubular stent were performed with PLA or PLGA. Although the new design shows a lower mass of polymeric material and its threads are three times thinner than the spiral stent, it fails to prevent the formation of urothelial hyperplasia [51]. The braided urethral BUS stent did not show any migration in experimental studies. Another improvement is that it does not require the use of a cystoscope, as it is released through an sheath [52].

Despite the advances shown during the first years of development of these stents, they still show weaknesses that preclude their use in patients. The two main problems relate to their limited efficacy in collapsing under pressure and their manifest inability to inhibit the initial fibrosis and polyposis associated with urothelial hyperplasia. One noteworthy fact is that, a biodegradable stent should be designed considering therapeutic force rather than initial force.

One of the suggested options to improve urethral stents is the addition of anti-inflammatory and anti-proliferative drugs. In vitro and animal model studies have been developed to evaluate drug-eluting stents with Dexamethasone, Indomethacin, Simvastatin, Ciprofloxacin and Sirolimus [52]. The latest study of a drug-eluting BUS is the use of Sirolimus to suppress granulation tissue formation after stent placement in a rat urethral model. The animal model study demonstrated suppression of urothelial hyperplasia formation secondary to urethral stent placement [5].

The tissue-engineered repair of urethral strictures with biodegradable stents is a recent research possibility and is perhaps the best approach to reduce complications in the treatment of urethral strictures. Previous studies have shown that cellularised BUS matrices are more effective than acellularised ones [53]. For this reason, Fu et al. developed a PLA-coated bioresorbable stent with autologous urothelial cells for urethral wall regeneration. At the end of the animal model study, 24 weeks, the regenerated urethral mucosa was indistinguishable from the control group and urodynamically there were no differences either [54].

This BUS–DES stent design represents the future in one of the urethral diseases with the worst prognosis, urethral strictures, as it will allow the delivery of cells and modulatory factors that facilitate healthy urethral healing [55].

6 Conclusions

The need to introduce these stents for hospital applications is crucial because of the benefits they provide to patients and the benefits in terms of reduced healthcare costs. Unfortunately, despite the significant progress that has been made recently, there are still limitations that need to be overcome, such as control of degradation rate and mechanical properties. The development of biodegradable metallic stents may be a line of research to overcome the current limitations of these stents. As well as the coating of stents to release drugs as they degrade in the urinary tract. Despite the necessary development that BUSs need, their future is very positive and near.

References

1. Wang L, Yang G, Xie H, Chen F. Prospects for the research and application of biodegradable ureteral stents: from bench to bedside. J Biomater Sci Polym Ed. 2018;29:1657–66.

2. Zong X, Ran S, Kim K-S, Fang D, Hsiao BS, Chu B. Structure and morphology changes during in vitro degradation of electrospun poly(glycolide-*co*-lactide) nanofiber membrane. Biomacromolecules. 2003;4:416–23.
3. De Grazia A, Somani BK, Soria F, Carugo D, Mosayyebi A. Latest advancements in ureteral stent technology. Transl Androl Urol. 2019;8:S436–41.
4. Sancaktutar AA, Soylemez H, Bozkurt Y, Penbegul N, Atar M. Treatment of forgotten ureteral stents: how much does it really cost? A cost-effectiveness study in 27 patients. Urol Res. 2012;40:317–25.
5. Kim KY, Park JH, Kim DH, Tsauo J, Kim MT, Son WC, Kang SG, Kim DH, Song HY. Sirolimus-eluting biodegradable poly-*l*-lactic acid stent to suppress granulation tissue formation in the rat urethra. Radiology. 2018;286(1):140–8.
6. Isotalo T, Talja M, Hellström P, Perttila I, Välimaa T, Törmälä P, Tammela TLJ. A double-blind, randomized, placebo-controlled pilot study to investigate the effects of finasteride combined with a biodegradable self-reinforced poly L-lactide acid spiral stent in patients with urinary retention caused by bladder outlet obstruction from benign prostatic hyperplasia. BJU Int. 2001;88:30–4.
7. Soria F, de la Cruz JE, Budía A, Serrano A, Galán-Llopis JA, Sánchez-Margallo FM. Experimental assessment of new generation of ureteral stents: biodegradable and antireflux properties. J Endourol. 2020;34:359–65.
8. Soria F, Morcillo E, Lopez de Alda A, Pastor T, Sánchez-Margallo FM. Catéteres y stents urinarios biodegradables. ¿Para cuándo? Arch Esp Urol. 2016;69:553–64.
9. Beysens M, Tailly TO. Ureteral stents in urolithiasis. Asian J Urol. 2018;5:274–86.
10. Barros AA, Oliveira C, Lima E, Duarte ARC, Healy K, Reis RL. Ureteral stents technology: biodegradable and drug-eluting perspective, vol. 7. Amsterdam: Elsevier; 2017.
11. Peppas NA, Langer R. New challenges in biomaterials. Science. 1994;263:1715–20.
12. Pulieri E, Chiono V, Ciardelli G, Vozzi G, Ahluwalia A, Domenici C, et al. Chitosan/gelatin blends for biomedical applications. J Biomed Mater Res A. 2008;86:311–22.
13. Barros AA, Rita A, Duarte ARC, Pires RA, Sampaio-Marques B, Ludovico P, et al. Bioresorbable ureteral stents from natural origin polymers. J Biomed Mater Res Part B Appl Biomater. 2015;103:608–17.
14. Barros AA, Oliveira C, Ribeiro AJ, Autorino R, Reis RL, Duarte ARC, et al. In vivo assessment of a novel biodegradable ureteral stent. World J Urol. 2018;36:277–83.
15. Barros AA, Browne S, Oliveira C, Lima E, Duarte ARC, Healy KE, et al. Drug-eluting biodegradable ureteral stent: new approach for urothelial tumors of upper urinary tract cancer. Int J Pharm. 2016;513:227–37.
16. Gunatillake P, Mayadunne R, Adhikari R. Recent developments in biodegradable synthetic polymers. Biotechnol Annu Rev. 2006;12:301–47.
17. Wang X, Zhang L, Chen Q, Hou Y, Hao Y, Wang C, et al. A nanostructured degradable ureteral stent fabricated by electrospinning for upper urinary tract reconstruction. J Nanosci Nanotechnol. 2015;15:9899–904.
18. Osman Y, Shokeir A, Gabr M, El-Tabey N, Mohsen T, El-Baz M. Canine ureteral replacement with long acellular matrix tube: is it clinically applicable? J Urol. 2004;172:1151–4.
19. Fu W-J, Xu Y-D, Wang Z-X, Li G, Shi J-G, Cui F-Z, et al. New ureteral scaffold constructed with composite poly(L-lactic acid)-collagen and urothelial cells by new centrifugal seeding system. J Biomed Mater Res A. 2012;100:1725–33.
20. Li G, Wang Z-X, Fu W-J, Hong B-F, Wang X-X, Cao L, et al. Introduction to biodegradable polylactic acid ureteral stent application for treatment of ureteral war injury. BJU Int. 2011;108:901–6.
21. Lumiaho J, Heino A, Pietilainen T, Ala-Opas M, Talja M, Valimaa T, et al. The morphological, in situ effects of a self-reinforced bioabsorbable polylactide (SR-PLA 96) ureteric stent; an experimental study. J Urol. 2000;164:1360–3.
22. Talja M, Valimaa T, Tammela T, Petas A, Tormala P. Bioabsorbable and biodegradable stents in urology. J Endourol. 1997;11:391–7.

23. Yang G, Xie H, Huang Y, Lv Y, Zhang M, Shang Y, et al. Immersed multilayer biodegradable ureteral stent with reformed biodegradation: an in vitro experiment. J Biomater Appl. 2017;31:1235–44.

24. Zou T, Wang L, Li W, Wang W, Chen F, King MW. A resorbable bicomponent braided ureteral stent with improved mechanical performance. J Mech Behav Biomed Mater. 2014;38:17–25.

25. Jana A, Das M, Balla VK. In vitro and in vivo degradation assessment and preventive measures of biodegradable Mg alloys for biomedical applications. J Biomed Mater Res A. 2022;110(2):462–87.

26. Lock JY, Wyatt E, Upadhyayula S, Whall A, Nuñez V, Vullev VI, et al. Degradation and antibacterial properties of magnesium alloys in artificial urine for potential resorbable ureteral stent applications. J Biomed Mater Res Part A. 2014;102:781–92.

27. Lumiaho J, Heino A, Kauppinen T, Talja M, Alhava E, Valimaa T, et al. Drainage and antireflux characteristics of a biodegradable self-reinforced, self-expanding X-ray-positive poly-L,D-lactide spiral partial ureteral stent: an experimental study. J Endourol. 2007;21:1559–64.

28. Lumiaho J, Heino A, Tunninen V, Ala-Opas M, Talja M, Valimaa T, et al. New bioabsorbable polylactide ureteral stent in the treatment of ureteral lesions: an experimental study. J Endourol. 1999;13:107–12.

29. Lingeman JE, Schulsinger DA, Kuo RL. Phase I trial of a temporary ureteral drainage stent. J Endourol. 2003;17:169–71.

30. Lingeman JE, Preminger GM, Berger Y, Denstedt JD, Goldstone L, Segura JW, et al. Use of a temporary ureteral drainage stent after uncomplicated ureteroscopy: results from a phase II clinical trial. J Urol. 2003;169:1682–8.

31. Hadaschik BA, Paterson RF, Fazli L, Clinkscales KW, Shalaby SW, Chew BH. Investigation of a novel degradable ureteral stent in a porcine model. J Urol. 2008;180:1161–6.

32. Chew BH, Paterson RF, Clinkscales KW, Levine BS, Shalaby SW, Lange D. In vivo evaluation of the third generation biodegradable stent: a novel approach to avoiding the forgotten stent syndrome. J Urol. 2013;189:719–25.

33. Chew BH, Lange D, Paterson RF, Hendlin K, Monga M, Clinkscales KW, et al. Next generation biodegradable ureteral stent in a yucatan pig model. J Urol. 2010;183:765–71.

34. Wang X, Shan H, Wang J, Hou Y, Ding J, Chen Q, et al. Characterization of nanostructured ureteral stent with gradient degradation in a porcine model. Int J Nanomed. 2015;10:3055–64.

35. Barros AA, Oliveira C, Reis RL, Lima E, Duarte ARC. Ketoprofen-eluting biodegradable ureteral stents by CO$_2$ impregnation: in vitro study. Int J Pharm. 2015;495:651–9.

36. Soria F, Morcillo E, Serrano A, Rioja J, Budía A, Sánchez-Margallo FM. Preliminary assessment of a new antireflux ureteral stent design in swine model. Urology. 2015;86:417–22.

37. Soria F, Morcillo E, de la Cruz JE, Serrano A, Estébanez J, Sanz JL, et al. Antireflux ureteral stent proof of concept assessment after minimally invasive treatment of obstructive uropathy in animal model. Arch Esp Urol. 2018;71:607–13.

38. Soria F, Morcillo E, Serrano A, Budía A, Fernandez I, Fernández-Aparicio T, et al. Evaluation of a new design of antireflux-biodegradable ureteral stent in animal model. Urology. 2018;115:59–64.

39. Soria F, de La Cruz JE, Caballero-Romeu JP, Pamplona M, Pérez-Fentes D, Resel-Folskerma L, Sanchez-Margallo FM. Comparative assessment of biodegradable-antireflux heparine coated ureteral stent: animal model study. BMC Urol. 2021;21(1):32.

40. Soria F, de La Cruz JE, Budia A, Cepeda M, Álvarez S, Serrano Á, Sanchez-Margallo FM. Iatrogenic ureteral injury treatment with biodegradable antireflux heparin-coated ureteral stent-animal model comparative study. J Endourol. 2021;35(8):1244–9.

41. Soria F, de La Cruz JE, Fernandez T, Budia A, Serrano Á, Sanchez-Margallo FM. Heparin coating in biodegradable ureteral stents does not decrease bacterial colonization-assessment in ureteral stricture endourological treatment in animal model. Transl Androl Urol. 2021;10(4):1700–10.

42. Jin L, Yao L, Yuan F, Dai G, Xue B. Evaluation of a novel biodegradable ureteral stent produced from polyurethane and magnesium alloys. J Biomed Mater Res B Appl Biomater. 2021;109(5):665–72.

43. Tie D, Liu H, Guan R, Holt-Torres P, Liu Y, Wang Y, Hort N. In vivo assessment of biodegradable magnesium alloy ureteral stents in a pig model. Acta Biomater. 2020;15(116):415–25.

44. Tie D, Hort N, Chen M, Guan R, Ulasevich S, Skorb EV, Zhao D, Liu Y, Holt-Torres P, Liu H. In vivo urinary compatibility of Mg–Sr–Ag alloy in swine model. Bioact Mater. 2021;4(7):254–62.
45. Shan H, Cao Z, Chi C, Wang J, Wang X, Tian J, Yu B. Advances in drug delivery via biodegradable ureteral stent for the treatment of upper tract urothelial carcinoma. Front Pharmacol. 2020;17(11):224.
46. Ho DR, Su SH, Chang PJ, Lin WY, Huang YC, Lin JH, Huang KT, Chan WN, Chen CS. Biodegradable stent with mTOR inhibitor-eluting reduces progression of ureteral stricture. Int J Mol Sci. 2021;22(11):5664.
47. Na HK, Song HY, Yeo HJ, Park JH, Kim JH, Park H, Kim CS. Retrospective comparison of internally and externally covered retrievable stent placement for patients with benign urethral strictures caused by traumatic injury. AJR Am J Roentgenol. 2012;198:55–61.
48. Petas A, Talja M, Tammela T, et al. A randomized study to compare biodegradable self-reinforced polyglycolic acid spiral stents to suprapubic and indwelling catheters after visual laser ablation of the prostate. J Urol. 1997;157:173–6.
49. Petas A, Talja M, Tammela TL, Taari K, Valimaa T, Tormala P. The biodegradable self-reinforced poly-L-lactic acid spiral stent compared with a suprapubic catheter in the treatment of post-operative urinary retention after visual laser ablation of the prostate. Br J Urol. 1997;80:439–43.
50. Isotalo T, Nuutinen JP, Vaajanen A, Martikainen PM, Laurila M, Tormala P, Talja M, Tammela TL. Biocompatibility and implantation properties of two differently braided, biodegradable, self-reinforced polylactic acid urethral stents: an experimental study in the rabbit. J Urol. 2005;174:2401–4.
51. Isotalo T, Nuutine JP, Vaajanen A, Martikainen PM, Laurila M, Tormala P, Talja M, et al. Biocompatibility properties of a new braided biodegradable urethral stent: a comparison with a biodegradable spiral and braided metallic stent in the rabbit urethra. BJU Int. 2006;97:856–9.
52. Kotsar A, Nieminen R, Isotalo T, Mikkonen J, Uurto I, Kellomäki M, Talja M, et al. Biocompatibility of new drug-eluting biodegradable urethral stent materials. Urology. 2010;75:229–34.
53. De Filippo RE, Yoo JJ, Atala A. Urethral replacement using cell seeded tubularized collagen matrices. J Urol. 2002;168:1789–92.
54. Fu WJ, Zhang X, Zhang BH, Zhang P, Hong BF, Gao JP, Meng B, et al. Biodegradable urethral stents seeded with autologous urethral epithelial cells in the treatment of post-traumatic urethral stricture: a feasibility study in a rabbit model. BJU Int. 2009;104:263–8.
55. Rashidbenam Z, Jasman MH, Tan GH, Goh EH, Fam XI, Ho CCK, Zainuddin ZM, Rajan R, Rani RA, Nor FM, Shuhaili MA, Kosai NR, Imran FH, Ng MH. Fabrication of adipose-derived stem cell-based self-assembled scaffold under hypoxia and mechanical stimulation for urethral tissue engineering. Int J Mol Sci. 2021;22(7):3350.

New Double-J Stent Design for Preventing/ Reducing Irritative Bladder Symptoms and Flank Pain

Daniel Yachia

1 Introduction

Ureteral stents entered the urologists armamentarium after Finney described the first Double-J in the late 1970s [1]. Despite the problems they create, yearly 1.5–2 million ureteral stents are inserted world-wide, either in their original JJ shape or in their various modifications for short and long indwelling periods. About 15% of these stents are used in chronically obstructed ureters.

With their worldwide use came also reports on the problems they create which are very common and can affect nearly 60–80% of the patients [2]. Without taking into consideration the medical problems of infection, encrustation, migration, stent breakage etc. the patients complain of urinary *frequency* (up to 60%), *urgency*/u*rge incontinence* (up to 60%) and f*lank pain* (up to 35%). Most of these symptoms are caused by their inherent design flaws common in all JJ and pigtail stents being in close contact with certain areas of the bladder. Urinary *frequency, urgency and* urge *incontinence* are caused by mechanical irritation of the bladder trigone induced by the bladder-end coil of the stent, which is in almost constant contact with the trigone. Additionally, during respiration, the up and down movement of the kidney, moves the bladder-end of the stent back and forth in the bladder, creating continuous friction with the trigone. The bladder trigone is an anatomical entity formed by the two ureteral orifices and the bladder neck very rich in innervation. Maximal vertical motion of the kidney from the end-expiratory to its end-inspiratory position is 39 mm [3]. Thinking that this friction may be reduced by using a softer material at the bladder end of the stent, in my *Closing Remarks* of the *Second International*

D. Yachia (✉)
Innoventions Ltd, Or Akiva, Israel

Department of Urology, Hillel Yaffe Medical Center, Hadera, Israel

Bruce Rappaport Faculty of Medicine, Technion, Haifa, Israel
e-mail: dyachia@innovenions-med.com; yachia@zahav.net.il

© The Author(s) 2022
F. Soria et al. (eds.), *Urinary Stents*,
https://doi.org/10.1007/978-3-031-04484-7_30

Symposium on Urological Stents (*ISUS-2*) held in Belgrade in March 18–20, 1999, I asked theoretically if using a softer material at the bladder-end of a JJ stent could reduce the irritative symptoms. Although the more rigid stents caused more dysuria, flank and suprapubic pain, Lenon's study could find no significant differences in the incidence of urgency, frequency, nocturia and hematuria [4]. A few years later the Polaris Ureteral Stent made of dual durometer material come to the market. The bladder-end of this stent was made of softer polymer with the hope that it will be better tolerated by the patients. To check if material softness can make a difference in the irritative symptoms Joshi's group, about a decade later run a blinded, randomized controlled trial comparing the firmer (*Percuflex*) and the softer (*Contour*) stents. This study also could not find a statistical difference in the patient's comfort and overall ureteral stent experience [5]. *Dual durometer stents* with a smooth transition from a firm polymer for the kidney end to a softer polymer at the bladder end (Polaris]) were also compared with a firm polymer made stent [Inlay Stent], but no difference between these stents could be found in any of the measured parameters [6]. Even coating the softer bladder-end with a hydrophilic material to reduce the friction between the stents and the trigone could not prevent the irritative symptoms [7, 8].

Another culprit for stent related symptoms is the use of an inappropriate stent length. Studies showed that inappropriate stent length induces the most disturbing symptoms. Al-Kandari's study found that "*Symptoms were worst when the bladder end crossed the midline*" [9]. This was confirmed by a study done by Dellis group that also showed that stent symptoms are worsened if the bladder end of the stent crosses the midline of the bladder [10]. Another study done by Ho's group indicated that longer than needed stents are associated with significantly higher incidence and severity of frequency and urgency, but they found no difference in the incidence of hematuria, bladder and flank pain, nocturia and urge incontinence [11].

Even if seemingly an appropriate length is inserted, there is an additional cause for the irritative symptoms: Respiration. During respiration, the up and down movement of the kidney, moves the bladder-end of the stent back and forth in the bladder, creating continuous friction with the trigone inducing the irritation. The maximal vertical motion of the kidney from the end-expiratory to its end-inspiratory position was found to be 39 mm [3]. These "*up and down movements of the kidneys*" make measurement of the ureteral length a challenge.

Flank pain is usually caused by urine refluxing from the bladder to the renal pelvis through the stent when the bladder is full or during urination when the intra-vesical pressure increases, increasing also the intra-renal pressure. This is the period the patients experience most of the pain.

Drug eluting ureteric stents were also tried for reducing stent related symptoms. Ketorolac-loaded stents showed only limited benefit in younger male patients who required less pain medication on days 3 and 4 compared with controls.

Fig. 1 Common ureteral
double-J stent

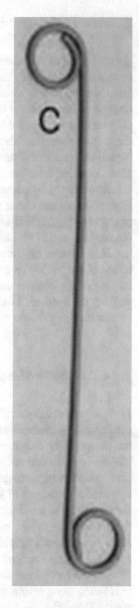

"Drug-coated stents have had only very limited success in reducing stent symptoms" [12].

The current, JJ or pig-tail ureteral stents have a 2-dimensional design, in which their renal- and bladder-ends are on the same plane but their curl in opposite directions (Fig. 1).

2   Are There Any Solutions?

By analyzing the JJ related symptoms in detail we concluded that by making certain changes in the design, the irritative and painful *ureteral stent related symptoms* can be prevented or significantly reduced by re-engineering the bladder-end of the JJ. A change of *shape* and/or in the *material* of the bladder segment or its *coating* probably can reduce/prevent its thrusting to the trigone caused during its "*in-* and *out-of-the-ureter movement*" during respiration. Comparison between loop-tail and regular pigtail ureteral stents on urination-related QoL showed that patients with loop tail stents emptied their bladder better than those with regular pigtails [13].

Accordingly, by accurately measuring the length of the ureter at inspiration and expiration we can chose the appropriate stent length. In addition, by modifying the position of the bladder-end of the stent we can prevent the constant contact between the bladder-end of the stent with the trigone. Also by adding a simple mechanism to the bladder end of the stent, we can create an anti-reflux mechanism. To these changes we can add a structural modification to allow its easy un-curling and re-curling of the bladder end of the stent during respiration, and by this, further preventing the friction of the in and out movement of the stent.

For reaching these goals we took the following steps.

2.1   Accurate Measurement of the Ureter

JJ stents are usually available in lengths between 20 and 28 cm to fit the length of the individual ureter of each patient. Urologists know that accurate measurement of the ureteral length is important for choosing the appropriate stent length to ensure patient comfort and reduce irritative symptoms. The reason for using the inappropriate stent length is mainly the empirical practice of deciding the length of the stent to be used, or the use of whatever length is available at the OR. Longer than needed stents will have a redundant part in the bladder, and shorter than needed ones may retract into the ureter, making their removal more difficult. Taking into consideration the patient's height as a predictor for choosing the appropriate stent length may work "*in the majority of ureters (grade 0 = 61%), with no stent being too short. In comparison, direct ureteric measurement oversized the stent in 83%, correctly predicting stent length in only 17%*" [14] where others chose different measuring means [15–17].

Easy and accurate ureteric length measurement for selecting the appropriate stent length is important. During respiration, the "up and down movements of the kidneys" makes accurate measurement of the ureteral length a challenge. At inspiration the distance between the kidney and the bladder is the shortest. The solution for this problem is to find a way for accurate measurement of the ureter. Even if we take the *average length* measured at inspiration (the kidney in its low position) + length at expiration [the kidney in its high position] the stent still will have a 2 cm of it moving up and down in the bladder (Fig. 2). The "*in-* and *out-of-the-ureter movement*"

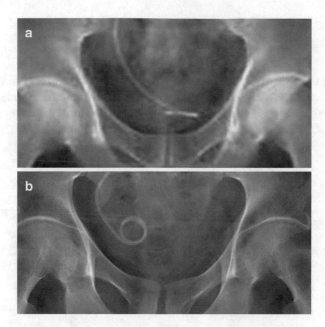

Fig. 2 X-ray view of the bladder end stent at inspiration (**a**) and expiration (**b**)

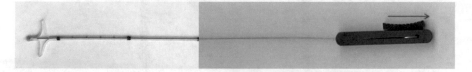

Fig. 3 Malecot-type ureteral length measuring ruler with a slider to open the Malecot wings

of the bladder-end of the stent during respiration causes continuous thrusting with the trigone 12–16 times every minute, meaning 17.280–23.040 *in* and *out* movements during 24 h.

That is the reason for accurate measurement of the ureteral length for choosing the appropriate stent length that can reduce this irritative cause. Flexible length ureteral stents with their distal parts made of softer material to allow easier furling and unfurling of its bladder-end were developed for this reason. Although these modifications somehow reduced the length related problems but still could not prevent the friction caused irritative symptoms.

A *Fogarty Balloon Catheter* with centimetric markings we designed can be used to measure the length of the ureter during the respiratory movements and decide the optimal double-J stent length. For further simplifying the making of an accurate measurement, we designed a simple *Ureteral Length Measuring Ruler* with a 2-flanged Malecot-type distal end activated by a slider handle (Fig. 3). This *ureteral ruler* allows measuring the ureteral length at inspiration, when the kidney is in its lowest position. The logic behind using this short distance will become clear when #4 will be presented.

2.2   Making Positioning Adjustment of the Bladder-End of the Stent

By rotating the axis of the bladder-end segment from flat to forward by 90°, the intravesical segment was positioned perpendicular to the trigone for minimizing its contact with the trigonal mucosa (Figs. 4a, b and 5a, b) This positioning adjustment requires separate stents for insertion to the right or the left ureter.

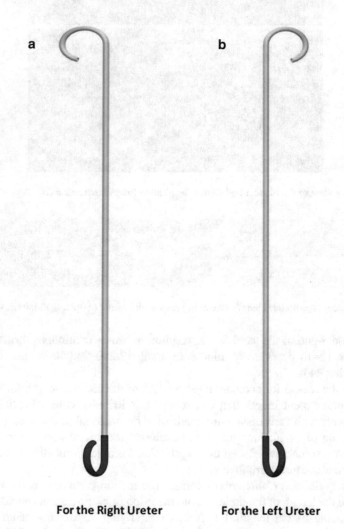

a

b

For the Right Ureter   For the Left Ureter

Fig. 4 90° forward direction of the bladder-end curl new double-J for the right (**a**) and left (**b**) ureter

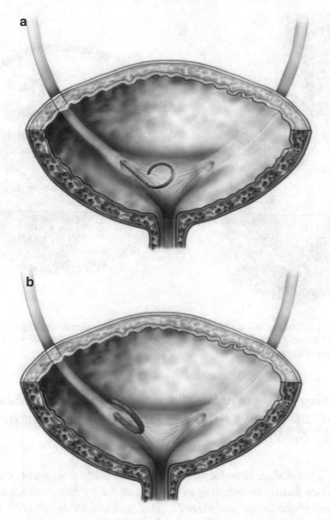

Fig. 5 (**a**) Continuous contact of the bladder-end curl of a common double-J stent with the trigone. (**b**) The 90° forward direction of the bladder-end curl of the new double-J stent, separating the curl from the trigone

2.3   Creating a Simple Anti-Reflux Mechanism

The place of the bladder-end opening of the stent was relocated to the side, creating a groove. This grove at the distal end of the bladder-end curl was covered with a pre-shaped soft silicone made sleeve-like tube to create an antireflux mechanism. The shape of the sleeve allows the guide-wire to pass along the lumen and the groove and then to pass between the stent tip and the sleeve by elevating the edge of the silicone sleeve. The soft silicone sleeve allows also the urine to drain into the bladder easily (Fig. 6a, b).

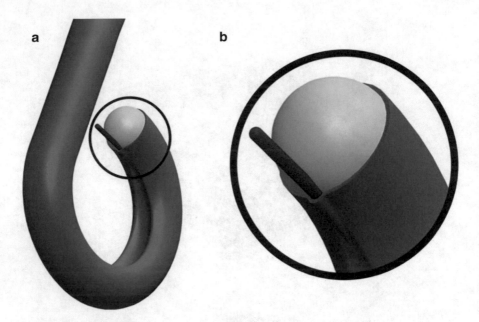

Fig. 6 Bladder-end of the new double-J stent with a soft silicone sleeve covering it for preventing reflux (**a**), and the way the guide-wire elevates the sleeve (**b**) similar to how urine will be drained into the bladder under the sleeve

2.4   Making Changes at the Bladder-End to Allow Its Easy Un-Curling and Re-Curling for Keeping the Stent Body in the Ureter

Additionally, we made a manufacturing change in the distal segment of the stent in order to reduce further its thrusting to the trigone during respiration, caused by its "*in-* and *out-of-the-ureter movement*". The manufacturing change was using multiple-durometer extrusion technology for producing a very soft bladder-end to allow its un-curling at expiration and re-curling at inspiration with the help of an embedded metal coil along the softer segment (Fig. 7a, b).

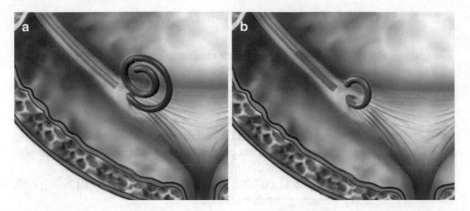

Fig. 7 At inspiration the bladder-end of the new double-J stent curve as a pig-tail but in a 90° forward direction distancing itself from the trigone (**a**), at expiration the bladder-end of the new double-J stent un-curls and allow its partial retraction into the ureter (**b**), again preventing contact with the trigone

3　The Way the New JJ Will Work

Since a double-J stent is a commodity used almost by all urologists it is important that the learning curve for the insertion and retrieval of the new stent design should be as easy and as near as possible to the insertion and retrieval of a common JJ.

With the new stent, the accurate ureteral measurement will be taken at the end of inspiration when the kidney is in its lowest position using the *Ureteral Length Measuring Ruler*.

The appropriate stent length for the appropriate side [right or left side] will be chosen for insertion.

The pre-inserted guide-wire's proximal end will be threaded from the renal end opening of the stent until it comes out between the side groove opening and the silicone sleeve at the bladder end as seen in Fig. 6.

Then the guide-wire will be threaded through the pusher's side opening to allow engaging the stent tip.

The stent will be pushed upward, until the bladder-end marker reaches the orifice and then it will be released by pulling out the guide wire and the pusher to allow curling of the bladder end.

After its release the un-curling and re-curling of the bladder-end of the stent will be observed during the respiratory movements.

3.1   Expected Advantages of the New Ureter JJ Stent

The general shape of the new stent is almost similar to current stents.

The learning curve for the physician will be quite short, because the insertion and retrieval of the new stent will be very similar to the current JJ stents, with the difference that the selected stent should be either for the *right* or *left* ureter.

The re-engineered features of bladder-end of the stent will minimize the contact between the new stent and the trigone and also prevent vesico-ureteral reflux.

With these changes in the design, the proprietary new JJ [*] is expected to prevent or significantly reduce most of the *ureteral stent related symptoms*.

[*] Patents Granted: USA: 11,007,046 B2 [2021]; EP: 3,297,573 [2020]; CN: 107847312 B.[2021]—Pending in other counties.

References

1. Finney R. Experience with new double-J ureteral catheter stents. J Urol. 1978;119:678–81.
2. Fischer KM, et al. Ureteral stent discomfort and its management. Curr Urol Rep. 2018;11(19):64.
3. Schwartz LH, et al. Kidney mobility during respiration. Radiother Oncol. 1994;32:84–6.
4. Lenon GM, et al. 'Firm' versus 'Soft' double pigtail ureteric stents: a randomised blind comparative trial. Eur Urol. 1995;28:1.
5. Joshi HB, Chitale SV, Nagarajan M, et al. A prospective randomized single-blind comparison of ureteral stents composed of firm and soft polymer. J Urol. 2005;174:2303.
6. Davenport K, et al. Prospective randomised trial comparing the Bard Inlay ureteric stent with the Boston Scientific Polaris ureteric stent using the validated Ureteric Stent Symptom Questionnaire. BJU Int Suppl. 2008;101:52.
7. Lee JN, Kim BS. Comparison of efficacy and bladder irritation symptoms among three different ureteral stents: a double-blind, prospective, randomized controlled trial. Scand J Urol. 2015;49:237–41.
8. Park HK, Paick SH, Kim HG, et al. The impact of ureteral stent type on patient symptoms as determined by the ureteral stent symptom questionnaire: a prospective, randomized, controlled study. J Endourol. 2015;29:367–71.
9. Al-Kandari AM, et al. Effects of proximal and distal ends of double-J ureteral stent position on postprocedural symptoms and quality of life: a randomized clinical trial. J Endourol. 2007;21:698.
10. Dellis A, et al. Relief of stent related symptoms: review of engineering and pharmacological solutions. J Urol. 2010;184:1267–72.
11. Ho CH, et al. Determining the appropriate length of a double-pigtail ureteral stent by both stent configurations and related symptoms. J Endourol. 2008;22:1427.
12. Krambeck AE, Walsh RS, Denstedt JD, et al. A novel drug eluting ureteral stent: a prospective, randomized, multicenter clinical trial to evaluate the safety and effectiveness of a ketorolac loaded ureteral stent. J Urol. 2010;183:1037–42.
13. Taguchi M, et al. Impact of loop-tail ureteral stents on ureteral stent-related symptoms immediately after ureteroscopic lithotripsy: comparison with pigtail ureteral stents. Investig Clin Urol. 2017;58:440.
14. Pilcher JM, Patel U. Choosing the correct length of ureteric stent: a formula based on the patient's height compared with direct ureteric measurement. Clin Radiol. 2002;57:59–62.

15. Barrett K, et al. Best stent length predicted by simple CT measurement rather than patient height. J Endourol. 2016;30:1029–32.
16. Hruby GW, et al. Correlation of ureteric length with anthropometric variables of surface body habitus. BJU Int. 2007;99:1119–22.
17. Taguchi M, et al. Simplified method using kidney/ureter/bladder X-ray to determine the appropriate length of ureteral stents. Int Braz J Urol. 2018;44:1224–33.

Drug Eluting Devices in the Urinary Tract

Panagiotis Kallidonis, Athanasios Vagionis, Despoina Liourdi, and Evangelos Liatsikos

1 Background

The obstruction of the upper urinary tract represents a common medical condition which could be related to significant and life-threating complications such acute renal insufficiency and urosepsis. Ureteral stents are commonly used to prevent and manage such complications. These stents provide non-surgical decongestion of the pelvicalyceal system by achieving unobstructed inflow of urine in the bladder. However, the use of conventional stents involves significant comorbidities, including stent-associated infection, encrustation, migration, hyperplastic urothelial reaction [1].

Urethral strictures represent a common cause of lower urinary tract obstruction with the characteristic of frequent recurrence. Patients suffering from urethral strictures can be treated by minimally invasive techniques [2] such as mechanical dilatation with balloon or placing of urethral stents [3].

In attempt to address the any stent-related complications, the urological research considered ideas and concepts used in interventional cardiology and radiology (Table 1). Percutaneous transluminal coronary angioplasty (PTCA) is the gold standard for coronary revascularization, even if restenosis complications exist in concerning rates. To address this complication, stents bearing pharmaceutical agents (most commonly immunosuppressive agents) have been used [4]. These drug-eluting stents (DESs) release single or multiple bioactive agents, which are deposited on adjacent tissues. The immunosuppressive substances reduce benign tissue proliferation and their use has significantly reduced restenosis rates after PTCA [5, 6]. In a similar fashion, the drug-coated balloons (DCBs) are used as a new

P. Kallidonis (✉) · A. Vagionis · E. Liatsikos
Department of Urology, University of Patras, Patras, Greece

D. Liourdi
Department of Internal Medicine, Ag. Andreas Hospital, Patras, Greece

© The Author(s) 2022
F. Soria et al. (eds.), *Urinary Stents*,
https://doi.org/10.1007/978-3-031-04484-7_31

Table 1 Summary of drug eluting devices used in experimental studies

Study group	Aim	Intervention	Results
Antimisiaris et al. Journal of Endourology 2000 [23]	In vitro preparation of liposome-covered metal stents and loading of liposomal drug formulations that will slowly release the drug in the vicinity of the stent	Apply to pieces of stent a large multi-lamellar (MLV) liposomes either empty or entrapping the corticosteroid anti-inflammatory-drug	$39.11 \pm 6.8\%$ of the lipid and $50.84 \pm 5.48\%$ of the drug was released from the stent pieces during 48 h of incubation in the presence of artificial urine
Cadieux et al. Journal of Urology 2006 [13]	Test of the effects of triclosan impregnated stent segments on the growth and survival of *Proteus mirabilis*	Instillation with 1×10^6 *P. mirabilis* 296 Randomised groups, intravesical stent: - Triclosan - Optima® - Percuflex Plus® UC: days 1, 3 and 7 Day 7: Incrustation and viable organisms in stents	UC: significantly less *P. mirabilis* in the triclosan group than in the Percuflex Plus® group at all time points and in the Optima® group on days 3 and 7
Chew et al. Journal of Endourology 2006 [9]	The bactericidal and bacteriostatic effect of a triclosan-eluting ureteral stent against common bacterial uropathogens in an in-vitro setting	Control stent and eluting stent with triclosan were suspended in artificial urine with bacterial pathogens to assess growth, virulence-promoter activity, and bacterial adherence	Triclosan stents had significantly fewer adherent viable bacteria than control stents Growth was inhibited in a dose-dependent fashion by Tcn eluate in all strains except *P. aeruginosa* and *Ent. faecalis*
Kotsar et al. Urology 2010 [25]	To assess the degradation process and the biocompatibility of biodegradable drug-eluting urethral stents	The effect of cytokines and other inflammatory mediators on control stents (bacterial lipopolysaccharide as a positive control) and biodegradable stent material (poly-96L/4D-lactic acid [PLA]) using the Human Cytokine Antibody Array	The increase in the production of inflammatory mediators with the PLA stent material was smaller than in the cells treated with lipopolysaccharide

Table 1 (continued)

Study group	Aim	Intervention	Results
Johnson et al. Urology 2010 [11]	Comparison of commercially available, antibiotic coated Foley catheters regarding activity, comparative potency and effect durability	An inhibition zone assay (diffusible inhibition) and an adherence assay was used to assess the inhibitory effect of coated urethral catheters, 2 with silver and 1 with nitrofurazone	The nitrofurazone coated catheter showed the greatest and most durable (through day 5) inhibitory activity One of the 2 silver coated catheters showed sparse but measurable inhibition zone activity on day 1 but not thereafter and no statistically significant activity on adherence assay. The other lacked detectable activity using either test system
Elayarajah et al. Pak J Biol Sci 2011 [10]	Evaluation of ureteral stents made of silicone impregnated with one or more antimicrobial agents (ofloxacin and ornidazole) to inhibit the growth of different bacterial pathogens that colonize the device surface	Stent pieces were impregnated in a polymer mixed antibiotic solution (ofloxacin and ornidazole) for uniform surface coating (drug-carrier-coated stents) to inhibit the growth of different bacterial pathogens that colonize the device surface	In qualitative test, the zone of inhibition around the coated stents showed sensitivity against the clinical isolates. In quantitative test, the number of adhered bacteria on the surface of coated stents was reduced to a significant level ($P < 0.05$)
Barros et al. International Journal of Pharmaceutics 2015 [19]	The evaluation of the in vitro elution profile of ketoprofen impregnated in the biodegradable ureteral stent during its degradation	To impregne with ketoprofen the biodegradable ureteral stents with each formulation: alginate-based, gellan gum-based	Ketoprofen impregnated stents were able to the release ketoprofen in the first 72 h in artificial urine solution

(continued)

Table 1 (continued)

Study group	Aim	Intervention	Results
Ma et al. Materials Science and Engineering 2016 [12]	To assess the degradation process and the biocompatibility of biodegradable ciprofloxacin-eluting ureteral stents	Poly(L-lactide-*co-ε*-caprolactone) (PLCL) with three different compositions as carriers for ciprofloxacin lactate (CIP) was coated on ureteral stents by the dipping method	Stage I: mainly controlled by chain scission instead of the weight loss or morphological changes of the coatings. Stage II: the release profile was dominated by erosion resulting from the hydrolysis reaction autocatalyzed by acidic degradation residues Ciprofloxacin loaded coatings displayed a significant bacterial resistance against *E. coli* and *S. aureus* without obvious cytotoxicity to human foreskin fibroblasts
Barros et al. Journal of Pharmaceutical Sciences 2017 [29]	The use of an ex vivo porcine model to assess the permeability of the anti-cancer drugs (paclitaxel, doxorubicin) delivered from BUS across porcine ureter	The permeability of the anticancer drugs (paclitaxel, doxorubicin) alone or released from the biodegradable ureteral stent (BUS) developed	Paclitaxel and doxorubicin drugs released from the BUS were able to remain in the ex vivo ureter and only a small amount of the drugs can across the different permeable membranes with a permeability of 3% for paclitaxel and 11% for doxorubicin. The estimated amount of paclitaxel remains in the ex vivo ureter tissue shown to be effective to affect the cancer cell and did not affect the non-cancer cells

alternative instead of DESs in selected cases and offer important advantages (Fig. 1). Their drug is released directly at the site of the stricture while avoiding any foreign material at the site of the stricture. Moreover, DCBs could manage vascular stricture sites inappropriate for stent placement [7].

The impressive impact of the DESs to avoid vascular restenosis proposed the drug-eluting idea to be used for the improvement of urological urinary stents. Thus, the effect of DESs to reduce the existing complications of the indwelling ureteral stents has been investigated [8] (Table 2). The possibility of using DCBs in endourology is also under research (Table 3).

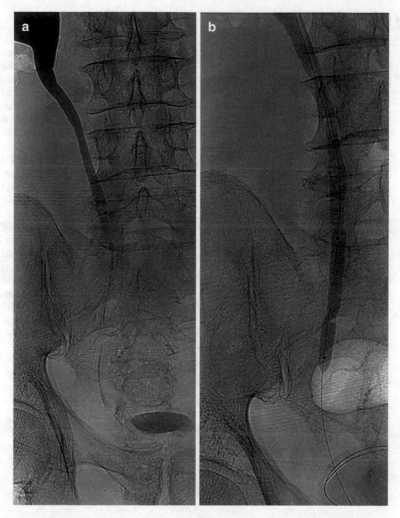

Fig. 1 Use of DCB in the ureter. (**a**) Ureter with stricture. (**b**) Use of DCB in the ureter to treat the stricture

Table 2 Summary of clinical studies using DES

Study group	Sample	Intervention	Method study	Results
Shin et al. Radiology 2005 [32]	20 Male dogs—urethra	20 Paclitaxel-eluting polyurethane-covered stents (DES) and 20 polyurethane-covered stents (control stents) were placed alternately between the proximal and distal urethra Group 1: n = 10 Sacrificed 4 weeks 1.1.: Drug stent in proximal urethra 1.2.: Control stent in distal urethra Group 2: n = 10 Sacrificed 8 weeks 2.1.: Control stent in proximal urethra 2.2.: Drug stent in distal urethra	Group 1: retrograde urethrography after sacrifice to evaluate percentage diameter of stenosis Group 2: retrograde urethrography at 4 weeks and 8 weeks before sacrifice The sectioned tissue samples were stained with hematoxylin–eosin: number of epithelial layers, thickness of granulation tissue, thickness of the papillary projection, and degree of submucosal inflammatory cell infiltration	Strong tendency toward a lower percentage diameter of stenosis and numeric mean values of the four histologic findings, which indicates less formation of tissue hyperplasia in the proximal urethra than in the distal urethra Thickness of the papillary projection was significantly less in drug stents than in control stents in the proximal urethra in the 8-week group (P ‹ 0.016)

Table 2 (continued)

Study group	Sample	Intervention	Method study	Results
Liatsikos et al. European association of Urology 2007 [31]	10 Female pigs—ureter	Randomly placed in either the right or left ureter in each of 10 study animals 1. n = 10 R-Stent 2. n = 10. Paclitaxel-eluting coronary stent Percutaneous nephrostomy was performed under ultrasonographic guidance and the collecting system was visualized. Peployment of the stent was finalized: nephrostomy tube was capped	Patency evaluation of ureteral lumen: Radiograph of the nephrostomy tract, intravenous urography and virtual endoscopy at 24 h and 21 days after the initial procedure, respectively Conventional ureteroscopy at 21 days Pathology examination of ureter: same pathologist minimizing possible bias	21 day follow-up: Group 1: 5 completely occluded 2 partially stenosed Group 2: no occluded stent Pathology examination 21 days: Obstructed R-Stents generated severe inflammation with metaplasia Paclitaxel-eluting MS generated a mild inflammatory response without hindering ureteral patency

(continued)

Table 2 (continued)

Study group	Sample	Intervention	Method study	Results
Cirioni et al. Antimicrobial Agents and Chemotherapy 2007 [17]	5 Adult female Wistar rats—ureter	2×10^7 CFU/mL *S. aureus*: inoculated into the bladder Control group C_0 without a bacterial challenge Challenged control group (C_1) without antibiotic prophylaxis i. 10 mg/kg of body weight teicoplanin intraperitoneally immediately after stent implantation ii. RIP-coated stents, in which 0.2-cm^2 sterile stents iii. Stents coated with intraperitoneal teicoplanin	Culturing serial tenfold dilutions (0.1 mL) of the bacterial suspension on blood agar plates. 37 °C for 48 h. Quantification: number of CFU per plate Toxicity: presence of any drug-related adverse effects	C0: None had microbiological evidence of stent infection C1: all presents infection. $6.6 \times 10 \pm 1.9 \times 10^6$ CFU/mL $3.8 \times 10 \pm 0.8 \times 10^3$ CFU/mL $6.7 \times 10^4 \pm 1.4 \times 10^3$ CFU/mL $p < 0.05$ iii. No bacterial counts ($P < 0.001$) None of the animals included in any group died or had any clinical evidence of drug-related adverse effects
Cauda et al. Journal of Endourology 2008 [18]	Five patients with bilateral obstructions ureter	For each patient heparin-coated Double J stent and a traditional polyurethane Double J stent for 1 month	Before placement and after removal stents were analyzed using field emission scanning electron microscopy (FESEM), energy dispersive spectroscopy (EDS) and micro-infrared spectrophotometry (Micro-IR) Comparison of thickness, extension, and composition of encrustation Analysis of two heparin-coated stent at 10 and 12 months	FESEM: significant differences between groups about encrustation thickness and extension EDS and Micro-IR: in heparinized stents the encrustations were not as uniform and compact as those in the uncoated stents 10–12 months: free of encrustations and had no changes in the heparin layer

Table 2 (continued)

Study group	Sample	Intervention	Method study	Results
Kotsar et al. BJUI 2009 [24]	16 Male rabbits urethra	4 Groups: the stents inserted into the prostatic urethra Drugs: indomethacin, dexamethasone and ciprofloxacine. 80L/20D-PLGA stents without a drug coating served as controls Four rabbits in each group, were killed after 1 month	The urethra surrounding the stent was dissected from the rabbits en bloc Tissue blocks: haematoxylin and eosin following routine techniques Biodegradation process evaluated by optic microscopic analyses Biological response eosinophilia, acute inflammatory changes (polymorphonuclear leucocytes), chronic inflammatory changes (lymphocytes, plasma cells) and the amount of fibrosis	Control stents and the dexamethasone-eluting stents degraded totally during the follow-up period Indomethacin- and ciprofloxacine-eluting stent groups, the degradation process was significantly delayed and they induced an increase in epithelial hyperplasia All the stents induced eosinophilia No significant differences in the intensity of acute or chronic inflammatory reactions and fibrosis
Cadieux et al. Journal of Endourology 2009 [14]	8 Humans-ureter	Each patient: Control stent 3 months with antibiotics preoperative and postoperative After this: change to triclosan-eluting stent 3 months with no antibiotics	Stent removal and processing: cut into three equal-length sections (bladder, ureteral, and kidney) encrustation and surface: blinded technician and air dried Stent-adherent organisms: brain heart Infusion agar susceptibility to triclosan was determined via duplicate plating on Mueller Hinton agar	Staphylococcus isolated more in control stents Enterococcus isolated more in triclosan stents Fewer antibiotics were used during triclosan stenting, coinciding with a slightly higher number of positive urine cultures and significantly fewer symptomatic infections

(continued)

Table 2 (continued)

Study group	Sample	Intervention	Method study	Results
Krambeck et al. J Urol. 2010 [20]	276 Patients—ureter	Randomization occurred 1:1 to KL or control stent groups Stents were removed by pull-string or cystoscopically. Patients were followed for 30 days after stent removal Primary study end point was intervention for pain Secondary end points included intervention due to stent, pain medication use, VAS assessed pain and patient satisfaction assessed using a 5-point scale	Blood and urine samples were obtained for routine chemistry studies, serum ketorolac levels and urinalysis on days 0, 1, 2, 4, 7 and 10 after placement, the day of stent removal, and days 2 and 30 after stent removal	None of the safety cohort had detectable serum ketorolac levels No difference in primary (9.0% ketorolac loaded vs 7.0% control, $p > 0.66$) or secondary (22.6% ketorolac loaded vs 25.2% control, $p > 0.67$) intervention rates Pain pill count at day 3: KL < Control ($p < 0.05$) Use no or limited pain medications: KL > Control Male KL > Female KL, male and female control. $P < 0.05$

Table 2 (continued)

Study group	Sample	Intervention	Method study	Results
Chew et al. Journal of Endourology 2010 [21]	92 Yorkshire pigs—ureter	Randomization in 5 groups Control: non-drug-eluting stent + oral Ketorolac. n = 12 Autopsy at 2, 5, 15 days Control: non-drug-eluting stent n = 20 15% Ketorolac-loaded stent n = 20 13% Ketorolac-loaded stent n = 20 7% Ketorolac-loaded stent n = 20 Groups 2, 3, 4, 5: Necropsies at 2, 5, 15, 30, 60 days	Percutaneous aspiration of urine and venipuncture were obtained immediately before the autopsy Ketorolac levels were measured in plasma, urine, and tissue sampled from ureters, bladder, kidneys, and liver using high performance liquid chromatography (HPLC, Waters Alliance Separations Module, Model 2695, Waters Corporation, Milford, MA) Remainder of the genitourinary organs and liver: fixed and processed for histopathologic analysis and analyzed for any abnormality by a veterinarian pathologist blinded to the treatment group	majority of ketorolac first 30 days Highest levels of ketorolac: Group 1 Highest levels of ketorolac in ureter and bladder tissues: Ketorolac stent dose-dependent fashion Gastric ulcerations: Group 1
Kallidonis et al. Journal of Endourology 2011 [37]	10 Pigs and 6 rabbits—ureter	A zotarolimus-eluting stent (ZES) and a bare metal stent (BMS) were inserted in each ureter in the contralateral ureter as a control	Evaluation Porcine: CT every week/4 weeks Rabbit: IVU every week/8 weeks Renal scintigraphies were performed before stent insertion and during the third week in all animals Optical coherence tomograph (OCT): evaluation of the luminal and intraluminal condition of the ureters with stents Histological examination: glycol-methacrylate	Hyperplastic reaction in both groups 7 Porcine ureter: BMSs completely obstructed Porcine ureters with ZES stents without obstruction 2 Rabbit ureter: BMSs completely obstructed No rabbit ureter obstruction in with ZES stent OCT: hyperplastic reaction in the ureters with BMS > ureters with ZESs

(continued)

Table 2 (continued)

Study group	Sample	Intervention	Method study	Results
Wang et al. Journal of Bioactive and Compatible Polymers 2011 [33]	34 Male New Zealand White rabbits with urethral strictures 4 Male New Zealand White rabbits, without urethral strictures and stents Urethra	Group 1: n = 17 control stents and strictures Group 2: n = 17 drug paclitaxel-stents and strictures Group 3: n = 4 without urethral strictures and stents	Changes in the stent and the urethral stent-area: examined with pediatric urethroscope at 4, 8, and 12 weeks after stent implantation 12 weeks: Retrograde urethrography to assess the urethral lumen Urodynamics: bladder capacity and urethral pressure Histological analysis: hematoxylin and eosin (HE) Biological changes were assessed for drug-eluting stent and compared to control stent groups	Retrograde urethrography and urodynamic results at 12 weeks showed no comparable differences among the three groups urethroscopic and histological follow-up indicated that the drug stents had minimized the stent-related inflammatory responses, urothelial hyperplasia, and scar formation compared with the drug-free stents
Krane et al. Journal of Endourology 2011 [28]	12 Sprague–Dawley Rats—Urethra	Formation urethral scars via electrocautery Groups: n = 6 Coated with Halofungione (HF) n = 6 uncoated First inserting the silicone catheter, then placing a 30-gauge needle transversely completely through the corpora spongiosum and catheter and applying 10 W of electrocautery to the needle for 3 s At 2 weeks: euthanized and excision pene with urethral stent	Histopathological analysis: Masson trichrome stain or anti–alpha-1 collagen and then examined with bright-field microscopy Drug levels: tissue specimens— > HF concentration analysis via spectrophotometry Blood: HF concentration via spectrophotometry absorption at 243 nm on a standard curve	Group 1: Local urethral concentration of HF was tenfold higher than serum concentration Had no new type I collagen depo- sition after urethral injury Group 2: had increased periurethral collagen type I deposition, typical of urethral stricture formation

Table 2 (continued)

Study group	Sample	Intervention	Method study	Results
Kotsar et al. Journal of Endourology 2012 [26]	24 Male New Zealand White rabbits— Urethra	4 Groups Biodegradable braided pattern poly(lactic-*co*-glycolic acid) (PLGA) urethral stents coated with racemic 50L/50D PLA with two different concentrations of indomethacin were inserted into the prostatic urethra Half of the animals in each group were sacrificed after 3 weeks and the other half after 3 months	Histologic analyses (hematoxylin and eosin) Following biologic response parameters: inflammatory changes (neutrophil infiltration), chronic inflammatory changes (lymphocyte and plasma cell infiltration), foreign body reaction, fibrosis, calcification, and eosinophil infiltration The degradation process of the stent and the development of epithelial hyperplasia (polyposis) was evaluated by scanning electron microscopy SEM	SEM analysis revealed that indomethacin coating had no effect on the degradation process of the stents. Histologic analyses at 3 weeks: indomethacin-eluting stents caused more calcification but no significant differences in other tissue reactions 3 months: the indomethacin-eluting stents caused less inflammatory reaction and calcification compared with the control stents

(continued)

Table 2 (continued)

Study group	Sample	Intervention	Method study	Results
Mendez et al. BJUI 2012 [15]	20 Subjects requiring short-term stenting (7–15 days)—ureter	Group 1: n = 10. Percuflex Plus® non-eluting stent (control) Group 2: n = 10. Triumph® triclosan eluting stent Group 1: 3 days of levofloxacin prophylaxis (500 mg once daily) Group 2: did not received atb	Midstream urine samples were collected from each subject just prior to both stent placement and removal Urine culture Stents: cut into three equal length sections, brain heart infusion agar supplemented with 0.5% yeast extract Stent isolates were sent for identification and standard antibiotic susceptibility testing	Stent placement after: Group 1: 9 Ureteroscopic and 1extracorporeal shock wave lithotripsy Group 2: 8 ureteroscopic and 2 extracorporeal shock wave lithotripsy No significant differences were observed for culture Group 2: reductions in lower flank pain scores during activity (58.1% reduction, $P = 0.017$) and urination (42.6%, $P = 0.041$), abdominal pain during activity (42.1%, $P = 0.042$) and urethral pain during urination (31.7%, $P = 0.049$)
Kim et al. Radiology 2018 [38]	36 male Sprague–Dawley rats—urethra	Randomization equally: Group A: control biodegradable stents Group B: stents coated with 90 μg/cm² sirolimus Group C: stents coated with 450 μg/cm² sirolimus Each group: 6 rates sacrificed after 4 weeks, the remaining after 12 weeks	Retrograde urethrography and histologic examination (hematoxylin–eosin stained slices)	Urethrographic and histologic examination: Granulation tissue formation Groups B, C < A ($P < 0.05$ for all). No significant differences between B and C Number of epithelial layers B > C at 4 weeks after stent placement ($P < 0.001$) Apoptosis C > B,A ($P < 0.05$)

Table 2 (continued)

Study group	Sample	Intervention	Method study	Results
Han et al. PLoS ONE 2018 [27]	Six dogs—urethra	12 EW-7197-eluting nanofiber-covered stent (NFCS) were placed in the proximal and distal urethras in each dog Control stent group n = 3 received NFCSs Drug-stent group n = 3 received EW-7197 (1000 μg)-eluting NFCSs All dogs were sacrificed 8 weeks after stent placement	Urethrography: 4–8 weeks after stent's placement The histological samples were longitudinally sectioned at the three different portions of the segment with the stent Hematoxylin and eosin (H&E) and Masson's trichrome (MT) stains were used to study the samples The items were submucosal inflammatory cell infiltration, the number of epithelial layers, the thickness of submucosal fibrosis, and the thickness of papillary projection	Urethrographic analysis: mean luminal DS group > CS group at 4 and 8 weeks after stent placement (all $p < 0.001$) Histological examination: thicknesses of the papillary projection, thickness of submucosal fibrosis, number of epithelial layers, and degree of collagen DS group < CS group (all $p < 0.001$) Degree of inflammatory cell infiltration was not significantly different

(continued)

Table 2 (continued)

Study group	Sample	Intervention	Method study	Results
Kram et al. Urolithiasis 2018 [30]	48 Male 9-week-old Sprague–Dawley rats—ureter	3 Groups: n = 16: dissection of the left ureter without uretero-ureteral anastomosis but blunt manipulation of the ureter n = 16. Transsection of the left ureter and end-to-end anastomosis with insertion of either an uncoated ureteral stent n = 16. Transsection of the left ureter and end-to-end anastomosis with insertion of either an pacitaxel-coated ureteral stent	Daily intraperitoneal injections of 5-bromo-2-deoxyuridine the first eight postoperative days, sacrificed on day 28 Healing of the ureteral anastomosis and proliferation of urothelial cells was examined histologically (hematoxylin–eosin staining) and immunohistochemically	Both types of stents shown: inflammation, fibrosis and urothelial changes Proliferation of urothelial cells was significantly lower in animals with paclitaxel-coated stents compared to those with uncoated stents (LI 41.27 vs. 51.58, p < 0.001)
Lin et al. Journal of Nanomaterials 2018 [22]	Five New Zealand white rabbits—ureter	5 cm segment of the analgesic (ketorolac and lidocaine)-eluting nanofiber-incorporated ureter stent was inserted Urine and blood samples were collected 1, 3, 7, 14, 21, and 28 days	Infrared spectra of the analgesic-loaded nanofibrous matrix were evaluated employing Fourier transform infrared (FTIR) spectrometry Elution behavior characteristics of lidocaine and ketorolac from the analgesic-eluting ureteral stents were evaluated using an in vitro release scheme	Analgesic-eluting ureteral stents could liberate high strengths of analgesics in vitro and in vivo for at least 50 and 30 days, respectively The blood levels were much lower throughout the study period

Table 3 Summary of clinical studies using DCB

Study group	Sample	Intervention	Method of study	Results
Barbalias et al. Journal of Endourology 2017 [3]	11 Rabbitsurethra	A. n = 2 Balloon without drug B. n = 3 Balloon without drug + PCB immediately C. n = 3 Balloon without drug + PCB 24 h D. n = 3 Balloon without drug + PCB 48 h	Hematoxylin and eosin and IHC with polyclonal anti-paclitaxel antibody in posterior urethra	Existence of ruptures across the urethras of all the animals Existence of ruptures across the urethras of all the animals A. No PTX no inflammation B. PTX distributing in all layers, no inflammation C. PTX distributing in all lauers, mild acute inflammation D. PTX distributing in all lauers, mild acute inflammation
Liourdi et al. Journal of Endourology 2014 [34]	9 Domestic pigs ureter	Right ureter of each pig: PBE dilation Left ureter of each pig: CB dilation Ureter removal: immediately after 12 h After 24 h	A, B, C: Two samples from each ureter First sample investigated by Nuclear Magnetic Resonance Spectroscopy (NMR) The other: histology and IHC using a specific for paclitaxel polyclonal antibody	Group B, C: Reduced inflammation in comparison to their controls PTX present in urothelial, submucosal and muscle layer concentration of the paclitaxel C < B Group A: PTX present in urothelium and submucosal layer

(continued)

Table 3 (continued)

Study group	Sample	Intervention	Method of study	Results
Visasoro et al. Canadian Urological Association journal 2020 [35]	53 Patients urethra	Mechanical balloon dilation or direct visualization internal urethrotomy prior to drug-coated balloon treatment	Patient evaluation at 2–5 days, 14 days, 3, 6, and 12-months after treatment	Anatomic success defined as urethral lumen $\geq$ 14 Fr at 12 months Anatomic success achieved in 70% The 14 failures included 7 cystoscopic recurrences, 5 retreatments patients, 2 who exited the study early due to symptom recurrence Baseline IPSS improved. Quality of life, flow rate, and post-void residual urine volumes improved significantly
Mann et al. Canadian Urological Association journal 2021 [36]	53 Patients urethra	Mechanical balloon dilation or direct visualization internal urethrotomy prior to drug-coated balloon treatment	Patient evaluation at 24 months after treatment	Anatomic success achieved in 70%, and baseline IPSS improvement from a mean of 25.2–6.9 at 24 months ($p < 0.0001$) Quality of life, flow rate, and post-void residual urine volumes improved significantly

2 Drug Eluting Devices

Drug eluting devices can be classified in three major categories based on the pharmaceutical agent they carry: antibiotic, anti-inflammatory agents and drugs inhibiting the cell proliferation.

2.1 DES Delivering Antibiotics

Infections of the urinary tract are related with the presence of foreign materials such as catheters and nephrostomy tubes. These cases consist the most frequent hospital infections. Any foreign bodies (catheters or urinary stent) offer a suitable surface for the formation of a highly resistant biofilm [9–12]. Coating the ureteral stents with antibiotics could limit bacterial growth on the foreign bodies and prevent urinary infections. Thus, several antibiotic agents have proposed for urinary stents [9–12].

2.1.1 Triclosan

The antimicrobial agent Triclosan inhibits the fatty acids synthesis and disrupts the integrity of the bacterial cell's wall. Chew et al. tested the efficiency of Triclosan eluting stents against common uropathogens in artificial urine. In terms of bacterial growth and adherence, Triclosan DESs was efficient against most of the uropathogens apart from *P. aeruginosa* [9]. An ex vivo study, Cadieux et al., using the curls of a Triclosan-eluting stent sutured in a rabbit urethra verified the *in vitro* result, showing also reduced inflammation in comparison to the control group [13]. The same research team tested the long-term effect of using the Triclosan-eluting stent in a small patient group. The patients kept the DES for three months and received oral antibiotics when having UTI symptoms [14]. The results showed no significant difference in the number of the bacteria in the urine cultures. The encrustation rate of the Triclosan-eluting stents was compared to conventional stents in a randomized control trial including 20 patients. These patients were treated with short duration stenting [15]. No significant difference in encrustation rate was observed between the two groups but the Triclosan-eluting stent was associated with reduced incidents of symptomatic UTIs, abdominal and urethral pain and subsequently a reduced need for antibiotic therapy. Overall, the promising results of the in vitro and preclinical in vivo models were not observed in patients. Only the overall antibiotic need and patient discomfort were reduced. Despite the beneficial effects observed in the primary experience of this DES, it has been removed from the market.

2.1.2 Quinolones

Quinolones are commonly used for the management of urinary tract infections. The effect of quinolone-eluting stents has been examined. Stents with a mixture of ofloxacin and ornidazole were evaluated in terms of efficacy against *E. coli* and *S. epidermidis* in a study performed by Balasubramanian et al. [16]. The stents were found to be effective against these uropathogens in an agar diffusion test and microbial adhesion was significantly reduced on them in artificial urine environment compared to conventional stents. Studies with DESs containing ciprofloxacin showed that they have reliable antibacterial effect against common uropathogens such as *S. aureus* and *E. coli* without damaging the Human Foreskin Fibroblasts [12].

2.1.3 Silver and Nitrofurazone

Urethral catheters containing silver or nitrofurazone were evaluated for their efficacy in the inhibition of resistant *E. coli* and *P. aeruginosa* [11]. Nitrofurazone-coated stents offered longer inhibition of all E.coli strains compared to conventional stents, while the silver-coated showed no significant inhibition. Neither the nitrofurazone-coated, nor the silver-coated stent had any effect against *P. aeruginosa*. The fact that silver has antimicrobial effect but the silver-coated stents did not have any effect, perhaps indicates that the concentration of silver released in the urethra was not high enough to reach its antimicrobial potential. This indicates that while the ability of a stent to release a substance from its surface is important, high enough concentrations are necessary so that the drug eluting stent is effective.

2.1.4 RNA-Inhibiting Peptides and Teicoplanin

Researchers using combination of RNAIII-inhibiting peptides and teicoplanin in a drug-eluting stent managed to significantly reduce the microbial colonization. Interestingly, urine cultures were negative for bacterial growth [17].

2.1.5 Heparin

Stents coated with heparin were used to examine the possibility of decreasing the encrustation of the stent. Because heparin is a negatively charged molecule, an assumption was made that the negatively charged crystals would repel each other resulting in less encrustation. The layer of encrustation on the heparin-eluting stents was thinner and more restricted than the encrustation on the conventional ones, Nonetheless, the two groups did not differ significantly in terms of bacterial adhesion on the stents [18].

2.2 DES Delivering Anti-Inflammatory Substances

The patient discomfort that follows the insertion of a stent is mainly caused by the inflammatory response of the tissue in contact with the stent. Several anti-inflammatory agents have been embedded on stents in an attempt to prevent patient discomfort.

2.2.1 Ketorolac

Several studies involved devices that contained Ketorolac to ease the pain and reduce the inflammation [19–22]. While the in vitro and animal in vivo studies showed promising results, in the clinical trials Ketorolac stents failed to show significant difference in pain management compared to conventional stents. Only in the category of men under 45 years, significant difference was identified. Ketorolac did not have detectable plasma levels of the patients and led to the assumption that the concentrations were not high enough to achieve the therapeutic levels.

2.2.2 Indomethacin, Dexamethasone and Simvastatin

Dexamethasone was one of the first anti-inflammatory drugs that has been used to cover stents. Antimisiaris et al. [23] applied large multi-lamellar liposomes containing dexamethasone to metallic stents to evaluate in vitro the rate of release of dexamethasone. Absorbable urethral stents containing indomethacin, dexamethasone and simvastatin were used in rabbit urethras to examine the potential reaction of the components and their potential effect in the degradation process [24]. In vivo animal studies using absorbable indomethacin-eluting stents revealed that the delivery of the drug did not intervene with the degradation of the stent and the use of the stents led to lower inflammation and calcification rate during the degradation [25, 26]. The potential role of the indomethacin-stent after urethrotomy should be examined.

2.2.3 EW-7197

Han et al. investigated a nano fiber-self expendable stent that contained the TGF-β type 1 inhibitor EW-7197 in a canine model [27]. The aim of the study was to compare the formation of granulation tissue between a control and a DES stent after an 8-week period. The use of DES resulted in wider urethral luminal diameters, thinner layers submucosal fibrosis and papillary projection and less epithelial layers and collagen deposition in comparison to the control group.

2.2.4 Halofungione (HF)

Krane et al. [28] eluted halofungione on a urethral stent. This alkaloid acts as a selective inhibitor of collagen type I. the stent was inserted in in rat urethras with strictures created by electrocautery. The use of halofungione prevented the formation of new type I collagen in the rat urethra.

2.3   DES and DCB Containing Anti-Cancer Drugs

Stents releasing anti-proliferative agents has been used in great extent in interventional cardiology. The combination of limiting the cell proliferation and avoiding the formation of fibrosis made this drug category especially suitable for preventing coronary vessel restenosis. The advantages in treating restenosis led to the creation of ureteral and urethral stents and balloons.

2.3.1   Paclitaxel

Paclitaxel inhibits the mitosis by stabilizing the microtubules of the cell. It is the most commonly used antiproliferative drug in studies evaluating devices for urinary stenosis.

Aiming to investigate the ability of antiproliferative drugs to permeate membrane models, Barros et al. [29] used ureteral stents with doxorubicin and paclitaxel. The researchers concluded that both drugs were restricted in the ureter and only a fraction of the total drug passed all the layers. Kram et al. [30] used a DES containing paclitaxel in rat ureters to examine its inhibitory effect in hyperplastic proliferation. The rats underwent ureteroureterostomy followed by the insertion of a drug-eluting or a conventional stent. The DES was found significantly more effective in reducing the cell proliferation in the side of the anastomosis. In a similar manner, Liatsikos et al. [31] compared DES to conventional stents in terms of inflammation and the tissue hyperplasia occurring in porcine ureter. The ureters with the indwelling DES showed increased patency in urography compared to the ureters with the conventional stent. Shin et al. came to the same conclusions after examining a custom made paclitaxel stent in canine urethra [32] (Fig. 2).

Biodegradable stents have been also evaluated in an experimental study. Wang et al. used a biodegradable paclitaxel DES in rabbit urethra and observed the absorption of the stent in 12 weeks. Moreover, the treated urethral mucosa showed no signs of fibrosis while the urethras of the control group showed signs of fibrosis [33].

In addition to DES, DCBs with paclitaxel have been investigated (Fig. 3). Barbalias et al. [3] studied how paclitaxel is distributed in layers of rabbit urethra. The study included the dilation of the posterior urethra and subsequent dilation with a paclitaxel-coated balloon. Histological analysis showed that paclitaxel penetrates the urethral layers and especially the urothelial barrier. A similar study by Liourdi et al. [34] proved that dilation with DCBs containing paclitaxel resulted in distribution of the drug in every layer of the ureter. While the forementioned studies proved that paclitaxel could be distributed in through the urothelium to the all the layers of the urethra and the ureter, these experiments were performed in animal models which did not have strictures.

ROBUST I is a multi-centered study prospective study examining the safety and efficacy of Optilume™ Drug Coated Balloon (DCB; Urotronic, Plymouth, MN) in patients with recurrent bulbar strictures. Visasoro et al. published the first-year

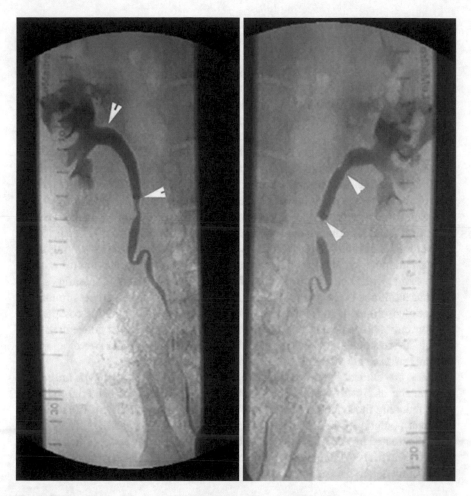

Fig. 2 DES vs bare metal stent efficacy comparison in a porcine model

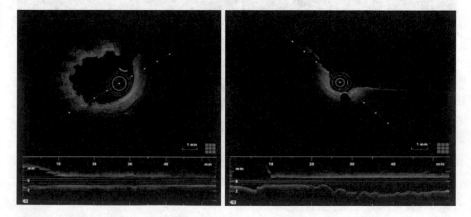

Fig. 3 Ureter optical coherence tomography before—after DCB

results results of 53 patients that have been treated in their center using the paclitaxel-coated balloon mentioning 70% anatomic success, which was defined as diameter of lumen equal or greater than 14 Fr [35]. The same research group published the 2 years results announcing 70% success in having at least 50% improved IPSS sore for 2 years after the surgery [36]. Flow rate and post-void residual urine volumes were also improved. There researchers did not encounter any severe adverse effects. The long-term results of the study are expected after a 5-year follow up has been completed. However, it is crucial to bear in mind that every patient in this study prior to use of the DCB balloon received either an uncoated balloon or direct visualization internal urethrotomy treatment until their urethral diameter was increased by 50%. Consequently, safe assumptions for the use of paclitaxel-balloons as monotherapy for the treatment of bulbar strictures cannot be made yet Fig. 4.

Apart from paclitaxel, the efficacy of other anti-proliferative agents such as zotarolimus and sirolimus have been evaluated. Kallidonis et al. [37] using DESs containing zotarolimus in pigs and rabbits showed that zotarolimus-eluting stents reduce inflammation and tissue hyperplasia in comparison to the control conventional stents. Kim et al. used two types of sirolimus-eluting stents containing different concentrations of the agent in male rat models [38]. The researchers found that the use of sirolimus stents reduced the formation of granulation tissue compared to the conventional stents and that the use of stents with sirolimus concentration of 450 $\mu g/cm^2$ resulted to less layers of epithelial growth and greater rate of apoptosis in comparison to the 90 $\mu g/cm^2$ stent and the conventional stent.

Many pre-clinical studies testing drug eluting devices have shown impressive results. The ability to prevent fibrosis, tissue proliferation or bacterial adhesion while reducing the symptoms and improving the patient's quality of life underline the great potential of these devices. That said, achieving a stable delivery of the drug, unaffected by the urine flow could be a key factor to lead to significant results in the human trials. Assumptions for the efficacy of the devices in humans cannot be made safely due to the lack of large clinical studies.

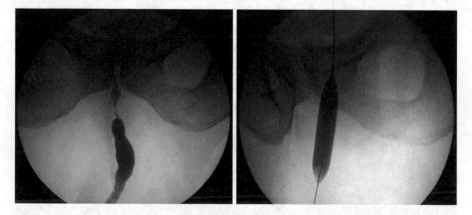

Fig. 4 Use of DCB in urethral strictures

References

2. Al-Aown A, Kyriazis I, Kallidonis P, Kraniotis P, Rigopoulos C, Karnabatidis D, et al. Ureteral stents: new ideas, new designs. Ther Adv Urol. 2010;2(2):85–92.
3. Vyas J, Ganpule A, Muthu V, Sabnis R, Desai M. Balloon dilatation for male urethral strictures "revisited". Urol Ann. 2013;5(4):245–8.
4. Barbalias D, Lappas G, Ravazoula P, Liourdi D, Kyriazis I, Liatsikos E, et al. Evaluation of the distribution of paclitaxel after application of a paclitaxel-coated balloon in the rabbit urethra. J Endourol. 2018;32(5):381–6.
5. Fattori R, Piva T. Drug-eluting stents in vascular intervention. Lancet. 2003;361(9353):247–9.
6. Ni L, Chen H, Luo Z, Yu Y. Bioresorbable vascular stents and drug-eluting stents in treatment of coronary heart disease: a meta-analysis. J Cardiothorac Surg. 2020;15(1):26.
7. Stefanini GG, Holmes DR Jr. Drug-eluting coronary-artery stents. N Engl J Med. 2013;368(3):254–65.
8. Nestelberger T, Kaiser C, Jeger R. Drug-coated balloons in cardiovascular disease: benefits, challenges, and clinical applications. Expert Opin Drug Deliv. 2020;17(2):201–11.
9. Kallidonis PS, Georgiopoulos IS, Kyriazis ID, Al-Aown AM, Liatsikos EN. Drug-eluting metallic stents in urology. Indian J Urol. 2014;30(1):8–12.
10. Chew BH, Cadieux PA, Reid G, Denstedt JD. In-vitro activity of triclosan-eluting ureteral stents against common bacterial uropathogens. J Endourol. 2006;20(11):949–58.
11. Elayarajah E, Rajendran R, Venkatrajah V, Sreekumar S. Biopolymer tocopherol acetate as a drug carrier to prevent bacterial biofilm formation on silicone ureteral stents. Int J Pharm Sci Rev Res. 2011;7(2):96–103.
12. Johnson JR, Johnston BD, Kuskowski MA, Pitout J. In vitro activity of available antimicrobial coated Foley catheters against *Escherichia coli*, including strains resistant to extended spectrum cephalosporins. J Urol. 2010;184(6):2572–7.
13. Ma X, Xiao Y, Xu H, Lei K, Lang M. Preparation, degradation and in vitro release of ciprofloxacin-eluting ureteral stents for potential antibacterial application. Mater Sci Eng C Mater Biol Appl. 2016;66:92–9.
14. Cadieux PA, Chew BH, Knudsen BE, Dejong K, Rowe E, Reid G, et al. Triclosan loaded ureteral stents decrease *Proteus mirabilis* 296 infection in a rabbit urinary tract infection model. J Urol. 2006;175(6):2331–5.
15. Cadieux PA, Chew BH, Nott L, Seney S, Elwood CN, Wignall GR, et al. Use of triclosan-eluting ureteral stents in patients with long-term stents. J Endourol. 2009;23(7):1187–94.
16. Mendez-Probst CE, Goneau LW, MacDonald KW, Nott L, Seney S, Elwood CN, et al. The use of triclosan eluting stents effectively reduces ureteral stent symptoms: a prospective randomized trial. BJU Int. 2012;110(5):749–54.
17. Balasubramanian E, Rajendran R, Venkatrajah SS. Biopolymer tocopherol acetate as a drug carrier to prevent bacterial biofilm formation on silicone ureteral stents. Int J Pharm Sci Rev Res. 2011;7:96–103.
18. Cirioni O, Ghiselli R, Minardi D, Orlando F, Mocchegiani F, Silvestri C, et al. RNAIII-inhibiting peptide affects biofilm formation in a rat model of staphylococcal ureteral stent infection. Antimicrob Agents Chemother. 2007;51(12):4518–20.
19. Cauda F, Cauda V, Fiori C, Onida B, Garrone E. Heparin coating on ureteral double J stents prevents encrustations: an in vivo case study. J Endourol. 2008;22(3):465–72.
20. Barros AA, Oliveira C, Reis RL, Lima E, Duarte AR. Ketoprofen-eluting biodegradable ureteral stents by CO_2 impregnation: in vitro study. Int J Pharm. 2015;495(2):651–9.
21. Krambeck AE, Walsh RS, Denstedt JD, Preminger GM, Li J, Evans JC, et al. A novel drug eluting ureteral stent: a prospective, randomized, multicenter clinical trial to evaluate the safety and effectiveness of a ketorolac loaded ureteral stent. J Urol. 2010;183(3):1037–42.
22. Chew BH, Davoudi H, Li J, Denstedt JD. An in vivo porcine evaluation of the safety, bioavailability, and tissue penetration of a ketorolac drug-eluting ureteral stent designed to improve comfort. J Endourol. 2010;24(6):1023–9.

23. Lin YC, Liu KS, Lee D, Li MJ, Liu SJ, Ito H. In vivo and in vitro elution of analgesics from multilayered poly(D,L)-lactide-*co*-glycolide nanofibers incorporated ureteral stents. J Nanomater. 2018;2018:8829.

24. Antimisiaris SG, Siablis D, Liatsikos E, Kalogeropoulou C, Tsota I, Tsotas V, et al. Liposome-coated metal stents: an in vitro evaluation of controlled-release modality in the ureter. J Endourol. 2000;14(9):743–7.

25. Kotsar A, Isotalo T, Uurto I, Mikkonen J, Martikainen P, Talja M, et al. Urethral in situ bio-compatibility of new drug-eluting biodegradable stents: an experimental study in the rabbit. BJU Int. 2009;103(8):1132–5.

26. Kotsar A, Nieminen R, Isotalo T, Mikkonen J, Uurto I, Kellomäki M, et al. Biocompatibility of new drug-eluting biodegradable urethral stent materials. Urology. 2010;75(1):229–34.

27. Kotsar A, Nieminen R, Isotalo T, Mikkonen J, Uurto I, Kellomaki M, et al. Preclinical evaluation of new indomethacin-eluting biodegradable urethral stent. J Endourol. 2012;26(4):387–92.

28. Han K, Park JH, Yang SG, Lee DH, Tsauo J, Kim KY, et al. EW-7197 eluting nano-fiber covered self-expandable metallic stent to prevent granulation tissue formation in a canine urethral model. PLoS One. 2018;13(2):e0192430.

29. Krane LS, Gorbachinsky I, Sirintrapun J, Yoo JJ, Atala A, Hodges SJ. Halofuginone-coated urethral catheters prevent periurethral spongiofibrosis in a rat model of urethral injury. J Endourol. 2011;25(1):107–12.

30. Barros AA, Oliveira C, Reis RL, Lima E, Duarte ARC. In vitro and ex vivo permeability studies of paclitaxel and doxorubicin from drug-eluting biodegradable ureteral stents. J Pharm Sci. 2017;106(6):1466–74.

31. Kram W, Rebl H, Wyrwa R, Laube T, Zimpfer A, Maruschke M, et al. Paclitaxel-coated stents to prevent hyperplastic proliferation of ureteral tissue: from in vitro to in vivo. Urolithiasis. 2018;48(1):47–56.

32. Liatsikos EN, Karnabatidis D, Kagadis GC, Rokkas K, Constantinides C, Christeas N, et al. Application of paclitaxel-eluting metal mesh stents within the pig ureter: an experimental study. Eur Urol. 2007;51(1):217–23.

33. Shin JH, Song HY, Choi CG, Yuk SH, Kim JS, Kim YM, et al. Tissue hyperplasia: influence of a paclitaxel-eluting covered stent—preliminary study in a canine urethral model. Radiology. 2005;234(2):438–44.

34. Wang ZX, Hong BF, Xu Z, Fu WJ, Cui FZ, Kun H. New biodegradable drug-eluting stents for urethral strictures in a rabbit model. J Bioact Compat Polym. 2011;26(1):89–98.

35. Liourdi D, Kallidonis P, Kyriazis I, Tsamandas A, Karnabatidis D, Kitrou P, et al. Evaluation of the distribution of paclitaxel by immunohistochemistry and nuclear magnetic resonance spectroscopy after the application of a drug-eluting balloon in the porcine ureter. J Endourol. 2015;29(5):580–9.

36. Virasoro R, DeLong JM, Mann RA, Estrella RE, Pichardo M, Lay RR, et al. A drug-coated balloon treatment for urethral stricture disease: Interim results from the ROBUST I study. Can Urol Assoc J. 2020;14(6):187–91.

37. Mann RA, Virasoro R, DeLong JM, Estrella RE, Pichardo M, Lay RR, et al. A drug-coated balloon treatment for urethral stricture disease: two-year results from the ROBUST I study. Can Urol Assoc J. 2021;15(2):20–5.

38. Kallidonis P, Kitrou P, Karnabatidis D, Kyriazis I, Kalogeropoulou C, Tsamandas A, et al. Evaluation of zotarolimus-eluting metal stent in animal ureters. J Endourol. 2011;25(10):1661–7.

39. Kim KY, Park JH, Kim DH, Tsauo J, Kim MT, Son WC, et al. Sirolimus-eluting biodegradable poly-*l*-lactic acid stent to suppress granulation tissue formation in the rat urethra. Radiology. 2018;286(1):140–8.

Methods and Materials for Drug Eluting Urinary Stents Design and Fabrication

Irene Carmagnola, Giulia Giuntoli, and Gianluca Ciardelli

1 Introduction

After urinary stenting, patients often suffer from mid- and long-term complications, such as infections, bacterial colonization, encrustations, or stent obstruction which are related to the design, materials and surface properties of the stent.

Drug eluting stents (DES) is an advance technology that can reduce the morbidity associated with stenting, by locally releasing loaded drugs in a time-controlled manner.

The first DES were introduced in the earlies'00 for cardiovascular applications to address the problems of restenosis associated with bare metal stents after coronary angioplasty [1]. In urology, DES could potentially solve or reduce a variety of stent-related and time-dependent complications, such as infections and obstruction, which are often related to encrustation and biofilm formation and which can dramatically result in stent failure [2]. Moreover, they could also find application for the management of cancer therapies [3] (Fig. 1).

Common stents are made of "inert" materials to minimize the foreign body reaction. Nonetheless, these stents are affected by several clinical problems. For instance, encrustation is caused by the deposition of urine constituents (such as

I. Carmagnola (✉) · G. Giuntoli
Department of Mechanical and Aerospace Engineering, Politecnico di Torino, Turin, Italy

PolitoBIOMed Lab, Politecnico di Torino, Turin, Italy
e-mail: irene.carmagnola@polito.it; giulia.giuntoli@polito.it

G. Ciardelli
Department of Mechanical and Aerospace Engineering, Politecnico di Torino, Turin, Italy

PolitoBIOMed Lab, Politecnico di Torino, Turin, Italy

Department for Materials and Devices of the National Research Council, Institute for the Chemical and Physical Processes (CNR-IPCF), Pisa, Italy
e-mail: gianluca.ciardelli@polito.it

© The Author(s) 2022
F. Soria et al. (eds.), *Urinary Stents*,
https://doi.org/10.1007/978-3-031-04484-7_32

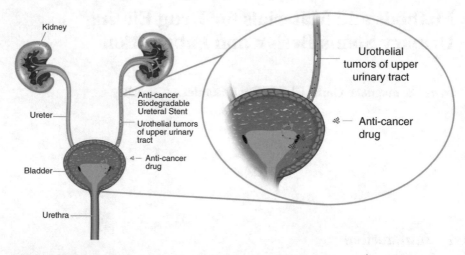

Fig. 1 Scheme of the concept of anti-cancer drug eluting biodegradable ureteral stent as a potential drug delivery system

proteins, ions and minerals) over the stent's surface [4]. This phenomenon occurs due to the physico-chemical characteristics of patient's urine, such as urine pH, composition and flow dynamics, as well as stent's constitutive materials or surface characteristics. Encrustation not only compromises stent drainage potential but also favor bacterial colonization and biofilm formation [5].

Different strategies can be applied to feature the stent with drug delivery systems able to reduce the incidence of encrustation and biofilm development by increasing the drug effectiveness and limiting any side effect associated with systemic delivery.

In this chapter is firstly reported an overview of the materials and manufacturing methods for conventional urinary stents, then are discussed the engineered strategies for the design and fabrication of drug eluting stents. These strategies can be divided into two main categories which are discussed in more detail in the next paragraphs: (1) DES obtained by surface functionalization and coating techniques, or (2) direct manufacturing.

2 Conventional Urinary Stents

2.1 Urinary Stent Materials

The constitutive materials of urinary stents have great influence on their performances and durability. Materials are selected based on several requirements such as biocompatibility, mechanical strength and flexibility, surface properties, ease processability and cost-effectiveness.

Non-biodegradable polymeric and metallic materials are the main constitutive materials used for urinary stenting. The first ureteral stent, described by Herdman in 1949, was made of polyethylene due to its desirable properties such as flexibility, strength, hydrophobicity and bio-inertness [6]. However, it was soon abandoned due to the occurrence of encrustations and the high risk of fracturing. Today, the most common polymeric non-biodegradable materials include silicones, polyurethanes, and other proprietary materials [7]. Between them, silicones have shown better performances in terms of encrustation resistance and ions deposition hindering [8].

Compared to polymeric stents, metallic stents made of titanium, nickel–titanium alloys (e.g. nitinol), or stainless steel have superior mechanical properties, and are often chosen to treat severe conditions, such as malignant ureteric strictures, or when long indwelling times are required [9]. Metallic stents suffer from encrustation as the polymeric ones but have higher migration rates and production costs.

More recently, biodegradable and/or bioresorbable stents have been introduced as novel class of temporary stents which can be dissolved or absorbed in the body [10]. These stents have the advantage of decreasing patient discomfort, eliciting fewer complications—for instance they are less prone to encrustation-, and reducing the healthcare costs (e.g. secondary procedures for stent replacement or removal). Biodegradable polymers include poly(L-lactide) acid (PLLA), polyglycolide (PGA) and polycaprolactone (PCL), whereas biodegradable metals include magnesium and its alloys [11]. Although very promising, no biodegradable nor bioresorbable stents have yet the U.S. Food and Drug Administration (FDA) regulatory approval for urological applications.

2.2 Conventional Stent Manufacturing

Extrusion is the most common technique for manufacturing polymeric hollow tubes from thermoplastic materials. Plastic materials, in the form of pellets, granules, flakes or powders, are fed from a hopper into the barrel of the extruder machine; the molten polymer is forced by a rotating screw into a die, which confers to the product its final shape. To obtain a hollow section, a pin or a mandrel is placed within the die, while, to prevent the tube from collapsing, a positive or negative pressure can be applied to the internal lumen or to the outside diameter of the tube, respectively. For tubes with multiple lumens, more than one pin can be inserted into the die.

Coextrusion is typically used to produce a multilayered tube by extruding simultaneously two or more discrete layers of different materials using the same die. This technique can be exploited, for instance, to encapsulate non-medical materials between two medical-material layers. Blow molding and die drawing are other hot process techniques employed for fabricating polymeric tubes. In the former, blown air expand the polymeric tube against a mold, while the latter, similarly to extrusion, forces the polymer through a conical die.

Metal based stents are obtained by extrusion or die casting, followed by surface treatments such as chemical or plasma etching, plasma treatment micro-electro discharge machining, and laser cutting [12]. Laser cutting is a rapid prototyping technique that ensures a high-precision, burr-free cut, reliability and flexibility of the design.

3 Drug Eluting Stents

Drug eluting stent is an effective means for local drug delivery to the urinary tract. It can potentially solve a variety of upper urinary tract problems, such as stent-related urinary tract infections and discomfort, ureteral stricture, and neoplastic diseases. There are many strategies for loading drugs, including: (1) hot melt extrusion; (2) soaking the polymers into drug solution (dipping); (3) CO_2 impregnation; (4) nanofibers; (5) nanoparticles. However, the release of drug elutes on the surface of biostable stents is often unsustainable and uncontrollable.

Some previous researches had coated drugs to the surface of biostable stents, and the results were not satisfactory due to the uncontrolled drug release. Alternatively, drugs or active agents can be continuously released in a controlled manner from a drug-eluting biodegradable stents (BUS), when the stent degrades. BUS are potentially a powerful tool to contrast the most frequent adverse effects reported by patients experiencing that are pain and difficulties in urinary tract.

Several surface engineering strategies have been applied to minimize encrustation and bacterial adherence over the stent surface, through antimicrobial (bactericidal), anti-fouling (bacteriostatic), lubricating or drug eluting coatings [13].

Natural antibacterial coatings include glycosaminoglycans and heparin—natural components of the urine that were found to delay encrustation; hydrophilic coatings such as phosphoryl-choline or hydrogels demonstrated the ability to inhibit biofilm formation thanks to the hydrophilic environment that hinders proteins adsorption, thus bacterial adhesion; similarly, chitosan is used for its intrinsic antibacterial properties. Other coatings, like diamond-like carbon or polytetrafluoroethylene, diminish the surface friction, facilitating stent insertion and placement while lowering patient discomfort.

3.1 Coating Strategies

Stents surface can be directly coated with active agents by several methods, such as impregnation by dipping or supercritical fluid technology [3], crystallization, spray-coating, or layer-by-layer techniques. The first are most traditional and used, instead layer-by-layer technique is quite innovative in the urinary stent fields.

Drugs immobilization by impregnation is a two-step procedure: first, a conventional polymeric or metallic stent is fully immersed into a solution containing the drug; subsequently the solvent evaporates leaving the surface coated with the drug.

Antibacterial agents/drugs can also be directly spray-coated onto the surface of the stent [14]. For example, Nasongkla et al. deposited chlorhexidine-loaded nanospheres on the surface by high-pressure emulsification-solvent evaporation technique. In detail nanosphere suspension was perpendicularly sprayed to the spinning silicone tubes for 10 s by air pump spray gun with the flow rate of 0.2 mL/s. Then silicone tubes were drained under air flow. The drug release ability of the coated silicone tubes were tested in artificial urine and the chlorhexidine was sustained release for 2 weeks. Additionally, nanoparticles based coating showed antibacterial activity against common bacteria causing urinary tract infections up to 15 days.

Similarly, direct crystallization allows to crystallize drug onto a substrate through temperature-dependent or microdrop spray, ensuring a slower release than amorphous drug layers due to lower dissolution rate and at the same time limiting the loaded drug amount [15]. However the direct crystallization method is characterized by burst drug release kinetics.

With solvent-based polymer spraying, a drug-eluting coating can be obtained with few steps, including [16]: drugs incorporation into the polymeric solution by mixing, drug/polymer formulation spraying onto the surface; solvent evaporation. Coating characteristics, such as thickness, can be easily tailored by controlling solvent evaporation kinetics or spaying parameters. DES with prolonged antibiotic action have been obtained by spray coating drug-loaded nanospheres solutions, obtaining a smooth and homogeneous coating after several spray cycles; a sustained drug release up to 30 days occurs after the initial burst release of the loaded drug [14].

Layer-by-layer technique was firstly proposed by Decher et al. in the beginning of 1990s and it based on the alternating exposure of a charged substrate to solutions of molecules with opposite charges. After each deposition step, the substrate is washed to avoid cross-contamination of the polyelectrolyte solutions and eliminate the excess polyelectrolytes. The LBL technique allows to obtain homogeneous coating with precise and tunable architecture. It is also applicable to substrates of any shape and dimension, it is environmentally friendly and all the deposition processes can be carried out in mild conditions with low-cost manufacturing. The coating features are easily tunable by adjusting the experimental parameters, such as pH, ionic strength and polyelectrolyte concentration [15–17]. Tzanov and co-workers proposed the layer-by-layer technique to modify the surface of silicone urinary catheters to achieve infection-preventive coatings, as summarized on Fig. 2. Aminocellulose nanospheres positively charged were combined with the hyaluronic acid (HA) polyanion to build a layer-by-layer construct on silicone surfaces. Silicone supports were previously functionalized by polymerizing 3-(aminopropyl) triethoxysilane, ensuring the deposition of the first negatively charged HA layer, the multilayer coating was build-up employing a multi-vessel automated dip coater system to obtain 5, 10 and 100 bilayers. LbL coating antibiofilm activity was tested against *P. aeruginosa*. The inhibition of biofilm formation was already

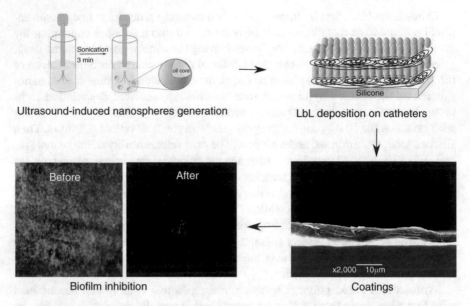

Fig. 2 Scheme of the antibacterial surfaces fabrication exploiting LbL techniques on silicone based surface. (From [18])

demonstrated with 5 bilayers coating. The antibiofilm efficiency of 10 bilayer multilayer coating on a Foley catheter was additionally validated under dynamic conditions using a model of the catheterized bladder in which the biofilm was grown during 7 days.

Although the manufacturing process is quite simple, DES obtained by direct coating methods are short term solutions and do not ensure sustained drug delivery. In fact, due to the rapid drug elution times, 90% of the drug is released within 2 days via burst release; once the thin biodegradable coatings are fully degraded or the drug content completely eluted, DES can be compared to conventional stents. To delay the complete depletion of the drug, additional coatings can be used for drug protection, among which the most common are hydrogels. Solutions employing drug delivery systems overcome the limited effectiveness of delivery observed for DES obtained by direct coating methods and provide the stent with sustained and controlled drug release over few weeks. The approach of using polymer coating layers has several functions: (1) delay the complete depletion of the active agent; (2) operate as drug loading system; (3) control drug release kinetics; (4) act as biocompatible coating after drug depletion.

Stents with a hydrophilic hydrogel coatings are currently commercially available (e.g., Universa® Soft Ureteral Stent-COOK® Medical). Hydrogel based coatings are design to reduce surface friction upon deployment which facilitates the placement of the stent and lowers patient discomfort and to be exploited for the controlled release of drugs and other biologically active compounds. For instance, antiproliferative drugs can be spray-coated onto the surface of the stent and be further covered with an additional hydrogel layer to protect them upon stent insertion and further prevent a burst release [19]. Similarly, hydrogel or other polymeric materials can also work as a carrier due to a direct or indirect incorporation of the targeted drug into the polymeric matrix. Indirect incorporation includes the use of nano-spheres/nanoparticles in which the drug can be loaded [20].

Drug-loaded nanoparticles can be prepared by several encapsulation methods which are reviewed by Pinto Reis et al., and others [21, 22]. Most of these procedures are simple and have industrial scale-up applicability, besides high encapsulation efficacy and improved pharmacokinetics and pharmacodynamics.

3.2 DES Direct Manufacturing

Drug eluting stents may be fabricated in a single process using direct manufacturing techniques. Drug delivery is a typical application of multilayered extruded tubes obtained by coextrusion [23]. In detail reservoir implants contain a drug loaded core encased in a rate controlling sheath. Co-extrusion to produce a core-sheath or multiple layer system requires multiple single screw extruders: centering and process adjustments to control dimensions can be difficult. The materials in the layers should stick together; generally chemical similarity predicts adhesion.

In the last decades additive manufacturing techniques have been emerged as alternative tool for the fabrication of drug-eluting implants combining the advantages of a targeted local drug therapy over longer periods of time with a manufacturing technique that easily allows modifications of the implant shape to comply with the individual needs of each patient [24]. Research until now has been focused on several aspects of this topic such as 3D-printing with different materials or printing techniques to achieve implants with different shapes, mechanical properties or release profiles.

3.3 DES Bioabsorbable Urinary Stents

Drug-eluting technologies can be successfully combined with completely biodegradable devices. A biodegradable stent would eliminate the need for the patient to undergo a stent removal procedure, the problems of chronic indwelling stents (encrustation, stone, formation, infection), as well as the complication feared by urologists knows as the forgotten stent.

Biodegradable urinary stents (BUS) include both bioabsorbable natural or synthetic polymers, or metals. Polymeric BUS are not yet in available for urological applications but represent an important area of investigation.

BUS present several benefits such as higher resistance to encrustation and elimination of stent removal/replacement procedures, with an overall reduction of healthcare costs. The most used biodegradable polymer is PLA. Polylactic acid (PLA) belongs to the family of aliphatic polyesters commonly made from α-hydroxy acids. It is both biocompatible and biodegradable and it is one of the most promising polymers in various applications, including biomedical field, due to its mechanical, thermoplastic and biological properties. PLA is a biodegradable polymer, which degrade in physiological environment by macromolecular scission into smaller fragments, and then into stable end-products. It is possible to produce PLA textile structures, by different techniques, such as extrusion of the polymer into mono- and multifilaments, which may be achieved by melt, dry, dry-wet-jet spinning or electrospinning.

Different techniques can be used to incorporate drugs/active agents on BUS. Freeze-casting has been proposed as a new fabrication method to obtain biodegradable porous stents with increased urine drainage and reduced risk of reflux [25]. This simple technique involves few steps: (1) preparation of a stable suspension or polymeric solution (usually water-based); (2) injection into a mold; (3) solidification by freezing within the mold; (4) solvent removal by sublimation (freeze-drying). Porous biodegradable DES could be further obtained by dispersing the selected drug in the polymeric solution using impregnation techniques. A method for obtaining drug-eluting BUS is supercritical CO_2-impregnation, reported by Barros et al. [26]. This technique has several advantages over conventional water- or solvent-based impregnation, since supercritical CO_2 shows high diffusivity and low viscosity, resulting in a fast diffusion of the solute molecules into the polymer matrix (Fig. 3). Moreover, CO_2 is chemically inert in a wide range of conditions, has low toxicity, environmental sustainability, besides being ready available and low-cost [27].

Nowadays, nanotechnologies are widely used in many fields, including biomedical applications. Among nanotechnologies, electrospinning (ES) is rapidly emerging as a simple, versatile, and cost-effective method for the fabrication of smooth non-woven fibers with controllable morphology and tunable porosity, from a charged polymer solution or melt. Electrospinning process involves the application of a high electric field to produce micro and nanofibers. The features of the end fibers depend both on solution properties, such as polymer molecular weight, concentration and conductivity, and operating parameters, such as flow-rate, applied voltage and tip-collector distance.

ES has high encapsulation efficiency for drug loading, controlled residence time, desirable delivery of encapsulated drug at a predictable rate, better stability, high surface contact area, degradability, and satisfactory softness and flexibility.

Chew et al. reported many studies about the fabrication of biodegradable eluting ureteral stent by using double-needle electrospinning [28, 29]. To address the main

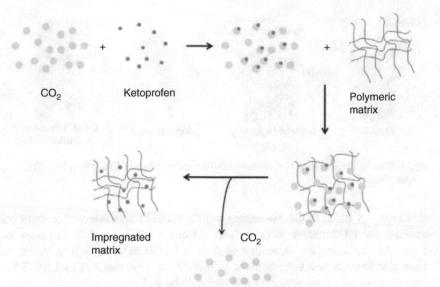

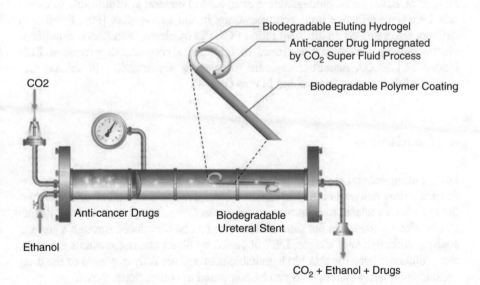

Fig. 3 Supercritical CO_2-impregnation process of ketoprofen into a polymeric matrix. (From [26])

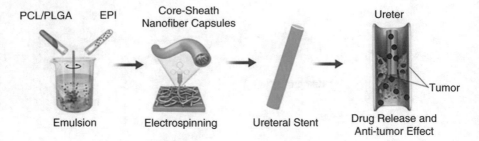

Fig. 4 Schematic illustration of preparation and antitumor effect of EPI-loaded PCL/PLGA electrospun fibers

challenges of BUS, PLGA degrading within 8 weeks was selected as stent basic material in combination with polycaprolactone (PCL) which degrades over 6 months. By using the technique of double nozzle electrospinning, researchers were able to produce a ureteral stent with different mass ratios of PCL/PLGA that degrade gradually from proximal end to the distal end.

PCL/PLGA based nanofibers can be exploited to have a controlled drug release. Ding et al. developed a biodegradable drug-loaded ureteral scaffolds able to maintain long-term effective drug concentrations in the lesion sites [30]. Epirubicin delivery was assessed on different ration PCL/PLGA electrospun fibers. Emulsion-electrospinning technology was used to fabricate a core–sheath structured EPI-loaded PCL/PLGA nanofiber capsules, displaying a sustained EPI release and controlled degradation *in vitro* and *in vivo* (Fig. 4).

4   Conclusions

Drug eluting ureteral stents, and in general urinary stents, were introduced to performed a drug delivery aiming to obtain a local treatment as well as to overcomes the main issues related to urinary stenting implantation. Drugs and/or active agents can be directly loaded in the stent structure or can be introduced through a surface coating. Although very simple, DES obtained by direct coating methods are short term solutions; once the thin biodegradable coatings are fully degraded or the drug content completely eluted, DES can be compared to conventional stents.

Drug-eluting technologies can then be combined with biodegradable bioabsorbable stents in order to eliminate the need for stent removal procedure. However some disadvantages remain still unsolved. In the last decades innovative manufacturing approaches and methods, such as nanotechnologies and additive manufacturing techniques, provide to scientists new tools for the design and fabrication on smart and custom-made urinary stents, able to go towards perfectly to patient needs.

References

1. Stone GW, Lansky AJ, Pocock SJ, Gersh BJ, Dangas G, Wong SC, et al. Paclitaxel-eluting stents versus bare-metal stents in acute myocardial infarction. N Engl J Med. 2009;360(19):1946–59.
2. Sali GM, Joshi HB. Ureteric stents: overview of current clinical applications and economic implications. Int J Urol. 2020;27:7–15.
3. Barros AA, Browne S, Oliveira C, Lima E, Duarte ARC, Healy KE, et al. Drug-eluting biodegradable ureteral stent: new approach for urothelial tumors of upper urinary tract cancer. Int J Pharm. 2016;513(1–2):227–37.
4. Elwood CN, Lo J, Chou E, Crowe A, Arsovska O, Adomat H, et al. Understanding urinary conditioning film components on ureteral stents: profiling protein components and evaluating their role in bacterial colonization. Biofouling. 2013;29(9).1115–22.
5. Barros AA, Oliveira C, Lima E, Duarte ARC, Healy K, Reis RL. Ureteral stents technology: biodegradable and drug-eluting perspective. In Comprehensive biomaterials II. Amsterdam: Elsevier; 2017. p. 793–812.
1. Herdman JP. Polythene tubing in the experimental surgery of the ureter. Br J Surg. 1949;37(145):105–6.
2. Todd AM, Knudsen BE. Ureteral stent materials: past, present, and future. In Ureteric stenting. New York: Wiley; 2017. p. 83–90.
3. Tunney MM, Keane PF, Jones DS, Gorman SP. Comparative assessment of ureteral stent biomaterial encrustation. Biomaterials. 1996;17(15):1541–6.
4. Liatsikos E, Kallidonis P, Kyriazis I, Constantinidis C, Hendlin K, Stolzenburg JU, et al. Ureteral obstruction: is the full metallic double-pigtail stent the way to go? Eur Urol. 2010;57(3):480–7.
5. Brotherhood H, Lange D, Chew BH. Advances in ureteral stents. Transl Androl Urol. 2014;3(3):314–9.
6. Eberhart RC, Su SH, Nguyen KT, Zilberman M, Tang L, Nelson KD, et al. Bioresorbable polymeric stents: current status and future promise. J Biomater Sci Polym Ed. 2003;14(4):299–312.
7. Kathuria YP. The potential of biocompatible metallic stents and preventing restenosis. Mater Sci Eng A. 2006;417(1–2):40–8.
8. Mosayyebi A, Manes C, Carugo D, Somani BK. Advances in ureteral stent design and materials. Curr Urol Rep. 2018;19(5):1–5.
9. Phuengkham H, Nasongkla N. Development of antibacterial coating on silicone surface via chlorhexidine-loaded nanospheres. J Mater Sci Mater Med. 2015;26(2):1–11.
10. Baquet M, Jochheim D, Mehilli J. Polymer-free drug-eluting stents for coronary artery disease. J Interv Cardiol. 2018;31(3):330–7.
11. McMahon S, Bertollo N, Cearbhaill EDO, Salber J, Pierucci L, Duffy P, et al. Bio-resorbable polymer stents: a review of material progress and prospects. Prog Polym Sci. 2018;83: 79–96.
12. Gentile P, Carmagnola I, Nardo T, Chiono V. Layer-by-layer assembly for biomedical applications in the last decade. Nanotechnology. 2015;26(42):422001.
13. Francesko A, Fernandes MM, Ivanova K, Amorim S, Reis RL, Pashkuleva I, et al. Bacteria-responsive multilayer coatings comprising polycationic nanospheres for bacteria biofilm prevention on urinary catheters. Acta Biomater. 2016;33:203–12. https://doi.org/10.1016/j. actbio.2016.01.020.
14. Lim WS, Chen K, Chong TW, Xiong GM, Birch WR, Pan J, et al. A bilayer swellable drug-eluting ureteric stent: localized drug delivery to treat urothelial diseases. Biomaterials. 2018;165:25–38. https://doi.org/10.1016/j.biomaterials.2018.02.035.
15. Laurenti M, Grochowicz M, Dragoni E, Carofiglio M, Limongi T, Cauda V. Biodegradable and drug-eluting inorganic composites based on mesoporous zinc oxide for urinary stent applications. Materials (Basel). 2020;13(17):3821.

16. Pinto Reis C, Neufeld RJ, Ribeiro AJ, Veiga F, Nanoencapsulation I. Methods for preparation of drug-loaded polymeric nanoparticles. Nanomed Nanotechnol Biol Med. 2006;2(1): 8–21.
17. Liu Y, Yang G, Jin S, Xu L, Zhao CX. Development of high-drug-loading nanoparticles. ChemPlusChem. 2020;85:2143–57.
18. Johnson AR, Forster SP, White D, Terife G, Lowinger M, Teller RS, et al. Drug eluting implants in pharmaceutical development and clinical practice. Expert Opin Drug Deliv. 2021;18(5):577–93. https://doi.org/10.1080/17425247.2021.1856072.
19. Domsta V, Seidlitz A. 3D-printing of drug-eluting implants: an overview of the current developments described in the literature. Molecules. 2021;26(13):4066.
20. Yin K, Divakar P, Wegst UGK. Freeze-casting porous chitosan ureteral stents for improved drainage. Acta Biomater. 2019;84:231–41.
21. Barros AA, Oliveira C, Reis RL, Lima E, Duarte ARC. Ketoprofen-eluting biodegradable ureteral stents by CO_2 impregnation: in vitro study. Int J Pharm. 2015;495(2):651–9.
22. Tadesse Abate M, Ferri A, Guan J, Chen G, Nierstrasz V. Impregnation of materials in supercritical CO_2 to impart various functionalities. In Advanced supercritical fluids technologies. London: IntechOpen; 2020.
23. Wang X, Shan H, Wang J, Hou Y, Ding J, Chen Q, et al. Characterization of nanostructured ureteral stent with gradient degradation in a porcine model. Int J Nanomed. 2015;10:3055–64.
24. Wang X, Zhang L, Chen Q, Hou Y, Hao Y, Wang C, et al. A nanostructured degradable ureteral stent fabricated by electrospinning for upper urinary tract reconstruction. J Nanosci Nanotechnol. 2015;15(12):9899–904.
25. Sun Y, Shan H, Wang J, Wang X, Yang X, Ding J. Laden nanofiber capsules for local malignancy chemotherapy. J Biomed Nanotechnol. 2019;15(5):939–50.

Preventing Biofilm Formation and Encrustation on Urinary Implants: (Bio)coatings and Tissue Engineering

Noor Buchholz, Petra de Graaf, Julia E. de la Cruz, Wolfgang Kram, Ilya Skovorodkin, Federico Soria, and Seppo Vainio

1 Introduction

Even though urinary stents and catheters have been commonly applied in medicine for several decades and still are constantly being modified and optimized, their structure and performance still requires further improvement. A major drawback of urinary implants is the deposition of organic and non-organic substances

N. Buchholz, P. de Graaf, Julia E. De la Cruz, W. Kram, I. Skovorodkin, F. Soria and S. Vainio contributed equally with all other contributors.

N. Buchholz (✉)
U-merge Scientific Office, London-Athens-Dubai, Athens, Greece

P. de Graaf
Department of Urology, University Medical Center Utrecht, Utrecht, The Netherlands
e-mail: pgraaf4@umcutrecht.nl

J. E. de la Cruz
U-merge Scientific Office, London-Athens-Dubai, Athens, Greece

Jesus Uson Minimally Invasive Surgery Centre Foundation, Caceres, Spain
e-mail: jecruz@ccmijesususon.com

W. Kram
Department of Urology, University Medical Center Rostock, Rostock, Germany
e-mail: wolfgang.kram@med.uni-rostock.de

I. Skovorodkin · S. Vainio
Laboratory of Developmental Biology, Disease Networks Research Unit, Faculty of Biochemistry and Molecular Medicine, Kvantum Institute, Infotech Oulu, University of Oulu, Oulu, Finland
e-mail: ilya.skovorodkin@oulu.fi; seppo.vainio@oulu.fi

F. Soria
Foundation, Jesús Usón Minimally Invasive Surgery Center, Cáceres, Spain
e-mail: fsoria@ccmijesususon.com

on their surface leading to biofilm formation resulting in encrustations, blockages, and infections.

In this chapter, we will present some modern biological research approaches to this problem. Promising research lines are stent coatings with antibodies, enzymes and various bioactive compounds. We will also discuss the possibility for making urinary implants more "tissue friendly" by designing biomimetic surfaces. Finally, in accordance with the paradigm "repair or regrow" we will touch on tissue engineering approaches to replace artificial urinary implants by those generated *in vitro* or *in vivo* from homologous tissue.

1.1   Antibody Coating

Despite significant differences between urine and blood as the extracellular environment, designing of urinary implants has always been inspired by research approaches in cardiovascular stent engineering.

Antibody stent coating is a technology that was successfully applied to improve clinical performance of cardiovascular stents and might be considered for further optimization of urinary stents.

Coating of vascular stents with certain types of antibodies (namely: CD34, CD133 and VEGFR2) enhances migration of endothelial progenitor cells (EPCs) circulating in the blood to the site of injury, thus accelerating the healing and regeneration of vascular tissue [1, 2]. At the same time, populating of the stent surface and surrounding tissue with EPCs prevents migration of inflammatory and smooth muscle cells which can cause neo-intimal hyperplasia, and re-stenosis and thrombosis of damaged blood vessels [1–3]. Antibody-coated cardiovascular stents showed promising results in preclinical trials [3]. Other antibodies with anti-inflammatory, anti-platelet and anti-proliferative effects also have shown their efficiency in reducing stenosis and neo-intimal hyperplasia *in vitro* [4, 5].

Despite the success of antibody stent-coating in cardiology, regrettably to our knowledge no preclinical or even experimental researches in this field have been presented for urinary implants to date. Hypothetically, antibodies of implant coatings could attract urinary and cell components that prevent biofilm formation and urothelial hyperplasia on one hand, and promote peri-implant tissue healing on the other hand in cases where such implants are used temporarily after injuries or operations to the urinary tract. As a prerequisite for such a research approach, efforts must be made to identify urinary and cellular components with the desired properties first.

2   Enzyme Coating

Antimicrobial enzymes (AE) have been tested as part of urinary catheter coatings. AE are found in immune systems of living organisms where their task is to attack pathogenic microbes. Hydrolytic AE destroy the structure of their foes, whereas oxidative AE trigger the production of antimicrobial molecules inside them. Quorum quenching AE interfere with bacterial quorum sensing which leads to inhibition of cell aggregation and virulent compounds [6].

AE can be attached to surfaces of medical devices, either permanently or ready to be released. Integrated methods for a controlled release include chelation or metal binding, disulfide [7], physical and ionic bonds [8].

Permanent or irreversible binding has however the advantage of better stability and decreased leaching. This can be achieved by crosslinking with linker molecules, entrapment, microencapsulation and covalent bonding [6].

For instance, cellobiose dehydrogenase (CDH), using cello-oligosaccharides as electron donors to produce H_2O_2, inhibited different urinary microbes including MRSA in the presence of either cellobiose or extracellular polysaccharides (EPS). The latter are essential in biofilm formation. Therefore, CDH could act as an antimicrobial agent "on demand" whenever beginning biofilm formation is triggering the reaction [9].

Oxalobacter formigenes is part of our gut microbiome and has been linked to non-infectious stone formation. It can degrade oxalate with the help of oxalate-degrading enzymes. These enzymes have been attached to stent coatings resulting in a 53% reduction in encrustation [10, 11].

When compared with current antibiotics or other antimicrobial agents used as active parts of urinary implant coatings, AE have certain advantages. They are highly specific targeting only a particular bacterium without disturbing the natural microbiome. Bacterial resistance to enzymes is very rare. Care must be taken not to overdose the enzymes though in order to prevent such resistance development. Enzymes are safe, natural, non-reactive and non-toxic to other than their target organisms.

Currently, AE are expensive to produce which puts them at a disadvantage to cheaper alternatives like silver and antibiotic coatings. And it has to be borne in mind that they are proteins. That means they can get denatured during i.e. sterilization, storage and transport [6].

3   Biomimetic Stents

Natural surfaces have been the envy of many researchers. However, they are difficult to mimic and usually outperform their artificial copies. If it comes to internal and external surfaces, researchers try to get as close to the properties of natural surfaces as possible. Natural surfaces are made to repel or let seep through whatever is physiologically required by their environment. Blood and blood vessels form such an environment. With cardiology leading the way for a long time in stent research, it is no surprise that the attempt to create biomimetic surfaces gets its push from cardiology as well.

Although stents have been used extensively in cardiology, they do have inherent problems such as inflammatory responses, thrombosis, endothelial hyperproliferation, delayed re-endothelialization, and ultimately stenosis and thrombotic obstruction [12]. An endothelium-like stent could alleviate many of these problems. A metal (copper)–catechol–(amine) (MCA) coated stent has thus been shown to facilitate a fast regeneration of a functional endothelium [12].

Earlier, a phosphorylcholine coating was effective in resisting platelet adhesion and prolong plasma recalcification time significantly. Contact angle measurements showed that the surface rearranged to become more hydrophilic at the polymer/water interface [13].

In blood vessels, biomimetic surfaces may create an enhanced anti-thrombogenic, anti-inflammatory and anti-proliferative micro-environment. In addition, such coatings could be made drug eluting [14]. Biomimetic stents will improve biocompatibility in the future [12]. Whether lessons learned from cardiology can be applied to a urinary environment will be the subject of future research. In theory, biomimetic surfaces have the ability to resist bacterial adhesion and consecutive biofilm formation.

4   Bioactive Nanocoating

As soon as urinary implants are inserted into a recipient, different biological materials start to accumulate on their surfaces. These substances, especially extracellular matrix (ECM) proteins, attract cells which migrate from surrounding tissue and form a biofilm thus affecting shape, mechanical properties and functionality of the implant. Application of nanomaterials [15, 16] can mimic cell—ECM interaction and, depending on what is required, can either suppress or induce cell migration.

To date, optimization of the structural and functional performance of the implants was mostly achieved by surface coating with different bioactive molecular substances such as growth factors and immunosuppressive and anti-inflammatory drugs.

Interaction between cells, tissues and implanted mechanical objects strongly depend on the surface to volume ratio and, consequently, varies significantly when the objects are represented at macro-, micro- or nano-scale size ranges. In particular, this concerns particles < 10–15 nm and irregular in size distribution which affects greatly such material properties as roughness, friction and surface dislocation [17].

Materials with a particular 3D nanostructure can be generated either by coating of the surface with nanoparticles or modification of the surface by chemical and physical treatments. Combining these methods is even more effective. A controllable release of nanoparticles to the surface of the implant creates an additional modality for surface coating which helps to reduce potential toxicity.

Different materials could be proposed for nanocoating of urinary implants with each of them possessing certain advantages and disadvantages as to their applicability and functionality. Polymer-based and lipid nanoparticles (i.e. liposomes) are usually biocompatible and can be easily biodegradable. They are suitable for transportation of biologically active compounds to the cells due to their similarity to natural nanoparticles—extracellular vesicles, which take part in cell-cell communication [18].

Carbon nanotubes and fullerenes likewise possess a high biocompatibility since carbon is one of the main components of living tissues. They are smaller in size and have a high surface-to-volume ratio. Since carbon nanoparticles can form complex three-dimensional structures, they are especially useful for targeted delivery of particular bioactive substances.

Metal-based nanoparticles produced usually from transition metals like zinc, gold, silver and copper, are described broadly in the scientific literature. However, despite demonstrated good antimicrobial properties their antifungal and anti-viral efficiencies have not been established.

Toxicity of nanocoating particles has not been a problem so far [19]. However, a deep understanding is required due to the wide range of nanomaterials proposed for medical application and the great variety of their physico-chemical properties and ensuing potential effects on biological tissues.

5   Tissue Engineering and Regenerative Medicine as Future Research Lines

This research line has preliminarily looked at urinary stents in the lower urinary tract. Stents were available for the treatment of lower urinary tract obstruction from the late 1980s. Despite initial enthusiasm, further studies questioned their usefulness as a primary treatment for urethral stricture disease [20]. Fibrotic tissue ingrowth is the main complication in permanently implanted stents but it can occur even in temporarily indwelling stents.

An ideal urinary stent should promote tissue healing, reduce fibrosis and scar formation, and maintain the physiological functions of the lower urinary tract. In addition, it would be desirable if they would be biodegradable and could stimulate their gradual replacement by regenerated autologous tissue.

Even though this is yet wishful thinking, some progress has been made in the field of vascular and coronary artery stenting where implantation of complex tissue composites rather than a simple stent is required. How can this be translated into urology, and more specifically into the treatment of lower urinary tract stricture disease?

There are few experimental trials on the designing of urethral stents using tissue engineering approaches [21, 22]. To our knowledge though, these clinical and preclinical applications have not proceeded beyond phase two trials.

The main problem of tissue engineered grafts or stents is the lack of appropriate acceptance by the host leading to fibrosis or rejection. If the wound bed consists of intact and viable tissue, transplantation of epithelium only might be sufficient [23]. In cases of fibrosis or developmental defects, vascularized grafts should be generated, e.g. by populating scaffolds with endothelial cells of endothelial progenitors [24–26].

In contrast to vascular stents, where the cells required for tissue regeneration can migrate from the blood, in urinary stents the recruitment of the cells from urine is rather unlikely though not impossible. If the urethral graft is well vascularized, blood flow might deliver important cells and cell progenitors to the sites of tissue regeneration. To make this approach clinically relevant, comprehensive studies on the role of inflammatory cells in tissue regeneration (which must be induced) and fibrosis (which must be prevented) are required.

In addition to *in situ* approaches where biodegradable urinary stents could be gradually replaced by regenerated tissue, we must consider cases where the tissue damage caused by trauma or disease is beyond the regenerative potential of the organism. In these cases, reconstruction of parts of the urinary tract must be done completely in vitro, using synthetic or naturally derived scaffolds [27, 28], manufactured by 3D printing [29] and electrostatic spinning [30], and populated by different types of cells (including autologous cells and progenitors) [31, 32]. Application of endothelial cell-attracting extracellular matrix into a graft scaffold and pre-vascularization of a transplant on vasculature-rich tissues (such as omentum) [31], as well as engineering of perfusable blood vessels of the transplant in vitro [33, 34] could be used for vascularization of the grafts. Combination of a "cell sheet technology" with bioprinting of cellularized scaffolds has a great potential for future perspectives of engineering of urinary stents.

Another completely different approach based on a "let mother nature do the job" paradigm can also be considered for designing urinary stents. The fundamental discovery of iPS cells [35] and the not yet that well-known tissue engineering technology of "blastocyst complementation" [36, 37] cumulatively might open the possibility to grow patient-specific organs (including different components of the lower urinary tract) in humanized animals. With this technique, certain gene modifications in the host organism prevents formation of the target organ during embryogenesis. Patient-derived iPS cells delivered to the blastocysts of immunocompromised animals will rescue the developmental program and form the target organ which will consist of human cells. After maturation in the animal host, the complete tissue/organ or its parts can be transplanted to the patient. As an alternative to the "blastocyst complementation" assay, based on the use of "humanized animals", it is also proposed to transplant specific human progenitor cells to actual sites of organogenesis thus leading to formation of target organs that consist of patient-derived cells [38]. These futuristic approaches, however, have not been tested in preclinical trials and can only be considered as a proof of concept to date.

6   Conclusions

In this chapter we have summarised modern biological approaches to improve the structure, function and performance of urinary stents. Some have been already applied in urinary stent production whilst others have been tested in the field of vascular stents, such as antibody or biomimetic coating. Bioengineering approaches aiming at the generation of complete analogs of damaged urinary tissue from autologous patient-derived cells represent a more futuristic outlook. Nevertheless, we hope that the rapid development of advanced multidisciplinary research platforms in modern biomedicine will make these approaches feasible in the near future.

References

1. Wawrzyńska M, Duda M, Wysokińska E, Strządała L, Biały D, Ulatowska-Jarża A, Kałas W, Kraszewski S, Pasławski R, Biernat P, Pasławska U, Zielonka A, Podbielska H, Kopaczyńska M. Functionalized CD133 antibody coated stent surface simultaneously promotes EPCs adhesion and inhibits smooth muscle cell proliferation—a novel approach to prevent in-stent restenosis. Colloids Surf B Biointerfaces. 2019;174(1):587–97.
2. Wawrzyńska M, Kraskiewicz H, Paprocka M, Krawczenko A, Bielawska-Pohl A, Biały D, Roleder T, Wojakowski W, O'Connor IB, Duda M, Michal R, Wasyluk Ł, Plesch G, Podbielska H, Kopaczyńska M, Wall JG. Functionalization with a VEGFR2-binding antibody fragment leads to enhanced endothelialization of a cardiovascular stent in vitro and in vivo. J Biomed Mater Res B Appl Biomater. 2020;108(1):213–24.
3. de Winter RJ, Chandrasekhar J, Kalkman DN, Aquino MB, Woudstra P, Beijk MA, Sartori S, Baber U, Tijssen JG, Koch KT, Dangas GD, Colombo A, Mehran R, MASCOT; REMEDEE Registry Investigators. 1-Year clinical outcomes of all-comer patients treated with the dual-therapy COMBO stent: primary results of the COMBO Collaboration. JACC Cardiovasc Interv. 2018;11(19):1969–78.
4. Cui S, Liu JH, Song XT, Ma GL, Du BJ, Lv SZ, Meng LJ, Gao QS, Li K. A novel stent coated with antibodies to endoglin inhibits neointimal formation of porcine coronary arteries. Biomed Res Int. 2014;2014:428619.
5. Lim KS, Jeong MH, Bae IH, Park JK, Park DS, Kim JM, Kim JH, Kim HS, Kim YS, Jeong HY, Song SJ, Yang EJ, Cho DL, Sim DS, Park KH, Hong YJ, Ahn Y. Effect of polymer-free TiO₂ stent coated with abciximab or alpha lipoic acid in porcine coronary restenosis model. J Cardiol. 2014;64(5):409–18.
6. Singha P, Locklin J, Handa H. A review of the recent advances in antimicrobial coatings for urinary catheters. Acta Biomater. 2017;50:20–40.
7. Cabral J, Novais J, Kennedy J. Immobilization studies of whole microbial cells on transition metal activated inorganic supports. Appl Microbiol Biotechnol. 1986;23(3–4):157–62.
8. Roig M. Immobilised cells and enzymes—a practical approach: Edited by J Woodward. Oxford: IRL Press; 1985. p. 177. ISBN-947946-21-7.
9. Thallinger B, Argirova M, Lesseva M, Ludwig R, Sygmund C, Schlick A, Nyanhongo GS, Guebitz GM. Preventing microbial colonisation of catheters: antimicrobial and antibiofilm activities of cellobiose dehydrogenase. Int J Antimicrob Agents. 2014;44(5):402–8.
10. Malpass CA, Millsap KW, Sidhu H, Gower LB. Immobilization of an oxalate-degrading enzyme on silicone elastomer. J Biomed Mater Res. 2002;63(6):822–9.
11. Watterson JD, Cadieux PA, Beiko DT, Cook AJ, Burton JP, Harbottle RR, Lee C, Rowe E, Sidhu H, Reid G, Denstedt JD. Oxalate-degrading enzymes from *Oxalobacter formigenes*: a novel device coating to reduce urinary tract biomaterial-related encrustation. J Endourol. 2003;17(5):269–74.
12. Yang Y, Gao P, Wang J, Tu Q, Bai L, Xiong K, Qiu H, Zhao X, Maitz MF, Wang H, Li X, Zhao Q, Xiao Y, Huang N, Yang Z. Endothelium-mimicking multifunctional coating modified cardiovascular stents via a stepwise metal-catechol-(amine) surface engineering strategy. AAAS Res. 2020;2020:9203906.
13. Fan D, Jia Z, Yan X, Liu X, Dong W, Sun F, Ji J, Xu J, Ren K, Chen W, Shen J, Qiu H, Gao R. Pilot study of a cell membrane like biomimetic drug-eluting coronary stent. Sheng Wu Yi Xue Gong Cheng Xue Za Zhi. 2007;24(3):599–602.
14. Elsawy MM, de Mel A. Biofabrication and biomaterials for urinary tract reconstruction. Res Rep Urol. 2017;9:79–92.
15. Webster TJ, Ahn ES. Nanostructured biomaterials for tissue engineering bone. In: Lee K, Kaplan D (eds) Tissue engineering II: basics of tissue engineering and tissue applications. 2007, Berlin: Springer. p. 275–308.
16. Brackman G, Coenye T. Quorum sensing inhibitors as anti-biofilm agents. Curr Pharm Des. 2015;21:5–11.

17. Rane GK, Welzel U, Meka SR, Mittemeijer EJ. Non-monotonic lattice parameter variation with crystallite size in nanocrystalline solids. Acta Mater. 2013;61(12):4524–33.
18. Jaggessar A, Shahali H, Mathew A, Yarlagadda PKDV. Bio-mimicking nano and micro-structured surface fabrication for antibacterial properties in medical implants. J Nanobiotechnol. 2017;15(1):64.
19. Raja IS, Song SJ, Kang MS, et al. Toxicity of zero- and one-dimensional carbon nanomaterials. Nanomaterials (Basel). 2019;9(9):1214.
20. Djordjevic ML. Treatment of urethral stricture disease by internal urethrotomy, dilatation, or stenting. Eur Urol Suppl. 2016;15(1):7–12.
21. de Kemp V, de Graaf P, Fledderus JO, Ruud Bosch JL, de Kort LM. Tissue engineering for human urethral reconstruction: systematic review of recent literature. PLoS One. 2015;10(2):e0118653.
22. Versteegden LRM, de Jonge PKJD, IntHout J, van Kuppevelt TH, Oosterwijk E, Feitz WFJ, de Vries RBM, Daamen WF. Tissue engineering of the urethra: a systematic review and meta-analysis of preclinical and clinical studies. Eur Urol. 2017;72(4):594–606.
23. Ram-Liebig G, Barbagli G, Heidenreich A, Fahlenkamp D, Romano G, Rebmann U, Standhaft D, van Ahlen H, Schakaki S, Balsmeyer U, Spiegler M, Knispel H. Results of use of tissue-engineered autologous oral mucosa graft for urethral reconstruction: a multicenter, prospective, observational trial. EBioMedicine. 2017;23:185–92.
24. de Graaf P, Ramadan R, Linssen EC, Staller NA, Hendrickx APA, Pigot GLS, Meuleman EJH, Bouman M, Özer M, Bosch JLHR, de Kort LMO. The multilayered structure of the human corpus spongiosum. Histol Histopathol. 2018;33(12):1335–45.
25. van Velthoven MJJ, Ramadan R, Zügel FS, Klotz BJ, Gawlitta D, Costa PF, Malda J, Castilho MD, de Kort LMO, de Graaf P. Gel casting as an approach for tissue engineering of multilayered tubular structures. Tissue Eng Part C Methods. 2020;26(3):190–8.
26. Zhang K, Fu Q, Yoo J, Chen X, Chandra P, Mo X, Song L, Atala A, Zhao W. 3D bioprinting of urethra with PCL/PLCL blend and dual autologous cells in fibrin hydrogel: an in vitro evaluation of biomimetic mechanical property and cell growth environment. Acta Biomater. 2017;50:154–64.
27. Wissing TB, Bonito V, Bouten CVC, Smits AIPM. Biomaterial-driven in situ cardiovascular tissue engineering—a multi-disciplinary perspective. NPJ Regen Med. 2017;16(2):18. https://doi.org/10.1038/s41536-017-0023-2.
28. Setayeshmehr M, Esfandiari E, Rafieinia M, Hashemibeni B, Taheri-Kafrani A, Samadikuchaksaraei A, Kaplan DL, Moroni L, Joghataei MT. Hybrid and composite scaffolds based on extracellular matrices for cartilage tissue engineering. Tissue Eng Part B Rev. 2019;25(3):202–24.
29. Kolesky DB, Truby RL, Gladman AS, Busbee TA, Homan KA, Lewis JA. 3D bioprinting of vascularized, heterogeneous cell-laden tissue constructs. Adv Mater. 2014;26(19):3124–30.
30. Fu WJ, Zhang X, Zhang BH, Zhang P, Hong BF, Gao JP, Meng B, Kun H, Cui FZ. Biodegradable urethral stents seeded with autologous urethral epithelial cells in the treatment of post-traumatic urethral stricture: a feasibility study in a rabbit model. BJU Int. 2009;104(2):263–8.
31. Zhao Z, Liu D, Chen Y, Kong Q, Li D, Zhang Q, Liu C, Tian Y, Fan C, Meng L, Zhu H, Yu H. Ureter tissue engineering with vessel extracellular matrix and differentiated urine-derived stem cells. Acta Biomater. 2019;88:266–79.
32. Chapple C. Tissue engineering of the urethra: where are we in 2019? World J Urol. 2020;38(9):2101–5.
33. Sakaguchi K, Shimizu T, Horaguchi S, Sekine H, Yamato M, Umezu M, Okano T. In vitro engineering of vascularized tissue surrogates. Sci Rep. 2013;3:1316.
34. Sekiya S, Shimizu T. Introduction of vasculature in engineered three-dimensional tissue. Inflamm Regen. 2017;37:25.
35. Takahashi K, Yamanaka S. Induction of pluripotent stem cells from mouse embryonic and adult fibroblast cultures by defined factors. Cell. 2006;126(4):663–76.

36. Stanger BZ, Tanaka AJ, Melton DA. Organ size is limited by the number of embryonic progenitor cells in the pancreas but not the liver. Nature. 2007;445(7130):886–91.
37. Yokoo T. Kidney regeneration with stem cells: an overview. Nephron Exp Nephrol. 2014;126(2):54.
38. Fujimoto T, Yamanaka S, Tajiri S, Takamura T, Saito Y, Matsumoto K, Takase K, Fukunaga S, Okano HJ, Yokoo T. In vivo regeneration of interspecies chimeric kidneys using a nephron progenitor cell replacement system. Sci Rep. 2019;9(1):6965.

Preventing Biofilm Formation and Encrustation on Urinary Implants: (Bio)molecular and Physical Research Approaches

Ali Abou-Hassan, Alexandre A. Barros, Noor Buchholz, Dario Carugo, Francesco Clavica, Filipe Mergulhao, and Shaokai Zheng

1 Introduction

Stents and catheters are used to facilitate urine drainage within the urinary system [1]. When such sterile implants are inserted into the urinary tract, ions, macromolecules and bacteria from urine, blood or underlying tissues accumulate on their surface. This often results in the formation of biofilm causing infections that can

A. Abou-Hassan, Barros, N. Buchholz, D. Carugo, F. Clavica, F. Mergulhao and S. Zheng contributed equally with all other contributors.

A. Abou-Hassan (✉)
Sorbonne Université, CNRS UMR 8234, PHysico-chimie des Électrolytes et Nanosystèmes InterfaciauX, Paris, France
e-mail: ali.abou_hassan@sorbonne-universite.fr

A. A. Barros
3B's Research Group, University of Minho, Barco Guimãraes, Portugal
e-mail: Alexandre.barros@i3bs.uninho.pt

N. Buchholz
U-Merge Scientific Office, London-Athens-Dubai, Athens, Greece

D. Carugo
Department of Pharmaceutics, UCL School of Pharmacy, University College London, London, UK
e-mail: d.carugo@ucl.ac.uk

F. Clavica · S. Zheng
ARTORG Center for Biomedical Engineering Research, Faculty of Medicine, University of Bern, Bern, Switzerland
e-mail: francesco.clavica@unibe.ch; shaokai.zheng@unibe.ch

F. Mergulhao
LEPABE, Faculty of Engineering, University of Porto, Porto, Portugal
e-mail: filipem@fe.up.pt

© The Author(s) 2022
F. Soria et al. (eds.), *Urinary Stents*,
https://doi.org/10.1007/978-3-031-04484-7_34

be responsible for discomfort and complications in patients [2]. Therefore, urinary tract implants may be considered as out-of-equilibrium systems where different phenomena acting at various times and length scales occur. This leads to their reshaping by deposition and encrustation of chemical and biological species on their surface and the formation of bacterial biofilms and mineral crystals. Due to the continuous nature of biological fluids, these phenomena are in perpetual dynamics and self-organization, which can complicate their study in the human body [3, 4]. Giving this complexity of the "system", a multidisciplinary input with different scientific approaches is needed to better understand and find solutions to this problem. In this chapter, we outline research strategies addressing biocompatibility, the use of antisense molecules, non-pathogenic bacteria and bacteriophages, and physical methods to prevent or inhibit biofilm formation and encrustation.

2   Biodegradable Metal Stents

Biodegradable metals are very appealing for urinary stent applications since they combine enhanced radial strength with a prolonged but controlled degradation time. Therefore, biodegradable metallic urinary stents (BMUS) constitute a promising research strategy overcoming some of the current stent limitations. The potential of biodegradable metals for urological applications was explored first by Lock et al., who investigated the efficacy of Magnesium–4%Yttrium (Mg–4Y), AZ31, and commercially pure Mg as antibacterial BMUS. They showed a significant decrease of *E. coli* viability in the presence of Mg alloys after 3 days compared with a commonly used commercially available polyurethane stent [5]. Zhang et al. explored the potential of the ZK60 Mg alloy and pure Mg for urinary applications in a rat model. ZK60 had a faster degradation rate than pure Mg and neither of the metals showed toxicity during the three weeks implantation time [6]. More recently, Tie et al. used a Mg alloy in a large animal model (*Guangxi Bama Minipig*) as a BMUS. The Mg alloy (ZJ31) presented a homogeneous degradation, excellent biocompatibility and antibacterial activity compared with stainless steel—a commonly used material for non-degradable metallic urinary stents [7].

Zinc (Zn) has a slower degradation time than Mg, with low tissue toxicity and good antibacterial activity. Champagne et al. compared pure Zn, Zn–0.5 Mg, Zn–1 Mg, Zn–0.5% aluminium (Zn–0.5Al), pure Mg and Mg–2Zn–1% manganese (Mg–2Zn1Mn), a commercially available Mg alloy. Zn-containing metals degraded more slowly, and more homogeneous corrosion was obtained for Zn–0.5Al [8].

Biodegradable metal stents in urology have only been explored by a few research groups to date, but these have shown good potential in terms of improved biocompatibility and antibacterial activity.

Mg has been studied the most, but Zn is another promising component. An alloy of both might combine the good biocompatibility and antibacterial properties of Mg with the slower degradation and increased homogeneity of Zn.

3   Molecular and Biological Approaches to Prevent Biofilm Formation and Encrustation

3.1   Antisense Molecules

Pathological protein synthesis, either as under- or overproduction, is a crucial part in many disease processes. Halting these abnormal syntheses might open the disease to effective therapies otherwise not available [9]. Antisense technology (AT) has been investigated for malignant, infectious, inflammatory and metabolic diseases [10]. It modulates protein synthesis by inhibiting gene expression through pairing an antisense nucleic acid sequence base with its complementary sense RNA strand. This stops translation into the target protein [9]. In addition, it can disturb other functions of RNA molecules such as splicing, folding, protein binding, microRNA activities, and RNA-mediated telomerase action [11]. AT is very target specific. For researchers, it is highly interesting since more and more underlying molecular pathways are getting identified for major diseases offering new opportunities to interfere in these. However, AT is not mature enough to overcome some inherent problems such as limited *in-vivo* stability, mode of application, and potential side effects [10]. AT may be used to address urinary implant contamination, infection, and biofilm formation (BF). Biofilms contain extracellular polysaccharides and nucleic acids. The presence of extracellular polysaccharides results in well-structured and strong biofilms [12], which in turn makes bacteria embedded within the biofilm up to 5000 times more antibiotic-resistant [13, 14]. Stopping the synthesis of extracellular polysaccharides can stop BF and/or weaken their bacteria-protective structure. AT would represent an early intervention whilst biofilm is still forming [15]. Especially in chronic infections with BF targeted by AT in its early stages, antibiotics can remain effective and remove or stop further biofilm activity [16].

Recently, it has been shown that the common urinary bacterium *Enterococcus faecalis* gene (efaA) is crucial in BF. Anti-sense *efaA* peptide nucleic acids could decrease it [17]. Research on AT to manipulate BF has only just begun. First the the genetic aspects governing bacterial BF processes need to be better understood [18]. Nevertheless, since one major drawback of urinary stents is the BF, antisense technology may be a promising approach to tackle this inherent stent problem in the future.

3.2   Non-Pathogenic Bacteria

Non-pathogenic bacteria can be used to reduce biofilm formation by pathogenic organisms using various mechanisms such as displacement, exclusion, and competition. In the displacement strategy, non-pathogenic cells or their metabolites disrupt the structure of a pre-formed pathogenic biofilm. Alternatively, pathogen exclusion can occur by blocking adhesion sites, and competition for nutrients or growth factors can inhibit the development of pathogenic strains [19]. Additionally, non-pathogenic bacteria can also modulate the immune system affecting pathogenic cells.

Non-pathogenic bacteria are able to produce a range of compounds, including biosurfactants, bacteriocins and extracellular polymeric surfaces (EPS), that can be detrimental to the development of pathogenic organisms or affect their adhesion to a surface. It has been shown that the production of biosurfactants may interfere with the microbial adhesion of pathogens, including those that are found in the urinary tract [20]. Bacteriocins were also shown to be useful given their high potency, stability, and low toxicity [21–23]. EPS comprises a large group of high-molecular-weight polymers produced by different metabolic pathways in various organisms with proven antibiofilm properties [24]. The production of a vast array of molecules, including lactic acid, fatty acids, enzymes, and hydrogen peroxide, with the potential to control pathogenic biofilms, has also been identified in non-pathogenic cells [19].

Compared to other coating strategies, the use of non-pathogenic cells to coat medical devices may be advantageous because the coating is alive. This allows for the self-renewal of the anti-pathogenic activity, whereas conventional coatings eventually become covered by biomass which may reduce their effectiveness [25].

A number of hurdles have to be overcome for the broad application of non-pathogenic bacteria to protect the surface of urological stent implants. For example, although it has been shown that a certain degree of protection can be obtained for short time periods, the stability and activity of the coating for longer periods of time must be carefully assessed. If the protective effect relies on the viability of the non-pathogenic bacteria (for instance, to produce interfering molecules), this can be an issue. Also, if translocation of the non-pathogenic biofilm occurs (for instance, due to shear forces caused by urine flow), the coating efficacy can be compromised.

3.3   Bacteriophages

Viruses that use bacteria as their hosts are called bacteriophages. Whilst duplicating in the bacteria, they disrupt the metabolism of their hosts in several ways. Lytic bacteriophages destroy the host cell membranes and cells. Lysogenic bacteriophages use the functioning bacterium to multiply whilst letting it live. Lytic bacteriophages can therefore function as antibacterial agents. They are readily available, selective as to their hosts, and non-toxic for surrounding tissue cells. As a consequence, they have been discussed as a coating constituent for medical implants [26]. In early experiments, bladder catheters were pre-treated with lytic *Staphylococcus epidermidis bacteriophage 456*. This led to a significant decrease in intraluminal biofilm formation [27].

As with antibiotics, bacteria can become resistant to bacteriophages. This may be overcome using a mixture of several lytic viruses [28–30]. Silicone bladder catheters coated with hydrogel and pre-treated with such a mixture were indeed efficient against multi-bacterial biofilms. It was proposed that such coating could tackle multi-bacterial biofilms by adapting the viral mixture [31].

Whilst the available evidence stems from experiments on bladder catheters only, the use of bacteriophages on urinary stents seems intuitive and promising. More importantly, since we live in an era of increasing and complex global bacterial resistance to antimicrobials, bacteriophages might represent an alternative approach in the future.

4   Physical Strategies to Prevent Biofilm Formation and Encrustation

4.1   Electrical Charges

The role of electrostatic charge is pivotal in bacterial adhesion. Most bacterial genera have a net negative charge as determined from quantification of their zeta-potential. Therefore, two types of engagement can be derived as antibacterial strategies, namely, material as repellent or as contact-killing agent. The first strategy implies that materials with high negative charge can be deployed as anti-bacterial stent material or coating to repel bacterial cells [32]. Heparin, having the highest negative charge density of known biological molecules [33], has been a popular candidate as stent coating material. However, its efficacy against biofilm formation has been controversial [33–35]. The second strategy relies on a positively charged surface and permeabilization of the bacterial cell membrane that leads to the leakage of intracellular material and eventual cell death. One approach involves grafting polyethyleneimine (PEI) [36] micro-brushes onto polyurethane stents followed by an alkylation process [37, 38]. The resulting micro-structure of PEI brushes with positive charges showed a reduction in both biofilm and encrustation development in *in vitro* and *in vivo* experiments [37]. Another choice of positively charged material is chitosan, which works as an antimicrobial against fungi, Gram-positive and Gram-negative bacteria through various modes of actions [39, 40]. A freeze-casting process was proposed to make entire ureteral stents from chitosan [41]. The best material and engagement strategy are yet to be concluded from further investigations.

4.2   Enhancing and Maintaining Ureteral Peristalsis

In physiological conditions, ureteral peristalsis moves the urine from the renal pelvis to the bladder. Although the insertion of ureteral stents can initially increase ureteral peristalsis, indwelling stents eventually lead to its cessation [42]. The mechanisms leading to aperistalsis in stented ureters are still unclear. A few models

[43] and experimental studies reported the possibility of artificially inducing ureteral peristalsis by: (1) electrical stimulation [44–46], (2) mechanical stimulation e.g. applying distension and/or (3) pharmacological treatment [45]. A possible strategy against encrustation and biofilm in stented ureters could be based on the 'flushing effect' of the ureteral peristalsis: if peristalsis can be preserved in stented ureters in the long term, the movements of the ureteral wall could eliminate encrustations and bacterial deposits from the stent surface. Haeberlin et al. demonstrated that peristalsis can be electrically induced in stented ureters. Catheters were inserted into *ex-vivo* ureters (the size of the catheters was comparable to conventional ureteral stents) and propagating contractions of the ureteral wall were observed after each electrical stimulation [46]. Since these experiments were only conducted in *ex-vivo* ureters in the short term (up to 3 h), *in-vivo* experiments are required to demonstrate the possibility of long-term preservation of the peristalsis by artificial electrical stimulation.

4.3   Ultrasound Waves

Ultrasound comprises longitudinal pressure waves with a frequency > 20 kHz. It represents a clinically viable modality of delivering mechanical stimulation within the body to achieve both therapeutic and diagnostic outcomes. It has also been demonstrated that ultrasound exposure can cause detachment of bacterial biofilms from different surface types and can promote the transport of antibiotics into planktonic or biofilm-forming bacterial cells [47]. Surface acoustic waves (SAW) are a type of sound waves that are transmitted along a surface, and the resulting vibrations have been identified as a factor reducing bacterial adhesion onto solid surfaces [48]. This approach has been adopted to counteract bacterial biofilm formation in bladder catheters, whereby an ultrasound transducer is coupled with the extracorporeal segment of the catheter. Upon activation, the transducer generates SAWs in the frequency range 100–300 kHz, resulting in surface oscillations with amplitudes of 0.2–2 nm that propagate over the catheter surface. In previous studies in a rabbit model, this method has been evaluated both *in vitro* and *in vivo* for inhibiting bacterial adhesion on Foley bladder catheters. It has been shown that SAW-activated catheters had a significantly lower biofilm load *in vitro,* and that this effect was greater when lower SAW intensities were employed (in the range 0.05–0.20 mW/cm²). These findings were confirmed *in vivo,* where the average number of days until the development of a urinary tract infection was extended to 7.3 ± 1.3 days in the SAW-catheter group, compared to 1.5 ± 0.6 days in a non-treated, control group [49].

A commercially available SAW-activated catheter (UroShieldTM) has been developed by NanoVibronix Inc. (USA). Zillich et al. investigated its efficacy and safety through a randomized, double blinded clinical study on 22 patients, in which catheters were deployed for an average of 9 days. Patients having the UroShieldTM catheter reported less pain and bladder spasm, and showed a marked reduction in biofilm formation [50]. More recently, a double blinded randomized controlled trial assessed 55 patients who had an indwelling urinary or suprapubic catheter for > 1-year, and had a treated urinary tract infection during 90 days prior to the commencement of the study. The large majority of patients having the SAW-activated UroShieldTM showed a significant reduction in bacterial load compared to the control group [51]. To the best of our knowledge, a similar approach has not yet been investigated for ureteric stents. Given the demonstrated efficacy of SAW on stent encrustation, this surely represents an interesting future research strategy. When developing such a strategy, there are some technical aspects to be considered. As we are dealing with fully intracorporeal devices, remote powering and control of the SAW activation, and a careful investigation into the propagation properties of the stent materials is needed. For the latter, geometrical features of a stent (e.g., presence of side holes) that may affect SAW propagation and the resulting surface displacement field must be considered, too.

4.4 Biosensors

One major problem of urinary stents and catheters is blockage by encrustation. If blockage occurs in a bladder catheter, it causes painful retention of urine and can provoke severe urinary tract infection and urosepsis. Often, the blockage results from urine infection with urease producing organisms, predominantly *Proteus mirabilis*. Urease generates ammonium which leads to an elevation of urinary pH. This leads to the precipitation of struvite and apatite, which then form a crystalline biofilm encrusting and blocking the urinary catheter. Biosensors are sensors that would alert patients and carers early of an ongoing encrustation and impending resulting blockage. A survey of the current literature shows that such sensors are mainly visual. A pH sensor based on a silicone-based strip incorporating a pH indicator (bromothymol blue) was integrated into an indwelling urinary catheter [52]. A change from yellow to blue indicating impending blockage occurred 19 days before the actual blockage in early human trials. Catheters can also be designed to integrate a pH dependent luminescent material [53]. A lanthanide (Eu) pH-responsive probe that can be incorporated in a hydrogel catheter coating was described. Upon elevation of pH in the presence of urease, the luminescence turns off. However, the system was not tested neither *in vivo* nor *in vitro*. Another approach to provide early warning of encrustation and blockage is to associate a 'trigger' layer, usually EUDRAGIT®S 100, on a hydrogel layer encapsulating a pH reporter or antibacterial agent [54, 55]. Upon elevation of the urinary pH, the upper layer dissolves, triggering the release of a pH indicator such as carboxyfluorescein or bacteriophages. Both approaches were tested in an *in vitro* bladder model, which provided a 12 h advanced warning of blockage and a 13–26 h advanced warning of delayed catheter blockage. The above are early and simple examples of pH-indicating visual biosensors. Because they are visual, they will only work on catheters where an extracorporeal part remains visible. However, the idea of biosensors to indicate early stent encrustation is an appealing one. Fully intracorporeal stents could be equipped with micro- or nano-technological wireless sensors for the same purpose.

5 Conclusions

In this chapter, we presented a brief but comprehensive overview of future research strategies in the prevention of urinary device encrustation with an emphasis on bio-degradability, molecular, microbiological and physical research approaches. The large and strongly associated field of stent coatings and tissue engineering is outlined elsewhere in this book.

There is still plenty of room for future investigations in the fields of material science, surface science, and biomedical engineering to improve and create the most effective urinary implants. In an era where material science, robotics and artificial intelligence have undergone great progress, futuristic ideas may become a reality. These ideas include the creation of multifunctional programmable intelligent urinary implants (core and surface) capable to adapt to the complex biological and physiological environment through sensing or by algorithms from artificial intelligence included in the implant. Urinary implants are at the crossroads of several scientific disciplines, and progress will only be achieved if scientists and physicians collaborate using basic and applied scientific approaches.

References

1. Lo J, Lange D, Chew BH. Ureteral stents and Foley catheters-associated urinary tract infections: the role of coatings and materials in infection prevention. Antibiotics (Basel). 2014;3:87–97.
2. Mosayyebi A, Manes C, Carugo D, Somani BK. Advances in ureteral stent design and materials. Curr Urol Rep. 2018;19:35.
3. Laffite G, Leroy C, Bonhomme C, Bonhomme-Coury L, Letavernier E, Daudon M, Frochot V, Haymann JP, Rouzière S, Lucas IT, Bazin D, Babonneau F, Abou-Hassan A. Calcium oxalate precipitation by diffusion using laminar microfluidics: toward a biomimetic model of pathological microcalcifications. Lab Chip. 2016;16:1157–60.
4. Rakotozandriny K, Bourg S, Papp P, Tóth Á, Horváth D, Lucas IT, Babonneau F, Bonhomme C, Abou-Hassan A. Investigating CaoX crystal formation in the absence and presence of polyphenols under microfluidic conditions in relation with nephrolithiasis. Cryst Growth Des. 2020;20:7683–93.
5. Lock JY, Wyatt E, Upadhyayula S, Whall A, Nuñez V, Vullev VI, Liu H. Degradation and antibacterial properties of magnesium alloys in artificial urine for potential resorbable ureteral stent applications. J Biomed Mater Res A. 2014;102:781–92.
6. Zhang S, Bi Y, Li J, Wang Z, Yan J, Song J, Sheng H, Guo H, Li Y. Biodegradation behavior of magnesium and Zk60 alloy in artificial urine and rat models. Bioact Mater. 2017;2:53–62.
7. Tie D, Liu H, Guan R, Holt-Torres P, Liu Y, Wang Y, Hort N. In vivo assessment of biodegradable magnesium alloy ureteral stents in a pig model. Acta Biomater. 2020;116:415–25.
8. Champagne S, Mostaed E, Safizadeh F, Ghali E, Vedani M, Hermawan H. In vitro degradation of absorbable zinc alloys in artificial urine. Materials (Basel). 2019;12:295.
9. Gupta S, Singh RP, Rabadia N, Patel G, Panchal H. Antisense technology. Int J Pharm Sci Rev Res. 2011;9:38–45.

10. Potaczek DP, Garn H, Unger SD, Renz H. Antisense molecules: a new class of drugs. J Allergy Clin Immunol. 2016;137:1334–46.

11. Goodchild J. Oligonucleotide therapeutics: 25 years agrowing. Curr Opin Mol Ther. 2004;6:120–8.

12. Hall-Stoodley L, Costerton JW, Stoodley P. Bacterial biofilms: from the natural environment to infectious diseases. Nat Rev Microbiol. 2004;2:95–108.

13. Costerton JW, Stewart PS, Greenberg EP. Bacterial biofilms: a common cause of persistent infections. Science. 1999;284:1318–22.

14. Neethirajan S, Clond MA, Vogt A. Medical biofilms—nanotechnology approaches. J Biomed Nanotechnol. 2014;10:2806–27.

15. Tursi SA, Tükel Ç. Curli-containing enteric biofilms inside and out: matrix composition, immune recognition, and disease implications. Microbiol Mol Biol Rev. 2018;82:e00028–18.

16. Zhang K, Li X, Yu C, Wang Y. Promising therapeutic strategies against microbial biofilm challenges. Front Cell Infect Microbiol. 2020;10:359.

17. Narenji H, Teymournejad O, Rezaee MA, Taghizadeh S, Mehramuz B, Aghazadeh M, Asgharzadeh M, Madhi M, Gholizadeh P, Ganbarov K, Yousefi M, Pakravan A, Dal T, Ahmadi R, Samadi Kafil H. Antisense peptide nucleic acids against*ftsZ* and*efaA* genes inhibit growth and biofilm formation of *Enterococcus faecalis*. Microb Pathog. 2020;139:103907.

18. Shirtliff ME, Mader JT, Camper AK. Molecular interactions in biofilms. Chem Biol. 2002;9:859–71.

19. Carvalho FM, Teixeira-Santos R, Mergulhão FJM, Gomes LC. The use of probiotics to fight biofilms in medical devices: a systematic review and meta-analysis. Microorganisms. 2021;9:27.

20. Morais IMC, Cordeiro AL, Teixeira GS, Domingues VS, Nardi RMD, Monteiro AS, Alves RJ, Siqueira EP, Santos VL. Biological and physicochemical properties of biosurfactants produced by *Lactobacillus jensenii* P(6a) and *Lactobacillus gasseri* P(65). Microb Cell Factories. 2017;16:155.

21. Al-Mathkhury HJF, Ali AS, Ghafil JA. Antagonistic effect of bacteriocin against urinary catheter associated *Pseudomonas aeruginosa* biofilm. N Am J Med Sci. 2011;3:367–70.

22. Vahedi Shahandashti R, Kasra Kermanshahi R, Ghadam P. The inhibitory effect of bacteriocin produced by *Lactobacillus acidophilus* ATCC 4356 and *Lactobacillus plantarum* ATCC 8014 on planktonic cells and biofilms of *Serratia marcescens*. Turk J Med Sci. 2016;46: 1188–96.

23. Sharma V, Harjai K, Shukla G. Effect of bacteriocin and exopolysaccharides isolated from probiotic on *P. aeruginosa* PAO1 biofilm. Folia Microbiol. 2018;63:181–90.

24. Abid Y, Casillo A, Gharsallah H, Joulak I, Lanzetta R, Corsaro MM, Attia H, Azabou S. Production and structural characterization of exopolysaccharides from newly isolated probiotic lactic acid bacteria. Int J Biol Macromol. 2018;108:719–28.

25. Chen Q, Zhu Z, Wang J, Lopez AI, Li S, Kumar A, Yu F, Chen H, Cai C, Zhang L, Probiotic E. Coli Nissle 1917 biofilms on silicone substrates for bacterial interference against pathogen colonization. Acta Biomater. 2017;50:353–60.

26. Singha P, Locklin J, Handa H. A review of the recent advances in antimicrobial coatings for urinary catheters. Acta Biomater. 2017;50:20–40.

27. Curtin JJ, Donlan RM. Using bacteriophages to reduce formation of catheter-associated biofilms by *Staphylococcus epidermidis*. Antimicrob Agents Chemother. 2006;50: 1268–75.

28. Carson L, Gorman SP, Gilmore BF. The use of lytic bacteriophages in the prevention and eradication of biofilms of *Proteus mirabilis* and *Escherichia coli*. FEMS Immunol Med Microbiol. 2010;59:447–55.

29. Fu W, Forster T, Mayer O, Curtin JJ, Lehman SM, Donlan RM. Bacteriophage cocktail for the prevention of biofilm formation by *Pseudomonas aeruginosa* on catheters in an in vitro model system. Antimicrob Agents Chemother. 2010;54:397–404.

30. Liao KS, Lehman SM, Tweardy DJ, Donlan RM, Trautner BW. Bacteriophages are synergistic with bacterial interference for the prevention of *Pseudomonas aeruginosa* biofilm formation on urinary catheters. J Appl Microbiol. 2012;113:1530–9.

31. Lehman SM, Donlan RM. Bacteriophage-mediated control of a two-species biofilm formed by microorganisms causing catheter-associated urinary tract infections in an in vitro urinary catheter model. Antimicrob Agents Chemother. 2015;59:1127–37.

32. Rzhepishevska O, Hakobyan S, Ruhal R, Gautrot J, Barbero D, Ramstedt M. The surface charge of anti-bacterial coatings alters motility and biofilm architecture. Biomater Sci. 2013;1:589–602.

33. Lange D, Elwood Chelsea N, Choi K, Hendlin K, Monga M, Chew Ben H. Uropathogen interaction with the surface of urological stents using different surface properties. J Urol. 2009;182:1194–200.

34. Appelgren P, Ransjo U, Bindslev L, Espersen F, Larm O. Surface heparinization of central venous catheters reduces microbial colonization in vitro and in vivo: results from a prospective, randomized trial. Crit Care Med. 1996;24:1482–9.

35. Riedl CR, Witkowski M, Plas E, Pflueger H. Heparin coating reduces encrustation of ureteral stents: a preliminary report. Int J Antimicrob Agents. 2002;19:507–10.

36. Lan T, Guo Q, Shen X. Polyethyleneimine and quaternized ammonium polyethyleneimine: the versatile materials for combating bacteria and biofilms. J Biomater Sci Polym Ed. 2019;30:1243–59.

37. Gultekinoglu M, Kurum B, Karahan S, Kart D, Sagiroglu M, Ertaş N, Haluk Ozen A, Ulubayram K. Polyethyleneimine brushes effectively inhibit encrustation on polyurethane ureteral stents both in dynamic bioreactor and in vivo. Mater Sci Eng C. 2017;71:1166–74.

38. Gultekinoglu M, Tunc Sarisozen Y, Erdogdu C, Sagiroglu M, Aksoy EA, Oh YJ, Hinterdorfer P, Ulubayram K. Designing of dynamic polyethyleneimine (Pei) brushes on polyurethane (Pu) ureteral stents to prevent infections. Acta Biomater. 2015;21:44–54.

39. Chang AKT, Frias RR, Alvarez LV, Bigol UG, Guzman JPMD. Comparative antibacterial activity of commercial chitosan and chitosan extracted from *Auricularia* sp. Biocatal Agric Biotechnol. 2019;17:189–95.

40. Verlee A, Mincke S, Stevens CV. Recent developments in antibacterial and antifungal chitosan and its derivatives. Carbohydr Polym. 2017;164:268–83.

41. Yin K, Divakar P, Wegst UGK. Freeze-casting porous chitosan ureteral stents for improved drainage. Acta Biomater. 2019;84:231–41.

42. Venkatesh R, Landman J, Minor SD, Lee DI, Rehman J, Vanlangendonck R, Ragab M, Morrissey K, Sundaram CP, Clayman RV. Impact of a double-pigtail stent on ureteral peristalsis in the porcine model: initial studies using a novel implantable magnetic sensor. J Endourol. 2005;19:170–6.

43. van Duyl WA. Theory of propagation of peristaltic waves along ureter and their simulation in electronic model. Urology. 1984;24:511–20.

44. van Mastrigt R, Tauecchio EA. Bolus propagation in pig ureter in vitro. Urology. 1984;23:157–62.

45. Teele ME, Lang RJ. Stretch-evoked inhibition of spontaneous migrating contractions in a whole mount preparation of the guinea-pig upper urinary tract. Br J Pharmacol. 1998;123:1143–53.

46. Haeberlin A, Schürch K, Niederhauser T, Sweda R, Schneider MP, Obrist D, Burkhard F, Clavica F. Cardiac electrophysiology catheters for electrophysiological assessments of the lower urinary tract—a proof of concept ex vivo study in viable ureters. Neurourol Urodyn. 2019;38:87–96.

47. LuTheryn G, Glynne-Jones P, Webb JS, Carugo D. Ultrasound-mediated therapies for the treatment of biofilms in chronic wounds: a review of present knowledge. Microb Biotechnol. 2020;13(3):613–28.

48. Wang H, Teng F, Yang X, Guo X, Tu J, Zhang C, Zhang D. Preventing microbial biofilms on catheter tubes using ultrasonic guided waves. Sci Rep. 2017;7:616.

49. Hazan Z, Zumeris J, Jacob H, Raskin H, Kratysh G, Vishnia M, Dror N, Barliya T, Mandel M, Lavie G. Effective prevention of microbial biofilm formation on medical devices by low-energy surface acoustic waves. Antimicrob Agents Chemother. 2006;50(12):4144.

50. Simon Z, Weber C, Ikinger U. Biofilm prevention by surface acoustic waves: a new approach to urinary tract infections—a randomized, double blinded clinical study. A report by NanoVibronix. Document: NV-US-WP-001. 2008.

51. Markowitz S, Rosenblum J, Goldstein M, Gadagkar HP, Litman L. The effect of surface acoustic waves on bacterial load and preventing catheter-associated urinary tract infections (CAUTI) in long term indwelling catheters. Med Surg Urol. 2018;7(4):1000210.
52. Malic S, Waters MG, Basil L, Stickler DJ, Williams DW. Development of an "early warning" sensor for encrustation of urinary catheters following *Proteus* infection. J Biomed Mater Res B Appl Biomater. 2012;100:133–7.
53. Surender EM, Bradberry SJ, Bright SA, McCoy CP, Williams DC, Gunnlaugsson T. Luminescent lanthanide cyclen-based enzymatic assay capable of diagnosing the onset of catheter-associated urinary tract infections both in solution and within polymeric hydrogels. J Am Chem Soc. 2017;139:381–8.
54. Milo S, Thet NT, Liu D, Nzakizwanayo J, Jones BV, Jenkins ATA. An in-situ infection detection sensor coating for urinary catheters. Biosens Bioelectron. 2016;81:166–72.
55. Milo S, Hathaway H, Nzakizwanayo J, Alves DR, Esteban PP, Jones BV, Jenkins ATA. Prevention of encrustation and blockage of urinary catheters by *Proteus mirabilis* via pH-triggered release of bacteriophage. J Mater Chem B. 2017;5:5403–11.

Ten Steps to Strategic Planning for the Urinary Stents of the Future

Federico Soria

1 Introduction

To summarise all the knowledge in the current book and to allow its use both at clinical practise and its application in patients, as well as in the improvement of urinary stents, the simplest way is to build a decalogue that provides a global vision of the requirements for the improvement of these medical devices.

2 Understanding the Side Effects and Complications Related to Urinary Stents

An in-depth knowledge of the side effects, complications, their pathophysiology and, above all, the etiopathogenesis associated with urinary stents is essential on the way to reduce the effects on patients, as well as to improve urinary stents. This knowledge allows urologists to identify symptoms early, as well as to arrange therapeutic measures to alleviate these symptoms [1]. Mainly antimicrobials, alpha-blockers or antimuscarinics to reduce discomfort in the lower urinary tract and, of course, analgesics. Knowledge and research into the etiopathogenesis of each of the adverse effects allows researchers to focus their research [2]. The detection of the cause of each adverse effect allows the identification of whether it is caused by the stent design itself, by the biomaterial or by a weak coating; these three factors are responsible for the majority of adverse effects related to urinary stents. We

F. Soria (✉)
Foundation, Jesús Usón Minimally Invasive Surgery Center, Cáceres, Spain
e-mail: fsoria@ccmijesususon.com

differentiate between adverse effects, which we consider inherent to the urinary stents themselves, such as vesicoureteral reflux, biofilm formation, and complications which, although related to the stents, are due to a malfunction of these medical devices. Among these complications, migrations, perforation, etc. are the most important. Therefore, the first factor to take into account is always knowledge of the adverse effects and complications produced by stents [3].

3   Proper Indication for the Use of Urinary Stents

It is clear that the simplest way to reduce the harmful effects associated with urinary stents is to reduce their use. This is the first choice in the face of the high percentage of associated complications. Since it is impossible to avoid their use due to their evident beneficial effects on patients, it would be necessary to determine in which type of patients their use outweighs the adverse effects. Unfortunately, this is currently the case with the use of metallic stents both at the ureteral or urethral area, with very high complication rates; their use is reduced to a very small number of patients and in many cases exclusively as a palliative treatment.

According to the current scientific literature, the use of ureteral stents after endourological treatment of ureteral or renal lithiasis is approximately 80%. This is a very high percentage, which means that the population susceptible to stent-related problems is very high. Unfortunately, both European and American guidelines cannot define with great scientific evidence the indications for urinary stenting. Stenting is well indicated in complicated ureteroscopies, but the difference between a complicated URS and a non-complicated URS always remains the surgeon's decision. As a result, since there is no criteria for deciding when it is mandatory to place a stent and, above all, when it is not mandatory, the use of these devices is on the rise. Although it is true that a great advance in this aspect is that stenting times have been reduced in an attempt to reduce adverse effects [4]. These effects and complications have been shown to be significantly related to the stenting time, increasing adversely in prolonged stenting times, generally longer than 6 weeks [5].

So a decrease in their use or at least a shortening of the stenting time, without delays in the removal date, would be associated with a better quality of life for patients.

4   Biomaterials

Another of the cornerstones on which the improvement of current urinary stents is based is the research being carried out on biomaterials that allow their use in the urinary tract. As can be seen, this point is critical, as the weaknesses demonstrated by the polymers, metals or their alloys currently in use are one of the main reasons for encrustation, bacterial and even fungal contamination, and sometimes stent fracture. The development of new biomaterials with better characteristics and suitable for the urinary environment will reduce these side effects. Certainly, the future of biomaterials to overcome the limitations they present in the urinary environment depends fundamentally on three factors. The first is to improve their mechanical properties in order to be effective in extrinsic strictures of malignant origin. Secondly, combining biomaterials in the same stent to combine the advantages of each, reducing their weaknesses. Finally, it is possible to coat the biomaterials so that they are not in contact with urine, so that only the coating is affected and the inner part keeps all its properties intact [6].

5 Coatings

This area of knowledge is probably where most resources are being allocated, as research into coatings that prevent or reduce biofilm formation is an issue that involves not only urinary stents, but virtually all implantable medical devices, catheters, prostheses, implants, catheters, etc. Thanks to coatings it is possible to isolate the rest of the biomaterials that make up the stent from the urine, as well as to combat the formation of biofilm that is associated with bacterial contamination as well as encrustation. Therefore, the search for new coatings is of great importance to improve the durability of urinary stents [7]. The aim of these coatings is to provide an "antibiotic free solution" to biofilm formation. To this end, a number of strategies have been developed, as described in the previous chapters. The use of agents with antimicrobial properties has been emphasised: metals such as Zn^{2+}, Ag^{1+}, CuO; superhydrophilic coatings, hydrogels [8]. Mainly in this section, AMPs, antimicrobial peptides, which are proteins with antimicrobial properties, stand out, especially CWR11, RK1 and RK2. Efforts are also being made to detect probiotics that compete against biofilm-forming bacteria and prevent their development. As well as agents with anti-adhesive properties that prevent bacterial adhesion to the stent surface by preventing the action of bacterial adhesins, thanks to bacteriocins [9].

6 New Designs

Another essential element in the improvement of stents and thus the decrease in the adverse effects associated with their use in the urinary tract is the development of new urinary stent designs. It is noteworthy that the design of pigtail ureteral stents has remained virtually unchanged over the last four decades, despite their obvious side effects. Many efforts have been made to reduce the effects related to the bladder pigtail, which is associated with dysuria and LUTS. Therefore modifications of this pigtail, reducing its size, changing its conformation, have been presented and evaluated in patient trials. Despite the decrease in patient discomfort, they have not demonstrated clear scientific evidence, and their use is currently not established in daily clinical practice [10]. To prevent vesicoureteral reflux, stents with anti-reflux systems have also been designed, which have not shown a clear improvement over conventional ureteral stents [11]. However, the development of intraureteral stents, or stents with a small bladder tip to facilitate their removal, has shown scientific evidence regarding the improvement in the quality of life of patients, making them a very interesting option for the present and future for certain patients [12, 13]. Magnetic ureteral stents for removal without the need for cystoscopy have also shown less painful and faster removal [14].

A further design innovation that have proven to be very useful and that were unthinkable decades ago is the possibility of removing metallic, ureteral or urethral stents. This design improvement is extremely attractive and broadens the indications for these stents in the urinary tract [15]. As has been seen in recent years and is expected in the coming years, design variability will reduce the discomfort associated with current designs. The goal is to personalise stents for each patient. The availability of more stent designs will allow choice, which with current plastic stents is almost impossible at the moment.

7 Biodegradable Stents (BUS)

One of the premises for the development of urinary stents is that they should all be biodegradable. In order to achieve the requirements that defines an ideal stent. It is difficult to understand that in the twenty-first century a surgical procedure is necessary to remove a stent. Avoiding cystoscopic removal of stents, avoiding anesthesia in pediatrics patients and avoiding the "forgotten stent" are short-term goals [16]. The development of BUS has expanded in recent years because the most important limitations in its development have been overcome. Firstly, the control of degradation, making this rate controllable thanks to the selection of polymers and copolymers, natural–synthetic or metallic, and above all the use of combinations of different biomaterials with different degradation rates [17]. On the other hand, the control of degradation fragments is a key limitation, since this is a major drawback, in particular when this type of stent is placed at the ureteral lumen level. BUSs must degrade gradually and fragment into small pieces smaller than 2 mm to ease their evacuation. A strategy that has been described for this type of stent and that is related to its design is the ability to degrade from distal to proximal, so that, despite degradation, the stent continues to perform its function as an internal scaffold [18, 19]. One of the most important current challenges is the preservation of the mechanical properties of the BUS, regardless of the nature of the biomaterials that comprise it. Therefore, a balance between the rate of degradation and the maintenance of the mechanical properties of the stents is necessary, which is of great importance in ureteral stents, but is completely mandatory for segmental stents at the urethral level, when used as an internal scaffold, cellularised or not, after treatment of ure-thral strictures.

8 Drug Eluting Stents (DES)

In an attempt to reduce lumen restenosis after vascular stenting, DESs were introduced. Neointimal hyperplasia resulted in in-stent reestenosis in 20–30% of cases after intervention with bare metallic stents. DES were developed not only to act as vascular scaffolds in the diseased coronary artery but also to reduce the relatively high rates of "in-stent reestenosis" and subsequent "target lesion revascularization" compared to its predecessor Bare Metallic stents. DESs have the potential of endoluminal release of pharmacological anti-proliferative substances and reduce the hyperplastic reaction by inhibiting the smooth muscle cell cycle and their proliferation. With the excellent background of vascular stents, applications in the urinary tract are a very encouraging field of development. The idea is to take advantage of the stent to add such an innovative and promising feature as local drug delivery. In this regard, local release of anti-inflammatory, analgesic, or even antiproliferative drugs to reduce urothelial hyperplasia related to urinary metallic stents, or chemotherapy in the upper urinary tract are some of the drugs that have been evaluated [20].

This delivery system would avoid systemic drugs side effects. Possibly reduce the total daily drug dose. As well as using drugs with a short half-life. An important factor is that this urinary delivery system avoids drug absorption, distribution and metabolism, as the urinary tract is a watertight system with low absorption capacity and the drugs are constantly eliminated through urination. A very important consideration is that with these delivery systems, there is the possibility of maintaining urine drug levels in the optimal therapeutic range [21, 22]. Compared to current bladder or pyeloureteral instillation systems, the improvement of patient satisfaction is to be expected.

9 Urine and Infection

The association between UTI and urinary stents, mainly ureteral stents, is one of the most common complications in patients. It should not be forgotten that the prevalence of bacterial colonisation of urinary stents is between 42 and 90%, leading to the development of bacteriuria and UTI [23]. One of the current problems, which needs urgent evaluation to allow for the improvement of stents, is related to the laboratory techniques used for the quantification or detection of urinary bacteria. Regarding the analysis of biofilm and bacteriuria associated with CDJs, despite a low sensitivity of 21–40% and a specificity of 46–64%, culture is the method of choice for detecting bacterial colonisation of the stent and asymptomatic bacteriuria. The first by direct culture of stent fragments and the latter by culture of urine samples [3, 23, 24]. As a result, there is currently no consensus on the ideal microbiological technique to make a fast and, above all, consensual determination that allows for the standardisation of clinical and experimental studies.

It is evident that the aim with current stents is that they remain in place for as long as necessary, since the rates of colonisation and bacteriuria increase considerably with time [3, 23–25]. With regard to biofilm formation, an incidence of 34–66% is found when the stent remains in place for less than 2 months, compared to 75–100% when the stent remains in place for more than 3 months [23, 25]. The incidence of asymptomatic bacteriuria ranges from 7 to 33% in patients with less than 1 month of stenting, 21–50% between 1 and 3 months and when the stent remains in place for more than 3 months, the incidence can reach up to 54% [24, 25]. With regard to the bacterial strains that make up the biofilm and those present in the urine, a large discrepancy has been demonstrated between stent cultures and urine cultures, showing that there is no direct correlation between the bacteria that colonise the stents and those that cause UTI [25].

Unfortunately, the source of colonisation is unlikely to be eradicated, as contamination is mainly at the time of insertion, through skin bacteria or the urethral microflora itself. This could justify the fact that in some series a double incidence of colonisation is observed in women compared to men, given the short length of their urethra and the risk of contamination; as well as the highly frequent presence of Gram+ bacteria in the stents, bacteria commonly present in the distal urethra and vaginal flora.

This susceptibility of urinary stents to contamination, being aware that urine has its own microbiome, must be taken into account in both clinical and research settings. The development of new biomaterials and coatings with antimicrobial properties is therefore one of the milestones for the development of safe and more effective stents. Especially since antibiotic prophylaxis has not shown clear scientific evidence in reducing colonisation of urinary stents. Therefore, only with contamination prevention and strategies to reduce formation is it possible to make progress on this issue, as bacteria in a biofilm can usually survive the presence of antimicrobial agents at a concentration, 1000–1500 times higher than the concentration that kills planktonic cells of the same species.

10 Drugs to Change the Composition of Urine

One of the promising strategies that may reduce the side effects of urinary stents, mainly related to encrustation and possibly also bacterial contamination, is the possibility of changing the composition of the medium in which the stent is placed, which is the urine. The main efforts are being made to alter the composition by oral administration of compounds that modify the urinary pH. Modification of the urinary pH alone causes a very important change as it affects both microorganisms and the precipitation capacity of compounds that are dissolved in the urine and which, due to their supersaturation, can precipitate and cause incrustation on the surface of urinary stents. In addition to pH modification, it is possible to administer crystallisation inhibitors that significantly reduce the risk of lithiasis formation or incrustation [26].

This strategy has begun to show encouraging results in clinical studies evaluating potassium sodium hydrogen citrate, or L-methionine and phytin, reducing the occurrence of stent encrustation. In addition, the synergistic ability of many compounds may allow combinations of these compounds to achieve better results in this area. It is clear that urinary stent fouling is multifactorial, but within these causes the composition of the urine is the main factor that triggers this phenomenon, along with the composition of the stent [27]. The availability of this tool and the fact that it is so easy to apply, usually orally, and safe, suggests that this is an important way to reduce the adverse effects of stents. Not only adverse effects, but also future designs with biodegradable materials that can be modulated in this sense or to activate drug release in DES.

11 Receptor-Based Stents and Tissue Engineering

Another future strategy for the development of urinary stents is, as with DES, to make more profit from the device in the urinary tract. This attempt to expand the benefits of stents is aimed on the one side at obtaining data from the urinary tract, and on the other at allowing the stents to be bio-coated and to facilitate tissue engineering applications.

The development of stents with nano pressure sensors, which can provide information on intrapyelic or intravesical pressure, or with other sensors capable of stimulating ureteral peristalsis. The miniaturisation of this type of sensors allows them to be incorporated into the surface of the stent and send wireless information of great interest.

The possibility of coating stents to promote tissue regeneration, or proper healing, is one of the future hopes of research. In particular, their use would be extremely useful as a scaffold after the treatment of complicated stenosis, mainly at the urethral level. Biocovered stents could reduce fibrosis and thus the formation of stricture scars. Biodegradable biocovered stents would allow their function as an internal scaffold and cellular vehicle to be followed by their controlled disintegration [7].

References

1. Tomer N, Garden E, Small A, Palese M. Ureteral stent encrustation: epidemiology, pathophysiology, management and current technology. J Urol. 2021;205(1):68–77. https://doi.org/10.1097/JU.0000000000001343.

2. Pecoraro A, Peretti D, Tian Z, Aimar R, Niculescu G, Alleva G, Piana A, Granato S, Sica M, Amparore D, Checcucci E, Manfredi M, Karakiewicz P, Fiori C, Porpiglia F. Treatment of ureteral stent-related symptoms. Urol Int. 2021;2:1–16. https://doi.org/10.1159/000518387.
3. Scotland KB, Lo J, Grgic T, Lange D. Ureteral stent-associated infection and sepsis: pathogenesis and prevention: a review. Biofouling. 2019;35(1):117–27. https://doi.org/10.1080/0892701 4.2018.1562549.
4. Saltzman B. Ureteral stents. Indications, variations, and complications. Urol Clin N Am. 1988;15(3):481–91.
5. Türk C, Petřík A, Sarica K, Seitz C, Skolarikos A, Straub M, Knoll T. EAU guidelines on interventional treatment for urolithiasis. Eur Urol. 2016;69(3):475–82. https://doi.org/10.1016/j.eururo.2015.07.041.
6. Domingues B, Pacheco M, de la Cruz JE, Carmagnola I, Teixeira-Santos R, Laurenti M, Can F, Bohinc K, Moutinho F, Silva JM, Aroso IM, et al. Future directions for ureteral stent technology: from bench to the market. Adv Ther. 2021;5(1):2100158. https://doi.org/10.1002/adtp.202100158.
7. Abou-Hassan A, Barros A, Buchholz N, Carugo D, Clavica F, de Graaf P, de La Cruz J, Kram W, Mergulhao F, Reis RL, Skovorodkin I, Soria F, Vainio S, Zheng S. Potential strategies to prevent encrustations on urinary stents and catheters—thinking outside the box: a European network of multidisciplinary research to improve urinary stents (ENIUS) initiative. Expert Rev Med Devices. 2021;18(7):697–705. https://doi.org/10.1080/17434440.2021.1939010.
8. Mosayyebi A, Manes C, Carugo D, Somani BK. Advances in ureteral stent design and materials. Curr Urol Rep. 2018;19(5):35. https://doi.org/10.1007/s11934-018-0779-y.
9. Forbes C, Scotland KB, Lange D, Chew BH. Innovations in ureteral stent technology. Urol Clin N Am. 2019;46(2):245–55. https://doi.org/10.1016/j.ucl.2018.12.013.
10. Taguchi M, Inoue T, Muguruma K, Murota T, Kinoshita H, Matsuda T. Impact of loop-tail ureteral stents on ureteral stent-related symptoms immediately after ureteroscopic lithotripsy: comparison with pigtail ureteral stents. Investig Clin Urol. 2017;58(6):440–6. https://doi.org/10.4111/icu.2017.58.6.440.
11. Ecke TH, Bartel P, Hallmann S, Ruttloff J. Evaluation of symptoms and patients' comfort for JJ-ureteral stents with and without antireflux-membrane valve. Urology. 2010;75(1):212–6. https://doi.org/10.1016/j.urology.2009.07.1258.
12. Yoshida T, Inoue T, Taguchi M, Matsuzaki T, Murota T, Kinoshita H, Matsuda T. Efficacy and safety of complete intraureteral stent placement versus conventional stent placement in relieving ureteral stent related symptoms: a randomized, prospective, single blind, multicenter clinical trial. J Urol. 2019;202(1):164–70. https://doi.org/10.1097/JU.0000000000000196.
13. Soria F, Morcillo E, Serrano A, Rioja J, Budia A, Moreno J, Sanchez-Margallo FM. Preliminary assessment of a new antireflux ureteral stent design in swine model. Urology. 2015;86(2):417–22. https://doi.org/10.1016/j.urology.2015.05.020.
14. Rassweiler MC, Michel MS, Ritter M, Honeck P. Magnetic ureteral stent removal without cystoscopy: a randomized controlled trial. J Endourol. 2017;31(8):762–6. https://doi.org/10.1089/end.2017.0051.
15. Morcillo E, Fernández I, Pamplona M, Sánchez-Margallo FM, Soria F. Metallic ureteral stents. Present and future. Arch Esp Urol. 2016;69(8):583–94.
16. Soria F, de la Cruz JE, Budia A, Serrano A, Galan-Llopis JA, Sanchez-Margallo FM. Experimental assessment of new generation of ureteral stents: biodegradable and antireflux properties. J Endourol. 2020;34(3):359–65. https://doi.org/10.1089/end.2019.0493.
17. Soria F, Morcillo E, Serrano A, Budia A, Fernández I, Fernández-Aparicio T, Sanchez-Margallo FM. Evaluation of a new design of antireflux-biodegradable ureteral stent in animal model. Urology. 2018;115:59–64. https://doi.org/10.1016/j.urology.2018.02.004.
18. Soria F, de La Cruz JE, Fernandez T, Budia A, Serrano Á, Sanchez-Margallo FM. Heparin coating in biodegradable ureteral stents does not decrease bacterial colonization-assessment in ureteral stricture endourological treatment in animal model. Transl Androl Urol. 2021;10(4):1700–10. https://doi.org/10.21037/tau-21-19.

19. Barros AA, Oliveira C, Ribeiro AJ, Autorino R, Reis RL, Duarte ARC, Lima E. In vivo assessment of a novel biodegradable ureteral stent. World J Urol. 2018;36(2):277–83. https://doi.org/10.1007/s00345-017-2124-3.
20. Kallidonis P, Kitrou P, Karnabatidis D, Kyriazis I, Kalogeropoulou C, Tsamandas A, Apostolopoulos DJ, Vrettos T, Liourdi D, Spiliopoulos S, Al-Aown A, Scopa CD, Liatsikos E. Evaluation of zotarolimus-eluting metal stent in animal ureters. J Endourol. 2011;25(10):1661–7. https://doi.org/10.1089/end.2011.0308.
21. Barros AA, Oliveira C, Reis RL, Lima E, Duarte AR. Ketoprofen-eluting biodegradable ureteral stents by CO_2 impregnation: in vitro study. Int J Pharm. 2015;495(2):651–9. https://doi.org/10.1016/j.ijpharm.2015.08.040.
22. Barros AA, Browne S, Oliveira C, Lima E, Duarte AR, Healy KE, Reis RL. Drug-eluting biodegradable ureteral stent: new approach for urothelial tumors of upper urinary tract cancer. Int J Pharm. 2016;513(1–2):227–37. https://doi.org/10.1016/j.ijpharm.2016.08.061.
23. Kehinde EO, Rotimi VO, Al-Hunayan A, Abdul-Halim H, Boland F, Al-Awadi KA. Bacteriology of urinary tract infection associated with indwelling J ureteral stents. J Endourol. 2004;18:891–6.
24. Farsi HM, Mosli HA, Al-Zemaity MF, Bahnassy AA, Alvarez M. Bacteriuria and colonization of double-pigtail ureteral stents: long-term experience with 237 patients. J Endourol. 1995;9:469–72.
25. Klis R, Korczak-Kozakiewicz E, Denys A, Sosnowski M, Rozanski W. Relationship between urinary tract infection and self-retaining double-J catheter colonization. J Endourol. 2009;23:1015–9.
26. Torrecilla C, Fernández-Concha J, Cansino JR, Mainez JA, Amón JH, Costas S, Angerri O, Emiliani E, Arrabal Martín MA, Arrabal Polo MA, García A, Reina MC, Sánchez JF, Budía A, Pérez-Fentes D, Grases F, Costa-Bauzá A, Cuñé J. Reduction of ureteral stent encrustation by modulating the urine pH and inhibiting the crystal film with a new oral composition: a multicenter, placebo controlled, double blind, randomized clinical trial. BMC Urol. 2020;20(1):65. https://doi.org/10.1186/s12894-020-00633-2.
27. Xue X, Liu Z, Li X, Lu J, Wang C, Wang X, Ren W, Sun R, Jia Z, Ji X, Chen Y, He Y, Ji A, Sun W, Zhang H, Merriman TR, Li C, Cui L. The efficacy and safety of citrate mixture vs sodium bicarbonate on urine alkalization in Chinese primary gout patients with benzbromarone: a prospective, randomized controlled study. Rheumatology (Oxford). 2021;60(6):2661–71. https://doi.org/10.1093/rheumatology/keaa668.

Printed in the United States
by Baker & Taylor Publisher Services